Prostate Cancer: Symptoms, Diagnosis & Treatment

Prostate Cancer: Symptoms, Diagnosis & Treatment

Topic Editors

Ana Faustino
Paula Oliveira
Lúcio Lara Santos

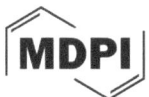

Basel • Beijing • Wuhan • Barcelona • Belgrade • Novi Sad • Cluj • Manchester

Topic Editors

Ana Faustino
University of Évora
Évora
Portugal

Paula Oliveira
University of Trás-os-Montes
and Alto Douro (UTAD)
Vila Real, Portugal
Portugal

Lúcio Lara Santos
Portuguese Institute of
Oncology
Porto
Portugal

Editorial Office
MDPI AG
Grosspeteranlage 5
4052 Basel, Switzerland

This is a reprint of the Topic, published open access by the journals *Cancers* (ISSN 2072-6694), *Current Oncology* (ISSN 1718-7729), *Life* (ISSN 2075-1729) and *Uro* (ISSN 2673-4397), freely accessible at: https://www.mdpi.com/topics/prostate_Cancer.

For citation purposes, cite each article independently as indicated on the article page online and as indicated below:

Lastname, A.A.; Lastname, B.B. Article Title. *Journal Name* **Year**, *Volume Number*, Page Range.

ISBN 978-3-7258-2781-7 (Hbk)
ISBN 978-3-7258-2782-4 (PDF)
https://doi.org/10.3390/books978-3-7258-2782-4

© 2024 by the authors. Articles in this book are Open Access and distributed under the Creative Commons Attribution (CC BY) license. The book as a whole is distributed by MDPI under the terms and conditions of the Creative Commons Attribution-NonCommercial-NoDerivs (CC BY-NC-ND) license (https://creativecommons.org/licenses/by-nc-nd/4.0/).

Contents

Nagjie Alijaj, Blaz Pavlovic, Paul Martel, Arnas Rakauskas, Valérie Cesson, Karim Saba, et al.
Identification of Urine Biomarkers to Improve Eligibility for Prostate Biopsy and Detect High-Grade Prostate Cancer
Reprinted from: *Cancers* **2022**, *14*, 1135, https://doi.org/10.3390/cancers14051135 1

Dirk Böhmer, Alessandra Siegmann, Sophia Scharl, Christian Ruf, Thomas Wiegel, Manuel Krafcsik and Reinhard Thamm
Impact of Dose Escalation on the Efficacy of Salvage Radiotherapy for Recurrent Prostate Cancer—A Risk-Adjusted, Matched-Pair Analysis
Reprinted from: *Cancers* **2022**, *14*, 1320, https://doi.org/10.3390/cancers14051320 21

Salvatore Cozzi, Lilia Bardoscia, Masoumeh Najafi, Andrea Botti, Gladys Blandino, Matteo Augugliaro, et al.
Adenoid Cystic Carcinoma/Basal Cell Carcinoma of the Prostate: Overview and Update on Rare Prostate Cancer Subtypes
Reprinted from: *Curr. Oncol.* **2022**, *29*, 1866–1876, https://doi.org/10.3390/curroncol29030152 . 32

Carsten Stephan, Bernhard Ralla, Florian Bonn, Max Diesner, Michael Lein and Klaus Jung
Vitamin D Metabolites in Nonmetastatic High-Risk Prostate Cancer Patients with and without Zoledronic Acid Treatment after Prostatectomy
Reprinted from: *Cancers* **2022**, *14*, 1560, https://doi.org/10.3390/cancers14061560 43

Juan Morote, Angel Borque-Fernando, Marina Triquell, Anna Celma, Lucas Regis, Manel Escobar, et al.
The Barcelona Predictive Model of Clinically Significant Prostate Cancer
Reprinted from: *Cancers* **2022**, *14*, 1589, https://doi.org/10.3390/cancers14061589 60

Anna-Lena Lemster, Elisabeth Sievers, Helen Pasternack, Pamela Lazar-Karsten, Niklas Klümper, Verena Sailer, et al.
Histone Demethylase KDM5C Drives Prostate Cancer Progression by Promoting EMT
Reprinted from: *Cancers* **2022**, *14*, 1894, https://doi.org/10.3390/cancers14081894 73

Yangyi Zhang, Bethany K. Campbell, Stanley S. Stylli, Niall M. Corcoran and Christopher M. Hovens
The Prostate Cancer Immune Microenvironment, Biomarkers and Therapeutic Intervention
Reprinted from: *Uro* **2022**, *2*, 74–92, https://doi.org/10.3390/uro2020010 93

Tânia Lima, António S. Barros, Fábio Trindade, Rita Ferreira, Adelino Leite-Moreira, Daniela Barros-Silva, et al.
Application of Proteogenomics to Urine Analysis towards the Identification of Novel Biomarkers of Prostate Cancer: An Exploratory Study
Reprinted from: *Cancers* **2022**, *14*, 2001, https://doi.org/10.3390/cancers14082001 112

Zoé Neviere, Elodie Coquan, Pierre-Emmanuel Brachet, Emeline Meriaux, Isabelle Bonnet, Sophie Krieger, et al.
Outcomes of Patients with Metastatic Castration-Resistant Prostate Cancer According to Somatic Damage DNA Repair Gene Alterations
Reprinted from: *Curr. Oncol.* **2022**, *29*, 2776–2791, https://doi.org/10.3390/curroncol29040226 . 138

Gordana Kocić, Jovan Hadzi-Djokić, Andrej Veljković, Stefanos Roumeliotis,
Ljubinka Janković-Veličković and Andrija Šmelcerović
Template-Independent Poly(A)-Tail Decay and RNASEL as Potential Cellular Biomarkers for
Prostate Cancer Development
Reprinted from: *Cancers* 2022, *14*, 2239, https://doi.org/10.3390/cancers14092239 . . . . **154**

Marcello Serra, Fortuna De Martino, Federica Savino, Valentina d'Alesio, Cecilia Arrichiello,
Maria Quarto, et al.
SBRT for Localized Prostate Cancer: CyberKnife vs. VMAT-FFF, a Dosimetric Study
Reprinted from: *Life* 2022, *12*, 711, https://doi.org/10.3390/life12050711 . . . . **168**

José Manuel Sánchez-Maldonado, Ricardo Collado, Antonio José Cabrera-Serrano, Rob Ter
Horst, Fernando Gálvez-Montosa, Inmaculada Robles-Fernández, et al.
Type 2 Diabetes-Related Variants Influence the Risk of Developing Prostate Cancer:
A Population-Based Case-Control Study and Meta-Analysis
Reprinted from: *Cancers* 2022, *14*, 2376, https://doi.org/10.3390/cancers14102376 . . . . **181**

Ahmad Abdelrazek, Ahmed M. Mahmoud, Vidhu B. Joshi, Mohamed Habeeb, Mohamed E.
Ahmed, Khaled Ghoniem, et al.
Recent Advances in Prostate Cancer (PCa) Diagnostics
Reprinted from: *Uro* 2022, *2*, 109–121, https://doi.org/10.3390/uro2020014 . . . . **204**

Hee Ryeong Jang, Kyoungyul Lee and Kyu-Hyoung Lim
Isolated Peritoneal Metastasis of Prostate Cancer Presenting with Massive Ascites: A Case
Report
Reprinted from: *Curr. Oncol.* 2022, *29*, 4423–4427, https://doi.org/10.3390/curroncol29070351 . **217**

Vlad Cristian Munteanu, Raluca Andrada Munteanu, Diana Gulei, Radu Mărginean, Vlad
Horia Schițcu, Anca Onaciu, et al.
New Insights into the Multivariate Analysis of SER Spectra Collected on Blood Samples for
Prostate Cancer Detection: Towards a Better Understanding of the Role Played by Different
Biomolecules on Cancer Screening: A Preliminary Study
Reprinted from: *Cancers* 2022, *14*, 3227, https://doi.org/10.3390/cancers14133227 . . . . **222**

Felice Crocetto, Gianluca Russo, Erika Di Zazzo, Pasquale Pisapia, Benito Fabio Mirto,
Alessandro Palmieri, et al.
Liquid Biopsy in Prostate Cancer Management—Current Challenges and Future Perspectives
Reprinted from: *Cancers* 2022, *14*, 3272, https://doi.org/10.3390/cancers14133272 . . . . **239**

Stergios Boussios, Elie Rassy, Michele Moschetta, Aruni Ghose, Sola Adeleke,
Elisabet Sanchez, et al.
BRCA Mutations in Ovarian and Prostate Cancer: Bench to Bedside
Reprinted from: *Cancers* 2022, *14*, 3888, https://doi.org/10.3390/cancers14163888 . . . . **257**

Alv A. Dahl and Sophie D. Fosså
High Neuroticism Is Related to More Overall Functional Problems and Lower Function Scores
in Men Who Had Surgery for Non-Relapsing Prostate Cancer
Reprinted from: *Curr. Oncol.* 2022, *29*, 5823–5832, https://doi.org/10.3390/curroncol29080459 . **286**

Ephraim E. Parent and Adam M. Kase
A Treatment Paradigm Shift: Targeted Radionuclide Therapies for Metastatic Castrate Resistant
Prostate Cancer
Reprinted from: *Cancers* 2022, *14*, 4276, https://doi.org/10.3390/cancers14174276 . . . . **296**

Jiazhou Liu, Shihang Pan, Liang Dong, Guangyu Wu, Jiayi Wang, Yan Wang, et al.
The Diagnostic Value of PI-RADS v2.1 in Patients with a History of Transurethral Resection of the Prostate (TURP)
Reprinted from: *Curr. Oncol.* **2022**, *29*, 6373–6382, https://doi.org/10.3390/curroncol29090502 . . 315

Jeremy Yuen-Chun Teoh, Alex Qinyang Liu, Violet Wai-Fan Yuen, Franco Pui-Tak Lai, Steffi Kar-Kei Yuen, Samson Yun-Sang Chan, et al.
Hemopatch to Prevent Lymphatic Leak after Robotic Prostatectomy and Pelvic Lymph Node Dissection: A Randomized Controlled Trial
Reprinted from: *Cancers* **2022**, *14*, 4476, https://doi.org/10.3390/cancers14184476 325

Alessio Paladini, Giovanni Cochetti, Alexandre Colau, Martin Mouton, Sara Ciarletti, Graziano Felici, et al.
The Challenges of Patient Selection for Prostate Cancer Focal Therapy: A Retrospective Observational Multicentre Study
Reprinted from: *Curr. Oncol.* **2022**, *29*, 6826–6833, https://doi.org/10.3390/curroncol29100538 . 335

Ryunosuke Nakagawa, Hiroaki Iwamoto, Tomoyuki Makino, Renato Naito, Suguru Kadomoto, Norihito Akatani, et al.
Development of a Prognostic Model of Overall Survival for Metastatic Hormone-Naïve Prostate Cancer in Japanese Men
Reprinted from: *Cancers* **2022**, *14*, 4822, https://doi.org/10.3390/cancers14194822 343

Tae Hyung Kim, Jason Joon Bock Lee and Jaeho Cho
Prostate-Specific Antigen Bounce after ^{125}I Brachytherapy Using Stranded Seeds with Intraoperative Optimization for Prostate Cancer
Reprinted from: *Cancers* **2022**, *14*, 4907, https://doi.org/10.3390/cancers14194907 355

August Sigle, Rodrigo Suarez-Ibarrola, Matthias Benndorf, Moritz Weishaar, Jonathan Morlock, Arkadiusz Miernik, et al.
Individualized Decision Making in Transperineal Prostate Biopsy: Should All Men Undergo an Additional Systematic Biopsy?
Reprinted from: *Cancers* **2022**, *14*, 5230, https://doi.org/10.3390/cancers14215230 366

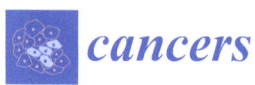 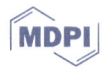

Article

Identification of Urine Biomarkers to Improve Eligibility for Prostate Biopsy and Detect High-Grade Prostate Cancer

Nagjie Alijaj [1,†], Blaz Pavlovic [1,†], Paul Martel [2], Arnas Rakauskas [2], Valérie Cesson [2], Karim Saba [3], Thomas Hermanns [3], Pascal Oechslin [3], Markus Veit [3], Maurizio Provenzano [3,‡], Jan H. Rüschoff [4], Muriel D. Brada [4], Niels J. Rupp [4,5], Cédric Poyet [3], Laurent Derré [2], Massimo Valerio [2], Irina Banzola [1,*,§] and Daniel Eberli [3,§]

1. Department of Urology, University Hospital of Zürich and University of Zürich, 8006 Zürich, Switzerland; nagjielaila.alijaj@usz.ch (N.A.); blaz.pavlovic@usz.ch (B.P.)
2. Department of Urology, Urology Research Unit and Urology Biobank, University Hospital of Lausanne, 1011 Lausanne, Switzerland; paul.martel@chuv.ch (P.M.); arnas.rakauskas@chuv.ch (A.R.); valerie.cesson@chuv.ch (V.C.); laurent.derre@chuv.ch (L.D.); massimo.valerio@chuv.ch (M.V.)
3. Department of Urology, University Hospital of Zürich, 8091 Zürich, Switzerland; sabakarim@gmail.com (K.S.); thomas.hermanns@usz.ch (T.H.); pascal.oechslin@usz.ch (P.O.); markus.veit@usz.ch (M.V.); maurizio.provenzano@gmail.com (M.P.); cedric.poyet@usz.ch (C.P.); daniel.eberli@usz.ch (D.E.)
4. Department of Pathology and Molecular Pathology, University Hospital of Zürich, 8091 Zürich, Switzerland; janhendrik.rueschoff@usz.ch (J.H.R.); murieldiana.brada@usz.ch (M.D.B.); niels.rupp@usz.ch (N.J.R.)
5. Faculty of Medicine, University of Zürich, 8032 Zürich, Switzerland
* Correspondence: irina.banzola@usz.ch; Tel.: +41762503737
† These authors contributed equally to this work as co-first authors.
‡ Current address: Praxiszentrum Lauématt, 5103 Wildegg, Switzerland.
§ These authors contributed equally to this work as co-last authors.

Citation: Alijaj, N.; Pavlovic, B.; Martel, P.; Rakauskas, A.; Cesson, V.; Saba, K.; Hermanns, T.; Oechslin, P.; Veit, M.; Provenzano, M.; et al. Identification of Urine Biomarkers to Improve Eligibility for Prostate Biopsy and Detect High-Grade Prostate Cancer. *Cancers* 2022, 14, 1135. https://doi.org/10.3390/cancers14051135

Academic Editors: Ana Faustino, Paula A. Oliveira and Lúcio Lara Santos

Received: 28 January 2022
Accepted: 18 February 2022
Published: 23 February 2022

Publisher's Note: MDPI stays neutral with regard to jurisdictional claims in published maps and institutional affiliations.

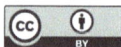

Copyright: © 2022 by the authors. Licensee MDPI, Basel, Switzerland. This article is an open access article distributed under the terms and conditions of the Creative Commons Attribution (CC BY) license (https://creativecommons.org/licenses/by/4.0/).

Simple Summary: The screening of prostate cancer (PCa), based on the serum prostate specific antigen (PSA), is characterized by a high number of false positives, leading to overdiagnosis of healthy men and overtreatment of indolent PCa. This clinical problem severely affects the quality of life of patients, who would benefit from more specific risk stratification models. By performing a mass spectrometry (MS) screening on urine samples collected prior to prostate biopsy, we identified novel biomarkers and validated them by ELISA. Here, we show that an upfront urine test, based on quantitative biomarkers and patient age, has a higher performance compared to PSA (AUC = 0.6020) and is a feasible method to improve the eligibility criteria for prostate biopsy, to detect healthy men (AUC = 0.8196) and clinically significant PCa, thereby reducing the number of unnecessary prostate biopsies.

Abstract: PCa screening is based on the measurements of the serum prostate specific antigen (PSA) to select men with higher risks for tumors and, thus, eligible for prostate biopsy. However, PSA testing has a low specificity, leading to unnecessary biopsies in 50–75% of cases. Therefore, more specific screening opportunities are needed to reduce the number of biopsies performed on healthy men and patients with indolent tumors. Urine samples from 45 patients with elevated PSA were collected prior to prostate biopsy, a mass spectrometry (MS) screening was performed to identify novel biomarkers and the best candidates were validated by ELISA. The urine quantification of PEDF, HPX, CD99, CANX, FCER2, HRNR, and KRT13 showed superior performance compared to PSA. Additionally, the combination of two biomarkers and patient age resulted in an AUC of 0.8196 (PSA = 0.6020) and 0.7801 (PSA = 0.5690) in detecting healthy men and high-grade PCa, respectively. In this study, we identified and validated novel urine biomarkers for the screening of PCa, showing that an upfront urine test, based on quantitative biomarkers and patient age, is a feasible method to reduce the number of unnecessary prostate biopsies and detect both healthy men and clinically significant PCa.

Keywords: eligibility for prostate biopsy; prostate cancer; PSA; screening; urine biomarker

1. Introduction

Prostate cancer (PCa) is one of the most frequently diagnosed cancers worldwide and a prominent reason for tumor-related deaths in men [1]. In past years, early detection of PCa and its clinical management became a controversial topic. On the one hand, implementation of the serum biomarker prostate specific antigen (PSA), as a standard for the screening of PCa in the early 1990s, resulted in an increased diagnosis of early-stage tumors and a reduction of PCa-specific mortality rates [2]. Additional refinements in the PCa screening procedure due to new biomarkers and technologies, such as magnetic resonance imaging (MRI), have further improved the predictive performances of PSA [3]. On the other hand, specificities of current diagnostic examinations remain low and still lead to a high number of false positives, resulting in unnecessarily performed prostate biopsies [4]. Therefore, overdiagnosis of healthy men and overtreatment of indolent PCa remains a clinical challenge with significant impact on the quality of life of patients due to possible severe side effects [5,6]. To overcome this problem, more specific risk stratification models that can complement PSA testing need to be developed, to distinguish clinically significant from indolent PCa, and to reduce the number of biopsies performed.

Urine is an ideal clinical specimen for diagnostic testing. Its easy collection is completely non-invasive and it allows the processing of large volumes, compared to tissue, blood or other biological materials. This enables the detection of biomarkers at any time point during patient care and facilitates not only diagnosis, but also the monitoring of the disease. The detection of biomarkers in urine has been studied for a wide range of cancers with ultrasensitive screening methods, such as nuclear magnetic resonance (NMR) spectroscopy and mass spectrometry (MS) [7,8]. Specific metabolites were examined for their potential to screen for cancers of the urological system, but also for non-urological tumors such as lung, breast, colorectal, gastric, hepatic, pancreatic, and renal cancer [9].

The prostate epithelium secretes cellular substances into the gland and prostate cancer cells can be shed into the prostatic fluids, where they exude into the urine [10,11]. Sensitive assays can then detect DNA, RNA, proteins, and exosomes of tumor origin [12,13]. MS proteomics can be a powerful tool for high-throughput screening of proteins in urine and can be used for the identification of new biomarkers [14,15]. The translation of such methods into the clinic for standard diagnostic screening is elusive because of the high cost of instruments and the need for specially trained personnel. Therefore, validation studies of biomarkers are often performed on larger patient cohorts with immunological assays such as ELISA, which is a well-established method for protein quantification.

The aim of this study was to discover novel urine biomarkers for the detection of PCa and investigate their potential as an improved diagnostic test. The goal was to select, with high sensitivity, men with unspecifically elevated PSA from men who could benefit from prostate biopsy, which remains the standard of care for the diagnosis of PCa. Since low-grade PCas are generally considered indolent, the aim of the study was also to identify biomarkers for the selection of men harboring high-grade PCa. Thus, by improving the eligibility criteria for prostate biopsy, we would reduce the number of unnecessary prostate biopsies performed. Additionally, it might offer the possibility of non-invasive disease monitoring. Tests that rely on the quantification of single biomarkers are often limited in their power to predict cancer, a disease that is hallmarked by its heterogenic biology [16,17]. Therefore, we focused on the quantification of multiple biomarkers to achieve an increased accuracy in predicting PCa.

We performed a MS screening on urine samples from 45 men with elevated PSA levels scheduled for prostate biopsy and identified 2.735 proteins across all samples, as well as potential biomarkers for the detection of all grades of PCa or high-grade tumors only. Top candidates were then validated by ELISA and a combinatory analysis predicted their performances as multiplexed diagnostic test for PCa screening.

2. Materials and Methods

2.1. Urine Collection and Processing

A total of 45 patients were enrolled in the study at the Urology Department of the University Hospital of Zürich (Zürich, Switzerland). Samples were collected as first-morning urine from men not subjected to prostatic massage, with high serum PSA levels (≥ 2 ng/mL) and/or abnormal digital rectal examination (DRE) results, before the performance of the prostate biopsy. Sample aliquots were then stored at $-80\ °C$ until use. Patients' recruitment, urine sample collection, and analysis were approved by the Ethics Committee of Kanton Zürich (BASEC n° 2016-00829).

2.2. Mass Spectrometry Analysis

Mass spectrometry (MS) analysis was performed by Biognosys AG (Schlieren, Switzerland). All solvents were HPLC-grade from Sigma Aldrich (Schaffhausen, Switzerland) and all chemicals, if not stated otherwise, were obtained from Sigma Aldrich (Schaffhausen, Switzerland).

2.2.1. Sample Preparation

After thawing, sample digestion was performed on single filter units (Sartorius Vivacon 500, 30.000 MWCO HY) following a modified FASP protocol (described by the Max Planck Institute of Biochemistry, Martinsried, Germany). Samples were denatured with Biognosys' Denature Buffer and reduced/alkylated using Biognosys' Reduction/Alkylation Solution for 1 h at 37 °C. Subsequently, digestion to peptides was carried out using 1 µg trypsin (Promega) per sample, overnight at 37 °C.

2.2.2. Clean-Up for Mass Spectrometry

Peptides were desalted using C18 Ultra Micro Spin columns (The Nest Group) according to the manufacturer's instructions and dried down using a SpeedVac system. Peptides were resuspended in 17 µL LC solvent A (1% acetonitrile, 0.1% formic acid (FA)) and spiked with the Biognosys iRT kit calibration peptides. Peptide concentrations were determined using a UV/VIS Spectrometer (SPECTROstar Nano, BMG Labtech, Ortenberg, Germany).

2.2.3. HPRP Fractionation

For HPRP fractionation of peptides, digested samples were pooled. Ammonium hydroxide was added to a pH value > 10. The fractionation was performed using a Dionex UltiMate 3000 RS pump (Thermo Scientific™) on an ACQUITY UPLC CSH C18 1.7 µm, 2.1 × 150 mm column (Waters). The gradient was 1% to 40% solvent B in 30 min, solvents were A: 20 mM ammonium formate in water, B: acetonitrile. Fractions were taken every 30 s and sequentially pooled to 12 fraction pools. These were dried down and resolved in 15 µL solvent A. Prior to mass spectrometric analyses, they were spiked with Biognosys' iRT kit calibration peptides. Peptide concentrations were determined using a UV/VIS Spectrometer (SPECTROstar Nano, BMG Labtech).

2.2.4. Shotgun LC–MS/MS for Spectral Library Generation

For shotgun LC–MS/MS measurements, 2 µg of peptides per fraction were injected to an in-house packed C18 column (Dr. Maisch ReproSil-Pur, 1.9 µm particle size, 120 Å pore size; 75 µm inner diameter, 50 cm length, New Objective) on a Thermo Scientific Easy nLC 1200 nano-liquid chromatography system connected to a Thermo Scientific™ Q Exactive™ HF mass spectrometer equipped with a standard nano-electrospray source. LC solvents were A: 1% acetonitrile in water with 0.1% FA; B: 15% water in acetonitrile with 0.1% FA. The nonlinear LC gradient was 1–52% solvent B in 60 min followed by 52–90% B in 10 s, 90% B for 10 min, 90–1% B in 10 s and 1% B for 5 min. A modified TOP15 method from Kelstrup was used [18]. Full MS covered the m/z range of 350–1650 with a resolution of 60.000 (AGC target value was 3×10^6) and was followed by 15 data dependent MS2 scans with a resolution of 15.000 (AGC target value was 2×10^5). MS2 acquisition precursor isolation width was 1.6 m/z, while normalized collision energy was centered at 27 (10% stepped collision energy) and the default charge state was 2+.

2.2.5. HRM Mass Spectrometry Acquisition

For DIA LC–MS/MS measurements, 2 µg of peptides and 1 IE of PQ500 reference peptides were injected per sample. For samples with less than 2 µg of total peptide available, the amount of reference peptides was adjusted accordingly. Peptides were injected into an in-house packed C18 column (Dr. Maisch ReproSil-Pur, 1.9 µm particle size, 120 Å pore size; 75 µm inner diameter, 50 cm length, New Objective) on a Thermo Scientific Easy nLC 1200 nano liquid chromatography system connected to a Thermo Scientific Q Exactive HF mass spectrometer equipped with a standard nano-electrospray source. LC solvents were A: 1% acetonitrile in water with 0.1% FA; B: 15% water in acetonitrile with 0.1% FA. The nonlinear LC gradient was 1–55% solvent B in 120 min followed by 55–90% B in 10 s, 90% B for 10 min, 90–1% B in 10 s, and 1% B for 5 min. A DIA method with one full range survey scan and 22 DIA windows was used.

2.2.6. Database Search of Shotgun LC–MS/MS Data and Spectral Library Generation

The shotgun mass spectrometric data were analyzed using Biognosys' search engine SpectroMine™, the false discovery rate on peptide and protein level was set to 1%. A human UniProt FASTA database (Homo sapiens, accessed on 1 July 2019) was used for the search engine, allowing for two missed cleavages and variable modifications (N-term acetylation, methionine oxidation, deamidation (NQ), carbamylation (KR)). The results were used for generation of a sample-specific spectral library.

2.2.7. HRM Data Analysis

HRM mass spectrometric data were analyzed using Spectronaut™ 14 software (Biognosys). The false discovery rate (FDR) on peptide and protein levels was set to 1% and data were filtered using row-based extraction. The spectral library generated in this study was used for the analysis. The HRM measurements analyzed with Spectronaut™ were normalized using global normalization.

2.2.8. Data Analysis

For testing of differential protein abundance, MS1 and MS2 protein intensity information was used [19]. Protein intensities for each protein were analyzed using a two sample Student's t-test, and p-values were corrected for overall FDR using the q-value approach [20]. The following thresholds were applied for candidate ranking: q-value < 0.05 and absolute average log2 ratio > 0.8074 (fold change > 1.75). After removal of proteins that were not identified in at least 90% of the samples, a selection based on ROC analysis was performed in order to identify the final list of the best performing 25 candidates (AUC > 0.670 and >10% specificity at 100% sensitivity).

2.3. ELISA Validation

Validation of mass spectrometry results was performed using commercially available ELISA kits and following the manufacturers' protocols (Table S1). Before use, urine sample aliquots were equilibrated to room temperature. Measurements were conducted using the Epoch 2 microplate reader (BioTek, Zürich, Switzerland) and data were analyzed with the Gen5 software (version 2.09, BioTek, Zürich, Switzerland).

2.4. Immunohistochemical Staining of Prostate Tissues

For immunohistochemical evaluation a representative tissue block of $n = 11$ prostate adenocarcinoma cases, including periurethral tumor manifestations if available, was selected and stained for specific antibodies (Table S2). Staining and detection was performed using an automated staining system (Ventana). Semi-quantitative evaluation for each antibody was performed by two experienced pathologists. For each tissue block a corresponding hematoxylin–eosin (HE)-stained slide was available for morphological identification of prostate cancer. For each immunohistochemical marker the expression in the tumor and normal prostatic tissue were evaluated separately by assigning a four-tiered score (0 = negative, 1 = weak, 2 = moderate, 3 = strong). The extent of stained benign and malignant glands was estimated in 10% increments. In addition, the cellular compartment of the staining for both tumor area and normal prostatic glands was specified, whereas in the normal prostatic glands further evaluation of the distinct stained cell type (luminal and basal cells) was recorded. The predominant staining pattern was assessed when considerable heterogeneity of the staining intensity was detected.

2.5. Statistics and Data Analysis

All statistical analyses (except for mass spectrometry data) were performed with the GraphPad prism software, version 9. Continuous variables were expressed as box-plots (from the 25th to the 75th percentile and median), with whiskers representing the minimum and the maximum values. Statistical significance was calculated with the unpaired non-parametric Mann–Whitney U test.

For the characterization of single biomarkers, ROC curve analysis was performed applying the Wilson/Brown method, whereas for combinatorial analysis of non-correlated proteins, a multiple logistic regression was applied. The correlation matrix was assessed with the Pearson correlation method.

An online tool was used to draw volcano plots (VolcaNoseR, https://huygens.science.uva.nl/VolcaNoseR/, accessed on 8 September 2021).

3. Results

3.1. Patient Characteristics

A total of 45 consecutive men with suspected PCa were enrolled in this study and underwent a prostate biopsy after urine sample collection. Their demographic and clinical characteristics are summarized in Table 1, including age, serum PSA and prostate volume. Biopsy results are classified according to the Gleason score (GS) and evaluated for diagnostic purposes by genitourinary pathologists at the University Hospital of Zürich. PCa was detected in 46.7% (21/45) and clinically significant PCa (GS 7–9) in 37.8% of the patients. More precisely, 8.9% of the patients were diagnosed with GS 6, 17.8% with GS 7a/b, and 20.0% harbored a GS 8 or GS 9 tumor. Gleason score follow-up at repeated biopsies or upon prostatectomy showed that only one patient was upgraded.

Table 1. Characteristics of the patients. Statistical analysis was performed using a Mann–Whitney U test, which showed age as the only variable significantly different between the tumor vs. non-tumor patients (age: $p = 0.048$; PSA: $p = 0.323$; prostate volume: $p = 0.164$). * Data available for only 41 patients.

	Number of Samples (% of Total)	Gleason Score	Median Age (Min–Max)	Median Serum PSA (Min–Max)	Prostate Volume (Min–Max) *
No Tumor	24 (53.3%)	0	63.5 (52–82)	6.60 (2.00–14.97)	60.19 (18.56–203.68)
Tumor	21 (46.7%)	6–9	65 (52–76)	7.22 (2.00–38.80)	48.59 (17.00–80.63)
	4 (8.9%)	6	65 (64–70)	8.53 (4.53–17.37)	60.54 (30.90–80.63)
	8 (17.8%)	7	65 (52–73)	4.94 (2.00–11.00)	50.00 (26.45–72.54)
	9 (20.0%)	8–9	74 (58–76)	12.41 (4.86–38.80)	47.17 (17.00–60.00)
Total	45 (100%)		65 (52–82)	6.90 (2.00–38.80)	52.00 (17.00–203.68)

Collected urine samples were then screened by MS and potential novel biomarkers analyzed by ELISA (Figure 1A).

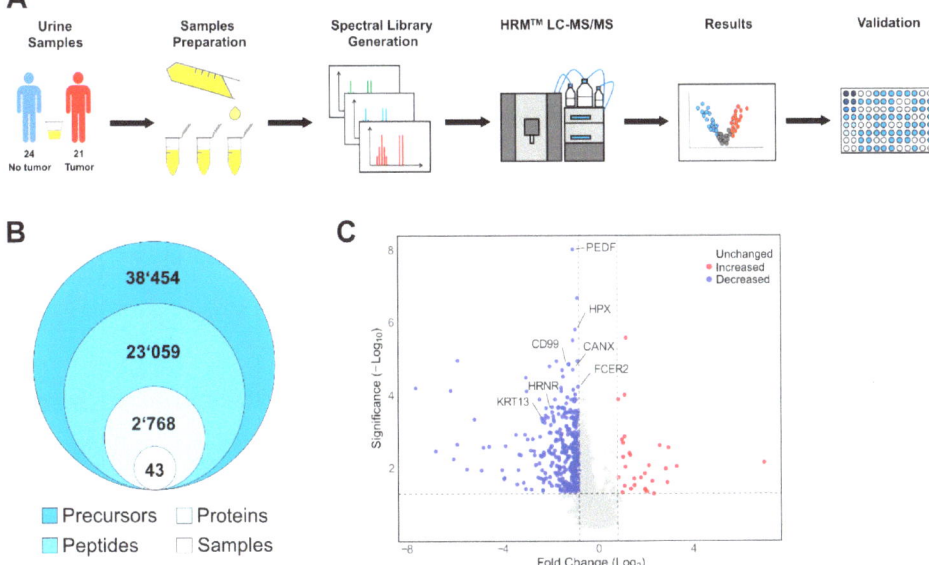

Figure 1. Identification of candidate urine biomarkers by mass spectrometry. (**A**) Schematic workflow overview of urine biomarker screening via mass spectrometry and validation with ELISA; (**B**) 2.768 proteins, 23.059 peptides, and 38.454 precursors were quantified across all 43 urine samples. (**C**) Volcano plot of 2.768 proteins quantified by mass spectrometry. The 351 differently distributed protein candidates are shown in blue (decreased in tumors) and red (increased in tumors) and were defined by: q-value < 0.05 and average fold change > 1.75. The seven candidates PEDF, HPX, CD99, CANX, FCER2, HRNR, and KRT13 are indicated.

3.2. Mass Spectrometry Screening and Selection of Urine Biomarkers for PCa Detection

For mass-spectrometry, a spectral peptide library was generated by shotgun LC–MS/MS of high-pH reversed-phase chromatography (HPRP) fractions from all 45 urine samples. Two samples showed a significant contamination with albumin, which led to the suppression of other peptide signals, and were therefore excluded from further analysis (data not shown). We identified a total of 38.454 precursors (peptides including different charges and modifications), corresponding to 23.059 unique peptides and 2.768 proteins across all 43 urine samples by using a false discovery rate of 1% (Figure 1B).

For the identification of candidate biomarkers to detect healthy men, we compared the abundance of 2.768 proteins in samples from patients not affected by tumor and those with PCa. Significantly dysregulated proteins were identified by setting the q-value below 0.05, at an average fold change of more than 1.75, resulting in 351 biomarker candidates (Figure 1C, Table S3). Strikingly, most of the candidates (321) displayed decreased levels in the urine of PCa patients compared to healthy men. In contrast, only 30 candidate biomarker candidates were found to have increased levels in the "tumor" group.

A key selection criterion for the best target molecules from the screening was the ability to discriminate healthy patients (with high specificity and accuracy), achieving a negligible number of false negatives (sensitivity > 90%). For this reason, all proteins that were not detected in more than three samples were excluded from further analysis. Additionally, proteins with low diagnostic performances, displaying a receiver operating characteristic (ROC) area under the curve (AUC) smaller than 0.670 and a specificity of less than 10% at 100% sensitivity, were removed. This ranking resulted in 43 biomarkers, with the top

25 candidates listed in Table S4. Among them, pigment epithelium-derived factor (PEDF), hemopexin (HPX), cluster of differentiation 99 (CD99), calnexin precursor (CANX), FCER2 (CD23, Fc fragment Of IgE receptor II), hornerin (HRNR), and keratin 13 (KRT13) showed remarkable diagnostic performance (Figure 2A,B; Table 2) and were selected for further validation by means of commercially available ELISA kits. Notably, all these biomarkers showed decreased levels in patients harboring prostate cancer.

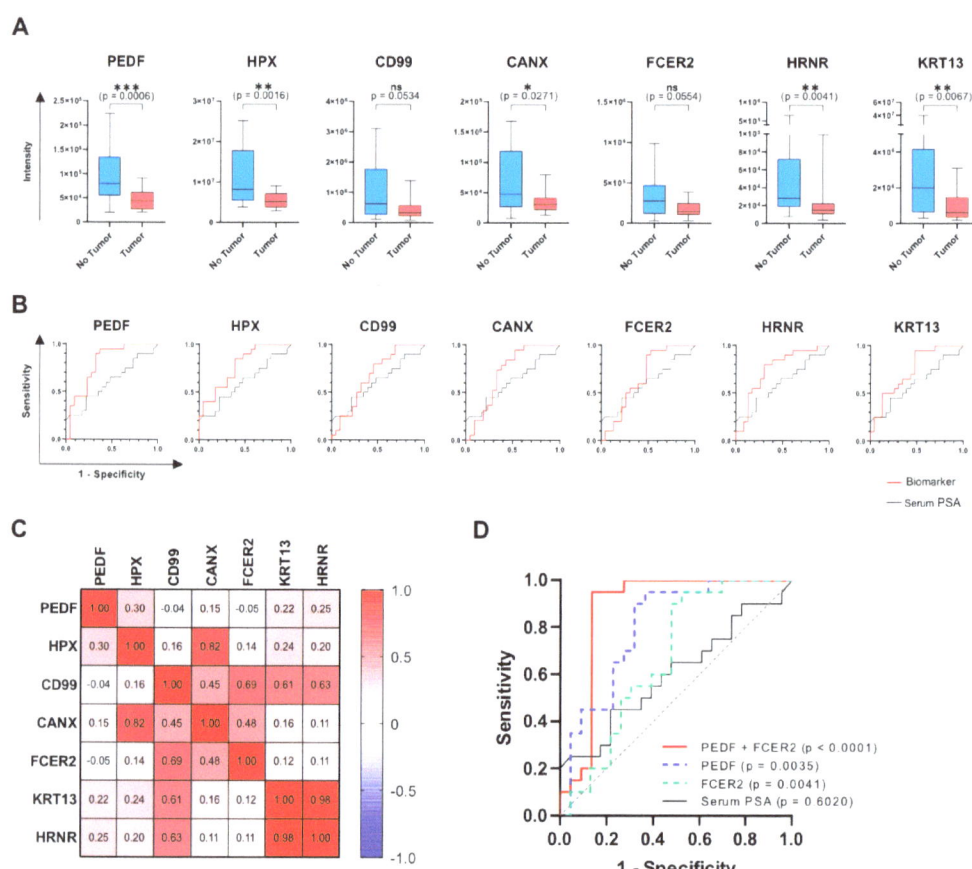

Figure 2. Potential candidate biomarkers for the detection of healthy men. Mass-spectrometry based quantification of the biomarkers (**A**) PEDF, HPX, CD99, CANX, FCER2, HRNR, and KRT13 in patients with and without PCa. Results are expressed as box-plots (from the 25th to the 75th percentile and median) with whiskers representing the minimum and the maximum values (Table S5). Statistical difference was assessed by the unpaired non-parametric Mann–Whitney U test with $p \leq 0.05$ defined as statistically significant (ns $p > 0.05$; * $p \leq 0.05$; ** $p \leq 0.01$; *** $p \leq 0.001$). (**B**) Diagnostic performances of the selected biomarkers assessed with the receiver operating characteristic (ROC). Each single biomarker (red curve) has a higher performance compared to serum PSA (black curve, AUC = 0.6020). (**C**) Correlation matrix assessed with the Pearson correlation method showing the correlation coefficients of the seven biomarkers with each other. A correlation between variables is defined as low for values up to ±0.3, medium for values up to ±0.5 and large for values up to ±1. (**D**) Combinatory analysis of non-correlating biomarkers via multiple logistic regression for the identification of tumor-free men. Coupling of PEDF and FCER2 resulted in the best performing biomarker combination, with an AUC of 0.8773 and a specificity of 72.7% at 100% sensitivity. Combined biomarkers displayed a higher performance compared to the single candidates and to serum PSA (black curve, AUC = 0.6020).

Table 2. ROC curve and multiple logistic regression analysis of the mass spectrometry results. The analysis was performed on the seven biomarker candidates and their possible non-correlating combinations for the identification of healthy men.

Biomarker	AUC	Std. Error	95% Confidence Interval	p-Value	Specificity at 90% Sensitivity	Specificity at 100% Sensitivity
PEDF	0.8023	0.070	0.6659 to 0.9386	0.0008	68.2	36.4
HPX	0.7761	0.070	0.6396 to 0.9125	0.0020	52.2	39.1
HRNR	0.7522	0.076	0.6033 to 0.9010	0.0047	47.8	13.0
KRT13	0.7391	0.075	0.5913 to 0.8869	0.0074	52.2	30.4
CANX	0.7043	0.085	0.5377 to 0.8708	0.0273	47.6	38.1
CD99	0.6750	0.083	0.5114 to 0.8386	0.0525	36.4	31.8
FCER2	0.6717	0.084	0.5075 to 0.8360	0.0544	52.2	30.4
PEDF + HPX	0.8977	0.050	0.7999 to 0.9956	<0.0001	72.7	50.0
PEDF + CD99	0.8786	0.056	0.7689 to 0.9883	<0.0001	76.2	66.7
PEDF + FCER2	0.8773	0.063	0.7530 to 1.000	<0.0001	86.4	72.7
PEDF + KRT13	0.8705	0.055	0.7618 to 0.9791	<0.0001	72.7	54.5
PEDF + HRNR	0.8568	0.058	0.7437 to 0.9699	<0.0001	77.3	54.5
PEDF + CANX	0.9105	0.053	0.8067 to 1.000	<0.0001	85.0	70.0
HPX + HRNR	0.8739	0.054	0.7682 to 0.9797	<0.0001	73.9	34.8
HPX + KRT13	0.8413	0.061	0.7211 to 0.9615	0.0001	60.9	56.5
HRNR + CANX	0.8496	0.062	0.7272 to 0.9720	0.0002	66.7	66.7
HPX + FCER2	0.8000	0.068	0.6670 to 0.9330	0.0008	60.9	60.9
HPX + CD99	0.7864	0.071	0.6462 to 0.9265	0.0015	63.6	54.5
KRT13 + CANX	0.7820	0.076	0.6322 to 0.9318	0.0023	61.9	61.9
KRT13 + FCER2	0.7652	0.074	0.6193 to 0.9111	0.0030	60.9	47.8
HRNR + FCER2	0.7457	0.076	0.5964 to 0.8949	0.0059	60.9	34.8

The illustrated box plots in Figure 2A show the intensities of the biomarkers in patients with and without PCa as quantified by MS. All biomarkers identify true negative patients that could be spared from performing an unnecessary prostate biopsy, although the p value was a borderline result in terms of statistical significance for two biomarkers. The ROC plots (Figure 2B) show the ability of the single biomarkers to detect all PCa (GS 6–9, red curves) in comparison to the current standard of care, which is serum PSA (black curves). Each of the seven biomarkers had a superior performance compared to PSA and was able to correctly classify 100% of patients with PCa, while detecting tumor free men at varying specificities (Table 2).

Taken together, these data demonstrate that urine is a reliable proteomic source of biomarkers for the early detection of PCa and that the seven selected biomarker candidates are capable of sparing a relevant number of men from unnecessary prostate biopsy while avoiding misdiagnosis of patients bearing a prostate tumor.

3.3. Increase of PCa Detection Performance through Combinatory Analysis of Biomarkers

To assess potential biomarker combinations via multiple logistic regression, we first performed a Pearson correlation analysis among biomarker levels in the patient cohort (Figure 2C). In fact, the combination of variables can improve the performance of a predictive model only if the variables are not correlated to each other. In our analysis, we therefore combined biomarkers with a correlation coefficient of up to 0.3. Since the size of the cohort is limited to 43 patients, combinations of a maximum of two biomarkers were taken into consideration, in order to prevent the generation of overfitted models. All possible 14 combinations of biomarkers revealed a significantly larger AUC compared to the null hypothesis of AUC = 0.5 (Table 2). Moreover, any combination of two proteins led to a superior diagnostic performance, with increased AUC and higher specificity at 90% and 100% sensitivity compared to the single biomarkers. As an example, Figure 2D illustrates the multiple logistic regression curve of the PEDF and FCER2 combination (red line), which reached the best specificity of 72.7% at 100% sensitivity. This indicates that potentially 72.7% of healthy men could be spared from performing an unnecessary biopsy.

Our data show that the combination of biomarkers markedly improves the diagnostic power of the model and leads to the superior detection of healthy patients who could be spared from a prostate biopsy.

3.4. Validation of Biomarker Performance by ELISA

The validation of the candidate proteins selected from the MS analysis was performed by ELISA. Conversely to MS, immunoassays are standardized techniques that can be easily performed in any laboratory and allow for easy comparison among cohorts. For the MS measurements, the different urine samples were normalized according to their total peptide concentration and a defined amount of 2 µg was injected for each run. This approach cannot be applied to ELISA. Nevertheless, normalization is necessary to compensate for variations due to diet, time of collection and physiological characteristics of patients. Therefore, we have chosen non-dysregulated molecules from the mass-spectrometry analysis, i.e., cluster of differentiation 44 (CD44) and ribonuclease A family member 2 (RNASE2) and used them as controls for ELISA quantification of the single biomarkers (Figure S1; Table S4). Consistent with the corresponding MS data, Mann–Whitney U analysis of the normalized ELISA data for each analyte showed a significant difference between patients diagnosed with PCa and healthy individuals (Figure 3A). Furthermore, ROC curve analysis is concurrent with each MS dataset, demonstrating that all biomarkers have the diagnostic potential to detect healthy men at 100% sensitivity (Table 3).

Table 3. ROC analysis of the ELISA results for the detection of healthy men and high-grade PCa. The table shows the diagnostic performance of ELISA results obtained normalizing the concentration of the seven candidates with two control molecules (CD44 and RNASE2). The "all PCa grades" analysis identifies healthy men (reaching 100% sensitivity at a specific threshold), whereas the "high-grade (GS 7–9) PCa" analysis identifies true negatives as either healthy men or patients harboring GS 6 PCa (reaching 100% sensitivity at a specific threshold).

	Biomarker	AUC	Std. Error	95% Confidence Interval	p-Value	Specificity at 90% Sensitivity	Specificity at 100% Sensitivity
All PCa grades	KRT13	0.8087	0.066	0.6797 to 0.9377	0.0005	43.5	43.5
	HPX	0.7696	0.071	0.6314 to 0.9077	0.0025	47.8	43.5
	PEDF	0.7609	0.073	0.6176 to 0.9041	0.0035	34.8	30.4
	CD99	0.7565	0.073	0.6136 to 0.8994	0.0041	52.2	47.8
	FCER2	0.7565	0.074	0.6114 to 0.9017	0.0041	47.8	13.0
	CANX	0.7457	0.076	0.5971 to 0.8942	0.0059	30.4	26.1
	HRNR	0.7120	0.080	0.5553 to 0.8686	0.0176	39.1	17.4
High-grade PCa	KRT13	0.7708	0.075	0.6247 to 0.9170	0.0033	40.7	37.1
	HPX	0.7546	0.074	0.6094 to 0.8998	0.0057	44.4	37.0
	PEDF	0.7292	0.079	0.5752 to 0.8831	0.0129	33.3	29.6
	FCER2	0.7269	0.081	0.5690 to 0.8847	0.0138	44.4	11.2
	CD99	0.7222	0.078	0.5688 to 0.8756	0.0159	40.7	40.7
	HRNR	0.6956	0.083	0.5321 to 0.8591	0.0337	37.0	14.8
	CANX	0.6528	0.086	0.4849 to 0.8207	0.0973	25.9	22.1

Detection of high grade PCa has a relevant clinical impact, as it allows differentiation between patients who would benefit from active surveillance and those who need active treatments. We therefore also tested the potential of our biomarkers to discriminate also

PCa GS ≥ 7. The quantitative analysis by ELISA shows that the seven biomarkers can detect high-grade PCa with high performance (Figure 3B, Table 3).

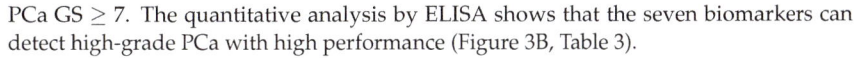

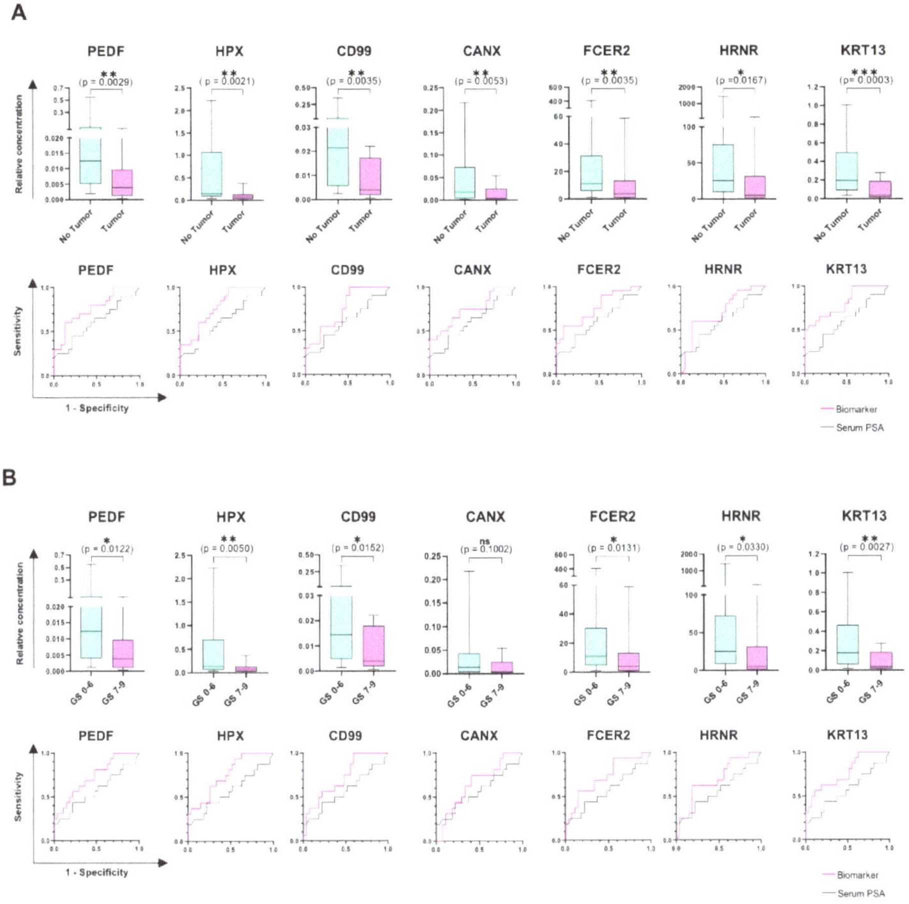

Figure 3. Validation of candidate biomarkers with ELISA for the detection of healthy men or high-grade PCa. Commercially available ELISA kits were used and results for PEDF, HPX, CD99, CANX, FCER2, HRNR, and KRT13 are represented as box-plots, where the relative concentration of the biomarkers normalized to two control molecules (CD44 and RNASE2) is compared for men with (**A**) no tumor to patients with any grade of PCa and (**B**) men with no tumor or low grade (GS = 6) PCa to patients harboring a high-grade tumor (GS ≥ 7). Significance was assessed with a statistical Mann–Whitney test (ns $p > 0.05$; * $p \leq 0.05$; ** $p \leq 0.01$; *** $p \leq 0.001$). Results are expressed as box-plots (from the 25th to the 75th percentile and median) with whiskers representing the minimum and the maximum values (Table S5). The diagnostic potential of the single biomarkers was investigated with receiver operating characteristic (ROC) analysis. All biomarkers (purple curve) showed a better performance compared to serum PSA (black curve, all grades AUC = 0.6020; high-grade PCa AUC = 0.5690).

When different biomarkers are normalized by the same controls, as in this study, their combinatory power is hampered by a highly correlated dataset (data not shown), driven by the identical normalization strategy. Hence, combinatorial analysis was performed by multiple logistic regression with non-normalized ELISA data. In this study, we excluded from the nomogram any clinical and demographic information with potentially high variability among individual clinics and cohorts. Prostate volume and digital rectal examination (DRE), for example, are known to be affected by the type of instrument used or by personnel expertise. We therefore included only the age of the patients as clinical variable to improve the predictive models. The Pearson correlation analysis of all variables is shown in Figure 4A. All combinations, including age, resulted in a significantly higher AUC compared to the null hypothesis and were able to detect all grades of PCa with 100% sensitivity (Table 4). As an example, the ROC curve of two of the best performing combinations, PEDF + FCER2 + age and KRT13 + FCER2 + age showed a specificity of 39.1% and 52.2% at 100% sensitivity, respectively (Figure 4B). Moreover, for the detection of high-grade tumors, the combination of uncorrelated analytes increased the overall performance of the single biomarkers. As model example, the ELISA quantification of KRT13, FCER2 + age showed a striking AUC of 0.7801 with a specificity of 48.1% at 100% sensitivity (Figure 4C).

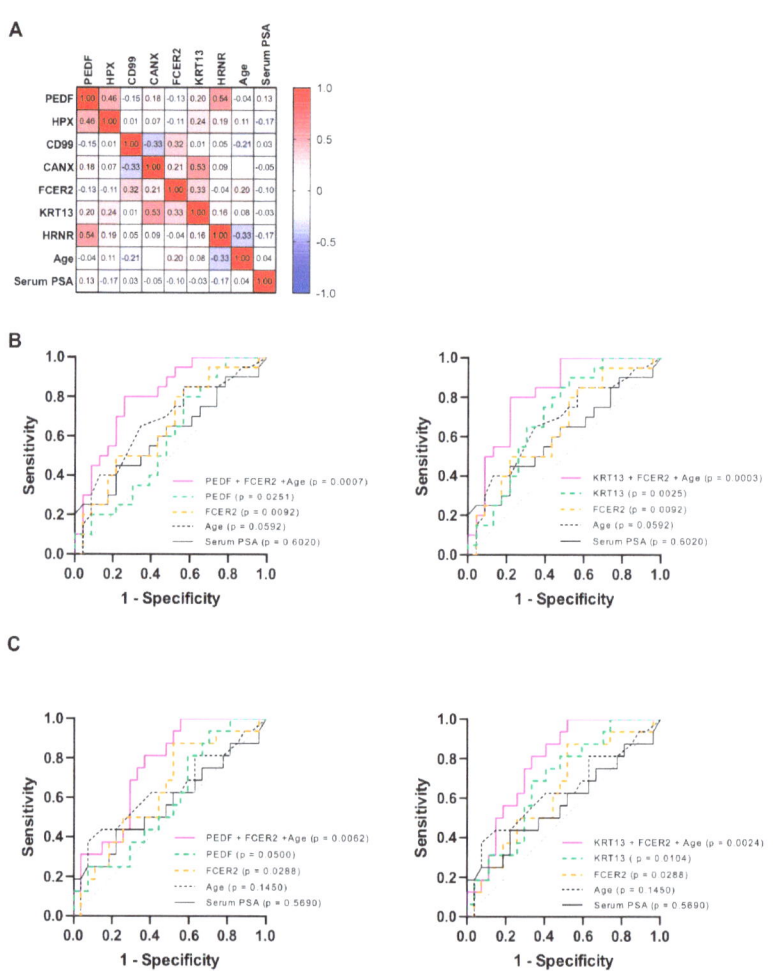

Figure 4. Multiple logistic regression analysis for the combination of biomarker levels (quantification by ELISA) with the patient's age. (**A**) Pearson correlation matrix showing the correlation coefficients of the seven biomarkers, age and serum PSA with each other. A correlation between variables is defined as low for values up to ±0.3, medium for values up to ±0.5 and large for values up to ±1. (**B**) Combinatory analysis of immunoassay validation for the detection of healthy men. The combination of PEDF and FCER2 resulted as best pair from mass spectrometry and, in addition to age, achieved a final AUC of 0.8022 and a 39.1% specificity at 100% sensitivity. ELISA results revealed that, with an AUC of 0.8196 and a specificity of 52.2%, the best performing combination of biomarker

was KRT13, FCER2, and age. Combined biomarkers showed a better performance compared to the single candidates and to serum PSA (black curve, AUC = 0.6020). (**C**) The combination of biomarkers with age can predict the presence of high-grade PCa. PEDF, FCER2, and age achieved a final AUC of 0.7523 and a 44.5% specificity at 100% sensitivity. By combining KRT13, FCER2, and age the performance reached an AUC of 0.7801 and a specificity of 48.1% (serum PSA is represented by the black curve, AUC = 0.5690).

Table 4. ROC curve and multiple logistic regression analysis of the ELISA results for the detection of healthy men or high-grade PCa. The seven single biomarkers (not normalized) and their combinations (including patients' age as variable) were analyzed. The "all PCa grades" analysis identifies healthy men (reaching 100% sensitivity at a specific threshold), whereas the "high-grade (GS 7–9) PCa" analysis identifies true negatives as either healthy men or patients harboring GS 6 PCa (reaching 100% sensitivity at a specific threshold).

	Biomarker	AUC	Std. Error	95% Confidence Interval	p-Value	Specificity at 90% Sensitivity	Specificity at 100% Sensitivity
All PCa grades	KRT13	0.7696	0.071	0.6298 to 0.9093	0.0025	52.2	30.4
	HRNR	0.7413	0.079	0.5865 to 0.8961	0.0069	52.2	8.7
	FCER2	0.7326	0.077	0.5813 to 0.8839	0.0092	52.2	39.1
	CANX	0.7043	0.080	0.5479 to 0.8608	0.0221	30.4	17.4
	PEDF	0.700	0.081	0.5404 to 0.8596	0.0251	30.4	30.4
	HPX	0.6978	0.081	0.5386 to 0.8570	0.0267	39.1	8.7
	CD99	0.6652	0.083	0.5032 to 0.8273	0.0642	34.8	21.7
	KRT13 + FCER2	0.8196	0.065	0.6927 to 0.9464	0.0003	52.2	52.2
	HPX + FCER2	0.8087	0.067	0.6767 to 0.9407	0.0005	43.5	30.4
	PEDF + FCER2	0.8022	0.067	0.6714 to 0.9329	0.0007	52.2	39.1
	HPX + KRT13	0.7826	0.070	0.6462 to 0.9190	0.0015	52.2	30.4
	HRNR + FCER2	0.7826	0.071	0.6429 to 0.9223	0.0015	56.5	13.0
	PEDF + KRT13	0.7804	0.070	0.6431 to 0.9178	0.0017	52.2	39.1
	KRT13 + CANX	0.7609	0.072	0.6189 to 0.9028	0.0035	47.8	30.4
	HPX + HRNR	0.7478	0.078	0.5960 to 0.8997	0.0055	43.5	8.7
	PEDF + CANX	0.7348	0.077	0.5844 to 0.8852	0.0085	47.8	26.1
	HRNR + CANX	0.7326	0.079	0.5781 to 0.8871	0.0092	43.5	8.7
	PEDF + CD99	0.7304	0.076	0.5808 to 0.8801	0.0099	43.5	34.8
	PEDF + HRNR	0.7283	0.080	0.5723 to 0.8842	0.0106	43.5	8.7
	HPX + CD99	0.7283	0.078	0.5753 to 0.8812	0.0106	39.1	17.4
	PEDF + HPX	0.7000	0.081	0.5417 to 0.8583	0.0251	26.1	13.0
High-grade PCa	KRT13	0.7361	0.077	0.5854 to 0.8868	0.0104	40.7	25.9
	HRNR	0.7199	0.084	0.5551 to 0.8847	0.0170	14.8	7.4
	FCER2	0.7014	0.079	0.5468 to 0.8560	0.0288	44.4	33.3
	HPX	0.6968	0.087	0.5262 to 0.8673	0.0327	7.4	7.4
	PEDF	0.6806	0.085	0.5141 to 0.8470	0.0500	33.3	18.5
	CD99	0.6644	0.086	0.4967 to 0.8320	0.0744	29.6	18.5
	CANX	0.6574	0.085	0.4907 to 0.8241	0.0875	22.2	14.8
	HPX + FCER2	0.7894	0.077	0.6376 to 0.9411	0.0017	33.3	33.3
	HPX + KRT13	0.7870	0.073	0.6432 to 0.9308	0.0018	33.3	18.5
	KRT13 + FCER2	0.7801	0.069	0.6447 to 0.9155	0.0024	51.8	48.1
	HPX + CD99	0.7662	0.078	0.6136 to 0.9188	0.0039	29.6	14.8
	PEDF + FCER2	0.7523	0.073	0.6090 to 0.8956	0.0062	48.1	44.5
	HRNR + FCER2	0.7523	0.076	0.6024 to 0.9022	0.0062	51.8	11.1
	HPX + HRNR	0.7500	0.084	0.5845 to 0.9155	0.0067	11.1	7.4
	PEDF + KRT13	0.7431	0.075	0.5964 to 0.8898	0.0083	44.5	33.3
	KRT13 + CANX	0.7384	0.076	0.5886 to 0.8882	0.0097	40.7	29.6
	PEDF + CD99	0.7176	0.078	0.5657 to 0.8695	0.0182	37.0	37.0
	PEDF + HPX	0.7083	0.083	0.5461 to 0.8705	0.0237	14.8	14.8
	HRNR + CANX	0.7014	0.083	0.5384 to 0.8644	0.0288	29.6	3.7
	PEDF + HRNR	0.6968	0.082	0.5358 to 0.8577	0.0327	33.3	11.1
	PEDF + CANX	0.6898	0.081	0.5303 to 0.8493	0.0394	44.4	18.5

Taken together, our data demonstrate that ELISA quantification of the biomarker candidates selected by MS is feasible and confirms the high diagnostic performance of the analytes, both as single and in combination for the detection of all PCa grades and clinically significant tumors (GS $\geq$ 7).

3.5. Immunohistochemical Analysis of Biomarker Expression in Malignant and Healthy Prostate Tissue

To investigate the possible origin of the biomarkers, we performed immunohistochemistry analysis on prostate tissues from 11 men (of the initial 45 patients) that underwent radical prostatectomy. Because it was not possible to analyze prostate tissue from healthy patients, the healthy tissue areas of the prostate were used as control for each patient who underwent prostatectomy. The stainings were performed on tissue blocks, including benign and malignant areas of the prostate to compare biomarker expression levels. In concordance with the MS and ELISA data, KRT13 staining showed a distinct expression in benign and low expression in malignant tissue areas (Figure 5A,B; Table S6). We observed basal cell staining for KRT13, PEDF, and HPX in benign regions of the gland, a cell type that is absent in acinar-type adenocarcinomas (Figure 5A–F). Immunohistochemical analysis of CD99, HRNR, and CANX confirmed the expression of these markers in the prostate but, due to high heterogeneity, with high- and low-expression areas in both healthy and tumor tissues, it was not possible to compare the two conditions (Figure S2). No expression of the B-cell specific antigen FCER2 was detected in the prostate (Figure S2).

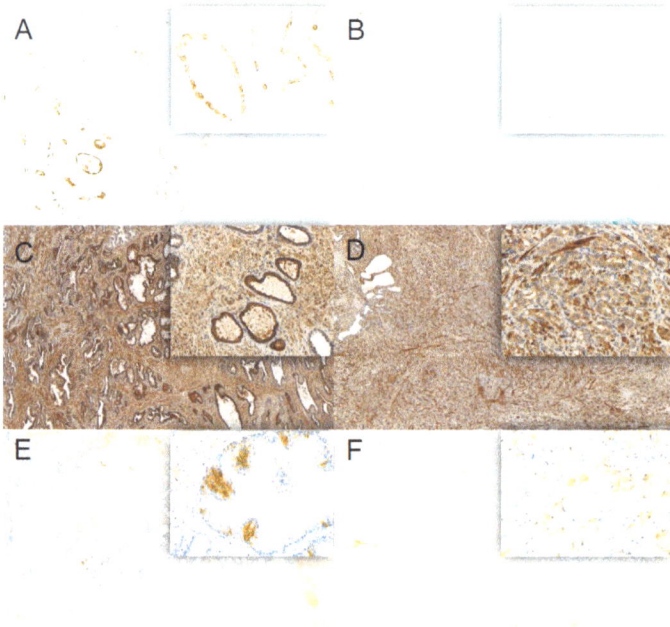

Figure 5. Immunohistochemical analysis of biomarker expression in benign and malignant prostate tissue. Overview (10× objective) of three biomarkers, which showed expression in basal cells, including respective magnifications (insets, 20× objective). (**A**) Positivity of KRT13 in basal cells of benign tissue, whereas (**B**) acinar adenocarcinoma shows loss of basal cells and KRT13 expression. (**C**) HPX showed in addition to expression in basal cells, reactivity in luminal cells of benign tissue, as well as obvious positivity in the fibromuscular stromal cells (background). (**D**) Prostate adenocarcinoma in comparison showed decreased expression of HPX. (**E**) PEDF showed reactivity in some of the basal cells, and weaker reactivity in luminal cells of the benign tissue. (**F**) In comparison, equally low expression in the (luminal) cells of the adenocarcinoma complexes.

4. Discussion

Despite continuous improvements in the reduction of overdiagnosis and overtreatment of men suspected of having PCa, the number of healthy men that are subject to invasive procedures remains high [6,21]. This trend is concordant with our cohort. For this study, patients were selected for prostate biopsy only due to abnormal DRE results and/or elevated PSA levels. Approximately half (53.3%) of patients resulted having no tumor and should have been spared from performing the biopsy (Table 1).

Thus, the aim of this study was to identify novel urine biomarkers to improve the eligibility criteria for prostate biopsy and to more specifically discriminate PCa at an early stage, reducing the number of unnecessary biopsies. Here, we demonstrated the feasibility of diagnostic tests for the screening of PCa relying on urine biomarkers that can be routinely quantified by standardized laboratory methods such as ELISAs.

Urine samples were collected from patients before performing the biopsy and subjected to proteomic screening by mass-spectrometry (MS) to select biomarker candidates that are dysregulated when a prostate tumor is present. Although MS results showed promising results, the application of mass-spectrometry for urine analysis as routine diagnostic test is not feasible, due to the lack of a standard method to compare different batches of samples. A more practical approach is the implementation of quantitative immune-assays such as ELISA, which represents the gold standard for biomarker assessment and validation [22]. Consequently, among the 25 most performant candidates, seven proteins (PEDF, HPX, CD99, FCER2 (CD23), CANX, HRNR, and KRT13) were subsequently quantified in the same urine samples by quantitative ELISA. Additionally, their performance for the diagnosis of PCa and prediction of high-grade tumors was assessed. Although the translation of targeted MS assays into the clinical diagnostic setting appears to be difficult due to high costs and specific expertise requirements [23], the validation by ELISA demonstrates the feasibility of a clinical implementation through standard techniques. MS results of the 25 top ranked biomarkers in this study showed a significant decrease in signal intensity when a prostate tumor is present and can identify PCa patients with better performance compared to the standard PSA test (Table S4).

PEDF showed the best performance as a single biomarker, with AUC of 0.8023 and specificity of 36.4% at 100% sensitivity (Figure 2A,B). On the other hand, as an example of the many possible options (Figure 2D), the best performing combination of PEDF and FCER2 markedly increase the AUC in predicting PCa compared to each individual marker and also to PSA. Specifically, with this combination 72.7% of unnecessary biopsies could be avoided, without missing any patient with PCa (100% sensitivity).

The proteomic content of urine is affected by many factors, such as individual lifestyle, diet and time of sampling. For this reason, absolute biomarker data need to be normalized with a different strategy compared to MS, in which normalization is based on the overall cohort protein content. Figure 3A shows normalized ELISA results of the biomarkers panel, where each single molecule shows a strong diagnostic performance, in concurrence with the MS data. By combining KRT13 and FCER2 with age, we reached an AUC of 0.8196 and a specificity 52.2% at 100% sensitivity (Figure 4B). Besides the early detection of PCa, risk stratification of patients to better select clinically significant tumors is important to support optimal treatment options. For this reason, we have assessed the ability of the seven biomarkers to also detect tumors with GS $\geq$ 7 as well. Figure 3B shows that all candidates can predict the presence of high-grade PCa more precisely than serum PSA. The combination of KRT13 and FCER2 with age for the detection of high-grade PCa reached an AUC of 0.7801 and a specificity of 48.1% at 100% sensitivity (Figure 4C), thus potentially reducing the number of unnecessary biopsies almost by half, without missing any patient with clinically relevant PCa. Depending on the clinic, region and patients' characteristics (e.g., age and expectation of life), men with low grade PCa (GS 6) will either be monitored or treated by local therapy options. In both cases, the novel biomarker panel can be applied to reduce unnecessary biopsies and monitor patients continuously and non-invasively. Therefore, by combining different biomarkers, we observed a relevant reduction of unnecessary biopsies, either performed on healthy individuals or on patients affected by clinically indolent tumors.

A relevant portion of the proteins identified in our study has already been described in other mass-spectrometry analyses of urine and to a lesser extent, in urinary extracellular vesicles, plasma or prostate tissue of patients. The seven biomarkers validated in our study were chosen exclusively based on their ability to predict PCa prior to biopsy and not considering their biological function. Nevertheless, some of them have been reported to be related to cancer. Although signal reduction in case of tumor progression as described for the seven biomarkers might be surprising, both literature and tissue analysis performed in this study support these findings. Hornerin (HRNR), a member of the fused-type S100 protein family, was shown to be expressed and to play a role in different tumor types [24–26]. Other members of the same protein family were examined in prostate tissue of PCa patients, demonstrating that the loss of S100A2 and increased expression of S100A4 are hallmarks of PCa progression [27]. Similarly, the prostate tissue analysis of the pigment epithelium-derived factor (PEDF), a natural angiogenesis inhibitor in prostate and pancreas [28,29], showed minimal expression in high grade PCa (GS 7–10), in contrast to healthy prostate tissue, where the staining shows high intensity [28]. The downregulation of CD99 was already shown to be essential for tumorigenesis. This has been described for several tumors [30–32], including prostate cancer [33]. In fact, the overexpression of CD99 in prostate cancer cells inhibited their migration and metastatic potential in both in vitro and in vivo experiments [31]. Hemopexin (HPX) has been described to be downregulated in urine from PCa patients compared to tumor free men, an observation that is in concordance with our findings [34]. Moreover, a bioinformatics analysis of multiple urinary and tissue proteomes revealed HPX downregulation in high-grade PCa compared to healthy tissue [35]. In contrast to our results, elevated levels in cancer have been reported for the remaining molecules. Increased levels of the Fc fragment of IgE receptor II (FCER2) have been implicated in different hematological malignancies and sarcomas [36–41]. In addition, FCER2 is expressed in subsets of B cells and in particular depicts follicular dendritic cell networks [42], whereas expression changes in urine could reflect an altered immune microenvironment in prostate adenocarcinoma patients. Keratin 13 (KRT13) belongs to the type I keratin family and its reduced expression has been associated with oral squamous cell carcinoma lesions [43–45] and bladder cancer [46]. In contrast to our results, a study in 2016 revealed a correlation between KRT13 tissue expression and prostate cancer metastasis [47]. However, as we could show expression of KRT13 in the basal cells of benign glands, and since the loss of basal cells is one hallmark of prostate adenocarcinoma [48], lower expression levels in urine could also be explained by increased tumoral occupation of the gland. The endoplasmic reticulum chaperone calnexin (CANX) is associated with newly synthesized glycoproteins and involved in correct protein folding [49]. So far, CANX has not been described in PCa but its altered expression has been associated with other cancers [50,51]. To the best of our knowledge, this is the first study to suggest a putative role in PCa for the above-described biomarkers in PCa, demonstrating their dysregulation at such an early stage (prior to biopsy) and the feasibility of their quantitative assessment in urine.

To investigate the possible origin of the biomarkers and their route to the urine, we performed a sequence-based analysis, predicting secretion pathways of proteins with the SecretomeP 2.0 server (http://www.cbs.dtu.dk/services/SecretomeP/, accessed on 5 October 2021). PEDF, HPX, CD99, and CANX are expressed with signal peptides and potentially traffic through the classical pathway (Golgi apparatus), whereas membrane protein FCER2 was predicted to traffic through a non-classical pathway. Conversely, KRT13 and HRNR do not appear to be secreted. This suggests that the proteins detected may be present in urine due to either the presence of cellular debris or particles deriving directly from the prostate or through blood filtration.

The prostate tissue analysis performed in this study confirms that six out of seven biomarkers validated by ELISA are expressed in prostatic adenocarcinomas. Intensity analysis shows that KRT13 levels are lower in tumor tissue compared to healthy prostate, in agreement with the MS and ELISA data. Tissue staining further revealed that KRT13, PEDF, and HPX are predominantly expressed in basal cells of the benign tissue, whereas they are not detected in tumor areas where basal cells have been lost. Notably, these findings are in support of the decreased levels detected in urine of PCa patients, as the basal cells might be responsible for the direct shedding or secretion of these biomarkers into the acinar lumen and thus the loss of expression of the biomarkers can be reflected in their dysregulated levels detected in the cohort. The heterogeneous expression of CD99, HRNR, and CANX in both healthy and tumor tissue hampered the quantitative comparison. FCER2 was not detected in prostate tissue and might derive from immune cells, as it is known to be expressed in B lymphocytes [52], thus suggesting that a relevant involvement of the immune system in PCa could be detected in urine at an early stage.

The present study has some limitations. First, it is a retrospective and single institution based study. Second, it relies on a small sample size, combining data of 43 patients for biomarker identification and validation. This became particularly evident when performing the multiple logistic regression analysis, as the cohort size determines the number of variables that can be combined to improve the model. To avoid false associations and large standard errors, a minimum number of five to ten events per predictor variable (EPV) has to be considered [53]. Since our cohort comprises 23 healthy men, we included no more than two to four predictor variables. Future studies investigating larger cohort sizes will allow the inclusion of higher numbers of variables and thereby improve their diagnostic performance. Nevertheless, for an explorative analysis of the biomarker candidates, the cohort provided a sufficient sample size and the combination of two to three variables yielded robust prediction models. Although it was currently not possible to validate the biomarkers in an independent cohort, their performance in this study was proved by use of two different and independent quantitative technologies, and the concordance of the findings underscores the importance of further validation of the targets.

5. Conclusions

In conclusion, here, we demonstrated that an upfront urine test based solely on the quantification of novel biomarkers is a feasible approach to improve eligibility criteria for a prostate biopsy and to detect the presence of high-grade PCa, independent of serum PSA, digital rectal examination, and clinical variables. The clinical implementation of a simple urine test represents one possible and safe way to reduce the overdiagnosis and overtreatment of PCa. Furthermore, since it is completely non-invasive, it could potentially be used for disease monitoring and active surveillance.

6. Patents

This study was submitted for patent application (applicant: University of Zürich; inventors: I. Banzola, N. Alijaj, B. Pavlovic, D. Eberli). The patent application was submitted to the European patent office (application number: EP 21/215742.4).

Supplementary Materials: The following supporting information can be downloaded at: https://www.mdpi.com/article/10.3390/cancers14051135/s1, Figure S1: Mass spectrometry analysis of two possible control molecules; Figure S2: Representative images of HRNR, CD99, CANX and FCER2 immunohistochemical stainings in one prostate adenocarcinoma patient (10× objective); Table S1: Commercial ELISA kits used for the validation of biomarker candidates; Table S2: Antibodies used for the immunohistochemical staining of prostate tissues; Table S3: Ranked candidate biomarkers from the MS screening for the detection of PCa; Table S4: Top 25 biomarkers and two control molecules resulted from mass spectrometry screening; Table S5: Statistical analysis of the biomarkers' mass-spectrometry and ELISA quantification results; Table S6: Immunohistochemical staining of eleven prostate adenocarcinoma cases.

Author Contributions: N.A., B.P., J.H.R., M.D.B. and N.J.R. acquired data. B.P. prepared the urine samples for mass spectrometry and ELISA measurements. N.A. and B.P. performed the ELISA experiments. M.D.B. and N.J.R. evaluated the immunohistochemical stainings of prostate tissues, which were comprehensively reviewed by J.H.R., N.A., B.P., M.D.B., J.H.R. and N.J.R., with contributions from D.E. and I.B. The collection of samples and clinical data were performed by A.R., K.S., C.P., T.H., P.O., V.C., M.P. and M.V. (Markus Veit). Substantial contributions to the conception, design, and intellectual content of the paper was made by N.A., B.P., P.M., L.D., M.V. (Massimo Valerio), D.E. and I.B. The paper was written by N.A., B.P. and I.B.; N.A. and B.P. contributed equally to this work as co-first authors; I.B and D.E. contributed equally to this work as co-last authors. All authors have read and agreed to the published version of the manuscript.

Funding: This work was supported by the "Gebert Rüf Stiftung" (GRS-039/18), the "Innosuisse-Swiss Innovation Agency" (40242.1 IP-LS), the "UZH Entrepreneur Fellowship" (University of Zurich, MEDEF 20018), and the "BRIDGE Proof of Concept programme" (Swiss National Science Foundation and Innosuisse, 40B1-0_203684/1).

Institutional Review Board Statement: The study was conducted according to the guidelines of the Declaration of Helsinki, and approved by the Ethics Committee of Canton Zürich, Switzerland (BASEC n° 2016-00829).

Informed Consent Statement: Informed consent was obtained from all subjects involved in the study.

Data Availability Statement: All data presented in this study are available in the manuscript and in the supplementary materials. Additional information are available for bona fide researchers who request it from the authors.

Acknowledgments: The authors would like to thank the SNSF and the Innosuisse programme for their support and Alexandra Veloudios for the collection of urine samples and the assistance in providing patient data. We are obliged to all patients for their dedicated collaboration.

Conflicts of Interest: N.J.R. discloses an advisory board function and receipt of honoraria from F. Hoffmann-La Roche AG. This study was submitted for patent application (applicant: University of Zürich; inventors: I. Banzola, N. Alijaj, B. Pavlovic, D. Eberli). The patent application was submitted to the European patent office (application number: EP 21/215742.4).

Abbreviations

PCa	prostate cancer
PSA	prostate specific antigen
MS	mass spectrometry
AUC	area under the curve
MRI	magnetic resonance imaging
NMR	nuclear magnetic resonance
ELISA	enzyme-linked immunosorbent assay
DRE	digital rectal examination
HPLC	high-performance liquid chromatography
FA	formic acid
UV/VIS	ultraviolet–visible
HPRP	high-pH reversed-phase chromatography
LC–MS	liquid chromatography–mass spectrometry
HRM	high resolution mass spectrometry
DIA	data-independent acquisition
FDR	false discovery rate
ROC	receiver operating characteristic
HE	Hematoxylin–eosin
GS	Gleason score
EPV	events per predictor variable
PEDF	pigment epithelium-derived factor
HPX	hemopexin

CD99	cluster of differentiation 99	
CANX	calnexin precursor	
FCER2	Fc fragment Of IgE receptor II	
HRNR	hornerin	
KRT13	keratin 13	
CD44	cluster of differentiation 44	
RNASE2	ribonuclease A family member 2	

References

1. Ferlay, J.; Colombet, M.; Soerjomataram, I.; Mathers, C.; Parkin, D.M.; Pineros, M.; Znaor, A.; Bray, F. Estimating the global cancer incidence and mortality in 2018: GLOBOCAN sources and methods. *Int. J. Cancer* **2019**, *144*, 1941–1953. [CrossRef] [PubMed]
2. Schroder, F.H.; Hugosson, J.; Roobol, M.J.; Tammela, T.L.; Zappa, M.; Nelen, V.; Kwiatkowski, M.; Lujan, M.; Maattanen, L.; Lilja, H.; et al. Screening and prostate cancer mortality: Results of the European Randomised Study of Screening for Prostate Cancer (ERSPC) at 13 years of follow-up. *Lancet* **2014**, *384*, 2027–2035. [CrossRef]
3. Osses, D.F.; Roobol, M.J.; Schoots, I.G. Prediction Medicine: Biomarkers, Risk Calculators and Magnetic Resonance Imaging as Risk Stratification Tools in Prostate Cancer Diagnosis. *Int. J. Mol. Sci.* **2019**, *20*, 1637. [CrossRef]
4. Bokhorst, L.P.; Zhu, X.; Bul, M.; Bangma, C.H.; Schroder, F.H.; Roobol, M.J. Positive predictive value of prostate biopsy indicated by prostate-specific-antigen-based prostate cancer screening: Trends over time in a European randomized trial. *BJU Int. Br. J. Urol.* **2012**, *110*, 1654–1660. [CrossRef] [PubMed]
5. Heijnsdijk, E.A.; Wever, E.M.; Auvinen, A.; Hugosson, J.; Ciatto, S.; Nelen, V.; Kwiatkowski, M.; Villers, A.; Paez, A.; Moss, S.M.; et al. Quality-of-life effects of prostate-specific antigen screening. *N. Engl. J. Med.* **2012**, *367*, 595–605. [CrossRef] [PubMed]
6. Van Poppel, H.; Hogenhout, R.; Albers, P.; van den Bergh, R.C.N.; Barentsz, J.O.; Roobol, M.J. Early Detection of Prostate Cancer in 2020 and Beyond: Facts and Recommendations for the European Union and the European Commission. *Eur. Urol.* **2021**, *79*, 327–329. [CrossRef] [PubMed]
7. Dinges, S.S.; Hohm, A.; Vandergrift, L.A.; Nowak, J.; Habbel, P.; Kaltashov, I.A.; Cheng, L.L. Cancer metabolomic markers in urine: Evidence, techniques and recommendations. *Nat. Rev. Urol.* **2019**, *16*, 339–362. [CrossRef]
8. Tanase, C.P.; Codrici, E.; Popescu, I.D.; Mihai, S.; Enciu, A.M.; Necula, L.G.; Preda, A.; Ismail, G.; Albulescu, R. Prostate cancer proteomics: Current trends and future perspectives for biomarker discovery. *Oncotarget* **2017**, *8*, 18497–18512. [CrossRef]
9. Bax, C.; Lotesoriere, B.J.; Sironi, S.; Capelli, L. Review and Comparison of Cancer Biomarker Trends in Urine as a Basis for New Diagnostic Pathways. *Cancers* **2019**, *11*, 1244. [CrossRef]
10. Fujita, K.; Nonomura, N. Urinary biomarkers of prostate cancer. *Int. J. Urol.* **2018**, *25*, 770–779. [CrossRef]
11. Albers, D.D.; Mc, D.J.; Thompson, G.J. Carcinoma cells in prostatic secretions. *J. Am. Med. Assoc.* **1949**, *139*, 299–303. [CrossRef] [PubMed]
12. Wang, G.; Zhao, D.; Spring, D.J.; DePinho, R.A. Genetics and biology of prostate cancer. *Genes Dev.* **2018**, *32*, 1105–1140. [CrossRef]
13. Filella, X.; Foj, L. Prostate Cancer Detection and Prognosis: From Prostate Specific Antigen (PSA) to Exosomal Biomarkers. *Int. J. Mol. Sci.* **2016**, *17*, 1784. [CrossRef] [PubMed]
14. Swensen, A.C.; He, J.; Fang, A.C.; Ye, Y.; Nicora, C.D.; Shi, T.; Liu, A.Y.; Sigdel, T.K.; Sarwal, M.M.; Qian, W.J. A Comprehensive Urine Proteome Database Generated From Patients With Various Renal Conditions and Prostate Cancer. *Front. Med.* **2021**, *8*, 548212. [CrossRef] [PubMed]
15. Wang, L.; Skotland, T.; Berge, V.; Sandvig, K.; Llorente, A. Exosomal proteins as prostate cancer biomarkers in urine: From mass spectrometry discovery to immunoassay-based validation. *Eur. J. Pharm. Sci.* **2017**, *98*, 80–85. [CrossRef]
16. Taube, S.E.; Clark, G.M.; Dancey, J.E.; McShane, L.M.; Sigman, C.C.; Gutman, S.I. A perspective on challenges and issues in biomarker development and drug and biomarker codevelopment. *J. Natl. Cancer Inst.* **2009**, *101*, 1453–1463. [CrossRef]
17. Fung, K.Y.; Tabor, B.; Buckley, M.J.; Priebe, I.K.; Purins, L.; Pompeia, C.; Brierley, G.V.; Lockett, T.; Gibbs, P.; Tie, J.; et al. Blood-based protein biomarker panel for the detection of colorectal cancer. *PLoS ONE* **2015**, *10*, e0120425. [CrossRef]
18. Kelstrup, C.D.; Young, C.; Lavallee, R.; Nielsen, M.L.; Olsen, J.V. Optimized fast and sensitive acquisition methods for shotgun proteomics on a quadrupole orbitrap mass spectrometer. *J. Proteome Res.* **2012**, *11*, 3487–3497. [CrossRef]
19. Huang, T.; Bruderer, R.; Muntel, J.; Xuan, Y.; Vitek, O.; Reiter, L. Combining Precursor and Fragment Information for Improved Detection of Differential Abundance in Data Independent Acquisition. *Mol. Cell Proteom.* **2020**, *19*, 421–430. [CrossRef]
20. Storey, J.D.; Tibshirani, R. Statistical significance for genomewide studies. *Proc. Natl. Acad. Sci. USA* **2003**, *100*, 9440–9445. [CrossRef]
21. Loeb, S.; Bjurlin, M.A.; Nicholson, J.; Tammela, T.L.; Penson, D.F.; Carter, H.B.; Carroll, P.; Etzioni, R. Overdiagnosis and overtreatment of prostate cancer. *Eur. Urol.* **2014**, *65*, 1046–1055. [CrossRef] [PubMed]
22. Jedinak, A.; Loughlin, K.R.; Moses, M.A. Approaches to the discovery of non-invasive urinary biomarkers of prostate cancer. *Oncotarget* **2018**, *9*, 32534–32550. [CrossRef] [PubMed]
23. Khoo, A.; Liu, L.Y.; Nyalwidhe, J.O.; Semmes, O.J.; Vesprini, D.; Downes, M.R.; Boutros, P.C.; Liu, S.K.; Kislinger, T. Proteomic discovery of non-invasive biomarkers of localized prostate cancer using mass spectrometry. *Nat. Rev. Urol.* **2021**, *18*, 707–724. [CrossRef] [PubMed]

24. Gutknecht, M.F.; Seaman, M.E.; Ning, B.; Cornejo, D.A.; Mugler, E.; Antkowiak, P.F.; Moskaluk, C.A.; Hu, S.; Epstein, F.H.; Kelly, K.A. Identification of the S100 fused-type protein hornerin as a regulator of tumor vascularity. *Nat. Commun.* **2017**, *8*, 552. [CrossRef] [PubMed]
25. Choi, J.; Kim, D.I.; Kim, J.; Kim, B.H.; Kim, A. Hornerin Is Involved in Breast Cancer Progression. *J. Breast Cancer* **2016**, *19*, 142–147. [CrossRef]
26. Fu, S.J.; Shen, S.L.; Li, S.Q.; Hua, Y.P.; Hu, W.J.; Guo, B.; Peng, B.G. Hornerin promotes tumor progression and is associated with poor prognosis in hepatocellular carcinoma. *BMC Cancer* **2018**, *18*, 815. [CrossRef] [PubMed]
27. Gupta, S.; Hussain, T.; MacLennan, G.T.; Fu, P.; Patel, J.; Mukhtar, H. Differential expression of S100A2 and S100A4 during progression of human prostate adenocarcinoma. *J. Clin. Oncol.* **2003**, *21*, 106–112. [CrossRef] [PubMed]
28. Doll, J.A.; Stellmach, V.M.; Bouck, N.P.; Bergh, A.R.; Lee, C.; Abramson, L.P.; Cornwell, M.L.; Pins, M.R.; Borensztajn, J.; Crawford, S.E. Pigment epithelium-derived factor regulates the vasculature and mass of the prostate and pancreas. *Nat. Med.* **2003**, *9*, 774–780. [CrossRef]
29. Halin, S.; Wikstrom, P.; Rudolfsson, S.H.; Stattin, P.; Doll, J.A.; Crawford, S.E.; Bergh, A. Decreased pigment epithelium-derived factor is associated with metastatic phenotype in human and rat prostate tumors. *Cancer Res.* **2004**, *64*, 5664–5671. [CrossRef]
30. Kim, S.H.; Shin, Y.K.; Lee, I.S.; Bae, Y.M.; Sohn, H.W.; Suh, Y.H.; Ree, H.J.; Rowe, M.; Park, S.H. Viral latent membrane protein 1 (LMP-1)-induced CD99 down-regulation in B cells leads to the generation of cells with Hodgkin's and Reed-Sternberg phenotype. *Blood* **2000**, *95*, 294–300. [CrossRef]
31. Manara, M.C.; Bernard, G.; Lollini, P.L.; Nanni, P.; Zuntini, M.; Landuzzi, L.; Benini, S.; Lattanzi, G.; Sciandra, M.; Serra, M.; et al. CD99 acts as an oncosuppressor in osteosarcoma. *Mol. Biol. Cell* **2006**, *17*, 1910–1921. [CrossRef] [PubMed]
32. Jung, K.C.; Park, W.S.; Bae, Y.M.; Hahn, J.H.; Hahn, K.; Lee, H.; Lee, H.W.; Koo, H.J.; Shin, H.J.; Shin, H.S.; et al. Immunoreactivity of CD99 in stomach cancer. *J. Korean Med. Sci.* **2002**, *17*, 483–489. [CrossRef] [PubMed]
33. Scotlandi, K.; Zuntini, M.; Manara, M.C.; Sciandra, M.; Rocchi, A.; Benini, S.; Nicoletti, G.; Bernard, G.; Nanni, P.; Lollini, P.L.; et al. CD99 isoforms dictate opposite functions in tumour malignancy and metastases by activating or repressing c-Src kinase activity. *Oncogene* **2007**, *26*, 6604–6618. [CrossRef] [PubMed]
34. Davalieva, K.; Kiprijanovska, S.; Maleva Kostovska, I.; Stavridis, S.; Stankov, O.; Komina, S.; Petrusevska, G.; Polenakovic, M. Comparative Proteomics Analysis of Urine Reveals Down-Regulation of Acute Phase Response Signaling and LXR/RXR Activation Pathways in Prostate Cancer. *Proteomes* **2018**, *6*, 1. [CrossRef] [PubMed]
35. Lima, T.; Henrique, R.; Vitorino, R.; Fardilha, M. Bioinformatic analysis of dysregulated proteins in prostate cancer patients reveals putative urinary biomarkers and key biological pathways. *Med. Oncol.* **2021**, *38*, 9. [CrossRef]
36. Sarfati, M.; Bron, D.; Lagneaux, L.; Fonteyn, C.; Frost, H.; Delespesse, G. Elevation of IgE-binding factors in serum of patients with B cell-derived chronic lymphocytic leukemia. *Blood* **1988**, *71*, 94–98. [CrossRef]
37. Caligaris-Cappio, F.; Ghia, P. The normal counterpart to the chronic lymphocytic leukemia B cell. *Best Pract. Res. Clin. Haematol.* **2007**, *20*, 385–397. [CrossRef]
38. Barna, G.; Reiniger, L.; Tatrai, P.; Kopper, L.; Matolcsy, A. The cut-off levels of CD23 expression in the differential diagnosis of MCL and CLL. *Hematol. Oncol.* **2008**, *26*, 167–170. [CrossRef]
39. Schlette, E.; Fu, K.; Medeiros, L.J. CD23 expression in mantle cell lymphoma: Clinicopathologic features of 18 cases. *Am. J. Clin. Pathol.* **2003**, *120*, 760–766. [CrossRef]
40. Walters, M.; Olteanu, H.; Van Tuinen, P.; Kroft, S.H. CD23 expression in plasma cell myeloma is specific for abnormalities of chromosome 11, and is associated with primary plasma cell leukaemia in this cytogenetic sub-group. *Br. J. Haematol.* **2010**, *149*, 292–293. [CrossRef]
41. Soriano, A.O.; Thompson, M.A.; Admirand, J.H.; Fayad, L.E.; Rodriguez, A.M.; Romaguera, J.E.; Hagemeister, F.B.; Pro, B. Follicular dendritic cell sarcoma: A report of 14 cases and a review of the literature. *Am. J. Hematol.* **2007**, *82*, 725–728. [CrossRef] [PubMed]
42. Peter Rieber, E.; Rank, G.; Köhler, I.; Krauss, S. Membrane Expression of FcϵRII/CD23 and Release of Soluble CD23 by Follicular Dendritic Cells. In *Dendritic Cells in Fundamental and Clinical Immunology*; Kamperdijk, E.W.A., Nieuwenhuis, P., Hoefsmit, E.C.M., Eds.; Springer: New York, NY, USA, 1993; pp. 393–398.
43. Ida-Yonemochi, H.; Maruyama, S.; Kobayashi, T.; Yamazaki, M.; Cheng, J.; Saku, T. Loss of keratin 13 in oral carcinoma in situ: A comparative study of protein and gene expression levels using paraffin sections. *Mod. Pathol.* **2012**, *25*, 784–794. [CrossRef]
44. Sakamoto, K.; Aragaki, T.; Morita, K.; Kawachi, H.; Kayamori, K.; Nakanishi, S.; Omura, K.; Miki, Y.; Okada, N.; Katsube, K.; et al. Down-regulation of keratin 4 and keratin 13 expression in oral squamous cell carcinoma and epithelial dysplasia: A clue for histopathogenesis. *Histopathology* **2011**, *58*, 531–542. [CrossRef] [PubMed]
45. Naganuma, K.; Hatta, M.; Ikebe, T.; Yamazaki, J. Epigenetic alterations of the keratin 13 gene in oral squamous cell carcinoma. *BMC Cancer* **2014**, *14*, 988. [CrossRef] [PubMed]
46. Marsit, C.J.; Houseman, E.A.; Christensen, B.C.; Gagne, L.; Wrensch, M.R.; Nelson, H.H.; Wiemels, J.; Zheng, S.; Wiencke, J.K.; Andrew, A.S.; et al. Identification of methylated genes associated with aggressive bladder cancer. *PLoS ONE* **2010**, *5*, e12334. [CrossRef] [PubMed]
47. Li, Q.; Yin, L.; Jones, L.W.; Chu, G.C.; Wu, J.B.; Huang, J.M.; Li, Q.; You, S.; Kim, J.; Lu, Y.T.; et al. Keratin 13 expression reprograms bone and brain metastases of human prostate cancer cells. *Oncotarget* **2016**, *7*, 84645–84657. [CrossRef] [PubMed]

48. Rüschoff, J.H.; Stratton, S.; Roberts, E.; Clark, S.; Sebastiao, N.; Fankhauser, C.D.; Eberli, D.; Moch, H.; Wild, P.J.; Rupp, N.J. A novel 5x multiplex immunohistochemical staining reveals PSMA as a helpful marker in prostate cancer with low p504s expression. *Pathol. Res. Pract.* **2021**, *228*, 153667. [CrossRef]
49. Schrag, J.D.; Bergeron, J.J.; Li, Y.; Borisova, S.; Hahn, M.; Thomas, D.Y.; Cygler, M. The Structure of calnexin, an ER chaperone involved in quality control of protein folding. *Mol. Cell* **2001**, *8*, 633–644. [CrossRef]
50. Dissemond, J.; Busch, M.; Kothen, T.; Mörs, J.; Weimann, T.K.; Lindeke, A.; Goos, M.; Wagner, S.N. Differential downregulation of endoplasmic reticulum-residing chaperones calnexin and calreticulin in human metastatic melanoma. *Cancer Lett.* **2004**, *203*, 225–231. [CrossRef]
51. Ryan, D.; Carberry, S.; Murphy, Á.C.; Lindner, A.U.; Fay, J.; Hector, S.; McCawley, N.; Bacon, O.; Concannon, C.G.; Kay, E.W.; et al. Calnexin, an ER-induced protein, is a prognostic marker and potential therapeutic target in colorectal cancer. *J. Transl. Med.* **2016**, *14*, 196. [CrossRef]
52. Hibbert, R.G.; Teriete, P.; Grundy, G.J.; Beavil, R.L.; Reljic, R.; Holers, V.M.; Hannan, J.P.; Sutton, B.J.; Gould, H.J.; McDonnell, J.M. The structure of human CD23 and its interactions with IgE and CD21. *J. Exp. Med.* **2005**, *202*, 751–760. [CrossRef] [PubMed]
53. Vittinghoff, E.; McCulloch, C.E. Relaxing the Rule of Ten Events per Variable in Logistic and Cox Regression. *Am. J. Epidemiol.* **2006**, *165*, 710–718. [CrossRef] [PubMed]

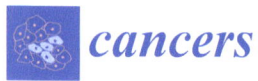 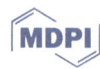

Article

Impact of Dose Escalation on the Efficacy of Salvage Radiotherapy for Recurrent Prostate Cancer—A Risk-Adjusted, Matched-Pair Analysis

Dirk Böhmer [1,*], Alessandra Siegmann [1], Sophia Scharl [2], Christian Ruf [3], Thomas Wiegel [2], Manuel Krafcsik [2] and Reinhard Thamm [2]

1 Department of Radiation Oncology, Charité University Medicine, Campus Benjamin Franklin, 12203 Berlin, Germany; alessandra.siegmann@charite.de
2 Department of Radiation Oncology, University Hospital Ulm, 89081 Ulm, Germany; sophiascharl@yahoo.de (S.S.); thomas.wiegel@uniklinik-ulm.de (T.W.); manuel.krafcsik@uniklinik-ulm.de (M.K.); reinhard.thamm@uniklinik-ulm.de (R.T.)
3 Department of Urology, Bundeswehrkrankenhaus Ulm, 89081 Ulm, Germany; bwkrhsulmurologie@bundeswehr.org
* Correspondence: dirk.boehmer@charite.de; Tel.: +49-30-450-627601

Simple Summary: This study evaluated 554 patients who underwent radical surgery for prostate cancer and later presented with persisting or rising PSA levels which required salvage radiotherapy. Our results showed that increasing the radiation dose during radiotherapy could reduce the risk of a second PSA relapse. These findings suggested that patients with failed prostatectomies might benefit from dose-escalated salvage radiotherapy to improve tumor control and postpone secondary treatments, such as hormonal or chemotherapy.

Abstract: Previous randomized trials have not provided conclusive evidence about dose escalations and associated toxicities for salvage radiotherapy (SRT) in prostate cancer. Here, we retrospectively analyzed whether dose escalations influenced progression-free survival in 554 patients that received salvage radiotherapy for relapses or persistently elevated prostate cancer antigen (PSA) after a radical prostatectomy. Patients received SRT between 1997 and 2017 at two University Hospitals in Germany. We compared patient groups that received radiation doses <7000 cGy (n = 225) or $\geq$7000 cGy (n = 329) to analyze the influence of radiation dose on progression-free survival. In a second matched-pair analysis of 216 pairs, we evaluated prognostic factors (pT2 vs. pT3–4, Gleason score [GS] $\leq$ 7 vs. GS $\geq$ 8, R0 vs. R1, and pre-SRT PSA <0.5 vs. $\geq$0.5 ng/mL). After a median follow-up of 6.8 (4.2–9.2) years, we found that escalated doses significantly improved progression-free survival (p = 0.0042). A multivariate analysis indicated that an escalated dose, lower tumor stages (pT2 vs. pT3/4), and lower GSs ($\leq$7 vs. 8–10) were associated with improved progression-free survival. There was no significant effect on overall survival. Our data suggested that escalating the radiation dose to $\geq$7000 cGy for SRT after a prostatectomy significantly improved progression-free survival. Longer follow-ups are needed for a comprehensive recommendation.

Keywords: prostate cancer; radical prostatectomy; salvage radiotherapy; dose-escalation; matched-pair analysis

1. Introduction

Among patients that undergo a radical prostatectomy (RP) for pT3 prostate cancer, persistent or rising prostate-specific antigen (PSA) levels occur in approximately 50% of those without and 70% of those with positive surgical resection margins [1–4]. Recent data have revealed that persistent PSA after an RP could significantly impact metastasis-free survival, overall survival (OS), and cancer-specific survival [3]. In non-randomized trials, the value of Prostate-Specific-Membrane-Antigen Positron-Emission-Tomography (PSMA-PET) imaging was evaluated in patients with PSA relapses [5]. Those results led to the current European Association of Urology (EAU) guideline recommendation that a PSMA-PET-CT should be offered to men with persistent PSA after RP and to men with biochemical recurrences [6].

International guidelines recommend salvage radiotherapy (SRT) for patients with persistent PSA values above 0.1 ng/mL, rising PSA values in subsequent PSA tests, or any PSA value above 0.1 ng/mL [7,8]. SRT should preferably commence before the PSA level reaches 0.5 ng/mL to ensure a high probability of achieving undetectable PSA values [9]. However, currently, we cannot rule out the possibility that there might be other indicators for SRT.

Despite new study results on SRT after RP for patients with persistent or rising PSA levels, four substantial questions remain controversial and are currently unresolved: the role of hormonal therapy, additional irradiation of pelvic lymphatics, the overall treatment dose for SRT, and the optimal fractionation scheme. Two randomized trials evaluated the addition of androgen deprivation therapy (ADT) to SRT, but the results were inconclusive [10,11]. Additionally, to date, there is no clear evidence to support the optimal treatment strategy for a PSA relapse, because there is no distinction between local, regional, distant, or both local and distant disease. Recently, a systematic review evaluated many factors to facilitate discriminations among different relapse sites [12]. Indeed, distinguishing local from distant disease is particularly important in making individual treatment decisions. Moreover, studies have shown that a high Gleason score (8–10) and a short PSA doubling time (<12 months) could significantly impact survival. Those findings may assist radiation oncologists in treatment decisions [2,12–14].

The role of dose escalation in SRT is currently under investigation. From primary radiotherapy, we know well that a radiation dose escalation improves oncological outcome measures, but at the expense of increased late toxicity. The Radiation Therapy Oncology Group 0126 trial confirmed these results, and furthermore, they demonstrated in a separate analysis that using appropriate intensity-modulated radiotherapy (IMRT) plans could reduce gastrointestinal or genitourinary late toxicities [15,16]. However, the oncological outcome results of two dose-escalation trials showed no significant difference between treatment arms for the primary endpoint [17,18].

In the present retrospective study, we aimed to evaluate whether dose-escalated SRT could provide an improved oncological outcome compared to lower-dose SRT. Additionally, we aimed to identify factors that could influence the oncological results.

2. Materials and Methods

Between 1997 and 2017, 554 patients from two university hospitals in Germany received SRT for biochemical failure after RP. We defined biochemical failure after surgery as persistent PSA levels >0.1 ng/mL or intermittent PSA elevations after undetectable PSA that rise above 0.1 ng/mL The median SRT dose was 7020 cGy, with an interquartile range (IQR) of 6660–7200 cGy. The clinical target volume comprised the prostatic fossa. When the tumor was pT3b or pT4 stage, the seminal vesicle bed was included in the SRT. Pelvic lymph nodes were not irradiated. More than half of all patients received modern radiotherapy techniques, namely IMRT. Patients were excluded when they had received a hormonal treatment before or during SRT or when they had lymph node involvement. Table 1 shows the baseline characteristics of all 554 patients.

Table 1. Baseline characteristics of 554 patients with failed RP that received low-dose (<70 Gy) or high-dose (≥70 Gy) SRT.

Characteristic	<70 Gy (N = 225)	≥70 Gy (N = 329)	All (N = 554)
Age at RP, years; median (IQR)	63 (59–67)	64 (60–68)	64 (59–68)
Pre-RP PSA *, ng/mL; median (IQR)	10.00 (7.00–15.16)	8.87 (5.98–14.4)	9.40 (6.28–14.7)
Tumor stage			
pT2	107 (48%)	182 (55%)	289 (52%)
pT3	114 (50%)	142 (43%)	256 (46%)
pT4	4 (2%)	5 (2%)	9 (2%)
Gleason score *			
GS ≤ 6	92 (41%)	96 (29%)	188 (34%)
GS = 7	87 (39%)	167 (51%)	254 (46%)
GS ≥ 8	46 (20%)	66 (20%)	112 (20%)
Surgical margins *			
R0	101 (45%)	201 (61%)	302 (55%)
R1	124 (55%)	128 (39%)	252 (45%)
Pre-SRT PSA, ng/mL; median (IQR)	0.294 (0.140–0.690)	0.290 (0.180–0.516)	0.292 (0.160–0.568)

Values are the number of patients (%), unless indicated otherwise. RP = radical prostatectomy; PSA = Prostate Specific Antigen; IQR = inter-quartile range; GS = Gleason score; * significant difference between groups.

The Cox proportional hazards regression model was used in multivariate analyses to determine and evaluate factors that could influence biochemical PFS (progression free survival). The significant risk factors were used for propensity matching [19]. The impact of dose-escalation was analyzed with the Kaplan-Meier method and univariable Cox regression [19,20].

To analyze the influence of risk factors on the outcome, we applied an adapted propensity-matching procedure with the following risk-factor groups: pT2 vs. pT3–4, GS ≤ 7 vs GS ≥ 8, R0 vs R1, and pre-SRT PSA < 0.5 vs. ≥ 0.5 ng/mL. This procedure identified 216 matched pairs.

Overall survival was defined from study initiation to death from any cause. PFS was defined as death, local or distant recurrence, initiation of any secondary anti-tumor treatment (e.g., ADT), or biochemical relapse (defined as PSA rising to more than 0.2 ng/mL above the post-SRT nadir).

3. Results

The median time from RP to the start of SRT was 23 months (range: 1.7–176 months). The pre-SRT PSA levels ranged from 0.04–8.87 ng/mL, with a median of 0.28 ng/mL.

After a median follow-up of 6.8 years (IQR: 4.2–9.2 years), the five-year PFS rates were 52% for patients that received <7000 cGy and 65% for patients that that received ≥7000 cGy (Figure 1). This difference was statistically significant ($p = 0.0042$).

In addition, the multivariable Cox regression analysis showed that a lower pT-stage, a lower Gleason score, a positive surgical resection status (R1), and a lower pre-SRT PSA level were significantly associated with an improved outcome (Table 2).

Figure 2a shows the PFS of propensity-matched patients. The dose-escalated SRT provided significantly higher PFS than lower-dose SRT within the group of 216 matched patient pairs (hazard ratio [HR] = 0.675; $p = 0.0054$). We found the same result after a repeated random combination of compatible match pairs, though the HRs and significance levels varied considerably. The same result was observed when the GS-matching criteria were changed from GS ≤ 7 vs. GS ≥ 8 to GS ≤ 6 vs. GS ≥ 7, which yielded 195 patient pairs (HR = 0.628, $p = 0.0017$, Figure 2b).

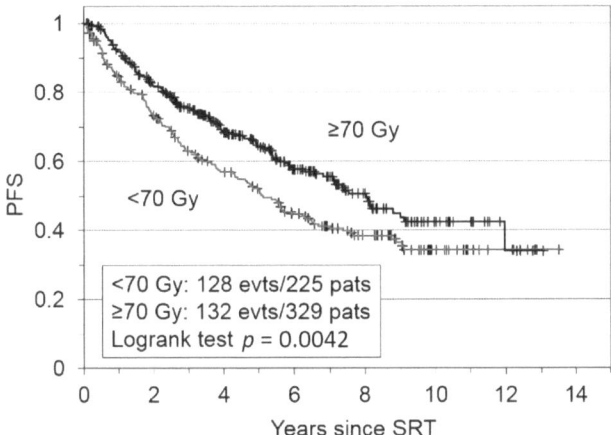

Figure 1. Kaplan-Meier plot shows progression-free survival (PFS) for the entire cohort of patients with failed prostatectomies (N = 554), after receiving salvage radiotherapy (SRT). Patients were grouped according to whether they received ≥70 Gy or <70 Gy.

Table 2. Multivariable Cox regression analysis of potential risk factors for PFS in patients with failed RP that received SRT. Significant factors were used for propensity score matching.

Risk Factors	HR (95% CI)	p
Pre-RP PSA < 10 * vs. ≥10 ng/ml	1.14 (0.88–1.47)	0.3278
pT2 * vs. pT3–4	2.13 (1.62–2.79)	<0.0001
GS ≤ 7 * vs. GS 8–10	1.60 (1.20–2.14)	0.0015
Surgical margin R0 * vs. R1	0.68 (0.53–0.88)	0.0031
Pre-SRT PSA < 0.5 * vs. ≥0.5 ng/ml	1.56 (1.21–2.02)	0.0007

PFS = progression-free survival; SRT = salvage radiotherapy; RP = radical prostatectomy; PSA = Prostate Specific Antigen; HR = hazard ratio; GS = Gleason score; * State used for reference.

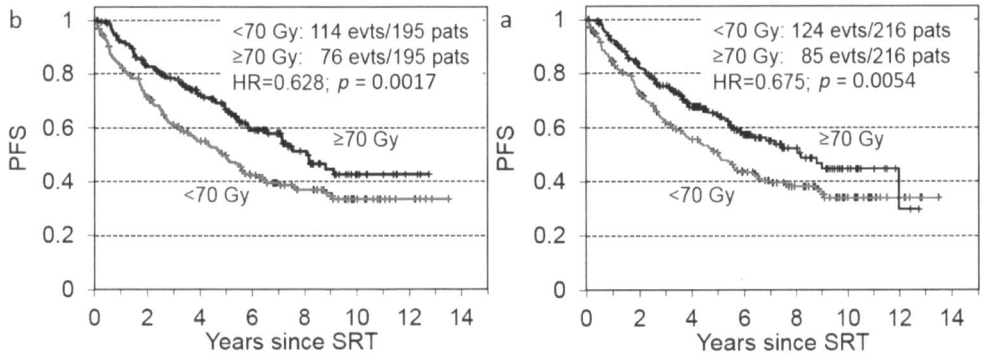

Figure 2. Progression-free survival (PFS) of propensity-matched patients with failed prostatectomies, after receiving salvage radiotherapy (SRT) delivered at ≥70 Gy or <70 Gy. Patients were propensity-matched 1:1 based on the following risk factors: pT2 vs. pT3–4, surgical margin status R0 vs. R1, and (a) Gleason score ≤ 7 vs. ≥8 (n = 216) or (b) Gleason score ≤ 6 vs. ≥7 (n = 195).

We then compared the different SRT doses in 387 patients (Figure 3a) that had received early SRT (PSA < 0.5 ng/mL). We found that the ≥7000 cGy dose improved the PFS (HR = 0.751) for patients with the significant risk factors identified in the multivariable Cox model (pT3–4, GS 8–10, R1), but the result was not statistically significant ($p = 0.154$). However, when we performed the analysis with propensity-matched patients (150 matched patient pairs, Figure 3b) we found a plausible improvement in PFS (HR = 0.719), with a trend towards significance ($p = 0.059$).

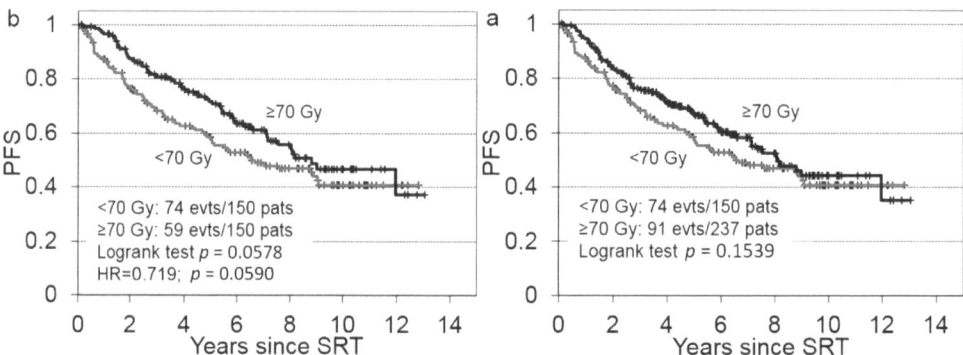

Figure 3. Progression-free survival (PFS) of patients with failed prostatectomies, after receiving early salvage radiotherapy (SRT) at a PSA < 0.5 ng/mL. SRT dosing groups ($\geq$70 Gy or <70 Gy) were compared (**a**) before (n = 387 patients) and (**b**) after (n = 300 patients) propensity matching 1:1 for the following significant risk factors: pT2 vs. pT3–4, Gleason score $\leq$ 7 vs. $\geq$8, and surgical margins R0 vs. R1.

Next, we evaluated factors that might influence OS with a multivariate analysis. We found that only age $\geq$64 years (HR = 2.16, p = 0.0051) and pT3–4 (HR = 1.97, p = 0.0133) could significantly adversely impact OS. Figure 4 shows the OS for the total patient cohort, stratified by (a) pT-stage and (b) SRT dose; only the pT stage impacted the OS. When we compared the pT2 and pT3–4 subgroups separately, we found that the different SRT doses did not significantly impact OS (Figure 4c,d).

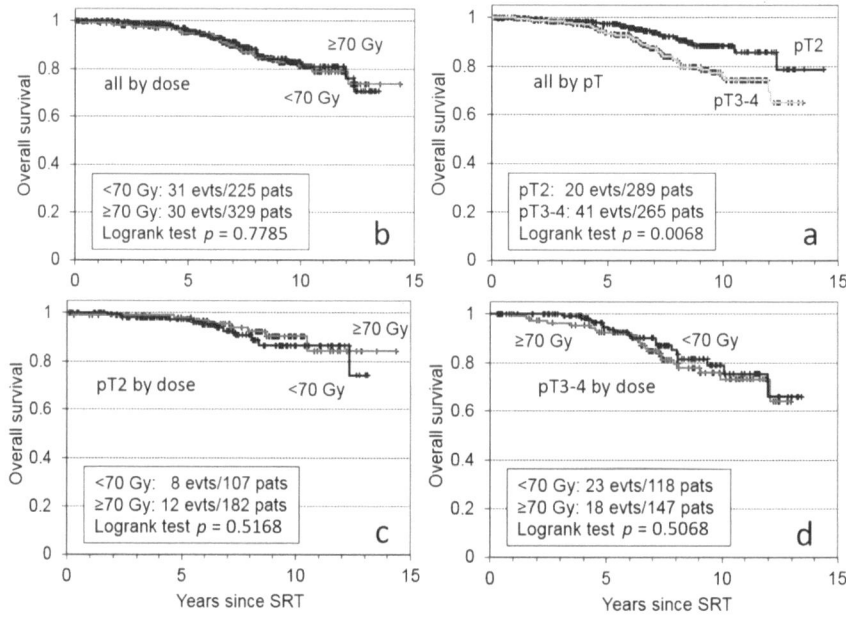

Figure 4. Kaplan-Meier plot shows overall survival of 554 patients with failed prostatectomies that received salvage radiotherapy (SRT). All 554 patients were stratified by (**a**) tumor stage (pT) and (**b**) SRT dose. Specific tumor-stage subgroups, (**c**) pT2 and (**d**) pT3–4, were stratified by SRT dose.

4. Discussion

After a failed RP, due to PSA persistence or relapse, escalating the SRT dose to >7000 cGy provided a significant advantage in PFS. We demonstrated this effect after adjusting for risk factors in a propensity-matched group of 432 patients. However, among patients with a pre-SRT PSA level < 0.5 ng/mL, we only observed a trend towards improved PFS with the escalated SRT dose. This lack of significance might have been due to the small number of patients in our subgroup.

We found that dose escalations did not significantly improve OS. These results were consistent with several previous retrospective studies. However, a large systematic review of more than 10,000 patients found that, for every 100 cGy dose escalation, the freedom from biochemical recurrence improved by 2%. Therefore, those authors concluded that the applied SRT dose should be above 7000 cGy [21,22]. Nevertheless, there were substantial biases among the analyzed publications. For example, in 60 out of 71 studies, the median radiation dose was <7000 cGy; the patient characteristics were inhomogeneous, due to the inclusion of patients with positive lymph nodes; and a mean of 11% of patients (range: 0–90%) received ADT.

Early results are available from two randomized trials that investigated the effect of escalated radiation doses in SRT [17,18]. In both trials, biochemical progression was set as the primary endpoint.

In the SAKK 09/10 trial of the Swiss Cancer Foundation, 350 patients with biochemical progression after an RP were randomized to receive SRT, with either 6400 cGy (32 fractions) or 7000 cGy (35 fractions) delivered with an external beam and directed to the prostate bed [18]. The primary endpoint was freedom from biochemical progression (FFBP). The intent-to-treat analysis was performed for 344 patients. The authors defined PSA progression after surgery as two consecutive PSA rises, with a final PSA > 0.1 ng/mL, or three sequential PSA elevations. In addition, all patients had a post-operative PSA nadir of $\leq$0.4 ng/mL and a pre-randomization PSA of $\leq$2 ng/mL. After a median follow-up of 6.2 years, the dose-escalated SRT was not associated with improved outcome for any of the oncological endpoints, including the primary endpoint, the clinical PFS, the time to hormonal treatment, or the OS. The late toxicity analysis showed a significant increase in late grades 2 and 3 gastrointestinal toxicities ($p = 0.009$) in the dose-escalated group. Although no differences were found in terms of quality of life, the authors argued that patients with dose-escalated SRT were at risk of higher late GI toxicity without any oncologic benefit.

It remains unclear why the 6-Gy dose increase did not provide a measurable difference in PFS. According to the study by King et al., the dose escalation should have improved PFS by 2% per Gy of dose increment [21]. In that case, the SAKK trial should have observed a 12% improvement in PFS with the 6-Gy increase in SRT dose. One reason for the lack of a difference between groups may have been an insufficient follow-up. It is known that many local recurrences occur more than eight years after SRT. Therefore, it was possible that, after the median follow-up of six years, the 64-Gy dose may have postponed tumor progression, and the 70-Gy dose might have provided a local cure.

Differences in patient characteristics between our cohort and the cohort of the SAKK 09/10 trial and the Chinese trial are summarized in Table 3.

Table 3. Patient characteristics comparing the available randomized trails and our data.

	SAKK 09/10 [18]	Chinese Trial [17]	Own Data
Type of study	Open-label, multicenter Phase III trial	Randomized controlled Phase III trial	Retrospective cohort
Inclusion criteria	Biochemical failure after RP 3 PSA rises or 2 rises with last being 0.1 ng/mL Postoperative PSA-Nadir $\leq$ 0.4 ng/mL No ADT before or during SRT pT2a-3b No macroscopic relapse Nodal negative	Biochemical failure or PSA persistence after RP (ART/SRT = 48/96) Postoperative PSA-Nadir $\leq$ 0.4 ng/mL No ADT before or during SRT pT3-4 positive margin Nodal negative	Biochemical failure after RP PSA rise above 0.1 ng/mL No ADT before or during SRT pT3-4 positive margin Nodal negative
Treatment groups	6400 cGy vs. 7000 cGy Target volume: prostatic bed Technique: 3D CRT (44%), IMRT (57%) Assignment to treatment by randomization	6600 cGy vs. 7200 cGy Target volume: prostatic bed (RTOG-guideline) Technique: IG-IMRT/IG-VMAT High Risk patients: pelvic RT (88%)	<7000 cGy vs. $\geq$7000 cGy Target volume: prostatic bed +/− seminal vesicle bed (T3/4) Technique: 3D CRT (74.9%), IMRT (25.1%) Matched-Pair-Analysis
Primary endpoint	Freedom from biochemical Progression: Definition: PSA-increase $\geq$ 0.4 ng/mL beyond post-SRT-Nadir	Biochemical PFS: secondary therapy Definition: PSA-increase > 0.2 ng/mL beyond post-SRT-Nadir (x2), OS: death of any cause	PFS, secondary therapy Definition: PSA-increase > 0.2 ng/mL beyond post-SRT-Nadir OS: death of any cause
Secondary endpoints	Clinical PFS Time to hormonal therapy, OS Acute and late toxicity Quality of life	Acute and late toxicity Toxicity of hormonal treatment	n.s.
Number of patients	350 Conv. D.: 175 (170 ITT) Escal. D.: 175 (174 ITT)	144 Conv. D.: 71 Escal. D.: 73	554 low dose: 225 high dose: 329
Pre-SRT-PSA-level	0.3 ng/mL (0.03–1.61)	0.2 ng/ml	0.28 ng/mL (0.04–8.87)
Follow-Up	6.2 years (IQR 5.5–7.2)	48.5 months (14–79 months)	6.8 years (IQR 4.2–9.2)
Time RP–SRT	6400 cGy: 25.9 mo. (14.0–42.3) 7000 cGy: 30.3 mo. (15.8–50.8)	8 mo.	23 mo. (1.7–176)
Results	Reported: 6-year-results 6400 cGy: 62.3% (95% CI: 54.2–69.4) 7000 cGy: 61.3% (95% CI: 53.4–68.3) bPFS: p = 0.44 Hazard-ratio: 1.14 (95% CI: 0.82–1.6)	Reported: 4-year-results 66 Gy: 75.9%; 95% CI, 71.6–79.6% 72 Gy: 82.6%; 95% CI, 78.8–85.7% bPFS: p = 0.299	Reported: 5-year-results Conventional dose: 52% Escalated dose: 65% PFS: p = 0.0042 Multivariate Analysis: significant improvement favoring: lower pT stage lower Gleason sum positive resection status lower-pre-SRT PSA level

Abbreviations: RP—radical prostatectomy; PSA—prostatic specific antigen; ADT—androgen deprivation therapy; SRT—salvage radiotherapy; cGy—centiGray; RTOG—Radiotherapy Oncology Group; 3D CRT-three-dimensional conformal radiotherapy; IG—image guided; IMRT—intensity modulated radiotherapy; VMAT; RT—radiotherapy; PFS—progression free survival; OS—overall survival; Conv. D.—conventional dose; Escal. D.—escalated dose; ITT—intention-to-treat; IQR—inter quartile range; bPFS—biochemical progression free survival; mo.—months; CI—confidence interval.

However, the well-considered definitions of inclusion criteria in the SAKK 09/10 trial might have led to a preselected patient cohort with a lower risk of progression compared to our cohort. Therefore, compared to our cohort, a higher proportion of patients in the SAKK-trial might not have needed an escalated radiation dose to prevent biochemical failure. Moreover, the large range of times from RP to SRT in our analysis could have resulted from the larger number of surgeons and/or variations in operative expertise. Both factors might also have introduced a selection bias in our study. For patients matched for pT2 vs. pT3–4, Gleason score ≤ 7 vs. ≥ 8, and surgical margins R0 vs. R1, escalating radiotherapy dose provides a near significant advantage in PFS ($p = 0.059$).

Another relevant factor influencing survival is PSA doubling time, as demonstrated in the systematic review by van den Broek [12]. In our patient cohort, data on the PSA doubling times were available only for a small subgroup of patients. Thus, we could not evaluate this risk factor.

In a Chinese phase III trial, 144 patients were randomly assigned to receive either 6600 cGy or 7200 cGy as an adjuvant for patients with high-risk factors (pT3–4, R1) or as salvage treatment for patients with a rising postoperative PSA of ≥ 0.2 ng/mL [17]. In the SAKK 09/10 trial, a higher overall dose did not provide an advantage for bPFS in the entire group, after a median follow-up of 48 months. However, in contrast to the SAKK-trial, in the Chinese trial, a subgroup analysis of patients at high risk (Gleason score 8–10) showed a significant improvement in the four-year bPFS with a 6-Gy dose escalation to 72 Gy (bPFS in 79.7% vs. 55.7% for 72-Gy vs. 66-Gy arms, respectively). That result agreed well with our findings, which showed five-year PFS rates of 52% and 65% for the <70 and ≥ 70 Gy groups, respectively ($p = 0.0042$). Moreover, in our investigation, we showed that the dose escalation was significantly beneficial, both for patients with Gleason scores of 8–10 and in patients with Gleason scores of 7 or higher. However, it should be noted that the different study designs of the Chinese trial and our study could have confounded the comparison; for example, the Chinese trial design included a shorter follow-up, the use of whole pelvic radiotherapy (88%), and the application of adjuvant radiotherapy (33% of patients). Moreover, due to substantial differences in cohorts and the possible introduction of a selection bias, a direct comparison between the Chinese trial and our cohort study is difficult. The Chinese trial included 48 patients with risk factors (pT3/4 or R1) that received adjuvant radiotherapy after an RP, without measurable PSA. Moreover, most of their patients (87.5%) received whole pelvic radiotherapy, and R1-resections were more frequent among patients in the high-dose cohort (64.4%) than among those in the low-dose cohort (47.9%, $p = 0.064$).

Although the patients in our cohort were highly homogeneous regarding the exclusions of pN+ disease and ADT applications, several studies have provided substantial evidence to show that some other pathological features can increase the risk of a selection bias. For instance, a previous retrospective analysis of 8770 patients showed that positive surgical margins (PSM) represented an independent predictor of biochemical failure [4]. In that study, among 579 patients that harbored PSMs, the likelihood of biochemical failure increased when the Gleason score was ≥ 4 at the margin, when the PSM was ≥ 3 mm long, and when the patient had multifocal positive margins. In the present study, these pathological details were not available for analysis, and this lack of data may have led to a substantial selection bias. Nevertheless, there are currently no data from randomized trials that focused on these aspects. Therefore, our results may be helpful when counseling patients in selecting an appropriate therapy.

Improving tumor control with higher radiation doses must be weighed against an increase in the occurrence of late toxicities. In this regard, our retrospective analysis may add further aspects to the current knowledge about variables that can influence dose escalations in SRT.

Both randomized trials mentioned above completed patient recruitments in the pre-PSMA-PET-CT era; thus, they mainly performed conventional staging. The increasing implementation of advanced functional imaging, like PET-CT, might provide additional selection criteria for identifying patients with PSA progression after an RP and enhance the ability to detect risk factors that indicate the need for treatment intensification. For example, patients with local recurrence detected with PET-CT are likely to require a localized dose escalation in the future. Conversely, patients with no detection of macroscopic recurrent disease might be treated effectively with lower radiation doses. Thus, the available randomized data are of limited validity compared to data from patients staged with modern imaging.

In a recent retrospective study, 150 patients with local prostate cancer relapses detected in choline-PET-CT were treated with SRT. Radiation was delivered to the prostatic bed ± lymph nodes in 55% of patients, and the recurrent lesion received a local dose of 8000 cGy. Five- and seven-year relapse-free survival rates were 70% and 60%, respectively. Given the high radiation dose, grades 3 and 4 late toxicities were surprisingly low (2%) [23]. Those survival data were consistent with the survival rates we observed in the high-dose group in the present study, and both studies supported dose escalations.

The present study had several limitations. First, it was a retrospective study, with all the inherent limitations, compared to a randomized trial setting. Second, our data were not statistically suitable for correlation analyses with clinical outcome measures (e.g., metastasis-free survival), due to the limited number of patients with hematogenous metastases (n = 5, 1.7%). Third, for many patients (including patients with R1), irradiation was initiated when the PSA level was <0.2 ng/mL. This irradiation may indicate potential overtreatment, but only in a small number of patients that might have had benign, low-level, gradual PSA recurrences. Fourth, there is evidence that increasing the SRT radiation dose significantly increases the risk of late radiation GI toxicity. Yet, this difference was irrespective of treatment technique [18]. Due to the lack of toxicity data, our analysis could not assess the tradeoff between oncological benefits and radiation side effects. Fifth, the baseline PSA levels and GS values were significantly different between the two dose groups. Despite our attempt to minimize data distortions with propensity matching, there was a substantial risk of selection bias and systematic bias. Finally, there was also a risk of a treatment bias, due to the type of therapy; some patients received traditional 3-D conformal radiation, and others received modern IMRT.

This study also had some notable strengths. Despite the retrospective nature of our data, the matched pair analysis represented a decisive advantage. Moreover, we included a large patient cohort, with homogeneous patient characteristics, and homogeneous patient treatments. These factors reduced the biases inherent in retrospective data analyses. Furthermore, we excluded patients with positive lymph nodes and patients that received ADT or whole pelvic radiotherapy. In addition, we applied strict propensity-matching rules to the cohort.

5. Conclusions

This retrospective study demonstrated that a dose escalation above 7000 cGy had advantageous effects in patients with prostate cancer that underwent SRT for PSA persistence or relapse after an RP. Our findings contrasted with those of the SAKK-09/10 trial but were partly consistent with findings from a Chinese randomized phase III trial. Our additional risk-adjusted propensity analysis corroborated the finding that SRT had a beneficial impact on PFS. Differences between studies may be explained by different definitions regarding inclusion criteria, disease progression, or other patient-related characteristics. With longer follow-up times, the results of SRT dose escalations may become significant, as proposed by King et al. [21].

Future studies should focus on the evaluation of subgroups that may benefit from dose escalations, like high-risk patients, particularly when examined with advanced imaging methods, like PSMA-PET-CT or PET-MRI. With modern imaging, we may achieve a consensus definition of the 'true' relapse, which might change radiotherapy strategies substantially in the future. Moreover, studies should identify patient-related risk factors that might increase the risk of late toxicities. This knowledge will facilitate appropriate counseling for these patients by enabling a risk–benefit evaluation of dose-escalated SRT.

Author Contributions: Conceptualization, D.B. and T.W.; methodology, D.B., T.W. and R.T.; validation and interpretation, D.B., A.S., S.S., C.R., T.W.; formal analysis, M.K. and R.T.; writing—original draft preparation, D.B.; writing—review and editing, all authors; visualization, T.W. and R.T.; project administration, D.B., T.W. and R.T. All authors have read and agreed to the published version of the manuscript.

Funding: This research received no external funding. D.B. provided costs for professional proofreading.

Institutional Review Board Statement: The study was conducted in accordance with the Declaration of Helsinki and approved by the Institutional Ethics Committee of the University of Ulm Ethics Committee (Approval number: 391/15).

Informed Consent Statement: Informed consent was obtained from all subjects involved in the study.

Data Availability Statement: The datasets generated during and/or analyzed during the current study are available from the corresponding author on reasonable request.

Acknowledgments: We are profoundly grateful to all patients who participated in this study as well as their families.

Conflicts of Interest: The authors declare no conflict of interest.

References

1. Bartkowiak, D.; Siegmann, A.; Bohmer, D.; Budach, V.; Wiegel, T. The impact of prostate-specific antigen persistence after radical prostatectomy on the efficacy of salvage radiotherapy in patients with primary N0 prostate cancer. *BJU Int.* **2019**, *124*, 785–791. [CrossRef]
2. Bartkowiak, D.; Thamm, R.; Bottke, D.; Siegmann, A.; Bohmer, D.; Budach, V.; Wiegel, T. Prostate-specific antigen after salvage radiotherapy for postprostatectomy biochemical recurrence predicts long-term outcome including overall survival. *Acta Oncol.* **2018**, *57*, 362–367. [CrossRef]
3. Preisser, F.; Chun, F.K.H.; Pompe, R.S.; Heinze, A.; Salomon, G.; Graefen, M.; Huland, H.; Tilki, D. Persistent Prostate-Specific Antigen After Radical Prostatectomy and Its Impact on Oncologic Outcomes. *Eur. Urol.* **2019**, *76*, 106–114. [CrossRef] [PubMed]
4. Preisser, F.; Coxilha, G.; Heinze, A.; Oh, S.; Chun, F.K.; Sauter, G.; Pompe, R.S.; Huland, H.; Graefen, M.; Tilki, D. Impact of positive surgical margin length and Gleason grade at the margin on biochemical recurrence in patients with organ-confined prostate cancer. *Prostate* **2019**, *79*, 1832–1836. [CrossRef]
5. Fendler, W.P.; Calais, J.; Eiber, M.; Flavell, R.R.; Mishoe, A.; Feng, F.Y.; Nguyen, H.G.; Reiter, R.E.; Rettig, M.B.; Okamoto, S.; et al. Assessment of 68Ga-PSMA-11 PET Accuracy in Localizing Recurrent Prostate Cancer: A Prospective Single-Arm Clinical Trial. *JAMA Oncol.* **2019**, *5*, 856–863. [CrossRef]
6. Mottet, N.; van den Bergh, R.C.N.; Briers, E.; Van den Broeck, T.; Cumberbatch, M.G.; De Santis, M.; Fanti, S.; Fossati, N.; Gandaglia, G.; Gillessen, S.; et al. EAU-EANM-ESTRO-ESUR-SIOG Guidelines on Prostate Cancer-2020 Update. Part 1: Screening, Diagnosis, and Local Treatment with Curative Intent. *Eur. Urol.* **2021**, *79*, 243–262. [CrossRef] [PubMed]
7. Pisansky, T.M.; Thompson, I.M.; Valicenti, R.K.; D'Amico, A.V.; Selvarajah, S. Adjuvant and Salvage Radiotherapy after Prostatectomy: ASTRO/AUA Guideline Amendment 2018–2019. *J. Urol.* **2019**, *202*, 533–538. [CrossRef]
8. National Comprehensive Cancer Network. Prostate Cancer (Version 3.2022). 2022. Available online: https://www.nccn.org/professionals/physician_gls/pdf/prostate.pdf (accessed on 3 March 2022).
9. Mottet, N.; van den Bergh, R.C.N.; Briers, E.; Expert Patient Advocate (European Prostate Cancer Coalition/Europa UOMO); De Santis, M.; Gillessen, S.; Grummet, J.; Henry, A.M.; van der Kwast, T.H.; Lam, T.B.; et al. *EAU—EANM—ESTRO—ESUR—ISUP—SIOG Guidelines on Prostate Cancer*; EAU Guidelines Office: Arnhem, The Netherlands, 2021.
10. Carrie, C.; Magne, N.; Burban-Provost, P.; Sargos, P.; Latorzeff, I.; Lagrange, J.L.; Supiot, S.; Belkacemi, Y.; Peiffert, D.; Allouache, N.; et al. Short-term androgen deprivation therapy combined with radiotherapy as salvage treatment after radical prostatectomy for prostate cancer (GETUG-AFU 16). A 112-month follow-up of a phase 3, randomised trial. *Lancet Oncol.* **2019**, *20*, 1740–1749. [CrossRef]
11. Shipley, W.U.; Seiferheld, W.; Lukka, H.R.; Major, P.P.; Heney, N.M.; Grignon, D.J.; Sartor, O.; Patel, M.P.; Bahary, J.P.; Zietman, A.L.; et al. Radiation with or without Antiandrogen Therapy in Recurrent Prostate Cancer. *N. Engl. J. Med.* **2017**, *376*, 417–428. [CrossRef] [PubMed]
12. Van den Broeck, T.; van den Bergh, R.C.N.; Arfi, N.; Gross, T.; Moris, L.; Briers, E.; Cumberbatch, M.; De Santis, M.; Tilki, D.; Fanti, S.; et al. Prognostic Value of Biochemical Recurrence Following Treatment with Curative Intent for Prostate Cancer: A Systematic Review. *Eur. Urol.* **2019**, *75*, 967–987. [CrossRef]

13. Tendulkar, R.D.; Agrawal, S.; Gao, T.; Efstathiou, J.A.; Pisansky, T.M.; Michalski, J.M.; Koontz, B.F.; Hamstra, D.A.; Feng, F.Y.; Liauw, S.L.; et al. Contemporary Update of a Multi-Institutional Predictive Nomogram for Salvage Radiotherapy after Radical Prostatectomy. *J. Clin. Oncol.* **2016**, *34*, 3648–3654. [CrossRef] [PubMed]
14. Kishan, A.U.; Tendulkar, R.D.; Tran, P.T.; Parker, C.C.; Nguyen, P.L.; Stephenson, A.J.; Carrie, C. Optimizing the Timing of Salvage Postprostatectomy Radiotherapy and the Use of Concurrent Hormonal Therapy for Prostate Cancer. *Eur. Urol. Oncol.* **2018**, *1*, 3–18. [CrossRef]
15. Michalski, J.M.; Moughan, J.; Purdy, J.; Bosch, W.; Bruner, D.W.; Bahary, J.P.; Lau, H.; Duclos, M.; Parliament, M.; Morton, G.; et al. Effect of Standard vs Dose-Escalated Radiation Therapy for Patients With Intermediate-Risk Prostate Cancer: The NRG Oncology RTOG 0126 Randomized Clinical Trial. *JAMA Oncol.* **2018**, *4*, e180039. [CrossRef] [PubMed]
16. Moore, K.L.; Schmidt, R.; Moiseenko, V.; Olsen, L.A.; Tan, J.; Xiao, Y.; Galvin, J.; Pugh, S.; Seider, M.J.; Dicker, A.P.; et al. Quantifying Unnecessary Normal Tissue Complication Risks due to Suboptimal Planning: A Secondary Study of RTOG 0126. *Int. J. Radiat. Oncol. Biol. Phys.* **2015**, *92*, 228–235. [CrossRef] [PubMed]
17. Qi, X.; Li, H.Z.; Gao, X.S.; Qin, S.B.; Zhang, M.; Li, X.M.; Li, X.Y.; Ma, M.W.; Bai, Y.; Li, X.Y.; et al. Toxicity and Biochemical Outcomes of Dose-Intensified Postoperative Radiation Therapy for Prostate Cancer: Results of a Randomized Phase III Trial. *Int. J. Radiat. Oncol. Biol. Phys.* **2020**, *106*, 282–290. [CrossRef] [PubMed]
18. Ghadjar, P.; Hayoz, S.; Bernhard, J.; Zwahlen, D.R.; Holscher, T.; Gut, P.; Polat, B.; Hildebrandt, G.; Muller, A.C.; Plasswilm, L.; et al. Dose-intensified Versus Conventional-dose Salvage Radiotherapy for Biochemically Recurrent Prostate Cancer After Prostatectomy: The SAKK 09/10 Randomized Phase 3 Trial. *Eur. Urol.* **2021**, *80*, 306–315. [CrossRef]
19. Cox, D.R. Regression Models and Life-Tables. *J. R. Stat. Soc.* **1972**, *34*, 187–220. [CrossRef]
20. Kaplan, E.L.; Meier, P. Nonparametric estimation from incomplete observations. *J. Am. Stat. Assoc.* **1958**, *53*, 457–481. [CrossRef]
21. King, C.R. The dose-response of salvage radiotherapy following radical prostatectomy: A systematic review and meta-analysis. *Radiother. Oncol.* **2016**, *121*, 199–203. [CrossRef] [PubMed]
22. Shelan, M.; Abo-Madyan, Y.; Welzel, G.; Bolenz, C.; Kosakowski, J.; Behnam, N.; Wenz, F.; Lohr, F. Dose-escalated salvage radiotherapy after radical prostatectomy in high risk prostate cancer patients without hormone therapy: Outcome, prognostic factors and late toxicity. *Radiat. Oncol.* **2013**, *8*, 276. [CrossRef] [PubMed]
23. D'Angelillo, R.M.; Fiore, M.; Trodella, L.E.; Sciuto, R.; Ippolito, E.; Carnevale, A.; Iurato, A.; Miele, M.; Trecca, P.; Trodella, L.; et al. 18F-choline PET/CT driven salvage radiotherapy in prostate cancer patients: Update analysis with 5-year median follow-up. *Radiol. Med.* **2020**, *125*, 668–673. [CrossRef]

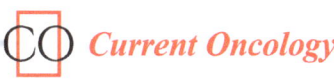

Review

Adenoid Cystic Carcinoma/Basal Cell Carcinoma of the Prostate: Overview and Update on Rare Prostate Cancer Subtypes

Salvatore Cozzi [1], Lilia Bardoscia [2,*], Masoumeh Najafi [3], Andrea Botti [4], Gladys Blandino [1], Matteo Augugliaro [1], Moana Manicone [1], Federico Iori [1], Lucia Giaccherini [1], Angela Sardaro [5], Cinzia Iotti [1] and Patrizia Ciammella [1]

[1] Radiation Oncology Unit, Azienda USL-IRCCS di Reggio Emilia, 42123 Reggio Emilia, Italy; salvatore.cozzi@hotmail.it or salvatore.cozzi@ausl.re.it (S.C.); gladys.blandino@ausl.re.it (G.B.); matteo.augugliaro@ausl.re.it (M.A.); moana.manicone@gmail.com (M.M.); federico.iori@ausl.re.it (F.I.); lucia.giaccherini@ausl.re.it (L.G.); cinzia.iotti@ausl.re.it (C.I.); patrizia.ciammella@ausl.re.it (P.C.)
[2] Radiation Oncology Unit, S. Luca Hospital, Healthcare Company Tuscany Nord Ovest, 55100 Lucca, Italy
[3] Department of Radiation Oncology Shohadaye Haft-e-Tir Hospital, Iran University of Medical Science, Teheran 1449614535, Iran; masy.najafi@gmail.com
[4] Medical Physics Unit, Azienda USL-IRCCS di Reggio Emilia, 42123 Reggio Emilia, Italy; andrea.botti@ausl.re.it
[5] Interdisciplinary Department of Medicine, Section of Radiology and Radiation Oncology, University of Bari Aldo Moro, 70124 Bari, Italy; angela.sardaro@uniba.it
* Correspondence: liliabardoscia@gmail.com

Abstract: Adenoid cystic carcinoma/basaloid cell carcinoma of the prostate (ACC/BCC) is a very rare variant of prostate cancer with uncertain behavior. Few cases are reported in the literature. Data on treatment options are scarce. The aim of our work was to retrospectively review the published reports. Thirty-three case reports or case series were analyzed (106 patients in total). Pathological features, management, and follow-up information were evaluated. Despite the relatively low level of evidence given the unavoidable lack of prospective trials for such a rare prostate tumor, the following considerations were made: prostate ACC/BCC is an aggressive tumor often presenting with locally advanced disease and incidental diagnosis occurs during transurethral resection of the prostate for urinary obstructive symptoms. Prostate-specific antigen was not a reliable marker for diagnosis nor follow-up. Adequate staging with Computed Tomography (CT) scan and Magnetic Resonance Imaging (MRI) should be performed before treatment and during follow-up, while there is no evidence for the use of Positron Emission Tomography (PET). Radical surgery with negative margins and possibly adjuvant radiotherapy appear to be the treatments of choice. The response to androgen deprivation therapy was poor. Currently, there is no evidence of the use of truly effective systemic therapies.

Keywords: adenoid cystic carcinoma; basaloid cell carcinoma; prostate cancer; surgery; radiotherapy; rare tumor variants

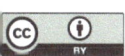

1. Introduction

Adenoid cystic carcinoma (ACC) of the prostate, also called basaloid carcinoma and adenoid cystic-like tumor, was first described in 1974 as a rare but distinctive variant of prostatic adenocarcinoma. It is histologically identical to adenoid cystic carcinoma of the salivary glands [1]. ACC is typically a salivary gland tumor that is composed of ductal and myoepithelial cells, but it can also arise in different sites, including the skin, cervix, and breast [2–5].

For a long time, two reasons have been considered for the independent existence of this tumor: first, myoepithelial cells are not indigenous to the prostate, and second, adenoid cystic morphology occurs along a spectrum of basaloid proliferations that encompass basal cell hyperplasia, basal cell adenoma, and basal cell carcinoma. Finally, in 2016, WHO

Classification of Tumours of the Urinary System and Male Genital Organs categorized adenoid cystic hyperplasia carcinoma and basaloid variants as malignant basal cell tumors (BCC) [6].

ACC/BCC is an extremely rare variant that is histologically difficult to detect, with uncertain behavior and about 100 cases reported in the literature compared to over 1 million acinar prostate cancer diagnoses every year. The age of onset ranges from 28 to 97 years, with peak incidence between 60 and 75 years; however, cases of young adults have been reported. When occurring in the prostate, these tumors predominantly show local infiltrative behavior.

Because of the rarity of this disease, therapeutic options for patients with ACC/BCC of the prostate are scarce. Most patients are treated with hormone therapy, radiotherapy, radical prostatectomy, or a combination of these treatments, although outcomes remain poor.

We retrospectively reviewed the published reports available in the literature until the present day. The used keywords for the literature research included "adenoid cystic", "adenoid cystic-like", "basaloid", "basal cell carcinoma", and "prostate". Available clinical information, management, outcomes, and follow-up data were extracted.

The management and follow-up data were also reviewed to ascertain the available treatment options for this rare type of prostate cancer.

2. Pathological Features

A wide range of basal cell lesions of the prostate gland have been described in the literature, from benign basal cell hyperplasia (BCH) to various infiltrative and invasive patterns. It is believed that, in contrast to usual prostate malignancies, they are originated from basal/reserve cells [7]. Grossly, ACC/BCC is commonly reported as a yellow specimen with a hard consistency. There are lobules separated by fibrous septa. There may be also hemorrhage, necrosis, and cystic changes [8]. Basophilic mucinous secretions are sometimes seen [7].

Histologically, prostate ACC has been identical to the usual head and neck ACCs, including the evidence of extensive perineural invasion [7–10]. Upon microscopic examination, the reported patterns are trabecular, glandular, cribriform, and variably sized solid nests. Early pathology reports already described ACC/BCC as irregular, variably sized nests of tumor cells, predominantly basaloid cells, and a lesser number of larger cells with pale eosinophilic cytoplasm, infiltrating the stroma with prominent cribriform architecture. Moreover, McKenny et al. observed an extensive intraglandular hyalinization completely replacing the glandular structures in some tumoral foci, different from the basaloid carcinoma that showed infiltration between normal glands, extraprostatic extension, and perineural invasion, but not with a cribriform pattern [11].

Tumoral cells have shown a high nuclear to cytoplasmic ratio, open chromatin, and scant cytoplasm with cytoplasmic vacuoles that resemble myoepithelial cells [7,8]. Basaloid characteristics in the reported cases are very prominent. Immunohistochemical examinations have shown a relationship among adenoid cystic carcinoma, basal cell hyperplasia, and adenoid basal cell tumors. Indeed, some authors have argued that it probably did not originate from the secretory epithelium of the prostate gland. Despite this, imaging, clinical, and pathologic evidence support ACC/BCC location to be within the prostate glandular tissue [9,10]. Beyond the perineural invasion (similar to head and neck ACCs), infiltrative pattern growth and extra-prostatic extension are also common features [7,8,10]. Since they originate from the basal cell layer, other than secretive, glandular epithelium, the almost or true negative Prostate-specific antigen (PSA) immunohistochemical staining is one of the usual features of ACC/BCC, except for some positive cases, especially in mixed-form ACC/BCC plus acinar adenocarcinoma [12,13].

From a molecular point of view, loss of PTEN expression and overexpression of EGFR are two frequent findings in ACC/BCC. The MYB translocation has often been described in true ACCs. In particular, the MYB–NFIB fusion protein has been reported to be associated with morphologic features reminiscent of adenoid cystic carcinoma in a cohort of basal cell carcinomas of the prostate [7]. Proliferative index, which is usually higher than 20% in

ACC, may be helpful to distinguish BCH from ACC. Diffuse Bcl-2 staining in ACC may also help to differentiate ACC and BCH or usual PCs in which such evidence is absent or scant. CK7 protein is positive in the luminal part of ACC, while high-molecular-weight cytokeratins (i.e., HMCK, 34βE12) are positive in the peripheral parts of the tumor mass. P63 protein usually also results strongly positive in ACCs. S100 and PSA markers may be positive, but not in all cases [7,14]. This tumor entity is probably not an homogenous tumor type comprised different subtypes and an in-depth molecular analysis could allow not only a better characterization of the disease but provide prognostic and predictive data of extreme importance. To date, from the data that emerged from our work, we are unable to state whether the presence of MYB translocation or HER2/PTEN alteration can allow different therapeutic approaches.

Compared to conventional acinar PCs, basal cell carcinoma usually shows little or no androgen receptor (AR) expression, with a very low percentage of patients or weak and patchy immunohistochemical staining reported in the literature [15]. The main pathological characteristics and hormonal reactions in ACC/BCC are summarized in Table 1.

Table 1. Summary of the main pathological features of ACC/BCC.

Morphologic Characters	Immunostaining	Molecular Characteristic
• Scare cytoplasm		
• High N/C ratio		
• Irregular and angulated nuclei with open chromatin		
• May exhibit nuclear and cytoplasmic micro vacuolation		
• Infiltration of adjacent parenchyma		
BCC pattern:	BCC pattern:	• loss of PTEN expression
• Variably sized, solid nests, cords or trabeculae, peripheral palisading of basaloid cell	• Basal cell markers, p63 or HMCK (34βE12)	• overexpression of EGFR • MYB–NFIB fusion
ACC pattern:	ACC pattern:	
• Prominent cribriform architecture	• CK 20-/CD7+ staining	
• Eosinophilic, hyaline, basement membrane-like material	• CK7 in pure solid form	
	• Basal cell nests	
	• Bcl-2 strongly and diffusely +	
	• High Ki67 nuclear staining	

Abbreviations: ACC: adenoid cystic carcinoma; BCC: basal cell carcinoma; N/C: nuclear-cytoplasmic ratio; HMCK: high-molecular-weight cytokeratins; CK cytokeratine; CD: cluster of differentiation; Bcl-2: B cell lymphoma-2; Ki67: marker of proliferation Ki67; ADT: androgen deprivation therapy.

3. Diagnosis and Staging

This rare form of prostate cancer tends to have non-specific symptoms that last for many years, showing an indolent course, for which it was originally suggested to be a potentially indolent disease. Most patients had symptoms of urinary tract obstruction, hematuria, nocturia, and pollakiuria or pelvic pain, often leading to incidental diagnosis by transurethral resection of the prostate (TURP). The initial step towards clinical diagnosis and staging was a digital rectal examination, which detected abnormalities in prostate glands. No preoperative imaging technique has provided sufficiently specific results. In some cases, anechoic lesions were observed by TRUS and typical of this cancer; however, these were not sufficient to establish a diagnosis between ACC/BCC and other prostate cancer subtypes or benign prostatic hyperplasia (BPH). Therefore, a pathologic examination of surgical or biopsy materials was required in order to obtain a certain diagnosis. It should be emphasized that, with the exception of a few cases (Table 2), the Prostate-specific antigen

(PSA) level remained within the normal range, so it cannot be considered an index of tumor aggressiveness. These findings suggest that ACC/BCC of the prostate lacks the capability of PSA production and concomitant acinar ADK of the prostate was found in patients with PSA elevation [8]. The low PSA value could support the idea that this rare variant should not be considered and treated as prostate cancer. In our opinion, this consideration is incorrect since the PSA value in patients diagnosed with rare forms of non-acinar prostate cancer, such as ductal carcinoma of the prostate, was often in the normal range.

Normal PSA values, in addition to mild symptoms, pushed urologists to use medical treatments for benign pathology, probably delaying the cancer diagnosis. From the analysis of the literature, in almost all cases it is presented with locally advanced disease, with encroachment beyond the prostate capsule and infiltration of the bladder, rectum, and sometimes the pelvic wall or pelvis bone. Less than 10% of patients had stage IV disease at onset; however, 30–40% of patients developed a recurrence or metastases early after radical treatment, predominantly to the bone, liver, and lung [16,17].

However, these data could be underestimated considering the lack of sufficient follow-up time (median 1 year). Dong et al. reported a case of massive lung metastases after one year of radical prostatectomy (RP) who underwent multiple chemotherapy lines and had stable disease after treatment with etoposide [18].

Because of this potential aggression and the risk of developing early metastases, many authors suggested pre-treatment staging with Computed Tomography (CT scan), Magnetic Resonance Imaging (MRI), and possibly bone scan, as well as a follow-up CT scan every 3–6 months. In the early stages of the disease, according to Zang's case report, MRI could be negative even when it is performed repeatedly [10].

There are no data available on the possible use of nuclear medicine tests for this tumor. Komura et al. described a case of stage IV ACC/BCC metastatic disease detected with 2-Fluoro-2-deoxy-D-glucose Positron Emission Tomography/Computed Tomography (PET/CT) [19]. Moreover, sporadic cases of positive metastases by ACC extra-prostatic tumors with 68 Ga-Prostate-Specific Membrane Antigen (PSMA) are reported. This could be a possible area for future investigation [20,21].

Table 2. Summary of case reports and case series published in the literature.

Author (Year)	N of Pts * (Tot: 106)	Age	PSA (ng/mL)	Symptoms	Diasease Stage	Treatment	Outcomes
Frankel, K. 1974 [22]	1	69	/	Acute urinary retention and nocturia	cT1c	TURP	36 m fup: NED
Tannenbaum, M. 1975 [23]	2	/	/	/	cT4	/	/
Kramer, S.A. 1978 [24]	1	55		Perineal pain and tenderness	cT4	TURP plus Pelvic exenteratio + RT (60 Gy)	/
Kuhajda, F.P. 1983 [25]	1	66		Urinary obstruction	/	TURP plus RT	NED
Gilrnour, A.M. 1986 [26]	1	76	/	5 y history of nocturia and poor stream	Organ confined disease	TURP plus RP	8 m fup: NED

Table 2. Cont.

Author (Year)	N of Pts * (Tot: 106)	Age	PSA (ng/mL)	Symptoms	Diasease Stage	Treatment	Outcomes
Ahn, K.S., 1991 [8]	1	38	/	Long history of nocturia and Dysuria	cT3b	RP	/
Denholm, S.W. 1992 [9]	1	28	Normal range	Urinary obstruction	cT4	TURP plus RT (45 Gy in 20 Fx) plus chemotherapy (5 Fluorouracil-Mitomycin C)	18 m fup: reduction of pelvic mass
Hasan, N. 1996 [22]	1	66	Normal range	Acute retention	Organ confined disease	TURP	4 m: NED
Pariente, J.L. 1998 [27]	1	73	168	/	/	TURP plus Androgen blockade	12 m fup: NED
Young, R.H. 1998 [28]	2	Case 1: 60 Case 2: 68	/	Acute retention	/	TURP and RP	8 y fup: NED
Minei, S. 2001 [29]	1	43	2	Urinary Obstruction	/	TURP	/
Schmid, H.P. 2002 [30]	1	43	Normal range	/	/	PR plus RT	8 y fup: local progression
Iczkowski, K.A. 2003 [16]	19	43–87	<9 ng/mL	Urinary Obstruction	4 cases: stage IV	TURP (10 pts), RP (2 pts), exenteratio, (2 pts) combined RP and RT (4 pts), biopsy (1 pts)	Mean fup 26 m (range 3–132): 10 pts: NED, 4 developed metastases 3 pts alive with tumor, 1 pt died of tumor
Mastropasqua, M.G. 2003 [14]	1	65	8.5	Nocturia, pelvic pain	pT3bN1	RP + LAD	8 mo fup: lung metastases
McKenney, J.K. 2004 [11]	4	36–60	/	/	Organ confined disease (1 pt) cT4 (3 pts)	RP (2 pts), TURP	1 died 3 mo after PR 9 m fup: NED
Fayyad, L.M. 2006 [31]	1	75	/	/	/	TURP + CT + ADT	5 y fup: died for metastases
Ali, T. 2007 [17]	29	42–89	/	Urinary Obstruction	/	TURP (16 pts), TURP + RP (5 pts) RP + RT + CT (4 pts) Biopsia (4 pts)	Mean fup 4.3 y: 14 pts NED 4 pts local recurrence 4 pts metastases

Table 2. Cont.

Author (Year)	N of Pts * (Tot: 106)	Age	PSA (ng/mL)	Symptoms	Diasease Stage	Treatment	Outcomes
Komura, K. 2010 [19]	1	67	Normal range	Urinary Obstruction, pelvic pain	IV	Docetaxel and Extramustine	Lung metastases after 3 m of treayment
Bohn, O.L. 2010 [32]	1	65	Normal range	Long history of dysuria and urinary outlet obstruction	Organ confined disease	RP	12 mo fup: NED
Ahuja, A. 2011 [33]	1	32	Normal range	Obstructive lower urinary tract symptoms	cT4	Bilateral orchidectomy and Bicalutamide	6 mo fup: Stable disease
Tuan, J. 2012 [34]	1	78	Normal range	Urinary tract symptoms, nocturia and gross hematuria	T4N1M0	TURP plus RT (45 Gy in 20 Fx) plus CT (5-Fluorouracil + Mitomycin C)	36 mo fup: NED
Stearns, G. 2012 [35]	1	69	Normal range	Hematuria	cT4N0	Etoposide and Cisplatin plus RP	Early progression
Chang, K. 2012 [36]	3	48–65	Normal range	Acute urinary retention	Cases 1 and 2: Organ confined disease Case 3: lung metastases	Cases 1 and 2: 50 Gy RT Case 3: Androgen blockade (Bicalutamide + Goserelin)	Cases 1 and 2: bone progression after 2 mo Case 3: died 5 mo after treatment
Tsuruta, K. 2012 [37]	1	48		Hematuria	cT4	Etoposide and Cisplatin plus pelvic exenteratio	Liver metastases after 3 mo
Bishop, J.A. 2015 [38]	12	65–86	/	/	/	TURP	/
Simper, N.B. 2015 [39]	9	57–97	/	/	Locoregional confined disease,	TURP (6 pts), Pelvic exenteratio (1 pt), RP (2 pts)	44 mo fup: 5 pts NED 4 pts local recurrence 1 pt metastases
Zang, M. 2016 [10]	1	73	1.9	Nine years of peritoneal pain	cT4	Pelvic exenteratio	22 mo fup: PSA:0
Bernhardt, D. 2018 [40]	2	Case 1: 65 Case 2: 44	Normal range	Perirectal pain	Case 1: pT2c pN0 M1, Case 2: cT4	TURP plus RP plus RT as photon IMRT plus C12 heavy ion boost	Case 1: 16 mo fup local and distant progression Case 2: NED
Shibuya, T. 2018 [41]	1	68	Normal range	/	cT1c	RP	1 y fup: NED

Table 2. Cont.

Author (Year)	N of Pts * (Tot: 106)	Age	PSA (ng/mL)	Symptoms	Diasease Stage	Treatment	Outcomes
Dong, S. 2020 [18]	1	62	Normal range	/	pT2	RP + RT	2 y fup: lung metastases
Julka, P.K. 2020 [13]	1	79	/	Hematuria	CT4N0M1(liver)	TURP plus CT (Carboplatin + Paclitaxel) then ADT (Degarelix)	16 mo fup: stable disease
Ridai, S. 2021 [42]	1	40	3.5	Obstructive lower urinary tract symptoms	cT3b	TURP plus concurrent CT (Cisplatin)-RT as photon IMRT	1 y fup: cerebellar metastases
He, L. 2021 [43]	1	92	<0.05 post-TURP	Urethral stricture, urinary retention	cT1c	TURP plus RT	4 mo fup: NED

* Abbreviations: N°: number; PTS: patients; PSA: Prostate-specific antigen; TURP: transurethral resection of prostate; RP: radical prostatectomy; fup: follow-up; MO: months; Y: years; RT: radiotherapy; C12: 12 carbon; IMRT: Intensity-modulated radiation therapy; NED: no evidence of disease, ADT: androgen deprivation therapy; CT: chemotherapy. The text continues here (Table 2).

4. Treatment Options and Outcomes

Given the rarity of ACC/BCC prostate cancer, there were no prospective trials to determine the optimal treatment. Thirty-three articles published in the literature, for a total of 106 patients, were evaluated with the aim of identifying the most suitable treatment and evaluating outcomes (Table 2). Various treatment approaches have been described in the literature. They are mainly based on tumor histology and/or borrowed from some more usual ACC/BCC tumor sites (e.g., head and neck), hence highlighting there is no uniformity in the management of such a rare prostate disease due to the lack of knowledge on its clinical and biological characteristics.

Follow-up data were reported in 28 of 30 articles (90 patients) and ranged from 3 to 136 months. Of these, four (4.4%) died from cancer-related causes, 41 (45.5%) were reported to be free of recurrence (NED), 21 (23.3%) were alive, but with evidence of disease, and 24 (26.6%) showed local progression or developed distant metastases mainly in the lungs, liver, and rarely bone.

In some patients, radical surgical resection was a treatment option for localized disease, ensuring free margins and a clear histological characterization of ACC/BCC. However, the extensive locally infiltrative pattern and perineural spread often cause difficulty in achieving high tumor control rates [24,38,44]. Prognostic factors such as advanced tumors, positive resection margins, and perineural infiltration drove the indication for postoperative radiotherapy [37]. Such findings were imported from the guidelines for acinar prostate cancer and ACC cancer of the head and neck region. In fact, most of the patients (38 patients, 36.5%) were treated with TURP, acting immediately on the clinical symptoms, while in five (4.8%) cases, only diagnostic biopsy was performed.

Aggressive surgical treatments, such as pelvic exenteration, that were initially applied (four patients, 3.8%) [16,22,39] were subsequently abandoned to give way to more conservative treatments, often characterized by the combination of two or more therapeutic approaches. Radical prostatectomy was adopted in 17 patients (16.4%), while postoperative radiotherapy, with a total dose of 66 Gy in 33 sessions or 45 Gy in 15 sessions, was added to RP in 11 cases (10.36%). Radical radiotherapy for a total dose of 45–50 Gy associated with hormone therapy or chemotherapy was administered in eight cases (7.9%).

The authors of this article believe it is important in the case of patients with urinary symptoms not to act immediately with TURP, but to opt for symptom control through the use of drugs since TURP could preclude the possibility of surgery or disallow escalation of the radiotherapy dose, compromising the patient's outcome.

Iczkowski et al. [16] reviewed and reported 19 cases of ACC/BCC neoplasm of the prostate, identifying young age, involvement of peripheral zone of the prostate, extra-prostatic spread, and perineural and peri-glandular invasion as important prognostic factors. Ali and colleagues also suggested potentially aggressive behavior attributable to the common presence of cancer cells in the periprostatic adipose tissue and extension to the thick muscle bundles of the bladder neck [17].

As far as systemic therapy is concerned, it is not possible to draw clear conclusions. Only six (5.7%) patients with advanced ACC/BCC disease received systemic approaches, with various drugs used, such as 5-Fluorouracil plus Mitomycin C; Docetaxel; Carboplatin plus Paclitaxel; Cisplatin; and ADT (Bicalutamide and/or LHRH analogues/antagonists), alone or combination strategies [9,13,29,36,37]. A case of locally advanced prostate BCC treated with concurrent chemoradiation was recently reported. A 70 Gy total target dose was delivered in 35 fractions with an intensity-modulated technique and concomitant, weekly cisplatin with evidence of complete local remission and disappearance of the lower urinary tract symptoms and pain at the one-year follow-up visit, but distant metastatic oligoprogression of the disease [42]. Of note, since ACC/BCC has proven to not express the AR, the impact of ADT remains unclear, even if luteinizing hormone-releasing hormone agonists and antiandrogen drugs are still considered the treatment of choice for inoperable cases or metastatic disease [15,39]. The question arises spontaneously whether the forms of ACC/BCC of the prostate can or should be treated as similar tumors of other sites (i.e., ACC tumors of the head and neck area). In the some reports, the authors report experiences in adding chemotherapy based on cisplatin or taxanes (as in head and neck pathologies), but there are very few cases and it is not possible to draw a conclusion [13,33,42].

5. Discussion

Adenoid cystic carcinoma/basal cell carcinoma is an extremely rare variant of prostate cancer first described in 1974. Just over 100 cases are currently reported in the literature worldwide. In view of the rarity and the lack of prospective studies, it is possible to define some features only based on few case reports. Despite this, it is possible to draw some important conclusions which may guide physicians to choose the best therapeutic approach. The correct identification of ACC/BCC from a pathological point of view is of extreme importance and therefore, when there is histological suspicion, the specimens should be referred to an expert pathologist. The serum PSA value does not represent a useful marker in this histological variant, so a clinical picture with persistent obstructive urinary symptoms unresponsive to medical therapy, even in the absence of a rise in PSA, necessitates investigation with a biopsy. Above all, serum PSA should not be used as the sole tool for follow up. Contrary to what has been hypothesized in the past, ACC/BCC has usually been shown not to present with an indolent character, rather it tends to have loco-regional spread with potential to metastasize. Given the potential aggressiveness of the tumor, owing to metastatic disease at presentation, an adequate radiological staging with CT scan plus bone scan and MRI should be performed prior to radical treatment, with curative intent and during the follow-up period. If necessary, the use of second-level functional imaging (i.e., Choline-PET or PSMA-PET) is desirable to complete the staging framework [13,43]. Moreover, TURP should also be avoided as an upfront treatment in cases of symptoms in order not to compromise subsequent treatment and preferred medical treatment.

Young age, involvement of the peripheral zone of the prostate, extra-prostatic spread, and perineural and peri-glandular invasion are important prognostic factors. The presence of these factors make radical prostatectomy alone insufficient to guarantee disease control, therefore a combined treatment including adjuvant radiotherapy should be considered as a standard of care. No conclusive data can be drawn on the best systemic treatment, nor on the efficacy of androgen deprivation therapy, especially as ACC/BCC has proven to be independent from androgen stimulation [19,33]. Recently, a phenotypic multi-dimensional assay testing the patient's tumor tissue against different drug combinations has been proposed, along with an accurate prediction of clinical outcome, thus offering a personalized way to select the most appropriate treatment option for the individual patient, especially with rare cancers [13,38]. A more accurate refinement of the histopathologic features of prostatic ACC/BCC can probably help tailor treatment based on tumor phenotypes and involved genetic pathways that includes various potential therapeutic targets [39]. Since prospective studies are not conceivable due to the rarity of ACC/BCC worldwide, the collection of real-world data, possibly with large international, retrospective databases is desirable to better understand the adequate management of ACC/BCC and the role of different therapeutic strategies.

Author Contributions: Conceptualization, S.C.; Methodology, S.C., L.B., and M.N.; Validation, A.S., C.I., and P.C.; Formal Analysis, A.B. and M.A.; Data Curation, M.M. and F.I.; Writing—Original Draft Preparation, S.C., G.B., and M.N.; Writing—Review and Editing, L.B. and L.G.; Supervision, C.I. and P.C.; Project Administration, S.C. All authors have read and agreed to the published version of the manuscript.

Funding: This research received no external funding.

Institutional Review Board Statement: Not applicable.

Informed Consent Statement: Not applicable.

Data Availability Statement: Not applicable.

Conflicts of Interest: The authors declare no conflict of interest.

References

1. Frankel, K.; Craig, J.R. Adenoid cystic carcinoma of the prostate. Report of a case. *Am. J. Clin. Pathol.* **1974**, *62*, 639–645. [CrossRef] [PubMed]
2. Woida, F.M.; Ribeiro-Silva, A. Adenoid cystic carcinoma of the Bartholin gland: An overview. *Arch. Pathol. Lab. Med.* **2007**, *131*, 796–798. [CrossRef] [PubMed]
3. Ramakrishnan, R.; Chaudhry, I.H.; Ramdial, P.; Lazar, A.J.; McMenamin, M.E.; Kazakov, D.; Brenn, T.; Calonje, E. Primary cutaneous adenoid cystic carcinoma: A clinicopathologic and immunohistochemical study of 27 cases. *Am. J. Surg. Pathol.* **2013**, *37*, 1603–1611. [CrossRef] [PubMed]
4. Bennett, A.K.; Mills, S.E.; Wick, M.R. Salivary-type neoplasms of the breast and lung. *Semin. Diagn. Pathol.* **2003**, *20*, 279–304. [CrossRef]
5. Moran, C.A.; Suster, S.; Koss, M.N. Primary adenoid cystic carcinoma of the lung. A clinicopathologic and immunohistochemical study of 16 cases. *Cancer* **1994**, *73*, 1390–1397. [CrossRef]
6. Moch, H.; Cubilla, A.L.; Humphrey, P.A.; Reuter, V.E.; Ulbright, T.M. The 2016 who classification of tumours of the urinary system and male genital organs-Part B: Prostate and bladder tumours. *Eur. Urol.* **2016**, *70*, 106–119. [CrossRef]
7. Li, J.; Wang, Z. The pathology of unusual subtypes of prostate cancer. *Chin. J. Cancer Res.* **2016**, *28*, 130–143. [CrossRef]
8. Ahn, S.K.; Kim, K.; Choi, I.J.; Lee, J.M. Adenoid cystic carcinoma of the prostate gland—Pathological review with a case report. *Yonsei Med. J.* **1991**, *32*, 74–78. [CrossRef]
9. Denholm, S.W.; Webb, J.N.; Howard, G.C.; Chisholm, G.D. Basaloid carcinoma of the prostate gland: Histogenesis and review of the literature. *Histopathology* **1992**, *20*, 151–155. [CrossRef]
10. Zhang, M.; Pettaway, C.; Vikram, R.; Tamboli, P. Adenoid cystic carcinoma of the urethra/Cowper's gland with concurrent high-grade prostatic adenocarcinoma: A detailed clinicopathologic case report and review of the literature. *Hum. Pathol.* **2016**, *58*, 138–144. [CrossRef]
11. McKenney, J.K.; Amin, M.B.; Srigley, J.R.; Jimenez, R.E.; Ro, J.Y.; Grignon, D.J.; Young, R.H. Basal cell proliferations of the prostate other than usual basal cell hyperplasia: A clinicopathologic study of 23 cases, including four carcinomas, with a proposed classification. *Am. J. Surg. Pathol.* **2004**, *28*, 1289–1298. [CrossRef] [PubMed]
12. Begnami, M.D.; Quezado, M.; Pinto, P.; Linehan, W.M.; Merino, M. Adenoid cystic/basal cell carcinoma of the prostate: Review and update. *Arch. Pathol. Lab. Med.* **2007**, *131*, 637–640. [CrossRef] [PubMed]
13. Julka, P.K.; Verma, A.; Gupta, S.; Gupta, K.; Rathod, R. Adenoid cystic carcinoma of the prostate: An unusual subtype of prostate cancer. *J. Transl. Genet. Genom.* **2020**, *4*, 455–463. [CrossRef]
14. Mastropasqua, M.G.; Pruneri, G.; Renne, G.; De Cobelli, O.; Viale, G. Basaloid cell carcinoma of the prostate. *Virchows Arch.* **2003**, *443*, 787–791. [CrossRef] [PubMed]

15. Segawa, N.; Tsuji, M.; Nishida, T.; Takahara, K.; Azuma, H.; Katsuoka, Y. Basal cell carcinoma of the prostate: Report of a case and review of the published reports. *Int. J. Urol.* **2008**, *15*, 557–559. [CrossRef]
16. Iczkowski, K.A.; Ferguson, K.L.; Grier, D.D. Adenoid cystic/basal cell carcinoma of the prostate clinicopathologic findings in 19 cases. *Am. J. Surg. Pathol.* **2003**, *27*, 1523–1529. [CrossRef]
17. Ali, T.Z.; Epstein, J.I. Basal cell carcinoma of the prostate: A clinicopathologic study of 29 cases. *Am. J. Surg. Pathol.* **2007**, *31*, 697–705. [CrossRef]
18. Dong, S.; Liu, Q.; Xu, Z.; Wang, H. An unusual case of metastatic basal cell carcinoma of the prostate: A case report and literature review. *Front. Oncol.* **2020**, *10*, 859. [CrossRef]
19. Komura, K.; Inamoto, T.; Tsuji, M.; Ibuki, N.; Koyama, K.; Ubai, T.; Azuma, H.; Katsuoka, Y. Basal cell carcinoma of the prostate: Unusual subtype of prostatic carcinoma. *Int. J. Clin. Oncol.* **2010**, *15*, 594–600. [CrossRef]
20. Klein Nulent, T.J.W.; Valstar, M.H.; Smit, L.A. Prostate-specific membrane antigen (PSMA) expression in adenoid cystic carcinoma of the head and neck. *BMC Cancer* **2020**, *20*, 519. [CrossRef]
21. Uijen, M.J.; van Boxtel, W.; van Herpen, C.M.; Gotthardt, M.; Nagarajah, J. 68Ga-prostate-specific membrane antigen-11-avid cardiac metastases in a patient with adenoid cystic carcinoma, a rare presentation of a rare cancer. *Clin. Nucl. Med.* **2020**, *45*, 716–718. [CrossRef] [PubMed]
22. Frankel, K.; Craig, J.R. Adenoid cystic carcinoma of the prostate. *Am. J. Clin. Pathol.* **1974**, *62*, 639–645. [CrossRef] [PubMed]
23. Tannenbaum, M. Adenoid cystic or "salivary gland" carcinomas of prostate. *Urology* **1975**, *6*, 238–239. [CrossRef]
24. Kramer, S.A.; Bredael, J.J.; Krueger, R.P. Adenoid cystic carcinoma of the prostate-report of a case. *J. Urol.* **1978**, *120*, 383–384. [CrossRef]
25. Kuhajda FPMann, R.B. Adenoid cystic carcinoma of the prostate. A case report with immunoperoxidase staining for prostate-specific acid phosphatase and prostate-specific antigen. *Am. J. Clin. Pathol.* **1984**, *81*, 257–260. [CrossRef]
26. Gilrnour, A.M.; Bell, T.J. Adenoid cystic carcinoma of the prostate. *Br. J. Urol.* **1986**, *58*, 105–106.
27. Pariente, J.L.; Hostyn, B.; Grenier, N.; Ferriere, J.M.; Le Guillou, M. Diagnosis and follow up of a prostate cystic carcinoma. *Br. J. Urol.* **1998**, *81*, 177. [CrossRef]
28. Young, R.H.; Frierson Jr, H.F.; Mills, S.E.; Kaiser, J.S.; Talbot, W.H.; Bham, A.K. Adenoid cystic-like tumor of the prostate gland. A report of two cases and review of the literature on 'adenoid cystic carcinoma' of the prostate. *Am. J. Clin. Pathol.* **1988**, *89*, 49–56. [CrossRef]
29. Minei, S.; Hachiya, T.; Ishida, H.; Okada, K. Adenoid cystic carcinoma of the prostate: A case report with immunohistochemical and in situ hybridization staining for prostate-specific antigen. *Int. J. Urol.* **2001**, *8*, S41–S44. [CrossRef]
30. Schmid, H.P.; Semjonow, A.; Eltze, E.; Wprtler, K.; Hertle, L. Late recurrence of Adenoid cystic carcinoma of the prostate. *Scand. J. Urol. Nephrol.* **2002**, *36*, 158–159. [CrossRef]
31. Fayyad, L.M.; Al-Jader, K.M.; Al-Hawwari, B.A. Asynchronous adenoid cystic carcinoma of the prostate and transitional cell carcinoma of the urinary bladder. *Saudi Med. J.* **2006**, *27*, 1060–1062. [PubMed]
32. Bohn, O.L.; Rios-Luna, N.P.; Navarro, L.; Duran-Peña, A.; Sanchez-Sosa, S. Basal cell carcinoma of the prostate gland: A case report and brief review of the basal cell proliferations of the prostate gland. *Ann. Diagn. Pathol.* **2010**, *14*, 365–368. [CrossRef] [PubMed]
33. Ahuja, A.; Das, P.; Kumar, N.; Saini, A.K.; Seth, A.; Ray, R. Adenoid cystic carcinoma of the prostate: Case report on a rare entity and review of the literature. *Pathol. Res. Pract.* **2011**, *207*, 391–394. [CrossRef] [PubMed]
34. Tuan, J.; Pandha, H.; Corbishley, C.; Khoo, V. Basaloid carcinoma of the prostate: A literature review with case report. *Indian J. Urol.* **2012**, *28*, 322–324. [CrossRef]
35. Stearns, G.; Cheng, J.S.; Shapiro, O.; Nsouli, I. Basal cell carcinoma of the prostate: A case report. *Urology* **2012**, *79*, e79–e80. [CrossRef]
36. Chang, K.; Dai, B.; Kong, Y.; Qu, Y.; Wu, J.; Ye, D.; Yao, X.; Zhang, S.; Zhang, H.; Zhu, Y.; et al. Basal cell carcinoma of the prostate: Clinicopathologic analysis of three cases and a review of the literature. *World J. Surg. Oncol.* **2013**, *11*, 193. [CrossRef]
37. Tsuruta, K.; Funahashi, Y.; Kato, M. Basal cell carcinoma arising in the prostate. *Int. J. Urol.* **2014**, *21*, 1072–1073. [CrossRef]
38. Bishop, J.A.; Yonescu, R.; Epstein, J.I.; Westra, W.H. A subset of prostatic basal cell carcinomas harbor the MYB rearrangement of adenoid cystic carcinoma. *Hum. Pathol.* **2015**, *46*, 1204–1208. [CrossRef]
39. Simper, N.B.; Jones, C.L.; MacLennan, G.T. Basal cell carcinoma of the prostate is an aggressive tumor with frequent loss of PTEN expression and overexpression of EGFR. *Hum. Pathol.* **2015**, *46*, 805–812. [CrossRef]
40. Bernhardt, D.; Sterzing, F.; Adeberg, S.; Herfarth, K.; Katayama, S.; Foerster, R.; Hoerner-Rieber, J.; Koning, L.; Debus, J.; Rieken, S.; et al. Bimodality treatment of patients with pelvic adenoid cystic carcinoma with photon intensitymodulated radiotherapy plus carbon ion boost: A case series. *Cancer Manag. Res.* **2018**, *10*, 583–588. [CrossRef]
41. Shibuya, T.; Takahashi, G.; Kan, T. Basal cell carcinoma of the prostate: A case report and review of the literature. *Mol. Clin. Oncol.* **2019**, *10*, 101–104. [CrossRef] [PubMed]
42. Ridai, S.; Moustakbal, C.; Lachgar, A.; Jouhadi, H.; Benider, A.; Regragui, M.; Marnissi, F. Prostatic basal cell carcinoma treated by chemoradiation with weekly cisplatine: Case report and literature review. *Afr. J. Urol.* **2021**, *27*, 79. [CrossRef]

43. He, L.; Metter, C.; Margulis, V.; Kapur, P. A review leveraging a rare and unusual case of basal cell carcinoma of the prostate. *Case Rep. Pathol.* **2021**, *2021*, 5520581. [CrossRef] [PubMed]
44. Ayyathurai, R.; Civantos, F.; Manoharan, M. Basal cell carcinoma of the prostate: Current concepts. *BJU Int.* **2007**, *99*, 1345–1349. [CrossRef] [PubMed]

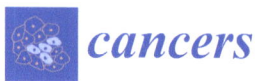

Article

Vitamin D Metabolites in Nonmetastatic High-Risk Prostate Cancer Patients with and without Zoledronic Acid Treatment after Prostatectomy

Carsten Stephan [1,2,*,†], Bernhard Ralla [1,†], Florian Bonn [3], Max Diesner [3], Michael Lein [4] and Klaus Jung [1,*]

1. Department of Urology, Charité-Universitätsmedizin Berlin, 10115 Berlin, Germany; bernhard.ralla@charite.de
2. Berlin Institute for Urologic Research, 10115 Berlin, Germany
3. Immundiagnostik AG, 64625 Bensheim, Germany; florian.bonn@immundiagnostik.com (F.B.); max.diesner@immundiagnostik.com (M.D.)
4. Department of Urology, Sana Medical Center Offenbach, 63069 Offenbach am Main, Germany; michael.lein@sana.de
* Correspondence: carsten.stephan@charite.de (C.S.); klaus.jung@charite.de (K.J.)
† These authors contributed equally to this paper.

Simple Summary: Recent research on prostate cancer and vitamin D is controversial. We measured three vitamin D_3 metabolites in 32 selected prostate cancer patients after surgery at four time points over four years. Within a large European study, half of the patients were prophylactically treated with zoledronic acid (ZA); the others received a placebo. After the study start, all the patients daily took calcium and vitamin D_3. The development of metastasis was not affected by ZA treatment. While two vitamin D metabolites had higher values after the study's start, with constant follow-up values, the $1,25(OH)_2$-vitamin D_3 concentrations remained unchanged. The latter form was the only metabolite that was higher in the patients with metastasis as compared to those without bone metastasis. This result is surprising. However, it is too premature to discuss possible prognostic value yet. Our results should be confirmed in larger cohorts.

Abstract: There are limited and discrepant data on prostate cancer (PCa) and vitamin D. We investigated changes in three vitamin D_3 metabolites in PCa patients after prostatectomy with zoledronic acid (ZA) treatment regarding their metastasis statuses over four years. In 32 patients from the ZEUS trial, $25(OH)D_3$, $24,25(OH)_2D_3$, and $1,25(OH)_2D_3$ were measured with liquid chromatography coupled with tandem mass spectrometry at four time points. All the patients received daily calcium and vitamin D_3. Bone metastases were detected in 7 of the 17 ZA-treated patients and in 5 of the 15 controls (without ZA), without differences between the groups ($p = 0.725$). While $25(OH)D_3$ and $24,25(OH)_2D_3$ increased significantly after the study's start, with following constant values, the $1,25(OH)_2D_3$ concentrations remained unchanged. ZA treatment did not change the levels of the three metabolites. $25(OH)D_3$ and $24,25(OH)_2D_3$ were not associated with the development of bone metastases. In contrast, $1,25(OH)_2D_3$ was also higher in patients with bone metastasis before the study's start. Thus, in high-risk PCa patients after prostatectomy, $25(OH)D_3$, $24,25(OH)_2D_3$, and $1,25(OH)_2D_3$ were not affected by supportive ZA treatment or by the development of metastasis over four years, with the exception of $1,25(OH)_2D_3$, which was constantly higher in metastatic patients. There might be potential prognostic value if the results can be confirmed.

Keywords: prostate cancer; prostatectomy; zoledronic acid treatment; vitamin D; circulating vitamin D metabolites; $25(OH)D_3$; $24,25(OH)_2D_3$; $1,25(OH)_2D_3$

Citation: Stephan, C.; Ralla, B.; Bonn, F.; Diesner, M.; Lein, M.; Jung, K. Vitamin D Metabolites in Nonmetastatic High-Risk Prostate Cancer Patients with and without Zoledronic Acid Treatment after Prostatectomy. *Cancers* **2022**, *14*, 1560. https://doi.org/10.3390/cancers14061560

Academic Editors: Ana Faustino, Paula A. Oliveira and Lúcio Lara Santos

Received: 22 February 2022
Accepted: 15 March 2022
Published: 18 March 2022

Publisher's Note: MDPI stays neutral with regard to jurisdictional claims in published maps and institutional affiliations.

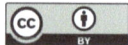

Copyright: © 2022 by the authors. Licensee MDPI, Basel, Switzerland. This article is an open access article distributed under the terms and conditions of the Creative Commons Attribution (CC BY) license (https://creativecommons.org/licenses/by/4.0/).

1. Introduction

Several international conferences in recent years have discussed, in detail, the current evidence and the ongoing controversies in vitamin D research [1–3]. Vitamin D_3 is mainly formed in the skin from 7-dehydrocholesterol upon ultraviolet B exposure. It is subsequently hydroxylated by two cytochrome-P450-mediated hydroxylation processes. In the liver, it is converted to 25-hydroxyvitamin D_3 (25(OH)D_3), released in the bloodstream and subsequently hydroxylated in the kidney, but also in other organs, including the prostate, to 1,25-dihydroxyvitamin D_3 (1,25(OH)$_2D_3$). The controversies concern both 25(OH)D_3 as the primary circulating vitamin D form reflecting the vitamin D status and 1,25(OH)$_2D_3$, the actual active metabolite that reacts with the vitamin D receptor. The controversial issues relate particularly to the extraskeletal actions of vitamin D and involve numerous diseases, such as various malignancies and cardiovascular, dermatologic, and immunological disorders [4]. Cell research and animal studies provide strong evidence of the potential molecular and cellular mechanisms underlying the actions of vitamin D and its metabolites [5–7]. However, corresponding observational and randomized controlled studies, probably due to their weak study designs, have frequently remained inconclusive and showed conflicting results concerning the hypothesized beneficial effect of vitamin D [3,8]. In this respect, prostate cancer (PCa) is no exception.

The complex biochemical and molecular relationship between PCa and vitamin D has been reviewed in numerous reports [9–11]. The limited and also partly discrepant data regarding the action of vitamin D in the treatment of PCa are exemplarily reflected by the results reported in some pertinent following studies. For example, a meta-analysis from 21 studies published until 2013 revealed a significant 17% higher risk of PCa in men with higher serum levels of 25(OH)D_3 [12]. In contrast, other studies reported that higher 25(OH)D_3 levels were associated with a 57% reduction in the risk of lethal PCa or improved prognosis [13–15]. A recently performed dose–response meta-analysis of 25(OH)D_3, which was based on seven relevant studies, supported the idea that a higher serum 25(OH)D_3 concentration was an important protective factor in PCa progression and was associated with reduced PCa mortality [16]. However, other studies showed that 25(OH)D_3 concentrations and vitamin D supplementation were not significantly associated with an increased PCa incidence and mortality rate [17–19]. An inverse association between the post-treatment plasma 1,25(OH)$_2D_3$ levels and all-cause and PCa-specific mortality in men with aggressive PCa suggested a possible beneficial effect of vitamin D supplementation in these men [20]. A recent study in 2021 found that men with PCa and vitamin D deficiency had higher overall and PCa-specific mortality, but there was no association between the risk of PCa (in biopsied men) and different vitamin D categories [21]. Our own data for 480 biopsied men also showed no correlation between 25(OH)D_3 and the pathological Gleason grade or differences between 222 men with and 258 without PCa [22].

It can be assumed that these contradictory results are mainly because basic principles for studies on the effect of vitamin D concerning health status have frequently been disregarded. Amrein et al. [8] defined four preconditions for an optimal study design in their seminal article "Vitamin D deficiency 2.0" as follows: (a) the measurement of the vitamin D status at baseline, (b) the consideration of vitamin D deficiency as a study inclusion criterion, (c) the application of an intervention capable of altering the vitamin D status, and (d) repeat measurements to verify the vitamin D status.

Considering these indispensable aspects for a valid study, it was therefore of interest to find out the possible changes in vitamin D status in patients after prostatectomy under the influence of the bisphosphonate zoledronic acid (ZA). ZA was shown to prevent bone loss due to antiandrogen-deprivation therapy, reduce morbidity and pain, and improve survival in castration-resistant PCa [23,24]. ZA induces the direct inhibition of PCa cells in vitro, inhibits tumor-mediated angiogenesis, enhances bone-mineral density, and suppresses bone markers [25–27]. Recent guidelines regarding PCa management recommend ZA and Denosumab as bone-protective agents in the supportive care of patients with castration-resistant PCa and skeletal metastases to prevent or reduce skeletal-related events [28–31]. However, data on the vitamin D status in follow-up measurements from patients receiving ZA are rare. They mostly refer to patients suffering from osteoporosis, while detailed data from PCa patients are lacking [32,33].

The basis for the study on vitamin D metabolites presented here was the availability of serum samples from a randomized, open-label study to evaluate the efficacy of ZA treatment for bone-metastasis prevention in high-risk PCa patients [34]. Thus, we were able to initiate this study in a small subset of 32 patients to largely meet the above-described requirements for a valid vitamin D study measuring the three metabolites $25(OH)D_3$, $24,25(OH)_2D_3$, and $1,25(OH)_2D_3$. With this study, we intended to obtain better insights into the following open issues: (a) the changes in vitamin D metabolites in PCa patients after prostatectomy over four years, (b) possible ZA-treatment effects on the profile of vitamin D metabolites, and (c) abnormalities in the metabolite profile with regard to metastasis during the study.

2. Materials and Methods

2.1. Patients and Samples

The study was based on vitamin D measurements performed on blood samples available from PCa patients after radical prostatectomy in the ZEUS trial (https://www.isrctn.com/ISRCTN66626762 accessed on 6 February 2022; https://doi.org/10.1186/ISRCTN66626762). This trial was a randomized, open-label study to evaluate the efficacy of ZA treatment for bone-metastasis prevention in high-risk PCa patients [34]. Ethical approval was obtained from local medical ethics committees for all the participating hospitals of this multicenter study, and the patients signed an informed consent form. The details and results of this trial were previously reported [34]. Briefly, the here-investigated subgroup consisted of nonmetastatic PCa patients with at least one of three high-risk factors: a Gleason score of 8–10, node-positive disease, or prostate-specific antigen (PSA) at diagnosis $\geq$20 ng/mL. No other prior PCa treatment (antiandrogen monotherapy, chemotherapy, and treatment with bisphosphonates) was allowed. All the patients were included in this study within 6 months after radical prostatectomy. The patients either received an intravenous infusion of 4 mg every three months or were without ZA treatment and served as controls. All the patients were prescribed concomitant therapy with a daily 500 mg dose of calcium and 400–500 IU of vitamin D_3. Blood samples were collected under standard conditions in BD Vacutainer tubes before the study began and at every three-month visit. Serum samples were prepared and frozen at $-80\ ^\circ$C until analysis. We analyzed samples from 32 patients at four time points, as further explained in the Results.

2.2. Analytics for Vitamin D Metabolites

The $25(OH)D_3$ and $24,25(OH)_2D_3$ concentrations were determined with the KM1320 assay, and the concentration of $1,25(OH)_2D_3$ was determined with a development version of the KM1400 assay, both from Immundiagnostik AG, Bensheim, Germany. The vitamin D metabolites were purified by immunoaffinity enrichment, with $1,25(OH)_2D_3$ additionally derivatized for improved detection, and subsequently analyzed by liquid chromatography–tandem mass spectrometry on a QTrap 5500 system coupled to an Exion LC (AB Sciex, Darmstadt, Germany). All the samples were analyzed in two replicates using individual 3-point linear calibration curves. All the calibrants and controls were prepared from certified reference material (Cerilliant Corp., Round Rock, TX, USA) and validated with NIST®SRM®972a samples, if available. For $1,25(OH)_2D_3$, reference samples are not available, but the calibrants were tested with samples from the Vitamin D External Quality Assessment Scheme (DEQAS). The reproducibility of the measurements was calculated as the within-run precision from the duplicate measurements using the root-mean-square method [35]. The coefficients of variation (and their 95% confidence intervals) were 3.28% (2.92 to 3.76%) for $25(OH)D_3$, 4.73% (3.30 to 5.82%) for $24,25(OH)_2D_3$, and 8.96% (6.90 to 10.6%) for $1,25(OH)_2D_3$.

2.3. Statistical Analysis

MedCalc 20.027 (MedCalc Software, Ostend, Belgium) and GraphPad Prism 9.3.1 (GraphPad Software, La Jolla, CA, USA) were used as statistical programs as previously described [36]. One-way and two-way analyses of variance (ANOVAs) were performed. Repeated-measures analyses of variances (ANOVAs) were used for a single-factor study without a grouping variable or for a two-factor study with a specified grouping variable. Holm and Sidak's multiple-comparison test was applied to account for multiple testing. Pearson correlation analysis was used to determine the strength of the associations between vitamin D_3 metabolites. Two-sided p-values < 0.05 were considered statistically significant. The values in the figures are presented as the means ± 95% confidence intervals (95% CIs).

3. Results
3.1. Patient Characteristics and Study Design

The study included a total of 32 patients after radical prostatectomy characterized by at least one of three high-risk factors: a Gleason score of 8–10, node-positive disease, and PSA of ≥20 ng/mL at diagnosis. The individual data of all the patients are summarized in Table S1. Nineteen patients exhibited one high-risk factor (2 × positive nodes, 5 × PSA, and 12 × Gleason score), twelve patients had two factors (2 × PSA plus Gleason, 3 × PSA plus positive nodes, and 7 × Gleason plus positive nodes), and one patient had all three factors. The study started for 16 patients each in winter/spring and summer/autumn (Figure 1). In every patient, repeated measurements of vitamin D metabolites were performed in serum samples taken at four time points: before the study entry as baseline, after 3 and 9 months, and between 27 and 47 months when the study ended or bone metastasis was diagnosed. ZA was administered to 17 patients; 15 patients were controls and did not receive ZA treatment. Bone metastases were detected in 7 of the 17 ZA-treated patients during the study and in 5 of the 15 controls, indicating no significant differences between the two patient groups (Fisher's exact test, $p = 0.725$). This result corresponded with that of the ZEUS trial [34].

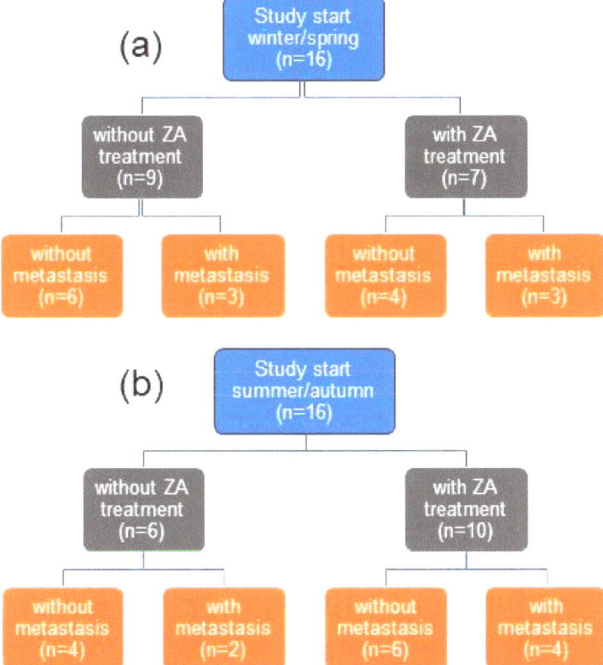

Figure 1. Overview of the study design and patient characteristics depending on the season of the study's start in winter/spring (**a**) and summer/autumn (**b**). Abbreviation: ZA = zoledronic acid.

The three vitamin metabolites $25(OH)D_3$, $24,25(OH)_2D_3$, and $1,25(OH)_2D_3$ were analyzed in detail. $25(OH)D_2$ and $1,25(OH)_2D_2$ were also measured, but in all 128 samples, the $25(OH)D_2$ concentrations were found to be under the lower limit of quantitation of 3.6 nmol/L, and $1,25(OH)_2D_2$ was not detectable. Thus, only the results for the three vitamin D_3 metabolites are reported here. The effects of the two abovementioned potential influencing factors "ZA treatment (yes/no)" and "bone metastasis during the study (yes/no)" as well as the seasonal dependency of the vitamin D_3 status were evaluated.

3.2. Vitamin D_3 Metabolites in the Total Study Cohort and Dependency on the Season of the Start of the Study

Figure 2a,c,e provide an overview of the concentration changes for the three metabolites in the total study cohort of the 32 patients during the study at four measuring points. Statistically significantly increased levels of $25(OH)D_3$ and $24,25(OH)_2D_3$ were observed within three months after the study's start, with approximately constant values at the two subsequent measuring points. In contrast, the $1,25(OH)_2D_3$ concentrations remained statistically unchanged over the entire study period.

As the seasonal dependency of the vitamin D_3 status, with lower concentrations in winter and spring in comparison to summer and autumn, is also well known for PCa patients [22,37,38], we subdivided the patients into two groups with respect to the season of their study entry (Figure 2b,d,f). Lower levels of $25(OH)D_3$ and $24,25(OH)_2D_3$ were detected in the patients who started their study in winter/spring in comparison to the patients with a study start in summer/autumn. While the patients with a study start in winter/spring showed distinctly increased concentrations of the two metabolites after three months of treatment, only moderately increased levels were found in the patients with summer/autumn study entry (Figure 2b,d). For $1,25(OH)_2D_3$, a subdivision of the patients did not have any effect on the influence of its concentration behavior over the entire study period (Figure 2f).

When evaluating the data, it must be taken into account that all the patients received vitamin D_3 supplementation. Thus, the data presented here demonstrate that, even after the first treatment interval of 3 months, an equalization of the $25(OH)D_3$ and $24,25(OH)_2D_3$ levels for the entire patient cohort over the study period was achieved, regardless of the season of the start of the study. Out of the 32 patients before the study entry, 17 (53%) patients had $25(OH)D_3$ concentrations below 50 nmol/L, which is the recommended threshold indicator of vitamin D deficiency in humans [3,8]. Fourteen of the sixteen patients who began the study in winter/spring had values below this threshold. After the first treatment interval of 3 months, only three (9.4%) patients of the total study group remained with values below that limit (Fisher's exact test, $p = 0.0003$).

3.3. Vitamin D_3 Metabolites in Relation to the ZA Treatment

The repeated measurements in ZA-treated and ZA-untreated patients resulted in different curves for the respective individual vitamin D_3 metabolite during the study (Figure 3). The $25(OH)D_3$ and $24,25(OH)_2D_3$ levels were significantly lower at study entry in comparison with the levels at the three subsequent study time points, but not significantly different between ZA-treated and ZA-untreated patients at all the time points (Figure 3a,b). Thus, repeated-measures ANOVA for these two-factor studies showed ZA treatment to be a non-significant source of variation (p-values of 0.219 and 0.240; Figure 3a,b) and the time interval to be a significant source of variation (p-values of 0.0001 and 0.0007; Figure 3a,b). In contrast, the $1,25(OH)_2D_3$ levels did not statistically differ between the ZA-treated and ZA-untreated patients at any of the measuring points (Figure 3c). These data prove that ZA treatment did not alter the levels of the three metabolites during the study. It can be concluded that the differences in the levels of $25(OH)D_3$ and $24,25(OH)_2D_3$ observed between the study's start and the subsequent measuring points were due to the concomitant supplementation of vitamin D_3 to all the study patients.

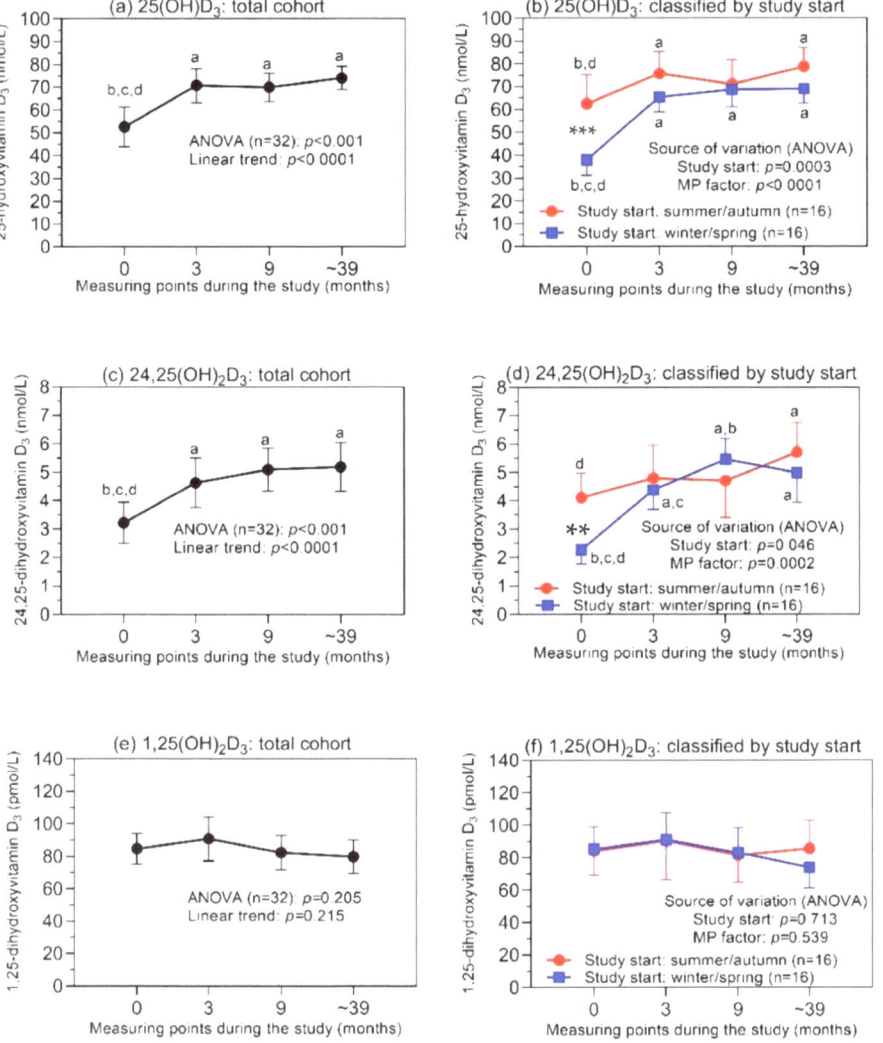

Figure 2. Levels of (**a**,**b**) 25(OH)D$_3$, (**c**,**d**) 24,25(OH)$_2$D$_3$, and (**e**,**f**) 1,25(OH)$_2$D$_3$ at different time intervals of the study in the total cohort, and dependence on the season of the start of the study. Subfigures (**a**,**c**,**e**) present the results of the repeated-measures ANOVA for a single factor study after treatment in the total cohort (n = 32). The corresponding subfigures (**b**,**d**,**f**) show the results of the two-factor study with repeated-measures ANOVA on the factor "study start" (winter/spring, n = 16, and summer/autumn, n = 16). Repeated measures were performed before the treatment (time point = 0) and 3 and 9 months after the treatment start. The last time point was 39 months (mean value) after the treatment start. Data at the time points are mean values with their 95% confidence intervals. At the error bars, the letters a, b, c, and d indicate statistically significant differences in the vitamin D$_3$ levels between the different measuring points (at least p < 0.05; corrected values according to Holm–Sidak test): a, compared to "before study"; b, compared to 3 months; c, compared to 9 months; d, compared to ~39 months. Statistically significant differences between the metabolite levels of the two study subgroups at the respective time points are characterized by asterisks: **, p < 0.01; ***, p < 0.001. Abbreviations: ANOVA = analysis of variance; MP factor = related to the time intervals of the measuring points.

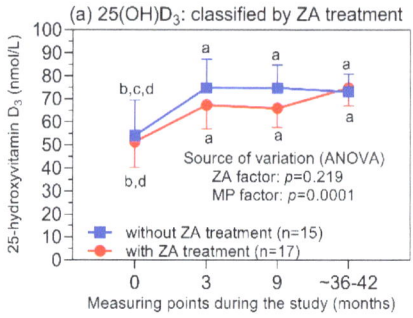
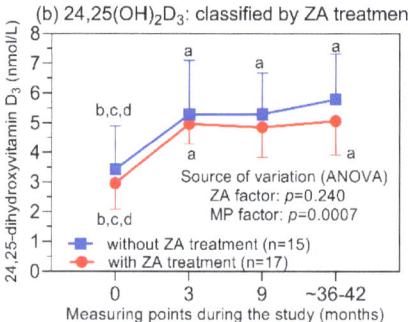
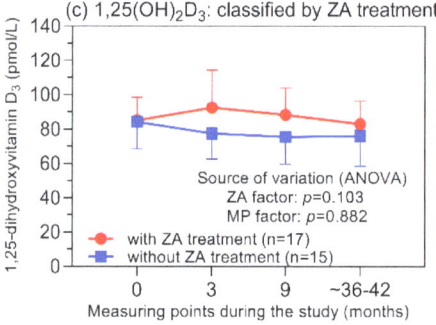

Figure 3. Levels of (**a**) 25(OH)D$_3$, (**b**) 24,25(OH)$_2$D$_3$, and (**c**) 1,25(OH)$_2$D$_3$ before and during the ZA treatment at different time intervals of the study. Repeated measures were performed before the treatment (time point = 0) and 3 and 9 months after the treatment start. The last measuring points were 36 and 42 months (mean values) for patients without and with ZA treatment, respectively. Results of the repeated-measures two-factor ANOVA classified according to the factor ZA treatment (without ZA, $n = 15$; with ZA, $n = 17$) are shown as mean values with their 95% confidence intervals. At the error bars, the letters a, b, c, and d indicate statistically significant differences in the vitamin D$_3$ levels between the different measuring points (at least $p < 0.05$; corrected values according to Holm–Sidak test): a, compared to "before study"; b, compared to 3 months; c, compared to 9 months; d, compared to ~36–42 months. No statistically significant differences for all three metabolite levels were found between the two ZA groups at the respective measuring points. Abbreviations: ANOVA = analysis of variance; ZA = zoledronic acid; MP factor = related to the time intervals of the measuring points.

3.4. Vitamin D$_3$ Metabolites in Relation to the Development of Bone Metastasis during the Study

The analysis of the concentrations of 25(OH)D$_3$ and 24,25(OH)$_2$D$_3$ regarding metastasis showed that they corresponded with those observed under the aspect of the ZA treatment (Figure 4). Neither metabolite was associated with the development of bone metastases in patients during the study, as the factor "metastasis" was not a significant variable of the source of variation (Figure 4a,b). The time-dependent changes can also be attributed to the concomitant vitamin D_3 supplementation. This is in contrast to the very striking $1,25(OH)_2D_3$ profile of the patients who did or did not suffer from bone metastasis during the study (Figure 4c). The patients who developed bone metastasis already had higher $1,25(OH)_2D_3$ values before the study's start compared to those without bone metastasis. This pattern remained throughout the study period. This observation suggests that $1,25(OH)_2D_3$ could be a possible factor associated with the metastatic process in PCa. Since our study was by no means designed to make prognostic statements, we have only compiled these indicative data in the supplement for interested readers (Figure S1).

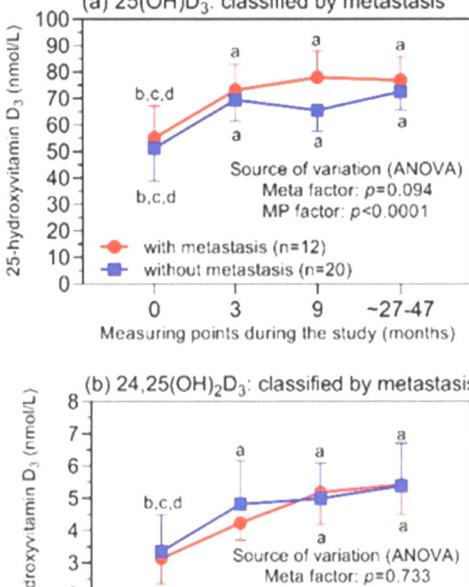

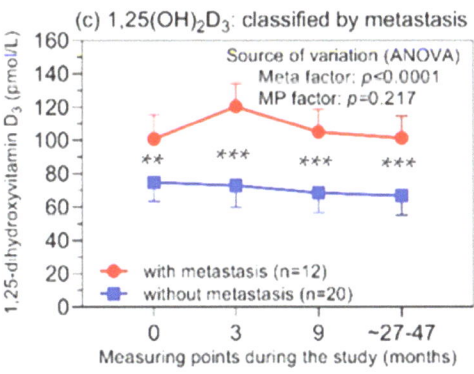

Figure 4. Levels of (**a**) $25(OH)D_3$, (**b**) $24,25(OH)_2D_3$, and (**c**) $1,25(OH)_2D_3$ in patients with and

without developed bone metastases during the study. Repeated measures were performed before the treatment (time point = 0) and 3 and 9 months after the treatment start. The last measuring points were 27 and 42 months (mean values) for the patients with ($n = 12$) and without ($n = 20$) bone metastasis, respectively. Results of the repeated-measures two-factor ANOVA classified according to the factor metastasis are shown as mean values with their 95% confidence intervals. At the error bars, the letters a, b, c, and d indicate statistically significant differences in the vitamin D_3 levels between the different measuring points (at least $p < 0.05$; corrected values according to Holm–Sidak test): a, compared to "before study"; b, compared to 3 months; c, compared to 9 months; d, compared to ~27–42 months. Statistically significant differences between the metabolite levels for the two study subgroups at the respective time points are characterized by asterisks: **, $p < 0.01$; *** $p < 0.001$. Abbreviations: ANOVA = analysis of variance; Meta factor = related to the developed bone metastasis; MP factor = related to the time intervals of the measuring points.

3.5. Correlations between Vitamin D_3 Metabolites

Strong correlations between the $25(OH)D_3$ and $24,25(OH)_2D_3$ levels were observed at the four measuring points, with correlation coefficients between 0.696 and 0.883 (mean ± SD; 0.776 ± 0.087) and p-values of <0.0001 in all cases. In this respect, the so-called vitamin D metabolite ratio (VMR), calculated as the ratio of $24,25(OH)_2D_3/25(OH)D_3 \times 100$, is of interest, as this ratio was suggested as an improved indicator of the vitamin D_3 status [39]. The close correlation between the two metabolites explains that a similar pattern was observed as for the two individual metabolites (Figure 5).

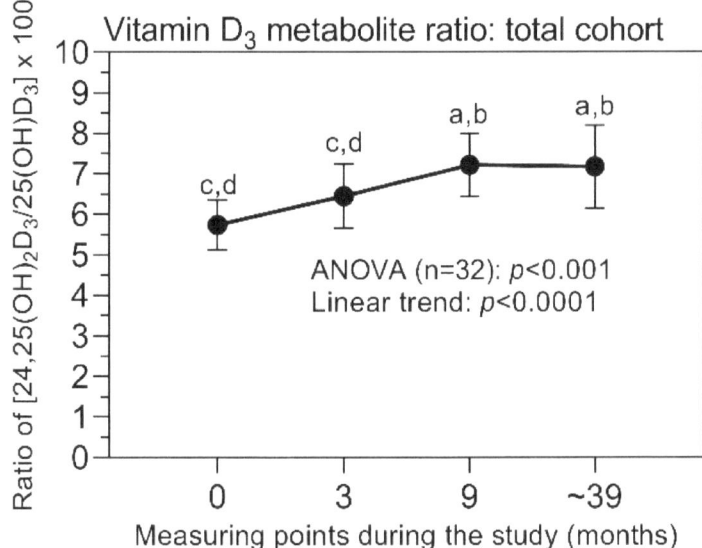

Figure 5. Change in the vitamin D_3 metabolite ratio (VMR) in the total cohort during the study. The ratio [$24,25(OH)_2D_3$ to $25(OH)D_3 \times 100$] defined as vitamin D_3 metabolite ratio increased during the study. Data at the time points are mean values with their 95% confidence intervals. At the error bars, the letters a, b, c, and d indicate statistically significant differences between the levels at the different measuring points (at least $p < 0.05$; corrected values according to Holm–Sidak test): a, compared to "before study"; b, compared to 3 months; c, compared to 9 months; d, compared to ~39 months. Further explanations are provided in the legend of Figure 2.

In contrast to the strong association between $25(OH)D_3$ and $24;25(OH)_2D_3$, the coefficients of the correlation between $25(OH)D_3$ and $1,25(OH)_2D_3$ as well as between $24,25(OH)_2D_3$ and $1,25(OH)_2D_3$ at the four measuring points were all non-significant, with values between -0.122 and 0.145 (-0.004 ± 0.148; p-values of 0.266 to 0.915) and -0.175 and 0.051 (-0.044 ± 0.174; p-values of 0.337 to 0.916), respectively.

4. Discussion

Our study showed that the main vitamin D metabolites $25(OH)D_3$, $24,25(OH)_2D_3$, and $1,25(OH)_2D_3$ were not affected in high-risk PCa patients who received ZA as supportive-care treatment over about 4 years. The ZA-treated patients and controls without ZA, who had $25(OH)D_3$ concentrations below the deficiency threshold of 50 nmol/L [1,40] due to a study start in winter/spring, achieved stable levels above this limit after 3 months with a daily concomitant supplementation of 400–500 IU of vitamin D cholecalciferol. These data additionally indicate good patient compliance with the supplement administration in contrast to other reports [41]. Simultaneously, stable $24,25(OH)_2D_3$ levels were also observed afterwards during the three subsequent time intervals. The occurrence of bone metastases also did not result in altered profiles for these two metabolites. The metabolite $1,25(OH)_2D_3$ also did not show profile changes during the entire observation time, but it was completely unaffected by the cholecalciferol supplementation, in contrast to $25(OH)D_3$ and $24,25(OH)_2D_3$. In addition, it was remarkable that patients with metastasis already had higher concentrations of $1,25(OH)_2D_3$ in comparison to those patients without metastasis at the study's beginning and during the entire study.

Thus, the results partly differed for $25(OH)D_3$ and $24,25(OH)_2D_3$, on the one hand, and for $1,25(OH)_2D_3$, on the other hand. Therefore, it is advisable to discuss the data for the metabolites separately.

It is currently generally accepted that the circulating $25(OH)D_3$ is the best indicator characterizing the vitamin D status [1]. However, a final consensus about the definition of vitamin D deficiency based on a cutoff level of $25(OH)D_3$ was not reached in the last International Conferences on Controversies in Vitamin D [1–3,8]. The Endocrine Task Force on Vitamin D defined a $25(OH)D_3$ level of 50 nmol/L as a deficiency cutoff [42]. This cutoff was also recommended by the Institute of Medicine, USA [40]. A higher threshold of 75 nmol/L was suggested by other expert groups [8]. This absence of consensus results mainly from the lack of traceability and harmonization/standardization of the various $25(OH)D_3$ assays that were applied in the different studies [3,43,44]. Our study revealed that, after treatment with vitamin D cholecalciferol, the high percentage of patients with deficient levels of $25(OH)D_3$ below 50 nmol/L at the start of the study could be reduced from 53 to 9.4%. In guidelines and comments, a daily supplement dosage of 10 to 50 µg (400–2000 IU) of vitamin D has been recommended to achieve at least this threshold of 50 nmol/L [8,40,45–49]. As the half-life of circulating $25(OH)D_3$ is estimated to be approximately 15 days [50], this daily supplementation results in a steady state of $25(OH)D_3$ after three to four months [48,51]. The increase in circulating $25(OH)D_3$ depends on the baseline level and the dose of the supplemented vitamin D. For an initial level of 25 nmol/L, an increase to more than 60 nmol/L was reported with a daily supplement of 400 IU for three months [52]. This corresponds with the observation in our study (Figure 2b). A similar pattern was visible for the metabolite $24,25(OH)_2D_3$. The first and second hydroxylation steps converting $25(OH)D_3$ to $24,25(OH)_2D_3$ and $1,25(OH)_2D_3$, respectively, are likely to be inversely regulated by the same effectors (parathormone, $1,25(OH)_2D_3$, and fibroblast growth factor 23/klotho) [53–55], but there remains a close relationship between the two metabolites $25(OH)D_3$ and $24,25(OH)_2D_3$ in the bloodstream. This is reflected in the strong Pearson correlation coefficients of 0.776 during the entire study period. The VMR, calculated as the ratio between $24,25(OH)_2D_3$ and $25(OH)D_3$, also confirms the increased levels of both metabolites after three months of the study compared with the baseline values at the study's beginning (Figure 5). VMR has been proposed as a more sensitive indicator for monitoring vitamin D intake [56–58], but some recent studies failed to confirm this advantage over the assessment based on $25(OH)D_3$ only [39,59,60].

Several studies in osteoporosis patients treated with ZA or other bisphosphonates have shown that there is a close relationship between the observed increased bone-mineral density and the circulating 25(OH) vitamin D concentration [33,61–64]. To achieve this treatment effect, different threshold levels of 25(OH) vitamin D have been reported. This is certainly because the assays used in various studies did not show clear traceability [3,33]. However, despite these conflicting data, studies concerning the usefulness of ZA in PCa patients have generally been performed with a concomitant supply of vitamin D both in the trial and placebo arms [27,34]. Follow-up data for vitamin D metabolites, however, are lacking. The less-satisfactory evidence for vitamin D in combination with bisphosphonates has been summarized in a meta-analysis [65]. Out of 27 randomized studies [65], the authors of one of only three studies with ZA monotherapy without the administration of vitamin D advised the prophylactic administration of vitamin D and the monitoring of the vitamin D levels for these patients [23]. In this respect, our follow-up data for the vitamin D metabolites support this recommendation. The data show that, with daily medication with 100 to 125 µg of cholecalciferol, a long-term level of $25(OH)D_3$ of >50 nmol/L can be achieved. In recent PCa guidelines, ZA has been recommended as a bone-protective agent and for pain relief in castration-resistant PCa patients and those with bone metastases [29,30]. Thus, ZA continues to be an important component of PCa management, even though the primary expectations of preventing bone metastases were not met [30,34].

For $1,25(OH)_2D_3$, the reference range (95% confidence interval) in the serum/plasma of healthy adults (between 20 and 70 years) has been determined to be 59 to 159 pmol/L [66]. The circulating $1,25(OH)_2D_3$ accounts for only approximately 0.1% of $25(OH)D_3$. A comparable proportion of the two metabolites was detected in prostate tissue, and their concentrations were correlated with serum levels [67,68]. The baseline concentrations of $1,25(OH)_2D_3$ in our PCa cohort were within this reference range, except for three patients with lower values. Moreover, the repeated measures in our study showed that the concentrations did not significantly change over the entire period. There were no increased $1,25(OH)_2D_3$ values due to the supplementation of cholecalciferol, in contrast to $25(OH)D_3$ and $24,25(OH)_2D_3$, particularly during the first treatment interval (Figure 2e,f) and for the subclassification with/without metastasis (Figure 4c). The circulating $1,25(OH)_2D_3$ is strictly controlled by a multiregulatory feedback system consisting of parathormone, fibroblast growth factor, calcium, phosphate, and $1,25(OH)_2D_3$ itself [69]. In consequence, normal circulating levels of $1,25(OH)_2D_3$ are largely ensured by the adequate synthesis of $1,25(OH)_2D_3$ from its precursor $25(OH)D_3$, even at moderately decreased concentrations of $25(OH)D_3$ [66,70]. This was also evident in our study and, likewise, explains the missing correlations between $1,25(OH)_2D_3$ and $25(OH)D_3$ or $24,25(OH)_2D_3$. Other studies with and without additional vitamin D intake also reported missing correlations or low coefficients for the correlation between $1,25(OH)_2D_3$ and $25(OH)D_3$ [38,70–75]. The peculiarity of sufficiently functioning $1,25(OH)_2D_3$ synthesis despite a limited $25(OH)D_3$ substrate supply as long as a severe vitamin deficiency is not present also makes it understandable that $1,25(OH)_2D_3$ is not considered a valid marker for global vitamin D deficiency [70,76].

However, our finding of higher $1,25(OH)_2D_3$ levels in patients with subsequent metastasis during the study compared with distinctly lower levels in patients without progression was apparently surprising. However, it should be pointed out that the higher values in the metastasized PCa group were always in the reference range of circulating $1,25(OH)_2D_3$ [66]. Significantly, the elevated baseline values were confirmed during the study. This is in contrast to other PCa and cancer studies in which increased levels of circulating $1,25(OH)_2D_3$ were associated with improved outcome data [20,67,77,78]. Numerous preclinical studies based on cell-culture experiments and animal studies showed that $1,25(OH)_2D_3$ inhibits the proliferation, migration, and invasion of cancer cells; suppresses angiogenesis; activates the apoptosis and differentiation of cells; or synergistically potentiates the antitumor activity of chemotherapeutic agents [5,79–86]. Since $1,25(OH)_2D_3$ is the actual active vitamin D metabolite, these experimental data are also used as arguments to confirm the hypothesis of an anticancer effect of vitamin D [5,87]. However, it is noticeable that the $1,25(OH)_2D_3$ concentrations used in the experiments are often 100–1000-fold higher than those detected in the bloodstream and target tissues [67,88–90]. This obvious contradiction has largely been ignored in the literature to date [91]. Furthermore, other experiments with a transgenic prostate mouse model showed enhanced distant metastasis upon prolonged treatment with $1,25(OH)_2D_3$ [92]. Increased metastasis in treatment experiments with $1,25(OH)_2D_3$ was also observed in a model of mammary-gland cancer in mice depending on the age of the mice [93,94].

We interpret the higher $1,25(OH)_2D_3$ in the subgroup of PCa patients with metastasis after prostatectomy as a possible reflection of the interrelated complex action of this vitamin metabolite. $1,25(OH)_2D_3$ not only directly influences tumor development via the vitamin D receptor as mentioned above but also indirectly modulates this process through crosstalk with the tumor microenvironment, different immunological pathways, and the functional interplay between the vitamin D and androgen receptors [6,7,9,95]. It is also conceivable that the higher serum levels of $1,25(OH)_2D_3$ in the case of the subsequently metastasized PCa subcohort led, through the C23 and C24 metabolic pathways for $1,25(OH)_2D_3$, to higher levels of their intermediates in cells [96]. These intermediates, for which very little is yet known [69], could favor direct or indirect cancerogenesis-promoting effects. Obviously, studies on their possible molecular mechanisms require experiments with biologically relevant concentrations, as already critically discussed above. On the other hand, this association between higher $1,25(OH)_2D_3$ levels and subsequent metastasis does not necessarily imply a causal relationship between the two observations. Due to the lack of corresponding follow-up data for the vitamin D metabolites in other studies, these particular results have likely not been captured to date. However, we think it is important to point out these findings so that they can be verified in other studies and provide potential prognostic decision support.

Some limitations of our study should be mentioned while interpreting the results. First, it was a retrospective study with a limited sample size of patients and without external validation. Second, only the three essential vitamin D metabolites could be measured due to the limited availability of the sample material. Third, all the patients in both the study and control arms received vitamin D and calcium. Despite these limitations, we consider the results of this study to provide interesting information for understanding open questions in the ongoing vitamin D debate in practice. The strength of our study is based on the use of sophisticated analytical methods with traceability and good analytical performance as well as the strict adherence to the requirements for valid vitamin D studies.

5. Conclusions

The two vitamin D metabolites $25(OH)D_3$ and $24,25(OH)_2D_3$ were not affected by supportive ZA treatment or the development of metastasis over four years in our selected cohort of high-risk PCa patients after prostatectomy. Surprisingly, the low-abundance metabolite $1,25(OH)_2D_3$ was already higher before the study's start in patients who developed bone metastasis compared to those without bone metastasis. Before potential prognostic decision support can be provided, verification in other studies is necessary.

Supplementary Materials: The following supporting information can be downloaded at: https://www.mdpi.com/article/10.3390/cancers14061560/s1. Figure S1: $1,25(OH)_2D_3$ level as prognostic indicator of subsequent bone metastasis after radical prostatectomy, Table S1: Clinicopathological risk factors of the study patients with and without zoledronic acid treatment and subsequent metastasis.

Author Contributions: Conceptualization, C.S., B.R., K.J. and M.L.; data curation, F.B., K.J. and M.D.; formal analysis, C.S., F.B. and K.J.; investigation, C.S., B.R. and K.J.; methodology, F.B., K.J. and M.D.; project administration, C.S., K.J. and M.L.; resources, F.B., B.R. and M.D.; software, F.B. and M.D.; supervision, C.S., K.J. and M.L.; validation, C.S., F.B., K.J. and M.D.; visualization, C.S. and K.J.; writing—original draft preparation, C.S., B.R., F.B. and K.J.; writing—review and editing, C.S., B.R., F.B., K.J., M.D. and M.L. All authors have read and agreed to the published version of the manuscript.

Funding: This research received no external funding.

Institutional Review Board Statement: The present study was part of the registered and approved trial "Effectiveness of Zometa® treatment for the prevention of bone metastases in high risk prostate cancer patients: a randomized, open-label, multicenter study of the European Association of Urology in Cooperation with the Scandinavian Prostate Cancer Group and the Arbeitsgemeinschaft Urologische Onkologie (ISRCTN66626762 https://doi.org/10.1186/ISRCTN66626762)". This substudy focused on secondary outcome measures of bone health, as indicated in the trial protocol. The study was conducted in accordance with the Declaration of Helsinki and received ethics approval from the local medical ethics committees of the participating study centers, as indicated in [34].

Informed Consent Statement: Informed consent was obtained from all the subjects involved in the study.

Data Availability Statement: The data presented in this study are available upon reasonable request from the corresponding author.

Acknowledgments: The authors thank Christien Caris and Wim Witjes for their helpful assistance with the patient data management.

Conflicts of Interest: F.B. and M.D. are employees of Immundiagnostik AG, Bensheim, Germany. All the authors declare that they have no conflicts of interest and no direct or indirect commercial incentives associated with publishing the manuscript.

References

1. Giustina, A.; Bouillon, R.; Binkley, N.; Sempos, C.; Adler, R.A.; Bollerslev, J.; Dawson-Hughes, B.; Ebeling, P.R.; Feldman, D.; Heijboer, A.; et al. Controversies in vitamin D: A statement from the Third International Conference. *JBMR Plus* **2020**, *4*, e10417. [CrossRef] [PubMed]
2. Giustina, A.; Adler, R.A.; Binkley, N.; Bouillon, R.; Ebeling, P.R.; Lazaretti-Castro, M.; Marcocci, C.; Rizzoli, R.; Sempos, C.T.; Bilezikian, J.P. Controversies in vitamin D: Summary Statement from an International Conference. *J. Clin. Endocrinol. Metab.* **2019**, *104*, 234–240. [CrossRef] [PubMed]
3. Giustina, A.; Adler, R.A.; Binkley, N.; Bollerslev, J.; Bouillon, R.; Dawson-Hughes, B.; Ebeling, P.R.; Feldman, D.; Formenti, A.M.; Lazaretti-Castro, M.; et al. Consensus statement from 2(nd) International Conference on Controversies in Vitamin D. *Rev. Endocr. Metab. Disord.* **2020**, *21*, 89–116. [CrossRef]
4. Bouillon, R.; Marcocci, C.; Carmeliet, G.; Bikle, D.; White, J.H.; Dawson-Hughes, B.; Lips, P.; Munns, C.F.; Lazaretti-Castro, M.; Giustina, A.; et al. Skeletal and extraskeletal actions of vitamin D: Current evidence and outstanding questions. *Endocr. Rev.* **2019**, *40*, 1109–1151. [CrossRef]
5. Ma, Y.; Johnson, C.S.; Trump, D.L. Mechanistic insights of vitamin D anticancer effects. *Vitam. Horm.* **2016**, *100*, 395–431. [CrossRef]
6. Bilani, N.; Elson, L.; Szuchan, C.; Elimimian, E.; Saleh, M.; Nahleh, Z. Newly-identified pathways relating vitamin D to carcinogenesis: A Review. *In Vivo* **2021**, *35*, 1345–1354. [CrossRef]
7. Jeon, S.M.; Shin, E.A. Exploring vitamin D metabolism and function in cancer. *Exp. Mol. Med.* **2018**, *50*, 1–14. [CrossRef]
8. Amrein, K.; Scherkl, M.; Hoffmann, M.; Neuwersch-Sommeregger, S.; Kostenberger, M.; Tmava Berisha, A.; Martucci, G.; Pilz, S.; Malle, O. Vitamin D deficiency 2.0: An update on the current status worldwide. *Eur. J. Clin. Nutr.* **2020**, *74*, 1498–1513. [CrossRef]
9. Ahn, J.; Park, S.; Zuniga, B.; Bera, A.; Song, C.S.; Chatterjee, B. Vitamin D in prostate cancer. *Vitam. Horm.* **2016**, *100*, 321–355. [CrossRef] [PubMed]
10. Trump, D.L.; Aragon-Ching, J.B. Vitamin D in prostate cancer. *Asian J. Androl.* **2018**, *20*, 244–252. [CrossRef] [PubMed]
11. Capiod, T.; Barry Delongchamps, N.; Pigat, N.; Souberbielle, J.C.; Goffin, V. Do dietary calcium and vitamin D matter in men with prostate cancer? *Nat. Rev. Urol.* **2018**, *15*, 453–461. [CrossRef]
12. Xu, Y.; Shao, X.; Yao, Y.; Xu, L.; Chang, L.; Jiang, Z.; Lin, Z. Positive association between circulating 25-hydroxyvitamin D levels and prostate cancer risk: New findings from an updated meta-analysis. *J. Cancer Res. Clin. Oncol.* **2014**, *140*, 1465–1477. [CrossRef] [PubMed]
13. Shui, I.M.; Mucci, L.A.; Kraft, P.; Tamimi, R.M.; Lindstrom, S.; Penney, K.L.; Nimptsch, K.; Hollis, B.W.; Dupre, N.; Platz, E.A.; et al. Vitamin D-related genetic variation, plasma vitamin D, and risk of lethal prostate cancer: A prospective nested case-control study. *J. Natl. Cancer Inst.* **2012**, *104*, 690–699. [CrossRef]
14. Fang, F.; Kasperzyk, J.L.; Shui, I.; Hendrickson, W.; Hollis, B.W.; Fall, K.; Ma, J.; Gaziano, J.M.; Stampfer, M.J.; Mucci, L.A.; et al. Prediagnostic plasma vitamin D metabolites and mortality among patients with prostate cancer. *PLoS ONE* **2011**, *6*, e18625. [CrossRef]
15. Brandstedt, J.; Almquist, M.; Manjer, J.; Malm, J. Vitamin D, PTH, and calcium in relation to survival following prostate cancer. *Cancer Causes Control* **2016**, *27*, 669–677. [CrossRef] [PubMed]
16. Song, Z.Y.; Yao, Q.; Zhuo, Z.; Ma, Z.; Chen, G. Circulating vitamin D level and mortality in prostate cancer patients: A dose-response meta-analysis. *Endocr. Connect.* **2018**, *7*, R294–R303. [CrossRef] [PubMed]
17. Shahvazi, S.; Soltani, S.; Ahmadi, S.M.; de Souza, R.J.; Salehi-Abargouei, A. The effect of vitamin D supplementation on prostate cancer: A systematic review and meta-Analysis of clinical trials. *Horm. Metab. Res.* **2019**, *51*, 11–21. [CrossRef] [PubMed]

18. Ordonez-Mena, J.M.; Schottker, B.; Fedirko, V.; Jenab, M.; Olsen, A.; Halkjaer, J.; Kampman, E.; de Groot, L.; Jansen, E.; Bueno-de-Mesquita, H.B.; et al. Pre-diagnostic vitamin D concentrations and cancer risks in older individuals: An analysis of cohorts participating in the CHANCES consortium. *Eur. J. Epidemiol.* **2016**, *31*, 311–323. [CrossRef]
19. Gilbert, R.; Metcalfe, C.; Fraser, W.D.; Donovan, J.; Hamdy, F.; Neal, D.E.; Lane, J.A.; Martin, R.M. Associations of circulating 25-hydroxyvitamin D with prostate cancer diagnosis, stage and grade. *Int. J. Cancer* **2012**, *131*, 1187–1196. [CrossRef]
20. Nair-Shalliker, V.; Bang, A.; Egger, S.; Clements, M.; Gardiner, R.A.; Kricker, A.; Seibel, M.J.; Chambers, S.K.; Kimlin, M.G.; Armstrong, B.K.; et al. Post-treatment levels of plasma 25- and 1,25-dihydroxy vitamin D and mortality in men with aggressive prostate cancer. *Sci. Rep.* **2020**, *10*, 7736. [CrossRef]
21. Stroomberg, H.V.; Vojdeman, F.J.; Madsen, C.M.; Helgstrand, J.T.; Schwarz, P.; Heegaard, A.M.; Olsen, A.; Tjonneland, A.; Struer Lind, B.; Brasso, K.; et al. Vitamin D levels and the risk of prostate cancer and prostate cancer mortality. *Acta Oncol.* **2021**, *60*, 316–322. [CrossRef] [PubMed]
22. Stephan, C.; Lein, M.; Matalon, J.; Kilic, E.; Zhao, Z.; Busch, J.; Jung, K. Serum vitamin D is not helpful for predicting prostate cancer aggressiveness compared with the Prostate Health Index. *J. Urol.* **2016**, *196*, 709–714. [CrossRef] [PubMed]
23. Denham, J.W.; Nowitz, M.; Joseph, D.; Duchesne, G.; Spry, N.A.; Lamb, D.S.; Matthews, J.; Turner, S.; Atkinson, C.; Tai, K.H.; et al. Impact of androgen suppression and zoledronic acid on bone mineral density and fractures in the Trans-Tasman Radiation Oncology Group (TROG) 03.04 Randomised Androgen Deprivation and Radiotherapy (RADAR) randomized controlled trial for locally advanced prostate cancer. *BJU Int.* **2014**, *114*, 344–353. [CrossRef] [PubMed]
24. Saad, F.; Gleason, D.M.; Murray, R.; Tchekmedyian, S.; Venner, P.; Lacombe, L.; Chin, J.L.; Vinholes, J.J.; Goas, J.A.; Chen, B.; et al. A randomized, placebo-controlled trial of zoledronic acid in patients with hormone-refractory metastatic prostate carcinoma. *J. Natl. Cancer Inst.* **2002**, *94*, 1458–1468. [CrossRef] [PubMed]
25. Lee, M.V.; Fong, E.M.; Singer, F.R.; Guenette, R.S. Bisphosphonate treatment inhibits the growth of prostate cancer cells. *Cancer Res.* **2001**, *61*, 2602–2608. [PubMed]
26. Wood, J.; Bonjean, K.; Ruetz, S.; Bellahcene, A.; Devy, L.; Foidart, J.M.; Castronovo, V.; Green, J.R. Novel antiangiogenic effects of the bisphosphonate compound zoledronic acid. *J. Pharmacol. Exp. Ther.* **2002**, *302*, 1055–1061. [CrossRef] [PubMed]
27. Ryan, C.W.; Huo, D.; Demers, L.M.; Beer, T.M.; Lacerna, L.V. Zoledronic acid initiated during the first year of androgen deprivation therapy increases bone mineral density in patients with prostate cancer. *J. Urol.* **2006**, *176*, 972–978. [CrossRef]
28. Lowrance, W.T.; Breau, R.H.; Chou, R.; Chapin, B.F.; Crispino, T.; Dreicer, R.; Jarrard, D.F.; Kibel, A.S.; Morgan, T.M.; Morgans, A.K.; et al. Advanced Prostate Cancer: AUA/ASTRO/SUO Guideline PART II. *J. Urol.* **2021**, *205*, 22–29. [CrossRef]
29. Mottet, N.; Cornford, P.; van den Bergh, R.C.N.; Briers, E.; De Santis, M.; Gillessen, S.; Grummet, J.; Henry, A.M.; van der Kwast, T.H.; Lam, T.B.; et al. EAU Guidelines. Edn. Presented at the EAU Annual Congress Milan. 2021. Available online: http://uroweb.org/guidelines/compilations-of-all-guidelines/ (accessed on 6 February 2022).
30. Prostate Cancer: Diagnosis and Management [A] Evidence Review for Bisphosphonates. NICE Guideline NG131, Published by National Institute for Health and Care Excellence, May 2019, Last Updated December 2021. Available online: http://www.nice.org.uk/guidance/ng131 (accessed on 6 February 2022).
31. Saylor, P.J.; Rumble, R.B.; Tagawa, S.; Eastham, J.A.; Finelli, A.; Reddy, P.S.; Kungel, T.M.; Nissenberg, M.G.; Michalski, J.M. Bone health and bone-targeted therapies for prostate cancer: ASCO Endorsement of a Cancer Care Ontario Guideline. *J. Clin. Oncol.* **2020**, *38*, 1736–1743. [CrossRef]
32. Bourke, S.; Bolland, M.J.; Grey, A.; Horne, A.M.; Wattie, D.J.; Wong, S.; Gamble, G.D.; Reid, I.R. The impact of dietary calcium intake and vitamin D status on the effects of zoledronate. *Osteoporos. Int.* **2013**, *24*, 349–354. [CrossRef]
33. Mosali, P.; Bernard, L.; Wajed, J.; Mohamed, Z.; Ewang, M.; Moore, A.; Fogelman, I.; Hampson, G. Vitamin D status and parathyroid hormone concentrations influence the skeletal response to zoledronate and denosumab. *Calcif. Tissue Int.* **2014**, *94*, 553–559. [CrossRef] [PubMed]
34. Wirth, M.; Tammela, T.; Cicalese, V.; Gomez Veiga, F.; Delaere, K.; Miller, K.; Tubaro, A.; Schulze, M.; Debruyne, F.; Huland, H.; et al. Prevention of bone metastases in patients with high-risk nonmetastatic prostate cancer treated with zoledronic acid: Efficacy and safety results of the Zometa European Study (ZEUS). *Eur. Urol.* **2015**, *67*, 482–491. [CrossRef] [PubMed]
35. Hyslop, N.P.; White, W.H. Estimating precision using duplicate measurements. *J. Air Waste Manag. Assoc.* **2009**, *59*, 1032–1039. [CrossRef]
36. Peters, R.; Stephan, C.; Jung, K.; Lein, M.; Friedersdorff, F.; Maxeiner, A. Comparison of PHI and PHI density for prostate cancer detection in a large retrospective Caucasian cohort. *Urol. Int.* **2021**, *in press.* [CrossRef]
37. Chesney, R.W.; Rosen, J.F.; Hamstra, A.J.; Smith, C.; Mahaffey, K.; DeLuca, H.F. Absence of seasonal variation in serum concentrations of 1,25-dihydroxyvitamin D despite a rise in 25-hydroxyvitamin D in summer. *J. Clin. Endocrinol. Metab.* **1981**, *53*, 139–142. [CrossRef]
38. Li, H.; Stampfer, M.J.; Hollis, J.B.; Mucci, L.A.; Gaziano, J.M.; Hunter, D.; Giovannucci, E.L.; Ma, J. A prospective study of plasma vitamin D metabolites, vitamin D receptor polymorphisms, and prostate cancer. *PLoS Med.* **2007**, *4*, e103. [CrossRef] [PubMed]
39. Aloia, J.; Fazzari, M.; Shieh, A.; Dhaliwal, R.; Mikhail, M.; Hoofnagle, A.N.; Ragolia, L. The vitamin D metabolite ratio (VMR) as a predictor of functional biomarkers of bone health. *Clin. Endocrinol.* **2017**, *86*, 674–679. [CrossRef] [PubMed]

40. Ross, A.C.; Manson, J.E.; Abrams, S.A.; Aloia, J.F.; Brannon, P.M.; Clinton, S.K.; Durazo-Arvizu, R.A.; Gallagher, J.C.; Gallo, R.L.; Jones, G.; et al. The 2011 report on dietary reference intakes for calcium and vitamin D from the Institute of Medicine: What clinicians need to know. *J. Clin. Endocrinol. Metab.* **2011**, *96*, 53–58. [CrossRef]
41. Link, H.; Diel, I.; Ohlmann, C.H.; Holtmann, L.; Kerkmann, M.; for the Associations Supportive Care in Oncology (AGSMO), Medical Oncology (AIO), Urological Oncology (AUO), within the German Cancer Society (DKG) and the German Osteooncological Society (DOG). Guideline adherence in bone-targeted treatment of cancer patients with bone metastases in Germany. *Support. Care Cancer* **2020**, *28*, 2175–2184. [CrossRef]
42. Holick, M.F.; Binkley, N.C.; Bischoff-Ferrari, H.A.; Gordon, C.M.; Hanley, D.A.; Heaney, R.P.; Murad, M.H.; Weaver, C.M.; Endocrine, S. Evaluation, treatment, and prevention of vitamin D deficiency: An Endocrine Society clinical practice guideline. *J. Clin. Endocrinol. Metab.* **2011**, *96*, 1911–1930. [CrossRef]
43. Sempos, C.T.; Heijboer, A.C.; Bikle, D.D.; Bollerslev, J.; Bouillon, R.; Brannon, P.M.; DeLuca, H.F.; Jones, G.; Munns, C.F.; Bilezikian, J.P.; et al. Vitamin D assays and the definition of hypovitaminosis D: Results from the First International Conference on Controversies in Vitamin D. *Br. J. Clin. Pharmacol.* **2018**, *84*, 2194–2207. [CrossRef] [PubMed]
44. Altieri, B.; Cavalier, E.; Bhattoa, H.P.; Perez-Lopez, F.R.; Lopez-Baena, M.T.; Perez-Roncero, G.R.; Chedraui, P.; Annweiler, C.; Della Casa, S.; Zelzer, S.; et al. Vitamin D testing: Advantages and limits of the current assays. *Eur. J. Clin. Nutr.* **2020**, *74*, 231–247. [CrossRef] [PubMed]
45. Bollerslev, J.; Rejnmark, L.; Marcocci, C.; Shoback, D.M.; Sitges-Serra, A.; van Biesen, W.; Dekkers, O.M.; European Society of, E. European Society of Endocrinology Clinical Guideline: Treatment of chronic hypoparathyroidism in adults. *Eur. J. Endocrinol.* **2015**, *173*, G1–G20. [CrossRef] [PubMed]
46. Hanley, D.A.; Cranney, A.; Jones, G.; Whiting, S.J.; Leslie, W.D.; Guidelines Committee of the Scientific Advisory Council of Osteoporosis Canada. Vitamin D in adult health and disease: A review and guideline statement from Osteoporosis Canada (summary). *CMAJ* **2010**, *182*, 1315–1319. [CrossRef]
47. Francis, R.M.; Aspray, T.J.; Bowring, C.E.; Fraser, W.D.; Gittoes, N.J.; Javaid, M.K.; Macdonald, H.M.; Patel, S.; Selby, P.L.; Tanna, N. National Osteoporosis Society practical clinical guideline on vitamin D and bone health. *Maturitas* **2015**, *80*, 119–121. [CrossRef]
48. EFSA Panel on Dietetic Products, Nutrition and Allergies (NDA). Dietary reference values for vitamin D. *EFSA J.* **2016**, *14*, 4547. [CrossRef]
49. Pilz, S.; Zittermann, A.; Trummer, C.; Theiler-Schwetz, V.; Lerchbaum, E.; Keppel, M.H.; Grubler, M.R.; Marz, W.; Pandis, M. Vitamin D testing and treatment: A narrative review of current evidence. *Endocr. Connect.* **2019**, *8*, R27–R43. [CrossRef]
50. Jones, G. Pharmacokinetics of vitamin D toxicity. *Am. J. Clin. Nutr.* **2008**, *88*, 582S–586S. [CrossRef]
51. Heaney, R.P.; Davies, K.M.; Chen, T.C.; Holick, M.F.; Barger-Lux, M.J. Human serum 25-hydroxycholecalciferol response to extended oral dosing with cholecalciferol. *Am. J. Clin. Nutr.* **2003**, *77*, 204–210. [CrossRef]
52. Lips, P.; Wiersinga, A.; van Ginkel, F.C.; Jongen, M.J.; Netelenbos, J.C.; Hackeng, W.H.; Delmas, P.D.; van der Vijgh, W.J. The effect of vitamin D supplementation on vitamin D status and parathyroid function in elderly subjects. *J. Clin. Endocrinol. Metab.* **1988**, *67*, 644–650. [CrossRef]
53. Petkovich, M.; Helvig, C.; Epps, T. CYP24A1 regulation in health and disease. In *Vitamin D*, 3rd ed.; Feldman, D., Pike, J.W., Adams, J.S., Eds.; Academic Press: New York, NY, USA, 2011; Volume 2, pp. 1525–1554.
54. Rubsamen, D.; Kunze, M.M.; Buderus, V.; Brauss, T.F.; Bajer, M.M.; Brune, B.; Schmid, T. Inflammatory conditions induce IRES-dependent translation of cyp24a1. *PLoS ONE* **2014**, *9*, e85314. [CrossRef]
55. De Paolis, E.; Scaglione, G.L.; De Bonis, M.; Minucci, A.; Capoluongo, E. CYP24A1 and SLC34A1 genetic defects associated with idiopathic infantile hypercalcemia: From genotype to phenotype. *Clin. Chem. Lab. Med.* **2019**, *57*, 1650–1667. [CrossRef] [PubMed]
56. Berg, A.H.; Powe, C.E.; Evans, M.K.; Wenger, J.; Ortiz, G.; Zonderman, A.B.; Suntharalingam, P.; Lucchesi, K.; Powe, N.R.; Karumanchi, S.A.; et al. 24,25-Dihydroxyvitamin d3 and vitamin D status of community-dwelling black and white Americans. *Clin. Chem.* **2015**, *61*, 877–884. [CrossRef] [PubMed]
57. Wagner, D.; Hanwell, H.E.; Schnabl, K.; Yazdanpanah, M.; Kimball, S.; Fu, L.; Sidhom, G.; Rousseau, D.; Cole, D.E.; Vieth, R. The ratio of serum 24,25-dihydroxyvitamin D_3 to 25-hydroxyvitamin D_3 is predictive of 25-hydroxyvitamin D_3 response to vitamin D_3 supplementation. *J. Steroid Biochem. Mol. Biol.* **2011**, *126*, 72–77. [CrossRef]
58. Cashman, K.D.; Hayes, A.; Galvin, K.; Merkel, J.; Jones, G.; Kaufmann, M.; Hoofnagle, A.N.; Carter, G.D.; Durazo-Arvizu, R.A.; Sempos, C.T. Significance of serum 24,25-dihydroxyvitamin D in the assessment of vitamin D status: A double-edged sword? *Clin. Chem.* **2015**, *61*, 636–645. [CrossRef]
59. Francic, V.; Ursem, S.R.; Dirks, N.F.; Keppel, M.H.; Theiler-Schwetz, V.; Trummer, C.; Pandis, M.; Borzan, V.; Grubler, M.R.; Verheyen, N.D.; et al. The effect of vitamin D supplementation on its metabolism and the vitamin D metabolite ratio. *Nutrients* **2019**, *11*, 2539. [CrossRef] [PubMed]
60. Kim, H.K.; Chung, H.J.; Le, H.G.; Na, B.K.; Cho, M.C. Serum 24,25-dihydroxyvitamin D level in general Korean population and its relationship with other vitamin D biomarkers. *PLoS ONE* **2021**, *16*, e0246541. [CrossRef]
61. Geller, J.L.; Hu, B.; Reed, S.; Mirocha, J.; Adams, J.S. Increase in bone mass after correction of vitamin D insufficiency in bisphosphonate-treated patients. *Endocr. Pract.* **2008**, *14*, 293–297. [CrossRef]
62. Carmel, A.S.; Shieh, A.; Bang, H.; Bockman, R.S. The 25(OH)D level needed to maintain a favorable bisphosphonate response is ≥ 3 ng/mL. *Osteoporos. Int.* **2012**, *23*, 2479–2487. [CrossRef]

63. Ishijima, M.; Sakamoto, Y.; Yamanaka, M.; Tokita, A.; Kitahara, K.; Kaneko, H.; Kurosawa, H. Minimum required vitamin D level for optimal increase in bone mineral density with alendronate treatment in osteoporotic women. *Calcif. Tissue Int.* **2009**, *85*, 398–404. [CrossRef]
64. Nakamura, Y.; Suzuki, T.; Kamimura, M.; Murakami, K.; Ikegami, S.; Uchiyama, S.; Kato, H. Vitamin D and calcium are required at the time of denosumab administration during osteoporosis treatment. *Bone Res.* **2017**, *5*, 17021. [CrossRef]
65. Alibhai, S.M.H.; Zukotynski, K.; Walker-Dilks, C.; Emmenegger, U.; Finelli, A.; Morgan, S.C.; Hotte, S.J.; Tomlinson, G.A.; Winquist, E. Bone health and bone-targeted therapies for nonmetastatic prostate cancer: A systematic review and meta-analysis. *Ann. Intern. Med.* **2017**, *167*, 341–350. [CrossRef] [PubMed]
66. Dirks, N.F.; Martens, F.; Vanderschueren, D.; Billen, J.; Pauwels, S.; Ackermans, M.T.; Endert, E.; Heijer, M.D.; Blankenstein, M.A.; Heijboer, A.C. Determination of human reference values for serum total 1,25-dihydroxyvitamin D using an extensively validated 2D ID-UPLC-MS/MS method. *J. Steroid Biochem. Mol. Biol.* **2016**, *164*, 127–133. [CrossRef]
67. Wagner, D.; Trudel, D.; Van der Kwast, T.; Nonn, L.; Giangreco, A.A.; Li, D.; Dias, A.; Cardoza, M.; Laszlo, S.; Hersey, K.; et al. Randomized clinical trial of vitamin D_3 doses on prostatic vitamin D metabolite levels and Ki67 labeling in prostate cancer patients. *J. Clin. Endocrinol. Metab.* **2013**, *98*, 1498–1507. [CrossRef] [PubMed]
68. Richards, Z.; Batai, K.; Farhat, R.; Shah, E.; Makowski, A.; Gann, P.H.; Kittles, R.; Nonn, L. Prostatic compensation of the vitamin D axis in African American men. *JCI Insight* **2017**, *2*, e91054. [CrossRef] [PubMed]
69. Tuckey, R.C.; Cheng, C.Y.S.; Slominski, A.T. The serum vitamin D metabolome: What we know and what is still to discover. *J. Steroid Biochem. Mol. Biol.* **2019**, *186*, 4–21. [CrossRef]
70. Lips, P. Relative value of 25(OH)D and 1,25(OH)2D measurements. *J. Bone Miner. Res.* **2007**, *22*, 1668–1671. [CrossRef] [PubMed]
71. Porojnicu, A.; Robsahm, T.E.; Berg, J.P.; Moan, J. Season of diagnosis is a predictor of cancer survival. Sun-induced vitamin D may be involved: A possible role of sun-induced Vitamin D. *J. Steroid Biochem. Mol. Biol.* **2007**, *103*, 675–678. [CrossRef]
72. Bouillon, R.A.; Auwerx, J.H.; Lissens, W.D.; Pelemans, W.K. Vitamin D status in the elderly: Seasonal substrate deficiency causes 1,25-dihydroxycholecalciferol deficiency. *Am. J. Clin. Nutr.* **1987**, *45*, 755–763. [CrossRef]
73. Hsu, S.; Prince, D.K.; Williams, K.; Allen, N.B.; Burke, G.L.; Hoofnagle, A.N.; Li, X.; Liu, K.J.; McClelland, R.L.; Michos, E.D.; et al. Clinical and biomarker modifiers of vitamin D treatment response: The multi-ethnic study of atherosclerosis. *Am. J. Clin. Nutr.* **2021**, *115*, 914–924. [CrossRef]
74. Shah, I.; Petroczi, A.; Naughton, D.P. Exploring the role of vitamin D in type 1 diabetes, rheumatoid arthritis, and Alzheimer disease: New insights from accurate analysis of 10 forms. *J. Clin. Endocrinol. Metab.* **2014**, *99*, 808–816. [CrossRef] [PubMed]
75. Tang, J.C.Y.; Jackson, S.; Walsh, N.P.; Greeves, J.; Fraser, W.D.; Bioanalytical Facility Team. The dynamic relationships between the active and catabolic vitamin D metabolites, their ratios, and associations with PTH. *Sci. Rep.* **2019**, *9*, 6974. [CrossRef] [PubMed]
76. Dirks, N.F.; Ackermans, M.T.; Lips, P.; de Jongh, R.T.; Vervloet, M.G.; de Jonge, R.; Heijboer, A.C. The when, what & how of measuring vitamin D metabolism in clinical medicine. *Nutrients* **2018**, *10*, 482. [CrossRef]
77. Corder, E.H.; Guess, H.A.; Hulka, B.S.; Friedman, G.D.; Sadler, M.; Vollmer, R.T.; Lobaugh, B.; Drezner, M.K.; Vogelman, J.H.; Orentreich, N. Vitamin D and prostate cancer: A prediagnostic study with stored sera. *Cancer Epidemiol. Biomark. Prev.* **1993**, *2*, 467–472. [PubMed]
78. Rosenberg, A.; Nettey, O.S.; Gogana, P.; Sheikh, U.; Macias, V.; Kajdacsy-Balla, A.; Sharifi, R.; Kittles, R.A.; Murphy, A.B. Physiologic serum 1,25 dihydroxyvitamin D is inversely associated with prostatic Ki67 staining in a diverse sample of radical prostatectomy patients. *Cancer Causes Control* **2019**, *30*, 207–214. [CrossRef] [PubMed]
79. Moreno, J.; Krishnan, A.V.; Feldman, D. Molecular mechanisms mediating the anti-proliferative effects of vitamin D in prostate cancer. *J. Steroid Biochem. Mol. Biol.* **2005**, *97*, 31–36. [CrossRef]
80. Sung, V.; Feldman, D. 1,25-Dihydroxyvitamin D_3 decreases human prostate cancer cell adhesion and migration. *Mol. Cell. Endocrinol.* **2000**, *164*, 133–143. [CrossRef]
81. Luo, W.; Yu, W.D.; Ma, Y.; Chernov, M.; Trump, D.L.; Johnson, C.S. Inhibition of protein kinase CK2 reduces Cyp24a1 expression and enhances 1,25-dihydroxyvitamin D_3 antitumor activity in human prostate cancer cells. *Cancer Res.* **2013**, *73*, 2289–2297. [CrossRef]
82. Swami, S.; Krishnan, A.V.; Wang, J.Y.; Jensen, K.; Horst, R.; Albertelli, M.A.; Feldman, D. Dietary vitamin D_3 and 1,25-dihydroxyvitamin D_3 (calcitriol) exhibit equivalent anticancer activity in mouse xenograft models of breast and prostate cancer. *Endocrinology* **2012**, *153*, 2576–2587. [CrossRef]
83. Bao, B.Y.; Yeh, S.D.; Lee, Y.F. 1alpha,25-dihydroxyvitamin D_3 inhibits prostate cancer cell invasion via modulation of selective proteases. *Carcinogenesis* **2006**, *27*, 32–42. [CrossRef]
84. Bao, B.Y.; Yao, J.; Lee, Y.F. 1alpha,25-dihydroxyvitamin D_3 suppresses interleukin-8-mediated prostate cancer cell angiogenesis. *Carcinogenesis* **2006**, *27*, 1883–1893. [CrossRef] [PubMed]
85. Ben-Eltriki, M.; Deb, S.; Guns, E.S.T. 1alpha,25-Dihydroxyvitamin D_3 synergistically enhances anticancer effects of ginsenoside Rh2 in human prostate cancer cells. *J. Steroid Biochem. Mol. Biol.* **2021**, *209*, 105828. [CrossRef]
86. Hershberger, P.A.; Yu, W.D.; Modzelewski, R.A.; Rueger, R.M.; Johnson, C.S.; Trump, D.L. Calcitriol (1,25-dihydroxycholecalciferol) enhances paclitaxel antitumor activity in vitro and in vivo and accelerates paclitaxel-induced apoptosis. *Clin. Cancer Res.* **2001**, *7*, 1043–1051. [PubMed]
87. Feldman, D.; Krishnan, A.V.; Swami, S.; Giovannucci, E.; Feldman, B.J. The role of vitamin D in reducing cancer risk and progression. *Nat. Rev. Cancer* **2014**, *14*, 342–357. [CrossRef] [PubMed]

88. Kovalenko, P.L.; Zhang, Z.; Cui, M.; Clinton, S.K.; Fleet, J.C. 1,25 dihydroxyvitamin D-mediated orchestration of anticancer, transcript-level effects in the immortalized, non-transformed prostate epithelial cell line, RWPE1. *BMC Genom.* **2010**, *11*, 26. [CrossRef] [PubMed]
89. McCray, T.; Pacheco, J.V.; Loitz, C.C.; Garcia, J.; Baumann, B.; Schlicht, M.J.; Valyi-Nagy, K.; Abern, M.R.; Nonn, L. Vitamin D sufficiency enhances differentiation of patient-derived prostate epithelial organoids. *iScience* **2021**, *24*, 101974. [CrossRef] [PubMed]
90. Giangreco, A.A.; Vaishnav, A.; Wagner, D.; Finelli, A.; Fleshner, N.; Van der Kwast, T.; Vieth, R.; Nonn, L. Tumor suppressor microRNAs, miR-100 and -125b, are regulated by 1,25-dihydroxyvitamin D in primary prostate cells and in patient tissue. *Cancer Prev. Res.* **2013**, *6*, 483–494. [CrossRef]
91. Milani, C.; Katayama, M.L.; de Lyra, E.C.; Welsh, J.; Campos, L.T.; Brentani, M.M.; Maciel Mdo, S.; Roela, R.A.; del Valle, P.R.; Goes, J.C.; et al. Transcriptional effects of 1,25 dihydroxyvitamin D_3 physiological and supra-physiological concentrations in breast cancer organotypic culture. *BMC Cancer* **2013**, *13*, 119. [CrossRef]
92. Ajibade, A.A.; Kirk, J.S.; Karasik, E.; Gillard, B.; Moser, M.T.; Johnson, C.S.; Trump, D.L.; Foster, B.A. Early growth inhibition is followed by increased metastatic disease with vitamin D (calcitriol) treatment in the TRAMP model of prostate cancer. *PLoS ONE* **2014**, *9*, e89555. [CrossRef]
93. Anisiewicz, A.; Pawlik, A.; Filip-Psurska, B.; Wietrzyk, J. Differential impact of calcitriol and its analogs on tumor stroma in young and aged ovariectomized mice bearing 4T1 mammary gland cancer. *Int. J. Mol. Sci.* **2020**, *21*, 6359. [CrossRef]
94. Pawlik, A.; Anisiewicz, A.; Filip-Psurska, B.; Nowak, M.; Turlej, E.; Trynda, J.; Banach, J.; Gretkierewicz, P.; Wietrzyk, J. Calcitriol and its analogs establish the immunosuppressive microenvironment that drives metastasis in 4T1 mouse mammary gland cancer. *Int. J. Mol. Sci.* **2018**, *19*, 2116. [CrossRef] [PubMed]
95. Szymczak, I.; Pawliczak, R. The active metabolite of vitamin D_3 as a potential immunomodulator. *Scand. J. Immunol.* **2016**, *83*, 83–91. [CrossRef] [PubMed]
96. Christakos, S.; Dhawan, P.; Verstuyf, A.; Verlinden, L.; Carmeliet, G. Vitamin D: Metabolism, molecular mechanism of action, and pleiotropic effects. *Physiol. Rev.* **2016**, *96*, 365–408. [CrossRef] [PubMed]

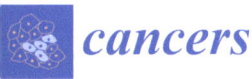

Article

The Barcelona Predictive Model of Clinically Significant Prostate Cancer

Juan Morote [1,2,*,†], Angel Borque-Fernando [3,†], Marina Triquell [1,2], Anna Celma [1,2], Lucas Regis [1,2], Manel Escobar [4], Richard Mast [4], Inés M. de Torres [5,6], María E. Semidey [5,6], José M. Abascal [7], Carles Sola [7], Pol Servian [8], Daniel Salvador [8], Anna Santamaría [9], Jacques Planas [1], Luis M. Esteban [10,‡] and Enrique Trilla [1,2,‡]

1. Department of Urology, Vall d'Hebron Hospital, 08035 Barcelona, Spain; mtriquell@vhebron.net (M.T.); acelma@vhebron.net (A.C.); lregis@vhebron.net (L.R.); jplanas@vhebron.net (J.P.); etrilla@vhebron.net (E.T.)
2. Department of Surgery, Universitat Autònoma de Barcelona, 08193 Barcelona, Spain
3. Department of Urology, Hospital Universitario Miguel Servet, IIS-Aragon, 50009 Zaragoza, Spain; aborque@comz.org
4. Department of Radiology, Vall d'Hebron Hospital, 08035 Barcelona, Spain; mescobar@vhebon.net (M.E.); rmast@vhebron.net (R.M.)
5. Department of Pathology, Vall d'Hebron Hospital, 08035 Barcelona, Spain; itorres@vhebron.net (I.M.d.T.); mesemidey@vehbron.net (M.E.S.)
6. Department of Morphological Sciences, Universitat Autònoma de Barcelona, 08193 Barcelona, Spain
7. Department of Urology, Parc de Salut Mar, 08003 Barcelona, Spain; jmabascalj@gmail.com (J.M.A.); csolamarques@psmar.cat (C.S.)
8. Department of Urology, Hospital Germans Trias I Pujol, 08916 Badalona, Spain; p.serviangermanstrias@gencat.cat (P.S.); dsalvadorhidalgo@gmail.com (D.S.)
9. Urology Research Group, Vall d'Hebron Research Institute, 08035 Barcelona, Spain; anna.santamaria@vhir.org
10. Department of Applied Mathematics, Escuela Universitaria Politécnica La Almunia, Universidad de Zaragoza, 50100 Zaragoza, Spain; lmeste@unizar.es
* Correspondence: jmorote@vhebron.net; Tel.: +34-9327-46009
† These authors contribute equally as co-first authors.
‡ These authors contribute equally as co-last authors.

Simple Summary: Magnetic-resonance-imaging-based predictive models (MRI-PMs) improve the MRI prediction of clinically significant prostate cancer (csPCa) in prostate biopsies. Risk calculators (RC) provide easy individual assessment of csPCa likelihood. MRI-PMs have been analysed in overall populations of men suspected to have PCa, but they have never been analysed according to the prostate imaging-report and data system (PI-RADS) categories. Therefore, the true clinical usefulness of MRI-PMs regarding the specific PI-RADS categories is unknown.

Abstract: A new and externally validated MRI-PM for csPCa was developed in the metropolitan area of Barcelona, and a web-RC designed with the new option of selecting the csPCa probability threshold. The development cohort comprised 1486 men scheduled to undergo a 3-tesla multiparametric MRI (mpMRI) and guided and/or systematic biopsies in one academic institution of Barcelona. The external validation cohort comprised 946 men in whom the same diagnostic approach was carried out as in the development cohort, in two other academic institutions of the same metropolitan area. CsPCa was detected in 36.9% of men in the development cohort and 40.8% in the external validation cohort ($p = 0.054$). The area under the curve of mpMRI increased from 0.842 to 0.897 in the developed MRI-PM ($p < 0.001$), and from 0.743 to 0.858 in the external validation cohort ($p < 0.001$). A selected 15% threshold avoided 40.1% of prostate biopsies and missed 5.4% of the 36.9% csPCa detected in the development cohort. In men with PI-RADS <3, 4.3% would be biopsied and 32.3% of all existing 4.2% of csPCa would be detected. In men with PI-RADS 3, 62% of prostate biopsies would be avoided and 28% of all existing 12.4% of csPCa would be undetected. In men with PI-RADS 4, 4% of prostate biopsies would be avoided and 0.6% of all existing 43.1% of csPCa would be undetected. In men with PI-RADS 5, 0.6% of prostate biopsies would be avoided and none of the existing 42.0% of csPCa would be undetected. The Barcelona MRI-PM presented good performance on the overall population; however, its clinical usefulness varied regarding the PI-RADS category. The selection of csPCa

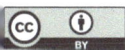

probability thresholds in the designed RC may facilitate external validation and outperformance of MRI-PMs in specific PI-RADS categories.

Keywords: clinically significant prostate cancer; magnetic resonance imaging; predictive model; risk calculator

1. Introduction

Prostate cancer (PCa) suspicion is established from prostate-specific antigen (PSA) serum elevation and/or abnormal digital rectal examination (DRE), while its diagnosis is confirmed with a prostate biopsy [1]. The classic approach based on systematic biopsies results in high rates of unnecessary biopsies and overdetection of insignificant PCa (iPCa) [2]. The detection of clinically significant prostate cancer (csPCa) has improved with the use of magnetic resonance imaging (MRI) and guided biopsies [3,4]. However, that approach can improve by emploting the proper selection of prostate biopsy candidates after MRI [5,6]. For this purpose, PSA density (PSAD) [7], MRI-based predictive models (MRI-PMs) [8], and modern markers [9] have been recommended. MRI-PMs share Prostate Imaging-Report and Data System (PI-RADS) scores and additional independent predictors as PSAD [8–10]. External validation is always required before implementing any predictive model in new population [11,12]. To date, at least fifteen MRI-PMs have been developed [11–25]. In 10 of them, MRI results were reported using the latest PI-RADS versions 2.0–2.1 [11,13,19–25]; 5 of them had any external validation [20–22,24,25]; and none had any associated web or smartphone risk calculator (RC). In addition, the performance of MRI-PMs regarding the PI-RADS categories has never been analysed.

Our main objective was to design a new web-RC for csPCa likelihood, derived from a developed MRI-PM in the metropolitan area of Barcelona, Spain. The RC calculator will provide the novel option of selecting the csPCa probability threshold to facilitate future external validations and outperformances in specific PI-RADS categories. The specific objectives were: i. to develop the Barcelona MRI-PM; ii. to externally validate the developed model in a representative cohort of the Barcelona metropolitan area; iii. to design a friendly and free available web-RC with the PCa probability threshold selection allowed; and iv. to analyse the MRI-PM performance regarding PI-RADS categories in the development and external validation cohorts.

2. Materials and Methods

2.1. Development Cohort

The development cohort was formed of 1987 men with suspected PCa who had serum PSA > 3 ng/mL and/or abnormal DRE and were referred to our early PCa detection program from the primary care system. All men were scheduled for pre-biopsy multiparametric MRI (mpMRI), and thereafter, underwent guided and/or systematic biopsies from 1 to 4 weeks later, between 1 January 2016 and 31 December 2019, in one academic institution (VHH) of the metropolitan area of Barcelona, Spain. Data were collected in a prospective database according to the standards of reporting for MRI-targeted biopsy studies (START) [26]. Written consent was provided by all participants, and the institutional review board approved the project (PR/AG-317/2017). Men excluded from the study were: those undergoing 5-alpha reductase inhibitors for symptomatic benign prostatic hyperplasia; those with a previous PCa diagnosis; those with previous findings of atypical small acinar proliferation or prostate-intraepithelial neoplasia with atypia; and those with an incomplete data set. Additionally, 183 men were also excluded because mpMRI was not carried out due to technical reasons (56 due to claustrophobia, 32 due to a heart pacemaker, and 95 due to any metal prosthesis). The final development cohort comprised 1486 men (Figure 1).

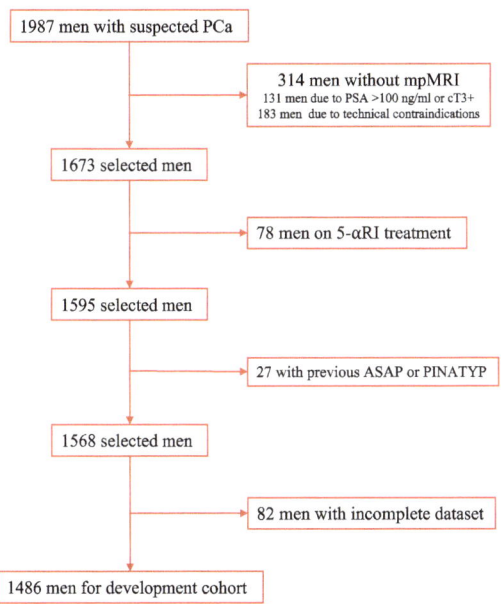

Figure 1. Flow chart of development cohort creation: inclusion and exclusion criteria.

2.2. External Validation Cohort

The external validation cohort comprised 946 men with suspected PCa who were retrospectively selected in two other academic institutions (PSM and GTIPH) and were representative of the metropolitan area of Barcelona, Spain. The criteria of PCa suspicion, the period of recruitment, and the diagnostic approach were the same as in the development cohort.

2.3. MRI Technique and Evaluation

MRI scans were acquired using a 3-tesla scanner with a standard surface phased-array coil. Magneto Trio (Siemens Corp., Erlangen, Germany) equipment was used for the development cohort and Diamond Select Achieva 3.0-TX (Phillips Corp., Eindoven, The Netherlands) and Nova Dual (Phillips Corp., Eindoven, The Netherlands) were used for the external validation cohorts. The acquisition protocol included T2-weighted imaging (T2W), diffusion-weighted imaging (DWI) and dynamic contrast-enhanced (DCE) imaging, according to the guidelines of the European Society of Urogenital Radiology. Two expert radiologists in each institution analysed images using the PI-RADSv.2.0, and in cases with multiple PI-RADS category lesions, the highest PI-RADS was selected for the model [27]. Prostate volume was assessed using MRI in all three institutions.

2.4. Prostate Biopsy Procedure

All men underwent a 2- to 4-core transrectal ultrasound (TRUS), cognitive-fusion guided biopsies for all PI-RADS > 3 lesions, and a 12-core TRUS systematic biopsy. Men with PI-RADS < 3 underwent a 12-core TRUS systematic biopsy. All biopsies were performed by one experienced urologist in each institution using the BK Focus 400 ultrasound scanner (BK Medical Inc., Herlev, Denmark) for the development cohort, and the Siemens Acuson 150 (Siemens Inc., Erlangen, Germany) and the Sonolite Antares (Siemens Inc., Erlangen, Germany) for the external validation cohort.

2.5. Pathologic Analysis and csPCa Definition

Biopsy samples were sent separately to local pathology departments, where two expert uro-pathologists analysed them, assigning them an International Society of Uro-Pathology (ISUP) grade group when PCa was detected. csPCa was defined when ISUP grade > 2 was founded [28].

2.6. Development of MRI-PM

The independent ability to predict csPCa of PI-RADSv.2.0 (1–5), age (years), ethnicity (Caucasian vs. others), serum PSA level (ng/mL), prostate volume (mL), DRE (normal vs. abnormal), PCa family history (no vs. first-degree relatives), and biopsy type (initial vs. repeat) was explored. PSAD was not directly included as a predictor because of the need for previous calculation, and due to having an area under the curve for csPCa detection of 0.892 and 0.897 when serum PSA and prostate volume were the predictors (data not shown).

2.7. Endpoint Measurements for the Performance Analysis of MRIPM

CsPCa detection rates and avoidable prostate biopsy rates.

2.8. Statistical Analysis

Descriptive statistics for the development and external validation cohorts were analysed and compared with the Chi-square and Mann–Whitney U tests. Binary logistic stepwise regression analysis of csPCa candidate predictors was performed for the model development. Continuous variables were modelled as linear or nonlinear predictors using restricted cubic splines. Calibration of the predictive model was assessed in both cohorts. Discrimination power was determined using the receiver operating characteristic (ROC) curve and the area under the curve (AUC), and clinical utility was determined using the clinical utility curve (CUC), which explored the potential rates of missed csPCa detection and avoidable prostate biopsies. The net benefit of the mpMRI- and MRI-based predictive model over biopsying all men was evaluated with a decision curve analysis (DCA). AUCs and specificities for 90% sensitivity to csPCa of the MRI and MRI-based predictive model in the development and external validation cohorts were compared with the DeLong and Chi-square tests, respectively. After selecting the threshold with 95% sensitivity to csPCa, the overall performances of the MRI and MRI-based predictive model were compared, and a sub-analysis—after stratifying by PI-RADS < 3, 3, 4 and 5—was performed. Sensitivity, specificity, positive and negative predictive values, and accuracy of rates of avoidable biopsies and potentially undetected csPCa were analysed. For the external validation, transparent reporting of a multivariable prediction model for individual prognosis or diagnosis (TRIPOD) statements were followed. Statistical analyses were computed using R programming language v.4.0.3 (The R Foundation for Statistical Computing, Vienna, Austria) and SPSS v.24 (IBM, statistical package for the social sciences, San Francisco, CA, USA).

3. Results

3.1. Characteristics of Development and External Validation Cohorts

The characteristics of development and external validation cohorts are summarised in Table 1. We noted a lower significant age and higher serum PSA in the development cohort than in the external validation cohort ($p < 0.001$). We also noted higher abnormal DRE, PCa family history, and repeat prostate biopsy rates in the external validation cohort ($p < 0.001$). The prostate volume was similar in both cohorts ($p = 0.559$). The Caucasian race was predominant in both cohorts ($p = 0.738$). Different case-mixes of PI-RADS categories existed between both cohorts ($p < 0.001$). We noted no significant increase in csPCa in the external validation cohort ($p = 0.054$), and a significant increase in iPCa ($p < 0.001$). The overall detection rate of csPCa was 36.9% in the development cohort, and regarding PI-RADS categories, 4.1% of men had PI-RADS < 3, 15.3% of men had PI-RADS 3, 52.4% of men had PI-RADS 4, and 83.4% of men had PI-RADS 5. The overall detection rate of csPCa was 40.8% in the external validation cohort, and regarding PI-RADS categories, 10.9% of men had PI-RADS < 3, 20.4% of men had PI-RADS 3, 51.9% of men had PI-RADS 4, and 84.0% of men had PI-RADS 5.

Table 1. Characteristics of men suspected to have PCa in development and external validation cohorts and comparisons between them.

Characteristic	Development Cohort	External Validation Cohort	p Value
Number of men	1486	946	-
Caucasian race, n (%)	1465 (98.6)	931 (98.4)	0.738
Median age at biopsy (IQR), years	69 (62–74)	67 (61–72)	<0.001
Median serum PSA (IQR), ng/mL	6.0 (4.4–9.2)	7.4 (5.5–10.9)	<0.001
Abnormal DRE, n (%)	329 (22.1)	283 (29.9)	<0.001
PCa family history, n (%)	127 (8.5)	34 (3.6)	<0.001
Median prostate volume (IQR), mL	55 (40–76)	55 (40–78)	0.559
Prior negative prostate biopsy, n (%)	388 (26.1)	293 (31.0)	0.010
PI-RADS v.2.0, n (%)			
1	242 (16.3)	185 (19.6)	
2	73 (4.9)	50 (5.3)	
3	444 (29.9)	201 (21.2)	<0.001
4	450 (30.3)	391 (41.3)	
5	277 (18.6)	119 (12.6)	
PCa detection, n (%)	693 (46.6)	521 (55.1)	<0.001
csPCa detection, n (%)	548 (36.9)	386 (40.8)	0.054
iPCa detection, n (%)	145 (9.8)	135 (14.3)	<0.001

IQR = interquartile range; n = number; PSA = prostate-specific antigen; DRE = digital rectal examination; PI-RADS = Prostate Imaging-Reporting and Data System; PCa = prostate cancer; csPCa = clinically significant PCa; iPCa = insignificant PCa.

3.2. MRI-Based Predictive Model Development and Performance

Logistic regression analysis showed age, serum PSA, DRE, prostate volume, PCa family history, type of biopsy, and PI-RADSv2.0 as independent predictors of csPCa (Table 2), and a forest plot ranking the odds ratios is presented in Figure S1.

Table 2. Logistic regression analysis of independent significant predictors of csPCa in prostate biopsies.

Predictor	Odds Ratio (95% CI)	p Value
Age at prostate biopsy, ref. prior year	1.056 (1.036–1.077)	<0.001
Serum PSA, ref. prior ng/mL	1.085 (1.056–1.114)	<0.001
DRE, ref. normal.	1.730 (1.195–2.503)	0.004
Prostate volume, ref. prior mL	0.970 (0.964–0.977)	<0.001
Family history of PCa, ref. no	1.788 (1.066–3.002)	0.028
Biopsy type, ref. initial	0.668 (0.478–0.934)	0.018
PI-RADS v.2.0 score, 2 to ref. 1	3.311 (1.008–10.879)	0.048
3 to ref. 1	6.551 (2.740–15.661)	<0.001
4 to ref. 1	32.088 (13.660–75.377)	<0.001
5 to ref. 1	75.673 (30.738–186.311)	<0.001

CI = confidence interval; PSA = prostate-specific antigen; DRE = digital rectal examination; PI-RADSv.2 = Prostate Imaging-Reporting and Data System v.2.; ref. = referenced to.

The ROC curves of mpMRI and MRI-PM in the development cohort are presented in Figure 2A. MRI-PM exhibited a net benefit of mpMRI over biopsying all men within the threshold, with a csPCa probability of 2%. MpMRI also exhibited a net benefit over biopsying all men (Figure 2B).

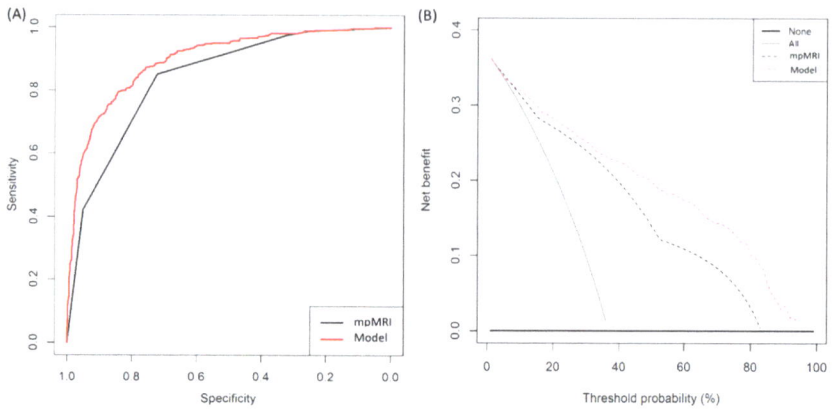

Figure 2. ROC curves showing the efficiency of MRI and MRI-PM in the development cohort (**A**). DCAs evaluating the net benefit of MRI and MRI-PM over biopsying all men belonging to the development cohort (**B**).

The AUC of the mpMRI increased from 0.842 (95% CI: 0.822–0.861) to 0.902 (95% CI: 0.880–0.914) of MRI-PM in the development cohort (p = 0.011). The efficacies of the mpMRI-PM were higher than those of mpMRI (p < 0.001) at 85%, 90%, and 95% sensitivities. At 90% sensitivity, the specificity of mpMRI was 56.8% (95% CI: 53.6–60.0) and that of MRI-PM was 69.5% (95% CI: 66.4–72.4; p < 0.001) (Table 3 (A)).

Table 3. Efficacy of mpMRI and MRI-based predictive model analysed from the AUCs and specificities corresponding to the 85%, 90% and 95% sensitivity thresholds for csPCa, in development cohort (A) and external validation cohort (B).

Predictor	Development Cohort (A)				External Validation Cohort (B)			
	AUC (95% CI)	Specificities According to Sensitivity			AUC (95% CI)	Specificities According to Sensitivity		
		85%	90%	95%		85%	90%	95%
mpMRI	0.842 (0.822–0.861)	72.4 (69.4–75.2%)	56.8 (53.6–60.0)	40.7 (37.5–43.9)	0.743 (0.711–0.776)	45.5 (41.3–49.7)	41.3 (32.9–48.3)	14.3 (11.6–17.5)
MRI-PM	0.897 (0.880–0.914)	78.1% (75.3–80.7)	69.5 (66.4–72.4)	55.7 (52.5–58.9)	0.858 (0.833–0.883)	67.7 (63.6–71.5)	52.3 (48.1–56.5)	32.3 (28.5–36.4)
p Value	=0.011	p = 0.005	<0.001	<0.001	<0.001	<0.001	<0.001	<0.001

mpMRI = multiparametric magnetic resonance imaging; MRI-PM = MRI-based predictive model; AUC = area under the curve; CI = confidence interval.

The MRI-PM derived nomogram is presented in Figure 3, and its calibration curve is presented in Figure S2A.

CUCs showing the rate of avoidable biopsies and the corresponding rate of potentially missed csPCa, regarding the continuous csPCa probability threshold, are presented in Figure 4.

Details of avoidable biopsies and the corresponding risk of missing csPCa detection, regarding the probability threshold for a development cohort of 1000 men with suspected PCa, are displayed with absolute values in Table S1 (A), and relative values in Table S2 (A). The 15% threshold was selected due to its 95% csPCa sensitivity, which corresponded with a 40% rate of avoidable biopsies. In PI-RADS 5, all csPCas would be correctly classified, and 0.5% of biopsies would be avoided. In PI-RADS 4, 0.6% of csPCas would be missed, and 4% of biopsies would be avoided. In PI-RADS 3, 28.2% of csPCa would be missed, and 61.9% of biopsies would be avoided. Finally, in PI-RADS < 3, an MRI-based predictive model would suggest biopsy in 4.3% of cases, and 33.3% of extremely infrequent csPCa in this scenario (4.2%) would be detected (Table 4 (A)). The discrimination ability of the

MRI-based predictive model regarding PI-RADS categories is shown in Figure S3A, and its net benefits over biopsying all men regarding PI-RADS are presented in Figure S4A.

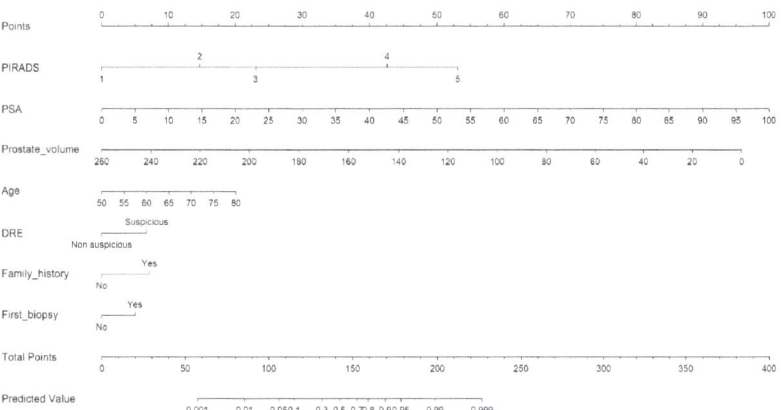

Figure 3. Nomogram derived from the developed MRI-PM model of csPCa in prostate biopsies.

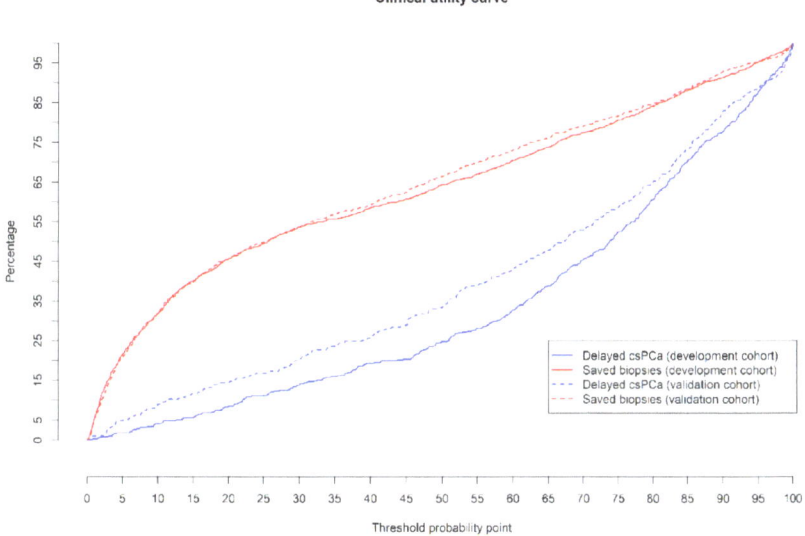

Figure 4. CUCs showing the rates of avoided biopsies (red lines) and corresponding missed csPCa (blue lines) regarding the continuous threshold of csPCa probability using MRI-PMs in development cohort (continuous lines) and external validation cohorts (interrupted lines).

3.3. External Validation of MRI-PM and Its Performance

The calibration curve of the MRI-PM shows how the nomogram slightly underestimated csPCa occurrence in the external validation cohort. For instance, for a 20% csPCa probability provided by the model (X axis), the real incidence is approximately 25%; thus, the model underestimates real csPCa occurrence. The intercept (0.261) and slope (0.815) show this disagreement, which is probably due to a 4% higher csPCa incidence (40.8 vs. 36.9%) in the cohort (Figure S2B).

Table 4. Clinical utility of MRI-based predictive model in terms of avoidable prostate biopsies and potentially missed csPCa in a 1000-sample-size development cohort (A) and external validation cohort (B), using the 15% threshold and regarding PI-RADS categories.

PI-RADS	Development Cohort (A)		External Validation Cohort (B)	
	Missed csPCa	Avoidable Biopsies	Missed csPCa	Avoidable Biopsies
1–2, n (%)	6/9 (66.7)	203/212 (95.7)	36/44 (81.8)	232/248 (93.5)
3, n (%)	13/46 (28.2)	185/299 (61.9)	6/43 (14.0)	134/212 (63.2)
4, n (%)	1/159 (0.6)	12/303 (4.0)	4/215 (1.9)	30/413 (7.3%)
5, n (%)	0/155 (0)	1/186 (0.5)	1/106 (0.9)	3/126 (2.4)
All, n (%)	20/369 (5.4)	401/1000 (40.1)	47/408 (11.5)	399/1000 (39.9)

The ROC curves of MRI-PM in the external validation cohort and development cohort are presented in Figure 5A and DCA, showing the net benefit of MRI-PM in both the external validation cohort and the development cohort (presented in Figure 5B, respectively). The AUC of mpMRI in the external validation cohort was 0.743 (95% CI: 0.711–0.776) compared to 0.842 (95% CI: 0.822–0.861) in the development cohort ($p < 0.001$). The AUC of MRI-PM in the external validation cohort was 0.858 (95% CI: 0.833–0.883) while it was 0.897 (95% CI: 0.880–0.914) in the development cohort ($p = 0.009$) (Table 3 (A) and (B)). At 90% sensitivity for csPCa, the specificity of MRI-PM decreased from 52.3% to 41.3% in the external validation cohort ($p < 0.001$) (Table 3 (B)).

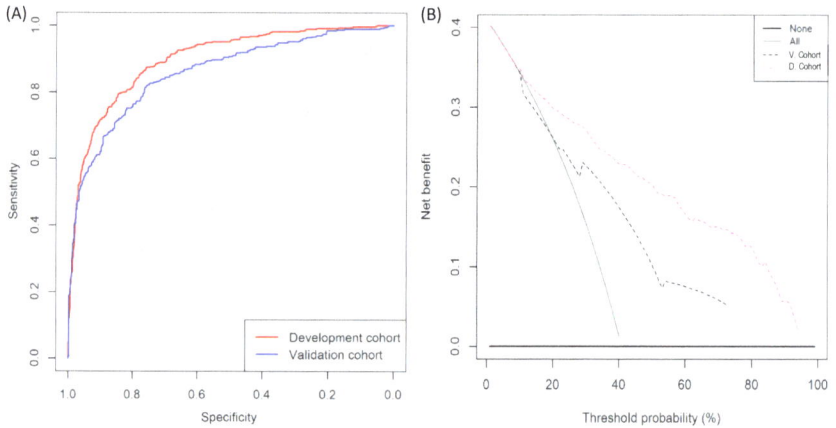

Figure 5. (**A**) ROC curves showing the efficacy of MRI-PM in development cohort and external validation cohort; (**B**) DCAs analysing the net benefit of MRI-PM in development (red interrupted line) and external validation (blue interrupted line) cohort over biopsying all men (continuous grey line).

The CUCs of MRI-PMs in the external validation cohort are presented in Figure 4, where those in the development cohort are also presented. Details of avoided prostate biopsies regarding the csPCa probability thresholds, and the corresponding risk of non-detected csPCa for an external validation cohort of 1000 men, are displayed with absolute and relative values in Tables S1 (B) and S2 (B). At the 15% threshold, MRI-PM avoided 39.9% of prostate biopsies and missed 11.5% of csPCas. In PI-RADS 5, 2.4% of prostate biopsies would be avoided and 0.9% of csPCa would be missed. In PI-RADS 4, 7.3% of prostate biopsies would be avoided and 18.6% of csPCa would be missed. In PI-RADS 3, 63.2% of prostate biopsies would be avoided and 14% of csPCas would be missed. Finally, in men with PI-RADS < 3, MRI-PM would suggest biopsying 6.5% of them, detecting 18.2% of existing csPCa (Table 4 (B)). The discrimination ability of MRI-PM regarding PI-RADS categories is shown in the ROC curves in Figure S4A, and the net benefits over biopsying all men regarding PI-RADS categories are presented in the DCA in Figure S4B.

3.4. Web-RC Design

The validated nomogram was implemented in a web-diagnostic tool using RStudio v.1.2.5001 (RStudio Team, 2015; RStudio: Integrated Development for RStudio, Inc., Boston, MA, USA; URL: http://www.rstudio.com/; accessed on 12 April 2020) and the shiny library. The designed RC incorporates the novel option of selecting the csPCa probability threshold, and it is freely available at https://mripcaprediction.shinyapps.io/MRIPCaPrediction/ (accessed on 23 November 2020).

4. Discussion

Early detection of csPCa can improve even after the spread of MRI and guided biopsies. The proper individualised selection of candidates for prostate biopsy is the current challenge [6]. The most recent MRI-PMs include the latest versions of PI-RADS as well as the prostate volume derived from MRI [11,19,20,24]. Our model was developed from PI-RADS v2.0, which was always reported from 3-tesla mpMRI. The clinical independent predictors finally included in the developed MRI-PM, without a limited range, were the age, serum PSA, and prostate volume. We aimed to design an RC covering real clinical practice in contrast with others that limit the range of these predictors [12]. Ethnicity was not part of our developed model, since it was not an independent predictor of csPCa, perhaps because only one race was prevalent in both the development and external validation cohorts, in contrast to others [16]. PSAD, which is the most powerful predictor of csPCa after PI-RADS, has undergone increased use following the spread of MRI, providing the most accurate measurement of prostate volume without the additional cost [5,6,10]. Furthermore, PSAD appears to be an ideal predictor of csPCa for MRI-PM sharing due to its dynamic behavior across PI-RADS categories [7]. PSAD can be directly incorporated into models as a ratio [11,16,17,19,23,24], or indirectly through the serum PSA and the prostate volume, which also are independent predictors of csPCa [12,13,15,18,21,25]. Due to the observation of similar odds ratios of the two ways of expressing PSAD, we used serum PSA and prostate volume to avoid any calculation before the introduction of data into the RC. PSAD has been compared with some MRI-PMs, showing good performances compared to those MRI-PMs with inadequate calibration in the external validation cohorts [29]. We also included in our MRI-PM the type of biopsy (initial or repeat), since it was also an independent predictor and it provided greater clinical applicability than MRI-PM developed exclusively in biopsy-naïve men [20,21] or in men with previous negative biopsies [13,19,23,24].

External validation of developed model is a key point. It was carried out in a cohort selected in two representative institutions of the same metropolitan area where the MRI-PM was developed, using the same criteria of suspected PCa and the same diagnostic approach to csPCa. Even so, a non-significant 4-percentage-point difference in csPCa incidence of 36.9% vs. 40.8% was observed. This was stressful for the developed model, although its ability to discriminate csPCa remained accurate in the external validation cohort only, with minimal underestimation. We selected the 15% probability threshold of csPCa from development cohort due to its 95% sensitivity and avoidance of 40% of prostate biopsies. The same threshold provided a chance of avoiding 39.9% of biopsies with an 11.5% lack of csPCa detection in the external validation cohort. The clinical utility and net benefit of developed MRI-PMs over biopsying all men with PI-RADS > 3 was low in both the development and external validation cohorts. The avoidable biopsies would be 4% in PI-RADS 4 and 0.5% in PI-RADS 5 in the development cohort, and 7.3% and 2.4%, respectively, in the external validation cohort. CsPCa would be undetected in 0.6% and 0%, and 1.9% and 0.9%, respectively, in the development and external validation cohorts. The performance and net benefit in men with PI-RADS < 3 was better. In men with PI-RADS 3, 61.9% and 62.3% of prostate biopsies would be avoided in the development and external validation cohorts, respectively, while 28.2% and 14% of the few existing csPCas would be undetected. Finally, in men with normal mpMRIs (PI-RADS < 3), 4.3% and 6.5% would be biopsied, respectively, in the developed and external validation cohorts, detecting 33.3% and 18.2% of existing csPCa, respectively. In these low and intermediate PI-RADS categories, the absolute number of undetected csPCa is low due to the limited number of existing csPCa that did not reach rates higher than 5–10% of all detected csPCa.

External validations in populations where predictive models are going to be used are essential, and accessible and friendly RC are needed to avoid the cumbersome and time-consuming use of nomograms [11,12]. A novelty of our designed RC is the option to select the csPCa probability threshold for the overall population or according to the PI-RADS categories. The threshold can be adapted to the overall csPCa incidence of external validation populations [30]. In addition, the threshold selection can also improve the usefulness of the model in specific PI-RADS categories. For example, if we find it unacceptable that 28% of existing csPCa in men with PI-RADS 3 are not detected, we can select the csPCa probability threshold of 7%, which results in 11% of csPCa missing; however, it will result in 26% avoided prostate biopsies instead of 62%. This is the first time that the behavior of any MRI-PM for csPCa has been analysed according to the PI-RADS categories. This analysis shows that the usefulness of MRI-PM is limited in men with PI-RADS >3, and especially in men with PI-RADS 5, in whom the biopsy must be always. High PI-RADS categories exhibit high rates of csPCa; therefore, loosing small rates of csPCa, in addition to their greater aggressiveness, is dangerous [27,31–35].

We developed a new MRI-PM for csPCa and externally validated it, initially in the same metropolitan area. An accessible and friendly RC was designed for its easy and widespread use. The novelty of selecting the csPCa probability threshold may be helpful in new external validations and to modulate the desired sensitivity to csPCa in each PI-RADS category. Rather than limitations, we believe that local reporting by experienced radiologists following PI-RADS v.2 [27]; local experienced pathologists reporting ISUP grades [28]; and local experienced urologist performing biopsies according to the recommended EAU scheme [1] are strengths, because they represent real-life early detection of csPCa. We believe a true limitation of our MRI-PM is the prediction of csPCa made in prostate biopsies, which do not represent the true pathology in whole prostate gland [36]. Our model cannot be implemented in populations where ethnicity predicts different risk of csPCa. The applicability of our developed predictive model in other contemporary populations is unknown and should be evaluated in future studies; these include non-academic populations or in referred populations for prostate biopsy centers with a different case-mix of PI-RADS and csPCa incidence. Performing guided biopsies using a cognitive-fusion technique does not seem to be a limitation, since all men in the development and validation cohorts underwent the same technique, and no difference with the software fusion-guided technique has been found [37]. Further validations in cohorts in which other biopsy schemes and fusion techniques are used are needed. Finally, genomics must report a deeper understanding of PCa aggressiveness, and will help to improve the current csPCa definition. Thus, in the near future, radiomics will be able to predict the newly redefined csPCa [38].

5. Conclusions

A new MRI-PM for csPCa was developed to improve and individualise the selection of candidates for prostate biopsy in the metropolitan area of Barcelona, Spain. An associated web-RC incorporates the option to select the csPCa probability threshold, which may improve further external validations and outperformances in specific PI-RADS categories. The developed MRI-PM was able to detect 95% of existing csPCa, avoiding 40% of prostate biopsies in our overall population. However, the analysis regarding PI-RADS categories shows that the developed MRI-PM outperforms in PI-RADS < 3.

Supplementary Materials: The following supporting information can be downloaded at: https://www.mdpi.com/article/10.3390/cancers14061589/s1, Figure S1: Forest plot of the odds ratios of independent predictors of csPCa in the development cohort; Figure S2: Calibration curve of MRI-PM in development cohort (A) and external validation cohort (B); Table S1: Estimation, in a 1000-case development cohort (A) and external validation cohort (B), of absolute missed csPCa and avoided biopsies for different thresholds and PI-RADS v.2.0 categories; Table S2: Estimation, in a 1000-case development cohort (A) and validation cohort (B), of relative values of missed csPCa and avoided biopsies for different thresholds and PI-RADS categories; Figure S3: Boxplots of the likelihoods of csPCa in men overall and regarding PI-RADS categories in development cohort (A) and external validation cohort (B); Figure S4: DCAs showing the net benefit of generated mpMRI-based predictive model over biopsying all men, according to the PI-RADS categories <3 (upper left), 3 (upper right), 4 (lower left), and 5 (lower right) in the development cohort (A), and the validation cohort (B).

Author Contributions: Conceptualization, J.M., A.B.-F. and L.M.E.; methodology, J.M., A.B.-F. and L.M.E.; software, L.M.E.; validation, L.M.E.; formal analysis, L.M.E.; investigation, J.M., A.B.-F. and L.M.E.; resources, J.M.; data curation, M.T., A.C., L.R., M.E., R.M., I.M.d.T., M.E.S., J.M.A., C.S., P.S., D.S., A.S. and J.P.; writing—original draft preparation, J.M.; writing—review and editing, J.M., A.B.-F. and L.M.E.; supervision, E.T.; project administration, J.M.; funding acquisition, J.M. All authors have read and agreed to the published version of the manuscript.

Funding: This research was funded by the Instituto de Salud Carlos III (ESP), grant number PI20/01666.

Institutional Review Board Statement: The study was conducted in accordance with the Declaration of Helsinki and approved by the Institutional Review of the Vall d´Hebron Hospital Campus (PR/AG-317/2017, approved on 28 August 2017).

Informed Consent Statement: Informed consent was obtained from all subjects involved in the study.

Data Availability Statement: The data presented in this study are available on request from the corresponding author.

Conflicts of Interest: The authors declare no conflict of interest.

References

1. Mottet, N.; van den Bergh, R.C.N.; Briesrs, E.; Briers, E.; Van den Broeck, T.; Cumberbatch, M.G.; De Santis, M.; Fanti, S.; Fossati, N.; Gandaglia, G.; et al. EAU-EANM-ESTRO-ESUR-SIOG Guidelines on Prostate Cancer-2020 Update. Part 1: Screening, Diagnosis, and Local Treatment with Curative Intent. *Eur. Urol.* **2021**, *79*, 243–262. [CrossRef] [PubMed]
2. Drazer, M.W.; Huo, D.; Eggener, S.E. National Prostate Cancer Screening Rates After the 2012 US Preventive Services Task Force Recommendation Discouraging Prostate-Specific Antigen-Based Screening. *J. Clin. Oncol.* **2015**, *33*, 2416–2423. [CrossRef] [PubMed]
3. Ahmed, H.U.; El-Shater Bosaily, A.; Brown, L.C.; Gabe, R.; Kaplan, R.; Parmar, M.K.; Collaco-Moraes, Y.; Ward, K.; Hindley, R.G.; Freeman, A.; et al. Diagnostic accuracy of multi-parametric MRI and TRUSbiopsy in prostate cancer (PROMIS): A paired validating confirmatory study. *Lancet* **2017**, *389*, 815–822. [CrossRef]
4. Schoots, I.G.; Padhani, A.R.; Rouvière, O.; Barentsz, J.O.; Richenberg, J. Analysis of Magnetic Resonance Imaging-directed Biopsy Strategies for Changing the Paradigm of Prostate Cancer Diagnosis. *Eur. Urol. Oncol.* **2020**, *3*, 32–41. [CrossRef]
5. Van Poppel, H.; Roobol, M.J.; Chapple, C.R.; Catto, J.W.F.; N'Dow, J.; Sønksen, J.; Stenzl, A.; Wirth, M. Prostate-specific Antigen Testing as Part of a Risk-Adapted Early Detection Strategy for Prostate Cancer: European Association of Urology Position and Recommendations for 2021. *Eur. Urol.* **2021**, *80*, 703–711. [CrossRef]
6. Van Poppel, H.; Hogenhout, R.; Albers, P.; van den Bergh, R.C.N.; Barentsz, J.O.; Roobol, M.J. A European Model for an Organised Risk-stratified Early Detection Programme for Prostate Cancer. *Eur. Urol. Oncol.* **2021**, *4*, 731–739. [CrossRef]
7. Morote, J.; Celma, A.; Diaz, F.; Regis, L.; Roche, S.; Mast, R.; Semidey, M.E.; de Torres, I.M.; Planas, J.; Trilla, E. Prostatic-specific antigen density behavior according to multiparametric magnetic resonance imaging result. *Urol. Oncol.* **2020**, *38*, 410–417. [CrossRef]
8. Schoots, I.G.; Roobol, M.J. Multivariate risk prediction tools including MRI for individualized biopsy decision in prostate cancer diagnosis: Current status and future directions. *World J. Urol.* **2020**, *38*, 517–529. [CrossRef]
9. Becerra, M.F.; Atluri, V.S.; Bhattu, A.S.; Punnen, S. Serum and urine biomarkers for detecting clinically significant prostate cancer. *Urol. Oncol.* **2021**, *39*, 686–690. [CrossRef]
10. Dianat, S.S.; Rancier Ruiz, R.M.; Bonekamp, D.; Carter, H.B.; Macura, K.J. Prostate volumetric assessment by magnetic resonance imaging and transrectal ultrasound: Impact of variation in calculated prostate-specific antigen density on patient eligibility for active surveillance program. *J. Comput. Assist. Tomogr.* **2013**, *37*, 589–595. [CrossRef]
11. Borque-Fernando, A.; Esteban, L.M.; Celma, A.; Regis, L.; de Torres, I.M.; Semidey, M.E.; Trilla, E.; Morote, J. How to implement magnetic resonance imaging before prostate biopsy in clinical practice: Nomograms for saving biopsies. *World J. Urol.* **2019**, *38*, 1481–1491. [CrossRef] [PubMed]
12. Alberts, A.R.; Roobol, M.J.; Verbeek, J.F.M.; Schoots, I.G.; Chiu, P.K.; Osses, D.F.; Tijsterman, J.D.; Beerlage, H.P.; Mannaerts, C.K.; Schimmöller, L.; et al. Prediction of High-grade Prostate Cancer Following Multiparametric Magnetic Resonance Imaging: Improving the Rotterdam European Randomized Study of Screening for Prostate Cancer Risk Calculators. *Eur. Urol.* **2019**, *75*, 310–318. [CrossRef] [PubMed]

13. Fang, D.; Zhao, C.; Ren, D.; Yu, W.; Wang, R.; Wang, H.; Li, X.; Yin, W.; Yu, X.; Yang, K.; et al. Could Magnetic Resonance Imaging Help to Identify the Presence of Prostate Cancer Before Initial Biopsy? The Development of Nomogram Predicting the Outcomes of Prostate Biopsy in the Chinese Population. *Ann. Surg. Oncol.* **2016**, *23*, 4284–4292. [CrossRef] [PubMed]
14. Kim, E.H.; Weaver, J.K.; Shetty, A.S.; Vetter, J.M.; Andriole, G.L.; Strope, S.A. Magnetic Resonance Imaging Provides Added Value to the Prostate Cancer Prevention Trial Risk Calculator for Patients With Estimated Risk of High-grade Prostate Cancer Less Than or Equal to 10. *Urology* **2017**, *102*, 183–189. [CrossRef]
15. Radtke, J.P.; Wiesenfarth, M.; Kesch, C.; Freitag, M.T.; Alt, C.D.; Celik, K.; Distler, F.; Roth, W.; Wieczorek, K.; Stock, C.; et al. Combined Clinical Parameters and Multiparametric Magnetic Resonance Imaging for Advanced Risk Modeling of Prostate Cancer-Patient-tailored Risk Stratification Can Reduce Unnecessary Biopsies. *Eur. Urol.* **2017**, *72*, 888–896. [CrossRef]
16. Bjurlin, M.A.; Rosenkrantz, A.B.; Sarkar, S.; Lepor, H.; Huang, W.C.; Huang, R.; Venkataraman, R.; Taneja, S. Prediction of Prostate Cancer Risk Among Men Undergoing Combined MRI-targeted and Systematic Biopsy Using Novel Pre-biopsy Nomograms That Incorporate MRI Findings. *Urology* **2018**, *112*, 112–120. [CrossRef]
17. Lee, S.M.; Liyanage, S.H.; Wulaningsih, W.; Wolfe, K.; Carr, T.; Younis, C.; Van Hemelrijck, M.; Popert, R.; Acher, P. Toward an MRI-based nomogram for the prediction of transperineal prostate biopsy outcome: A physician and patient decision tool. *Urol. Oncol.* **2017**, *35*, 66411–66418. [CrossRef]
18. Van Leeuwen, P.J.; Hayen, A.; Thompson, J.E.; James, E.; Moses, D.; Shnier, R.; Böhm, M.; Abuodha, M.; Haynes, A.M.; Ting, F.; et al. Multiparametric magnetic resonance imaging-based risk model to determine the risk of significant prostate cancer prior to biopsy. *BJU Int.* **2017**, *120*, 774–781. [CrossRef]
19. Niu, X.K.; Li, J.; Das, S.K.; Yang, C.B.; Peng, T. Developing a nomogram based on multiparametric magnetic resonance imaging for forecasting high-grade prostate cancer to reduce unnecessary biopsies within the prostate-specific antigen gray zone. *BMC Med. Imaging* **2017**, *17*, 11. [CrossRef]
20. Truong, M.; Wang, B.; Gordetsky, J.B.; Nix, J.W.; Frye, T.P.; Messing, E.M.; Thomas, J.V.; Feng, C.; Rais-Bahrami, S. Multi-institutional nomogram predicting benign prostate pathology on magnetic resonance/ultrasound fusion biopsy in men with a prior negative 12-core systematic biopsy. *Cancer* **2018**, *124*, 278–285. [CrossRef]
21. Huang, C.; Song, G.; Wang, H.; Li, J.; Chen, Y.; Fan, Y.; Fang, D.; Xiong, G.; Xin, Z.; Zhou, L. Multiparametric Magnetic Resonance Imaging-Based Nomogram for Predicting Prostate Cancer and Clinically Significant Prostate Cancer in Men Undergoing Repeat Prostate Biopsy. *Biomed. Res. Int.* **2018**, *2018*, 6368309. [CrossRef]
22. Mehralivand, S.; Shih, J.H.; Rais-Bahrami, S.; Oto, A.; Bednarova, S.; Nix, J.W.; Thomas, J.V.; Gordetsky, J.B.; Gaur, S.; Harmon, S.A.; et al. A Magnetic Resonance Imaging-Based Prediction Model for Prosate Biopsy Risk Stratification. *JAMA Oncol.* **2018**, *4*, 678–685. [CrossRef] [PubMed]
23. Boesen, L.; Thomsen, F.B.; Nørgaard, N.; Løgager, V.; Balslev, I.; Bisbjerg, R.; Thomsen, H.S.; Jakobsen, H. A predictive model based on biparametric magnetic resonance imaging and clinical parameters for improved risk assessment and selection of biopsy-naïve men for prostate biopsies. *Prostate Cancer Prostatic Dis.* **2019**, *2*, 311–319. [CrossRef] [PubMed]
24. Noh, T.I.; Hyun, C.W.; Kang, H.E.; Jin, H.J.; Tae, J.H.; Shim, J.S.; Kang, S.G.; Sung, D.J.; Cheon, J.; Lee, J.G.; et al. A Predictive Model Based on Bi-parametric Magnetic Resonance Imaging and Clinical Parameters for Clinically Significant Prostate Cancer in the Korean Population. *Cancer Res. Treat.* **2021**, *53*, 1148–1155. [CrossRef]
25. Chen, I.A.; Chu, C.H.; Lin, J.T.; Tsai, J.Y.; Yu, C.C.; Sridhar, A.N.; Sooriakumaran, P.; Loureiro, R.C.V.; Chand, M. Prostate Cancer Risk Calculator Apps in a Taiwanese Population Cohort: Validation Study. *J. Med. Internet Res.* **2020**, *22*, e16322. [CrossRef]
26. Bossuyt, P.M.; Reitsma, J.B.; Bruns, D.E.; Korevaar, D.A.; STARD Group. STARD 2015: An updated list of essential items for reporting diagnostic accuracy studies. *BMJ* **2015**, *351*, h5527. [CrossRef] [PubMed]
27. Weinreb, J.C.; Barentsz, J.O.; Choyke, P.L.; Choyke, P.L.; Cornud, F.; Haider, M.A.; Macura, K.J.; Margolis, D.; Schnall, M.D.; Shtern, F.; et al. PI-RADS Prostate Imaging—Reporting and Data System: 2015, Version 2. *Eur. Urol.* **2016**, *69*, 16–40. [CrossRef]
28. Epstein, J.I.; Egevad, L.; Amin, M.B.; Delahunt, B.; Srigley, J.R.; Humphrey, P.A.; Grading Committee. The 2014 International Society of Urological Pathology (ISUP) Consensus Conference on Gleason Grading of Prostatic Carcinoma: Definition of Grading Patterns and Proposal for a New Grading System. *Am. J. Surg. Pathol.* **2016**, *40*, 244–252. [CrossRef]
29. Deniffel, D.; Healy, G.M.; Dong, X.; Ghai, S.; Salinas-Miranda, E.; Fleshner, N.; Hamilton, R.; Kulkarni, G.; Toi, A.; van der Kwast, T.; et al. Avoiding Unnecessary Biopsy: MRI-based Risk Models versus a PI-RADS and PSA Density Strategy for Clinically Significant Prostate Cancer. *Radiology* **2021**, *300*, 369–379. [CrossRef]
30. Remmers, A.; Kasivisvanathan, V.; Verbeek, J.; Moore, C.M.; Roobol, M.J.; ERSPC Rotterdam Study Group and PRECISION Investigators Group. Reducing Biopsies and Magnetic Resonance Imaging Scans During the Diagnostic Pathway of Prostate Cancer: Applying the Rotterdam Prostate Cancer Risk Calculator to the PRECISION Trial Data. *Eur. Urol. Open Sci.* **2022**, *36*, 1–8. [CrossRef]
31. Mazzone, E.; Stabile, A.; Pellegrino, F.; Basile, G.; Cignoli, D.; Cirulli, G.O.; Sorce, G.; Barletta, F.; Scuderi, S.; Bravi, C.A.; et al. Positive Predictive Value of Prostate Imaging Reporting and DataSystem Version 2 for the Detection of Clinically Significant Prostate Cancer: A Systematic Review and Meta-analysis. *Eur. Urol. Oncol.* **2020**, *4*, 697–713. [CrossRef] [PubMed]
32. Schoots, I.G. MRI in early prostate cancer detection: How to manage indeterminate or equivocal PI-RADS 3lesions. *Transl. Urol.* **2018**, *7*, 70–82. [CrossRef] [PubMed]
33. Osses, D.F.; Roobol, M.J.; Schoots, I.G. Prediction Medicine: Biomarkers, Risk Calculators and Magnetic Resonance Imaging as Risk Stratification Tools in Prostate Cancer Diagnosis. *Int. J. Mol. Sci.* **2019**, *20*, 1637. [CrossRef] [PubMed]

34. Abreu-Gomez, J.; Wu, M.; McInnes, M.D.F.; Thornhill, R.E.; Flood, T.A.; Schieda, N. Shape Analysis of Peripheral Zone Observations on Prostate DWI: Correlation to Histopathology Outcomes After Radical Prostatectomy. *AJR. Am. J. Roentgenol.* **2020**, *214*, 1239–1247. [CrossRef]
35. Boschheidgen, M.; Schimmöller, L.; Arsov, C.; Ziayee, F.; Morawitz, J.; Valentin, B.; Radke, K.L.; Giessing, M.; Esposito, I.; Albers, P.; et al. MRI grading for the prediction of prostate cancer aggressiveness. *Eur. Radiol.* **2021**, *32*, 2351–2359. [CrossRef] [PubMed]
36. Rapisarda, S.; Bada, M.; Crocetto, F.; Barone, B.; Arcaniolo, D.; Polara, A.; Imbimbo, C.; Grosso, G. The role of multiparametric resonance and biopsy in prostate cancer detection: Comparison with definitive histological report after laparoscopic/robotic radical prostatectomy. *Abdom. Radiol.* **2020**, *45*, 4178–4184. [CrossRef] [PubMed]
37. Khoo, C.; Eldred-Evans, D.; Peters, M.; van Son, M.; van Rossum, P.S.N.; Connor, M.J.; Hosking-Jervis, F.; Tanaka, M.B.; Reddy, D.; Bass, E.; et al. Comparison of Prostate Cancer Detection between Visual Estimation (Cognitive Registration) and Image Fusion (Software Registration) Targeted Transperineal Prostate Biopsy. *J. Urol.* **2021**, *205*, 1075–10781. [CrossRef] [PubMed]
38. Ferro, M.; de Cobelli, O.; Vartolomei, M.D.; Lucarelli, G.; Crocetto, F.; Barone, B.; Sciarra, A.; Del Giudice, F.; Muto, M.; Maggi, M.; et al. Prostate Cancer Radiogenomics-From Imaging to Molecular Characterization. *Int. J. Mol. Sci.* **2021**, *22*, 9971. [CrossRef]

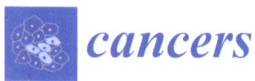

Article

Histone Demethylase KDM5C Drives Prostate Cancer Progression by Promoting EMT

Anna-Lena Lemster [1], Elisabeth Sievers [2], Helen Pasternack [1], Pamela Lazar-Karsten [1], Niklas Klümper [3], Verena Sailer [1], Anne Offermann [1], Johannes Brägelmann [4,5,6], Sven Perner [1,7] and Jutta Kirfel [1,*]

[1] Institute of Pathology, University Hospital Schleswig-Holstein, 23538 Luebeck, Germany; anna-lena.lemster@uksh.de (A.-L.L.); helen.pasternack@uksh.de (H.P.); pamela.lazar-karsten@uksh.de (P.L.-K.); verena-wilbeth.sailer@uksh.de (V.S.); anne.offermann@uksh.de (A.O.); sven.perner@uksh.de (S.P.)
[2] Institute of Pathology, University Hospital Bonn, 53127 Bonn, Germany; elisabeth.sievers@ukbonn.de
[3] Department of Urology and Pediatric Urology, University Hospital Bonn, 53127 Bonn, Germany; niklas.kluemper@ukbonn.de
[4] Department of Translational Genomics, Faculty of Medicine and University Hospital Cologne, University of Cologne, 50931 Cologne, Germany; johannes.braegelmann@uni-koeln.de
[5] Mildred Scheel School of Oncology Cologne, Faculty of Medicine and University Hospital Cologne, University of Cologne, 50931 Cologne, Germany
[6] Faculty of Medicine and University Hospital Cologne, Center for Molecular Medicine Cologne, University of Cologne, 50931 Cologne, Germany
[7] Institute of Pathology, Research Center Borstel, Leibniz Lung Center, 23845 Borstel, Germany
* Correspondence: jutta.kirfel@uksh.de

Citation: Lemster, A.-L.; Sievers, E.; Pasternack, H.; Lazar-Karsten, P.; Klümper, N.; Sailer, V.; Offermann, A.; Brägelmann, J.; Perner, S.; Kirfel, J. Histone Demethylase KDM5C Drives Prostate Cancer Progression by Promoting EMT. *Cancers* **2022**, *14*, 1894. https://doi.org/10.3390/cancers14081894

Academic Editors: Ana Faustino, Paula A. Oliveira and Lúcio Lara Santos

Received: 17 March 2022
Accepted: 7 April 2022
Published: 8 April 2022

Publisher's Note: MDPI stays neutral with regard to jurisdictional claims in published maps and institutional affiliations.

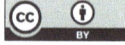

Copyright: © 2022 by the authors. Licensee MDPI, Basel, Switzerland. This article is an open access article distributed under the terms and conditions of the Creative Commons Attribution (CC BY) license (https://creativecommons.org/licenses/by/4.0/).

Simple Summary: Prostate cancer is the most common cancer in men and is one of the leading causes of cancer-related deaths. During prostate cancer progression and metastasis, the epithelial cells can undergo epithelial–mesenchymal transition (EMT). Here, we show that the histone demethylase KDM5C is highly expressed in metastatic prostate cancer. We establish that stable clones silence KDM5C in prostate cancer cells. Knockdown of KDM5C leads to a reduced migratory and invasion capacity. This is associated with changes by multiple molecular mechanisms. This signaling subsequently modifies the expression of various transcription factors like Snail, Twist, and Zeb1/2, which are also known as master regulators of EMT. Taken together, our results indicate the potential to therapeutically target KDM5C either alone or in combination with Akt/mTOR-inhibitor in prostate cancer patients by targeting the EMT signaling pathways.

Abstract: Prostate cancer (PCa) poses a major public health problem in men. Metastatic PCa is incurable, and ultimately threatens the life of many patients. Mutations in tumor suppressor genes and oncogenes are important for PCa progression, whereas the role of epigenetic factors in prostate carcinogenesis is insufficiently examined. The histone demethylase KDM5C exerts important roles in tumorigenesis. KDM5C has been reported to be highly expressed in various cancer cell types, particularly in primary PCa. Here, we could show that KDM5C is highly upregulated in metastatic PCa. Functionally, in KDM5C knockdown cells migratory and invasion capacity was reduced. Interestingly, modulation of KDM5C expression influences several EMT signaling pathways (e.g., Akt/mTOR), expression of EMT transcription factors, epigenetic modifiers, and miR-205, resulting in increased expression of E-cadherin and reduced expression of N-cadherin. Mouse xenografts of KDM5C knockdown cells showed reduced tumor growth. In addition, the Akt/mTOR pathway is one of the classic signaling pathways to mediate tumor metabolic homeostasis, which is beneficial for tumor growth and metastasis. Taken together, our findings indicate that a combination of a selective KDM5C- and Akt/mTOR-inhibitor might be a new promising therapeutic strategy to reduce metastatic burden in PCa.

Keywords: prostate cancer; CRPC; histone demethylase; KDM5C; epithelial-to-mesenchymal transition; signaling pathway

1. Introduction

Prostate cancer (PCa) is the most commonly diagnosed cancer in men worldwide and remains a leading cause of cancer-related mortality. Most PCa-related deaths are caused by development of metastatic disease and castration resistance. PCa frequently metastasizes to the bones, particularly the spine, where it can lead to pathological fractures with severe consequences. Once the cancer has spread to distant sites, including the bones, it is generally considered incurable. The occurrence of bone metastasis dramatically limits the patients' quality of life. Although the 5-year survival rate of PCa patients improved in the last ten years and is now at approximately 99% for localized PCa in the United States, this rate decreases to 32% in patients with distant metastasis [1]. The 10-year survival rate is at 18.5% in PCa patients with distant metastasis.

Metastatic spread is a step-wise process that involves loss of intercellular cohesion, cell migration, angiogenesis, access to systemic circulation, survival in circulation, evasion of local immune responses, and growth in distant organs. Cancer cells can accomplish multiple steps of the metastatic process at once through the engagement of a latent cellular program, the epithelial–mesenchymal transition (EMT) [2,3]. The induction of EMT is accompanied by a dynamic reprogramming of the epigenome involving changes in DNA methylation and several post-translational histone modifications. Histone lysine methylation is associated with either gene activation or silencing, depending on the site of the lysine residues. During TGFβ-mediated EMT, there is a global reduction in the heterochromatin mark H3 Lys9 dimethylation (H3K9me2), an increase in the euchromatin mark H3 Lys4 trimethylation (H3K4me3), and an increase in the transcriptional mark H3 Lys36 trimethylation (H3K36me3) [4].

Members of the KDM5 family (also known as JARID1) act as histone H3K4 demethylases. KDM5 family members have various biological functions; they can be crucial in the expression and repression of oncogenes and tumor suppressor genes, and can themselves serve as both. For instance, KDM5B is overexpressed in a variety of cancer types, and high levels of KDM5B have been observed in breast cancer and PCa (reviewed in [5]). Previously, we systematically investigated KDM5C expression patterns in two independent radical prostatectomy cohorts with a total of 761 primary PCas by immunohistochemistry and demonstrated that KDM5C was significantly overexpressed in primary PCa [6]. The oncogenic role of KDM5C was also observed in gastric cancer [7] and hepatocellular carcinoma [8]. Recent evidence indicates that members of the KDM5 cluster may also be involved in PCa metastasis. KDM5B, which is significantly overexpressed in localized and metastatic PCa, is an androgen receptor coactivator and may play an important role in controlling PCa cell invasion and metastasis [5]. It was demonstrated that KDM5D levels were highly downregulated in metastatic PCa. In addition, the KDM5D gene was frequently deleted in metastatic PCa [9]. However, the role of KDM5C in metastatic PCa has not been well studied.

Here, we show that KDM5C expression is enhanced in the metastatic tissue of lymph node-metastasized PCa and castration-resistant PCa (CRPC). Silencing of KDM5C in bone metastatic PCa cell line PC3 inhibited tumor growth in mouse xenografts. In addition, cellular depletion of KDM5C by shRNA inhibited PC3 cell migration, invasion, and epithelial–mesenchymal transition in vitro. Modulation of KDM5C expression influences several EMT signaling pathways (Hedgehog, Wnt, Notch, TGFβ, PI3K-AKT-mTOR), the expression of transcription factors (SNAI2, TWIST1, ZEB1, ZEB2), epigenetic modifiers (DNMT1, EZH2), and miR-205, resulting in increased expression of E-cadherin and reduced expression of N-cadherin.

Our findings provide a novel mechanistic role of KDM5C in PCa metastasis, suggesting that KDM5C may serve as a potential therapeutic target for advanced PCa patients.

2. Materials and Methods

2.1. Immunohistochemical Analysis and Quantification of Protein Expression

Formalin-fixed and paraffin-embedded prostatic tissue of lymph node metastasized PCa (N = 95) and castration-resistant PCa (CRPC) (N = 28) were provided from cohorts of the University Hospital of Luebeck. Our study was approved by the Ethics Committee of the University of Luebeck (17-313). These tissues and xenograft tumors were used to prepare tissue microarrays (TMA), as previously described in Shaikhibrahim et al. [10]. The following primary antibodies, KDM5C (34718, dilution 1:1000/1:2000, Abcam, Cambridge, UK), E-Cadherin (36, Ventana Medical System, Tucson, AZ, USA), Ki-67 monoclonal rabbit (30-9, Ventana Medical System), were used and detected with Ultra View Universal DAB Detection Kit (Ventana Medical System). Slides were then digitized using the Zeiss Panoramic Midi Scanner (3DHistech, Budapest, Hungary). The images of KI-67 staining were analyzed semi-quantitatively with the software Definiens Tissue Studio 2.1 (Tissue Studio v.2, Definiens AG, Munich, Germany) as previously described in Stein et al. [6]. KDM5C and CDH were analyzed through eyeball analyses, the definition of nuclear KDM5C and membranous CDH1 as negative or positive by two experienced observers. Samples with absence of carcinoma or lack of tissue were excluded.

2.2. Cell Culture and Lentiviral Transduction

PC3 cells were cultured in DMEM/F12 medium supplemented with 10% FBS, 100 U/ml Penicillin/Streptomycin, and 1% L-Glutamine (all from Invitrogen, Thermo Fisher Scientific, Waltham, MA, USA).

For lentiviral transduction, five individual clones from MISSION™ shRNA targeting JARID1C NM_001146702 (TRCN 0000358549, TRCN 0000234960, TRCN 0000234961, TRCN 0000022085, TRCN 0000022087) and one shControl clone (SHC004) (all from Sigma-Aldrich, St. Louis, MO, USA) were co-transfected with lentiviral packaging plasmids (psPAX2 plasmid 12,260 and pMD2.G plasmid 12,259 from Addgene, Teddington, UK) into HEK 293T cells. The resulting lentiviral particles were used to infect PC3 cells. Twenty-four h post infection, four µg/mL puromycin was added to select the infected cells. Infection efficiency was approximately 90%. Then, five days post-selection, cells of each clone were isolated by serial dilution in 96-well plates under puromycin selection to obtain single cell clones.

2.3. MTT Cell Proliferation Assay

MTT assay was performed, according to the manufacturer's protocol (Roche, Mannheim Germany) for the different time periods of 24 h, 48 h, and 72 h.

2.4. Migration and Invasion Assays

Cellular motility was analyzed by Transwell migration (Transwell Boyden chamber (#353097, Falcon/Corning, New York, NY, USA)) and Invasion chamber (Matrigel™ Invasion chamber (#354480, BD Biosciences, Heidelberg, Germany)) assays using cells prestarved in 2% FBS medium for 24 h as previously described in Sievers et al. [11].

2.5. RNA isolation and Quantitative Real-Time PCR (qRT-PCR)

RNA was extracted using PureLink® RNA Mini Kit (Ambion Life Technologies, Thermo Fisher Scientific), according to the manufacturer's protocol. Afterwards, cDNA synthesis was performed with 1 µg RNA using SuperScript III and Oligo (dT) 12-18 primers (Invitrogen, Thermo Fisher Scientific). Gene expression was quantified by real-time PCR as described by Lim et al. [12]. Each sample was run in triplicate and relative expression was determined by normalization to the TATA-binding protein (TBP) or Hypoxanthine-Guanine

Phosphoribosyl Transferase (HPRT) using the $2^{-\Delta\Delta Ct}$ method. Error bars indicate standard error of the mean (SEM). Primer sequences are available in the Supplementary Materials.

2.6. Isolation and TaqMan PCR Analyses of miRNA

MicroRNA from sh-transfected KDM5C knockdown and control cells was extracted using Invitrogen's mirVana miRNA Isolation Kit (#AM1560, Thermo Fisher Scientific), according to the manufacturer's specifications. Specific TaqMan™ advanced miRNA assays (TaqMan™ advanced miRNA cDNA Synthesis Kit (#A25576) and TaqMan™ Fast advanced Master Mix Kit (#4444556)) for the detection of hsa-miR-205-5p (#477967 mir) and the detection of endogenous control hsa-miR-361 (#478056 mir) were purchased from Invitrogen (Thermo Fisher Scientific) and used according to the manufacturer's specification. Each sample was run in triplicate in a 10 µL reaction. Relative expression was determined by normalization to endogenous miRNA control using the $2^{-\Delta\Delta Ct}$ method. Error bars indicate SEM.

2.7. Protein Extraction and Western Blot Analyses

Protein lysates were extracted from cells and blotted as described in Schulte et al. [13]. The following antibodies were used: KDM5C/JARID1C (1:1000, ab34718, Abcam); β-ACTIN (1:10.000, A5441; Sigma-Aldrich); E-cadherin (1:1000, #3195, Cell Signaling, Cambridge, UK); N-cadherin (1:1000, #14215, Cell Signaling); SNAI2/Slug (1:1000, #9585, Cell Signaling); α-TUBULIN (1:1000, #2144, Cell Signaling); SMAD1 (1:1000, #6944, Cell Signaling); SMAD4 (1:1000, #38454, Cell Signaling); H2Aub, (1:1000, #8240, Cell Signaling); H3K4me2, (1:1000, #035050, Diagenode); H3K4me3 (1:1000, ab1012, Abcam); STAT6 D3H4 (1:1000, #5397, Cell Signaling); Phospho-Smad1 Ser463/465/Smad5 Ser463/465/Smad9 Ser463/465 D5B10 (1:1000, #13820, Cell Signaling).

2.8. Kinase Activity Profiling

Tyrosine (PTK) and serine-threonine (STK) kinome activity profiling was performed using a PamStation®12 (PamGene, BJ's-Hertogenbosch, The Netherlands), according to the standard protocol provided by PamGene. Signal intensities for each peptide were analyzed with the PamGene BioNavigator Analysis software tool.

2.9. Growth of Xenograft Tumors in Mice

Mouse experiments were performed by Charles River Discovery Research Services Germany GmbH, Freiburg, Germany. PC3 wild-type cells were grown in RPMI 1640 with 10% FCS and 0.05 mg/mL gentamycin. Stable KDM5C knockdown cells were grown in DMEM high glucose with 10% FCS, 0.05 mg/mL gentamycin, and 200 mM L-glutamine. For each cell clone, 10 male NOD SCID mice were injected unilaterally into the flank with 5×10^6 cells in 100 µL volume (50% Matrigel). After injection, an aliquot of the cell suspension was used to verify the cell viability. Mice were weighed for 29 days, and tumors were measured twice a week. Mice were sacrificed and all tumors were collected, fixed in formalin, and embedded into paraffin.

2.10. Statistical Methods

For statistical analyses, unpaired Student's t-tests were performed. Results were considered significant when p-values were $p < 0.001$ ***; $p < 0.01$ **; $p < 0.05$ *, and n.s. for not significant. Functional protein association networks were generated in STRING DB V11.0 (https://string-db.org/, accessed on 8 September 2021). Network plots were generated in Cytoscape 3.8.1 (http://cytoscape.org/, accessed on 8 September 2021) and analyzed using Network Analyzer V4.4.6 and Omics Visualizer V1.3.0 (Cytoscape App Store-Omics Visualizer).

3. Results

3.1. KDM5C Expression Is Enhanced in Metastatic Prostate Cancer

Previously, we demonstrated that KDM5C was significantly overexpressed in primary PCa [6]. Here, we analyzed KDM5C expression in a PCa progression cohort. Both lymph node metastases and distant bone metastases showed nuclear KDM5C expression (Figure 1); however, distant metastases showed a much higher nuclear positivity. Of 95 cases of lymph node metastasis, 34% showed a nuclear KDM5C staining. Of 28 cases of distant metastasis, up to 75% showed a strong nuclear KDM5C staining.

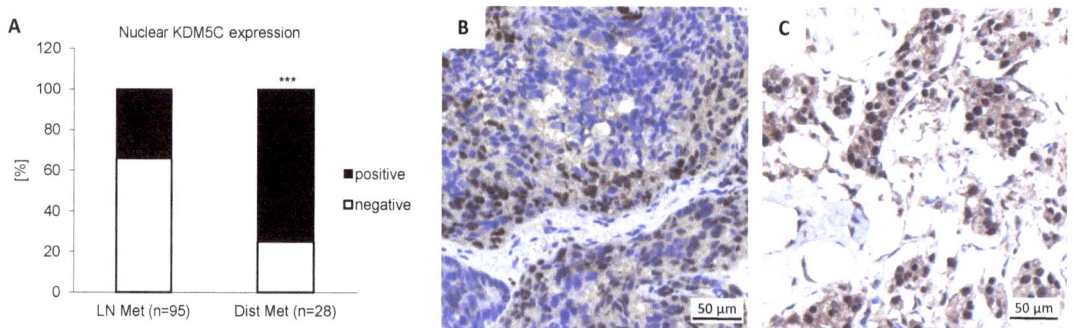

Figure 1. Immunohistochemical staining of KDM5C in a prostate cancer progression cohort. (**A**) Nuclear KDM5C expression in lymph node (LN) metastasis and bone (Dist) metastasis; (**B**) Representative sample of KDM5C protein expression in an invasive tumor edge in lymph node metastasis; (**C**) Representative sample of KDM5C protein expression in bone metastasis showing strong nuclear staining in tumor cells. (*** = $p < 0.001$).

3.2. KDM5C Knockdown Reduces Cell Migration and Invasion

To further study KDM5C expression different PCa cell types were used. KDM5C is strongly expressed in CRPC cells (PC3) and moderately expressed in metastatic androgen-sensitive cells (LNCaP), whereas KDM5C expression is low in benign prostatic BPH-1 cells (Figure 2A, uncropped Western blot in Figure S6).

Due to the lack of a selective and specific KDM5C inhibitor, we investigated the functional significance of KDM5C in PCa cells by downregulating KDM5C expression in PC3 cells (derived from a hormone-refractory PCa bone metastasis) using lentiviral short hairpin RNA (shRNA) technology (Figure 2A). Four single-cell derived clones showed particularly efficient knockdown of KDM5C. Two of them (PC3 shKDM5C 1.6 and 4.2), as well as two GFP control clones (shControl 1 and 4), were studied in more detail. The KDM5C gene expression was significantly reduced in the KDM5C knockdown cells compared to PC3 wild-type cells. KDM5C expression in shControl clones was not altered (Figure 2B).

As an initial step toward understanding the role of KDM5C in PCa events, we determined whether KDM5C expression alters cell phenotype and regulates PCa cell proliferation, migration, and invasion. Knockdown of KDM5C results in a minor impairment of proliferation measured by viability assay (Figure 2C). The phenotype of the KDM5C knockdown cells varied from that of the control cells (Figure 2D), and the KDM5C knockdown cells adhered less to the flask compared with control cells. Global levels of histone modifications were not affected by the knockdown of KDM5C (Figure S1, uncropped Western blot in Figure S7). This indicates its function through gene locus specific modifications.

Next, we investigated the migration and invasion capacity of KDM5C knockdown and control cells. Knockdown of KDM5C significantly reduces migration and invasion ability by approximately 75% (Figure 2E,F). These results suggest that KDM5C may act as an epigenetic modulator of migration and invasion.

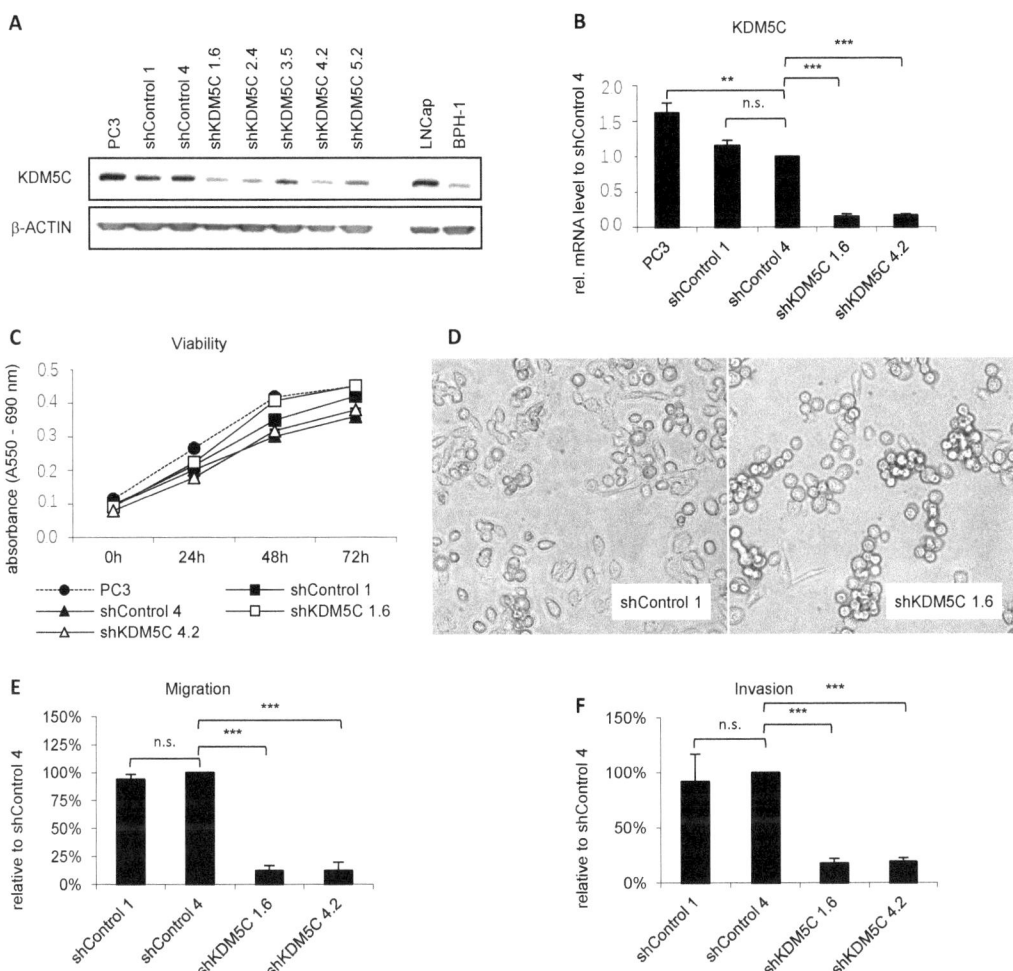

Figure 2. KDM5C expression after shRNA-mediated knockdown. (**A**) Representative Western blot of KDM5C expression in prostate cancer cell line PC3, different shRNA-transduced cell clones, LNCap, and BPH-1. ShControl clones with GFP serve as a control for the lentiviral transduction procedure. The loading control is β-ACTIN; (**B**) qRT-PCR analysis of KDM5C mRNA expression in prostate cancer cell line PC3 and different shRNA-transduced GFP control as well as KDM5C knockdown clones. mRNA expression was normalized to the nuclear housekeeper TBP and in relation to the shControl 4 clone. Error bars represent standard error of the mean from three independent experiments; (**C**) Viability of PC3 cells and several shRNA-transduced cell clones. One representative MTT assay of the parental cell line PC3 and its derived shRNA-controlled clones. Error bars represent standard error of the mean from the quintuplicates; (**D**) Phenotype of shControl clones compared to KDM5C knockdown clones. KDM5C knockdown cells were less adherent to the flask compared with control cells (15× magnification); (**E**) Migration and (**F**) Invasion of PC3 derived shRNA-transduced cell clones tested by Boyden and Invasion chamber assays. Error bars represent standard error of the mean from three independent experiments. (n.s. = not significant; ** = $p < 0.01$; *** = $p < 0.001$).

3.3. KDM5C-Mediated Changes in Epithelial-Mesenchymal Transition (EMT)

To investigate mechanisms by which KDM5C expression affects cell migration and invasion, we explored the effect of KDM5C knockdown on the expression of genes involved in EMT. The mesenchymal cell–cell adhesion molecule N-cadherin and SNAI2 promote EMT. In contrast, the epithelial cell–cell adhesion molecule E-cadherin inhibits this process. Knockdown of KDM5C led to increased expression of E-cadherin shown by qPCR (*CDH1*, Figure 3A) and Western blot (Figure 3D, uncropped Western blot in Figure S8). Knockdown also led to a reduced expression of N-cadherin (qPCR: *CDH2*, Figure 3B; Western blot: Figure 3D, uncropped Western blot in Figure S8). The qPCR (Figure 3C) and Western blot (Figure 3D, uncropped Western blot in Figure S8) showed reduced expression of SNAI2 after knockdown of KDM5C. Lymph nodes of PCa patients showed a negative correlation between KDM5C and E-cadherin expression (Figure S2). KDM5C expression was increased in the invasive tumor front whereas E-cadherin expression was reduced in this region.

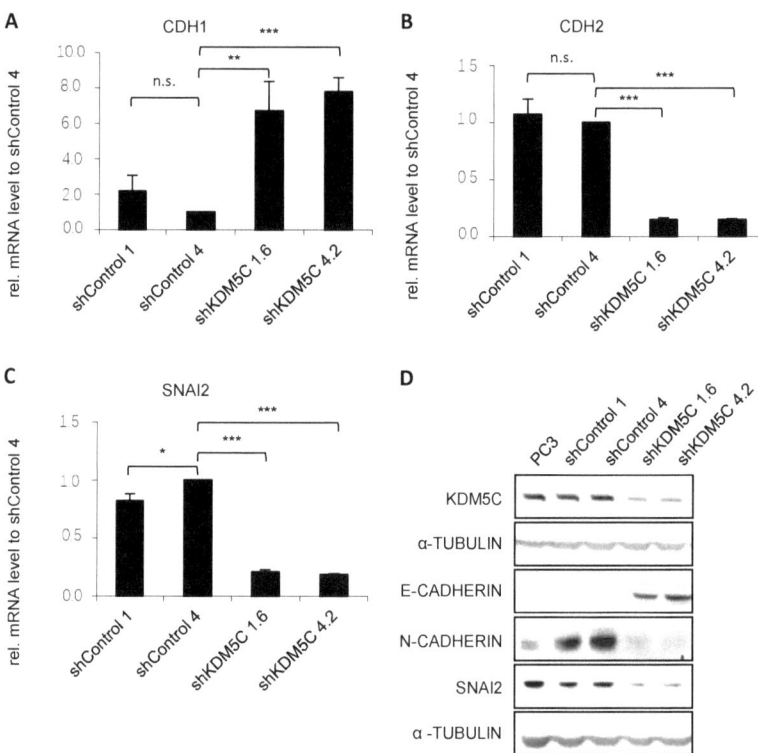

Figure 3. Differential expression of epithelial and mesenchymal markers ((**A**) CDH1; (**B**) CDH2; and (**C**) SNAI2) in PC3 and shRNA-transduced cell clones. qRT-PCR analysis of mRNA expression in GFP control as well as KDM5C knockdown clones. mRNA expression was normalized to the nuclear housekeeper *TBP* in (**A**,**C**) and *HPRT* in (**B**) and in relation to the shControl 4. Error bars represent standard error of the mean from three independent experiments. (**D**) Representative Western blot of the expression of KDM5C and EMT markers in PC3 cells and the shRNA-transduced cell clones. Western blot shows the expression of epithelial marker E-CADHERIN (CDH1) and its transcriptional repressor SNAI2 as well as the typical mesenchymal marker N-CADHERIN (CDH2) in GFP control and KDM5C knockdown clones. α-TUBULIN serves as a loading control. (n.s. = not significant; * = $p < 0.05$; ** = $p < 0.01$; *** = $p < 0.001$).

Several transcription factors respond to microenvironmental stimuli and function as molecular switches for the EMT program. We examined the transcription factors *TWIST1*, *TCF4*, *ZEB1*, and *ZEB2*, as well as *DNMT1* and *EZH2* by qPCR, and found that expression of all factors decreased significantly after knockdown of KDM5C (Figure 4A–F). Transcription factors can regulate EMT on the gene level. In addition, EMT is also regulated on the level of RNA. In particular, non-coding RNAs, known as microRNAs (miRNAs), can either exert a positive or a negative regulatory effect on EMT. In PCa, miR-205 exerts a tumor-suppressive effect by counteracting the epithelial-to-mesenchymal transition and reducing cell migration/invasion [14]. PC3 cells, known for their high metastatic ability, display low expression of miR-205. Knockdown of KDM5C leads to a robust increase in miR-205 (Figure 4G).

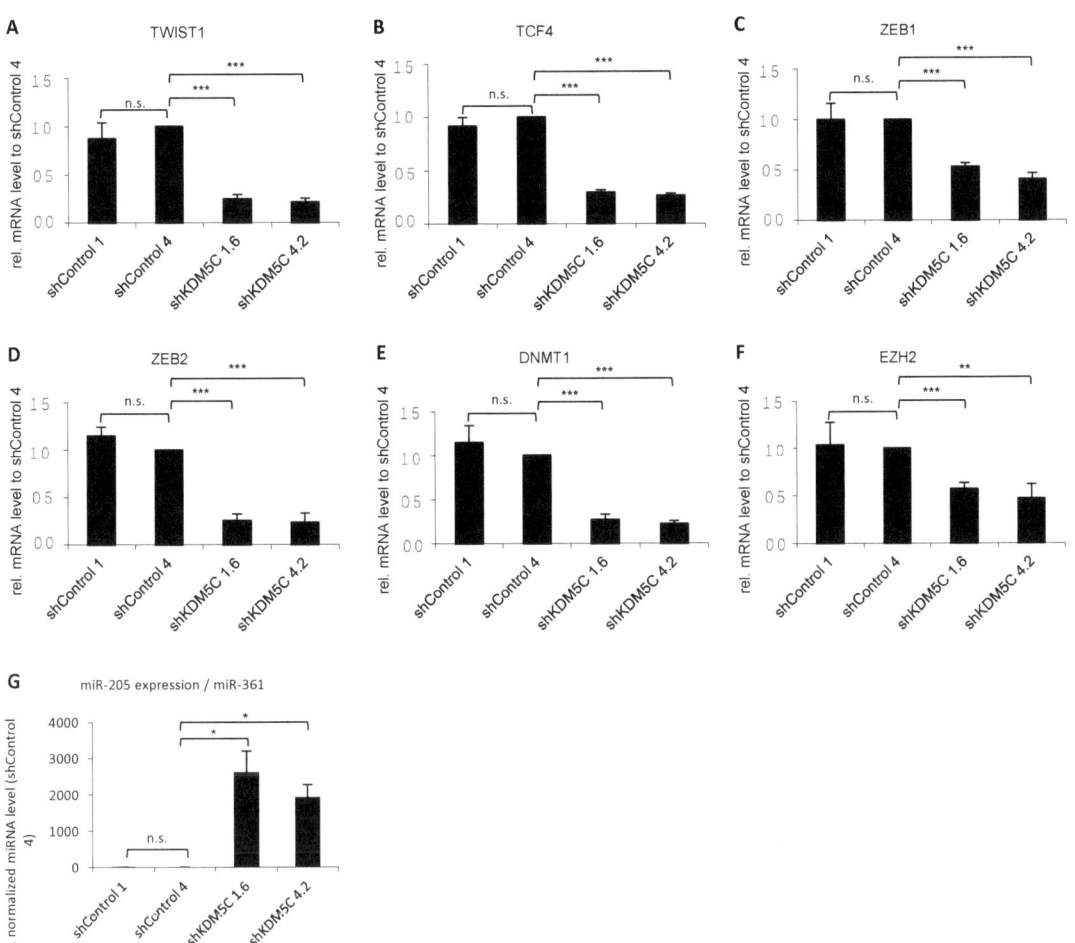

Figure 4. Expression of transcription factors ((**A**) *TWIST1*; (**B**) *TCF4*; (**C**) *ZEB1*; (**D**) *ZEB2*); epigenetic regulators (**E**) *DNMT1*; and (**F**) *EZH2*); and miR-205 (**G**), in stable KDM5C knockdown clones. qRT-PCR analysis of mRNA expression (**A–G**) in GFP control as well as KDM5C knockdown clones. mRNA expression (**A–F**) and microRNA expression (**G**) were normalized to the nuclear housekeeper *TBP* and to miR-361, respectively, and in relation to the shControl 4 clone. Error bars represent standard error of the mean from three independent experiments. (n.s. = not significant; * = $p < 0.05$; ** = $p < 0.01$; *** = $p < 0.001$).

3.4. KDM5C-Mediated Changes in Signaling Pathways

To determine whether KDM5C knockdown leads to changes in signaling pathways, we first analyzed the Wnt signaling pathway. While the ligands *WNT3A*, *WNT5A*, *WNT7A*, and *WNT11* of the Wnt pathway were significantly upregulated in KDM5C knockdown clones (Figure 5A–D) the receptor *FZD9* (Figure 5E) and the mediator *AXIN2* (Figure 5F) were significantly downregulated.

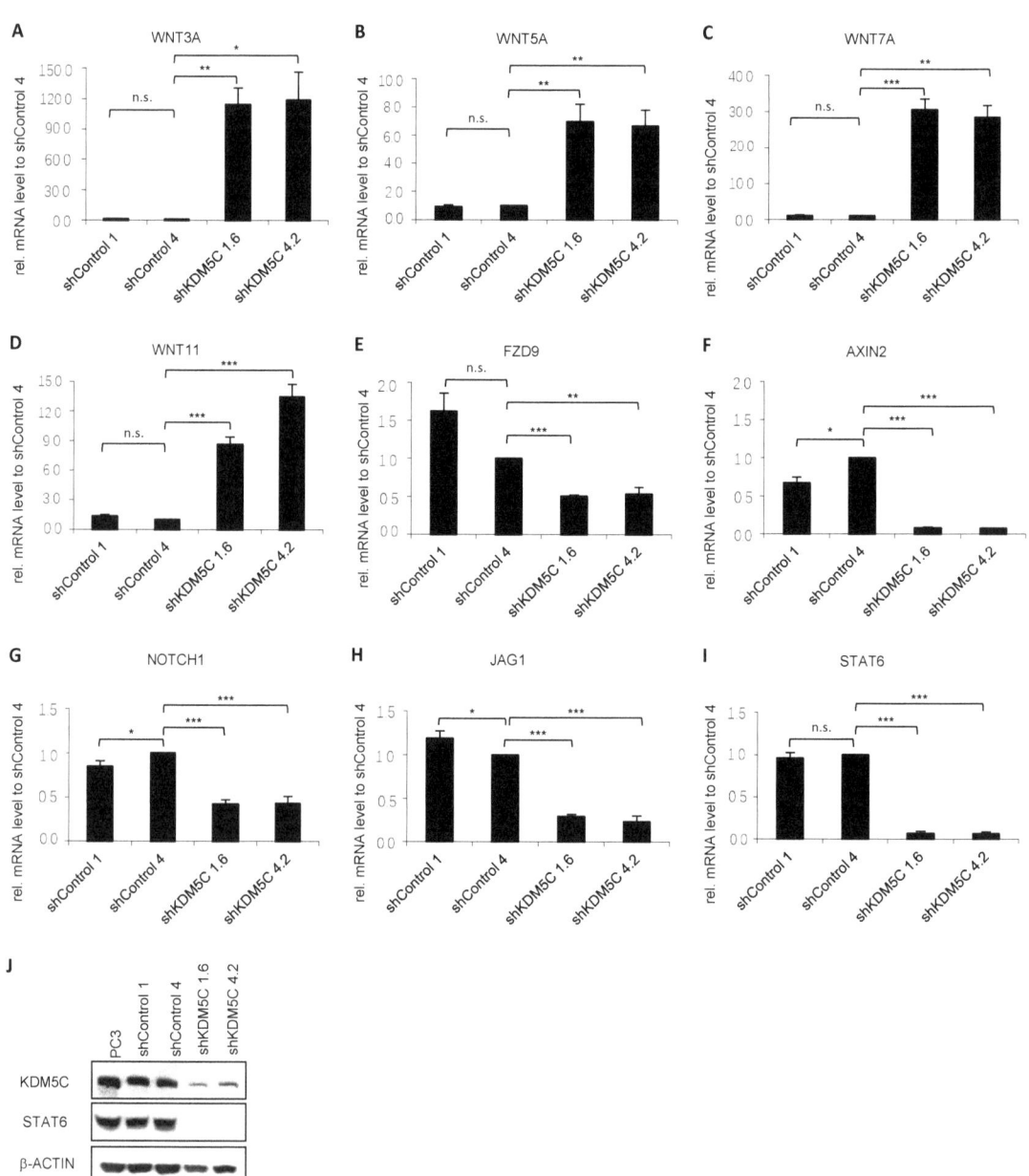

Figure 5. Expression of receptors, ligands, mediator, and target gene of the Wnt (**A**–**F**) and the Notch (**G**–**J**) signaling pathways associated with EMT progression. qRT-PCR analysis of mRNA expression in GFP control as well as KDM5C knockdown clones. Important ligands ((**A**) *WNT3A*; (**B**) *WNT5A*;

(**C**) *WNT7A*; and (**D**) *WNT11*); receptor ((**E**) *FZD9*); and mediator ((**F**) *AXIN2*) for the Wnt signaling were examined. For the Notch signaling important receptor ((**G**) *NOTCH1*), ligand ((**H**) *JAG1*), and its target gene ((**I**) *STAT6*) were examined. mRNA expression was normalized to the nuclear housekeeper *TBP* and in relation to the shControl 4 control clone. Error bars represent standard error of the mean from three independent experiments. (**J**) Representative Western blot of the expression of STAT6 in PC3 cells and the shRNA-transduced cell clones. β-ACTIN serves as a loading control. KDM5C shows the knockdown of KDM5C in shKDM5C 1.6 and shKDM5C4.2. (n.s. = not significant; * = $p < 0.05$; ** = $p < 0.01$; *** = $p < 0.001$).

The Notch signaling pathway is composed of four receptors (NOTCH1, 2, 3, 4) and five ligands (JAG1 and 2 and Delta-like 1, 3, and 4) [15]. Ligand *JAG1* (Figure 5G) and receptor *NOTCH1* (Figure 5H) were significantly downregulated after knockdown of KDM5C. The target gene STAT6 was also significantly downregulated after KDM5C knockdown, as shown by qPCR (Figure 5I) and Western blot (Figure 5J, uncropped Western blot in Figure S9).

Hedgehog pathway ligands, *SHH* and *DHH*, were significantly downregulated in KDM5C knockdown clones (Figure S3A,B). Mediators *GLI1*, *GLI2*, *GLI3*, and *HHIP* were also significantly downregulated in KDM5C knockdown clones (Figure S3C–F).

Finally, we examined mediators and ligands involved in the TGFβ signaling pathway. The ligands *BMP6* and *BMP7* were significantly upregulated (Figure S3G,H) whereas the ligand TGFB1 was significantly downregulated in stable KDM5C knockdown clones (Figure S3I). Knockdown of KDM5C resulted in significant upregulation of the mediator *SMAD1* (Figure S3J) and significant downregulation of the mediators *SMAD2*, *SMAD4*, and *SMAD7* (Figure S3K–M). Protein expression of SMAD1 was upregulated and SMAD4 was downregulated in knockdown clones (Figure S3N, uncropped Western blot in Figure S10).

3.5. KDM5C Knockdown Changes Kinase Activity Profile

We used PamGene's functional kinase assay to measure peptide phosphorylation by protein kinases in KDM5C knockdown and control cells. To measure the tyrosine (Tyr) and serine/threonine (Ser/Thr) kinase activity, we used the PamChips PTK (for Tyr) and STK (for Ser/Thr). Equal amounts of cell lysate from knockdown clones (shKDM5C 1.6 and shKDM5C 4.2) and control clones (shControl 1 and shControl 4) were analyzed. The mean signal intensity of each bait peptide of the stable knockdown clones was normalized to the corresponding peptide of the control clones and expressed as log2 fold change (LFC). We performed hierarchical clustering using Euclidean distance metrics for a graphical heat map (Figure 6A). We also determined the grouped *p*-values of the two stable knockdown clones shKDM5C 1.6 and shKDM5C 4.2 versus the grouped control clones by 2-grouped comparison (unpaired *t*-test) in the BioNavigator software. Figure 6B shows these results in volcano plots (PTK on the left side and STK on the right side) and Figure 6C shows a pathway analysis of the results in a high confidence interaction network.

Largely, the intensity of tyrosine substrate peptide phosphorylation was markedly reduced for most peptides in the knockdown clones. The intensity of phosphorylation was also decreased for most Ser/Thr peptide substrates (Figure 6A–C). We found that the activity of the kinases RPS6, PDPK1, PRKCB, MTOR, and PIK3R1 was reduced in KDM5C knockdown cells (Figure 6C). These are kinases that belong to the mechanistic target of the rapamycin (mTOR) signaling pathway. We also found kinases of the phosphoinositide-3-kinase (PI3K) signaling pathway that had an altered activity in KDM5C knockdown cells (Figure 6C), namely CDK2, CDK4, CDKN1A, RPS6, FOXO3, BAD, EPHA2, PDPK1, CREB1, ERBB2, MTOR, NOS3, PDGFRB, PIK3R1, NFKB1, JAK1, KIT, KDR, EPOR, CSF1R, VTN, and GYS2.

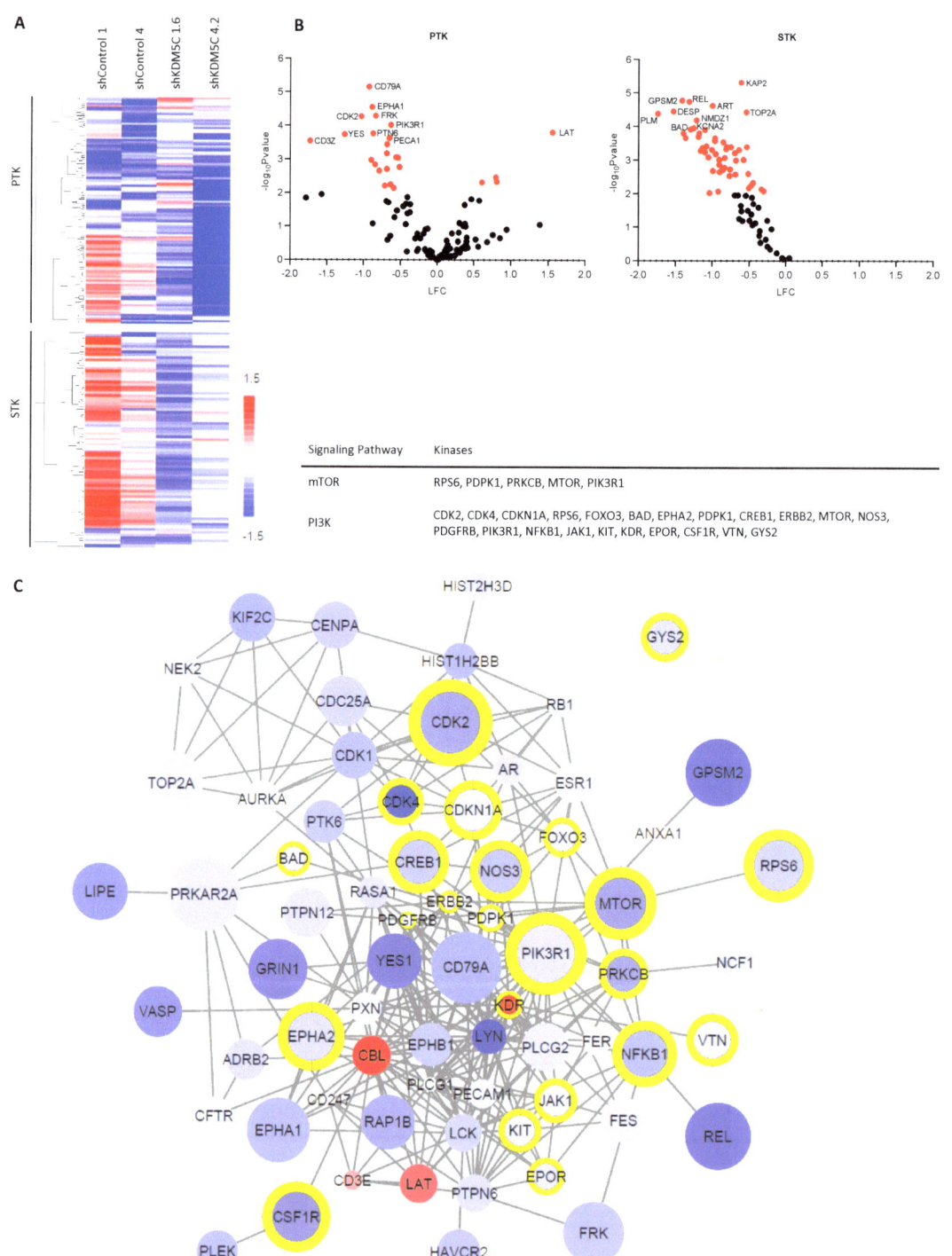

Figure 6. Kinase activity in KDM5C knockdown cells compared to control cells. (**A**) Clustered heat map of increased and decreased phosphorylation of Tyr (PTK, top) and Ser/Thr (STK, bottom) bait

peptides in control cells and stabile knockdown of KDM5C; (**B**) Volcano plots of the bait peptide phosphorylation from PTK (**left**) and STK (**right**) were assessed by student's *t*-test; (**C**) Pathway analysis of peptides from (**B**) ($p > 0.05$) in a high-confidence interaction network (edges) from STRING DB. Node color indicates increased and decreased phosphorylation of Tyr (PTK) and Ser/Thr (STK) bait peptides. Node size indicates $-\log_{10}(p$ value). Yellow border color indicates that the protein is involved in the PI3K-Akt-mTOR signaling pathway. KCNA1, KCNA3, RYR1, PPP1R1A, CACNA1C, GRIK2, DSP, FXYD1, TH, KCNA2, GPR6, ENO2, EPB42, STMN2, PFKFB3, SCN7A, GABRB2, EFS, PHKA1, and MYBPC3 are not shown in the network because they showed no interaction with the kinases in the network.

We also used a phosphokinase array with 37 different kinase phosphorylation sites as an independent experiment to investigate the kinase activity. There, we confirmed that CREB1 activity was not only downregulated in the PamGene's functional kinase assay but also in this independent experiment. We additionally identified a difference in three kinase phosphorylation sites in KDM5C knockdown clones compared to the PC3 wild type and the sh-transfected control 4. Knockdown of KDM5C resulted in decreased phosphorylation of GSK-3α/β (S21/S9), PLC-γ1 (Y783), and RSK1/2 (S221/S227) (Figure S4A,B).

3.6. KDM5C Knockdown Reduces Tumor Growth in Mice

To investigate KDM5C knockdown in mouse model, xenotransplants of PC3 and sh-transfected cells were studied. The growth of tumors with PC3 xenografts was significantly faster than the tumor growth of KDM5C knockdown cell xenografts over the course of 29 days (Figure 7A). Figure 7C shows exemplary samples of the xenograft tumors. Hematoxylin and eosin staining showed no morphologic differences in tissue. E-cadherin expression was high and N-cadherin expression was low in KDM5C knockdown xenograft, whereas the Ki-67 proliferation index was not altered (Figure 7B). Expression of KDM5C, CDH1 and CDH2 in xenografts was analyzed by qRT-PCR (Figure S5).

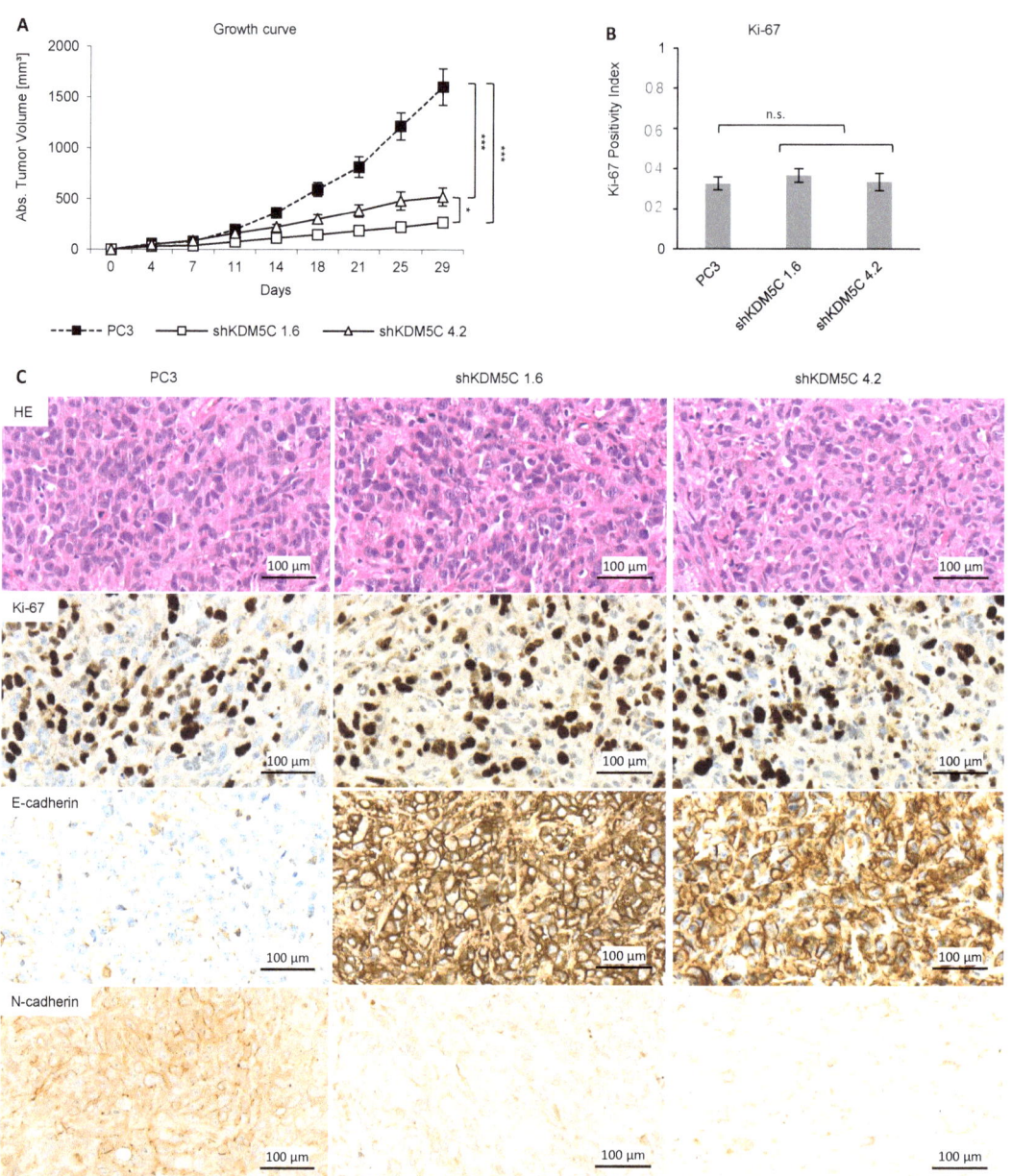

Figure 7. Comparison of mouse xenografts of PC3 wild type and KDM5C knockdown cells. (**A**) Growth curve of PC3 and shRNA-transduced cell tumors in mice xenografts. Error bars represent standard error of the mean from ten independent experiments. Tumors in mice receiving KDM5C knockdown cells were smaller than tumors of wild-type cells; (**B**) Index of Ki-67 positive cells in mice xenografts with PC3 and shRNA-transduced cells. Error bars represent standard error of the mean from eight independent experiments; (**C**) Representative samples of hematoxylin-eosin (HE) staining, as well as Ki-67, E-cadherin and N-cadherin protein expression in PC3 and shRNA-transduced cell mice xenografts. (n.s. = not significant; * = $p < 0.05$; *** = $p < 0.001$).

4. Discussion

Epithelial-to-mesenchymal transition (EMT) and its reverse mesenchymal-to-epithelial transition (MET) are paramount to the metastatic spread of carcinomas. There is a gradual transition between these phenotypic states. Therefore, carcinoma cells often exhibit a spectrum of epithelial/mesenchymal phenotype(s) [16–18].

KDM5C is significantly upregulated in primary [6] and metastatic PCa. Silencing of KDM5C in PCa cells inhibited cell migration and invasion. Knockdown of KDM5C results in modulation of several EMT-associated signaling pathways, thereby decreasing EMT-promoting factors and enhancing MET-promoting factors. Our findings are summarized in a model presented in Figure 8.

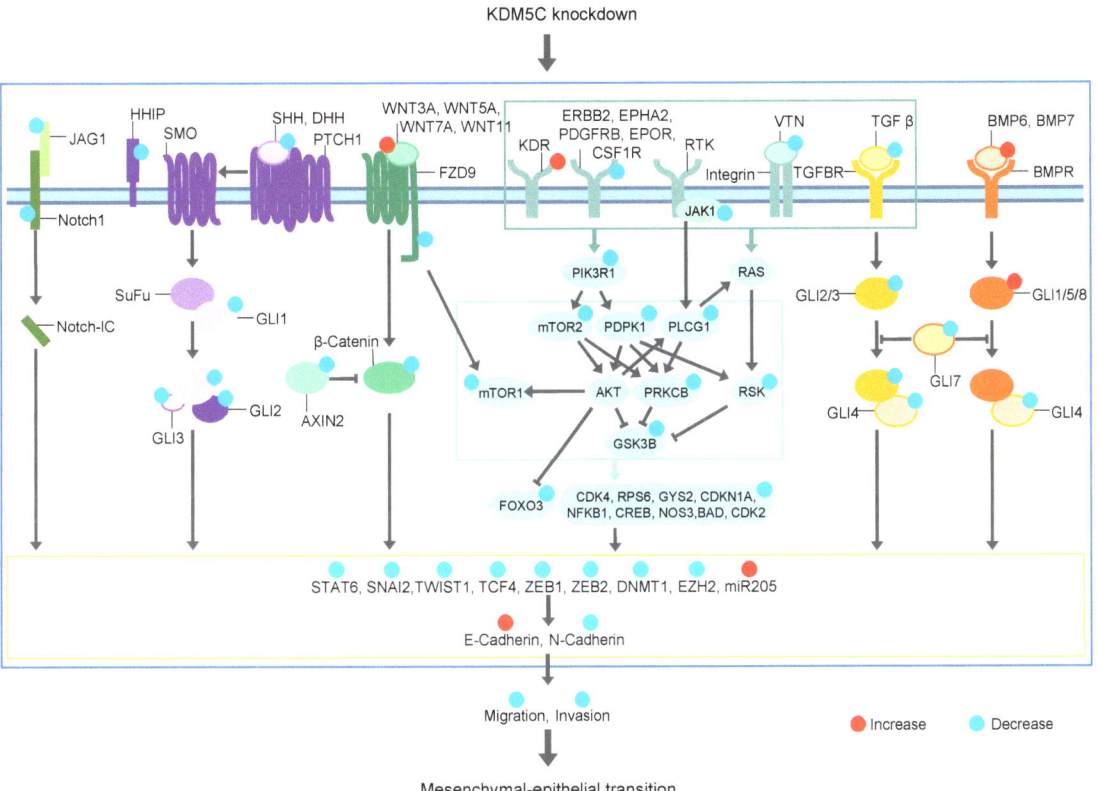

Figure 8. Simplified model of our results on the role of KDM5C in prostate cancer. KDM5C knockdown leads to downregulation of signaling pathways and transcription factors involved in EMT. E-cadherin expression is increased, and N-cadherin expression is decreased after KDM5C knockdown which results in MET.

An integrated and complex signaling network including transforming growth factor β (TGFβ), Wnt, Notch, and Hedgehog leads to the induction of EMT [19–22].

TGFβ is known to induce EMT in PCa [23], and BMP signaling, in turn, is involved in both EMT and MET [24]. We demonstrated that the expression of TFGB1, SMAD2, and SMAD4 (proteins of the TGFβ signaling [25]) is reduced and the expression of BMP6, BMP7, and SMAD1 (proteins of the BMP signaling pathway [25]) is increased after KDM5C knockdown. In epithelial kidney cells, BMP6 and BMP7 counteract TGFβ-induced EMT by reinducing E-cadherin [26,27]. In PCa, Buijs et al. showed that BMP7 expression is inversely related to tumorigenic and metastatic potential [28]. SMAD7 is part of a negative feedback loop regulating TGFβ signaling. Increased TGFβ signaling correlates with increased expression of SMAD7 [29]. Knockdown of KDM5C leads to decreased TGFβ signaling and decreased expression of SMAD7.

Wnt proteins can utilize signal transduction through the canonical β-catenin-dependent pathway and the noncanonical β-catenin-independent pathway, both of which are closely associated with EMT [30]. In PCa, WNT5A induced bone metastasis, and increased the activation of the WNT5A/FZD2 pathway leading to enhanced EMT [31,32]. We demonstrated that canonical Wnt ligands WNT3A and WNT7A and non-canonical Wnt ligands WNT5A and WNT11 are upregulated after KDM5C knockdown. However, the Wnt receptor FZD9, which is part of the canonical and non-canonical pathways, and AXIN2 are downregulated by KDM5C knockdown. AXIN2 serves as a negative regulator of the canonical Wnt signaling pathway and may act as a negative feedback loop to suppress the signaling pathway [33]. In addition, inhibition of FZD7 leads to decreased AXIN2 expression [34].

The Notch signaling pathway also participates in EMT [19], and its inhibition partially reverts EMT in lung adenocarcinoma cells and reduces their invasive behavior [35]. Silencing of the receptor NOTCH1 inhibits PCa cell invasion [36], whereas expression of the ligand JAG1 is associated with PCa progression, metastases, and recurrence [37]. We demonstrated that JAG1, NOTCH1, and STAT6 are downregulated by KDM5C silencing.

Several studies show that Shh signaling is associated with EMT and that inhibition of the signaling pathway results in suppression of EMT in PCa [38–40]. In the absence of Hedgehog pathway ligands, SHH, DHH, and Indian hedgehog (IHH), the pathway is in an "off" state [22]. We showed that SHH and DHH are downregulated after knockdown of KDM5C. In the presence of ligands, the pathway would be switched "on", resulting in the activation of the GLI family of transcription factors (GLI1, GLI2, and GLI3). GLI1 functions as a transcriptional activator, while GLI2 and GLI3 can be processed into transcriptional activators or repressors [41,42]. Silencing of KDM5C reduced the steady-state level of GLI1, GLI2, and GLI3. HHIP is a negative feedback regulator of hedgehog signaling [43] and was downregulated in our studies after KDM5C knockdown.

These findings strengthen the idea of a role for KDM5C in the regulation of TGFβ, Wnt, Notch, and Hedgehog leading to EMT.

We investigated the kinase activity profile of KDM5C knockdown cells compared to control cells. The PI3K and mTOR signaling pathways play an important role in the induction of EMT [44,45] and influence EMT in PCa [46,47]. We showed that the activity of several kinases e.g., CDK2, CREB1, RPS6, and mTOR is reduced in KDM5C knockdown cells. Other studies show that CREB1 is upregulated in metastases and its inhibition could reduce cell proliferation [48]. Inhibition of CDK2 is able to reduce cell invasion [49] and shows inhibitory effects on EMT [50], and suppression of RPS6 increases radiosensitivity in PCa [51]. Our phosphokinase array also showed that the activity of CREB1 and additionally GSK-3α/β, PLC-γ1, and RSK1/2 was downregulated in stable KDM5C knockdown clones. These kinases all play a role in tumors' metastasis [52–55] and may also play a role in the PI3K–Akt signaling pathway [56–60]. Therefore, a combination therapy with inhibition of KDM5C and the PI3K-Akt-mTOR signaling pathway might be beneficial for the patient.

All of the above-mentioned signaling pathways affect the expression of transcription factors and miRNAs, which then induce or repress E-cadherin and N-cadherin expression. The main function of EMT-related transcription factors is to repress epithelial-associated genes and induce mesenchymal genes [61]. Expression of the master EMT transcription factors is activated early in EMT [17,18]. SNAI1 and ZEB1 are expressed in epithelial cells and SNAI2 and ZEB2 are enriched in the early hybrid EMT state [18]. We could show that expression of ZEB1, SNAI2, and ZEB2 is downregulated in KDM5C knockdown cells. Decreased expression of these transcription factors is likely a consequence of the decreased activity of the above-mentioned signaling pathways in KDM5C knockdown. SNAI2 regulates cell proliferation and invasiveness in PCa through EMT [62]. ZEB1 and ZEB2 drive EMT by downregulation of E-cadherin in PCa [63]. TWIST1, which is also downregulated in KDM5C knockdown cells in our studies, suppresses E-cadherin and induces N-cadherin expression independently of SNAIL proteins [64]. In PCa, TWIST1/androgen receptor signaling mediates crosstalk between castration resistance and EMT [65]. TCF, DNMT1, and EZH2 are indirect repressors of E-cadherin, mediated by expression of ZEB1, ZEB2, and SNAI2, respectively [66–68]. We demonstrated that the expression of TCF4, DNMT1, and EZH2 is downregulated upon knockdown of KDM5C.

miR-205 also regulates EMT by targeting ZEB1 and ZEB2 [69] and inhibits cancer cell migration and invasion in PCa [70]. It has been observed that miR-205 is especially down-regulated in cells that have undergone EMT. This is accompanied by a pronounced decrease in E-cadherin and an increase in N-cadherin [69]. Inversely, ectopic expression of miR-205 in mesenchymal cell-initiated MET goes along with upregulation of E-cadherin and reduction of cell locomotion and invasion [69]. Knockdown of KDM5C results in an upregulation of miR-205 in our studies.

Pastushenko et al. discussed that co-expression of epithelial (e.g., E-cadherin) and mesenchymal markers (e.g., SNAI1) rather than either epithelial or mesenchymal states have been associated with poor clinical prognosis [71]. Simeonov et al. showed that in patients with epithelial EMT state, early EMT state and mesenchymal EMT state gene clusters had no association with disease prognosis, however, patients who had enriched late EMT state had a significantly increased risk of death [18]. In pancreatic cancer, the TGFβ signaling pathway is enriched in the late hybrid EMT state and tapered off in the mesenchymal state. Wnt and Notch are enriched only in the late hybrid EMT state and Hedgehog is enriched only in the mesenchymal state. The mTOR signaling pathway is enriched in the transition from the early to the late hybrid EMT state [18]. We found that these pathways were all active in PC3 cells and activity was downregulated in KDM5C knockdown cells. We demonstrated that reduction in viability of KDM5C knockdown cells is only minor in vitro. Therefore, the reduced tumor growth in mouse xenografts is not a result of the differential proliferation of these cells as shown by the unaltered Ki-67 expression in PC3 and KDM5C knockdown cells. Tumor growth might be reduced due to changes in the tumor microenvironment after KDM5C knockdown. Activation of the NF-kappaB pathway in the tumor milieu favors tumor survival and drives abortive activation of immune cells [72]. This pathway might be less active in KDM5C knockdown cells because NF-kappaB (NFKB1) activity was downregulated in these cells.

5. Conclusions

We found that the signaling pathways of the late EMT states are activated in PC3 wild-type and reduced after knockdown of KDM5C. This results in increased expression of E-cadherin, and a decreased expression of N-cadherin. The cells migrate less and are less invasive than PC3 wild-type cells. KDM5C knockdown also leads to reduced tumor growth in in vivo mouse xenografts. Therefore, we hypothesize that inhibition of KDM5C by a selective compound will hinder the process of EMT and delay progression of PCa.

Supplementary Materials: The following are available online at https://www.mdpi.com/article/10.3390/cancers14081894/s1, Table S1: qPCR primers used in this publication; Figure S1: Western blot of the expression of the global histone methylation in histone extracts from PC3 cells and the shRNA-transduced cell clones; Figure S2: Negative correlation between KDM5C and E-cadherin expression in metastatic PCa patient; Figure S3: Expression of ligand and mediator of the Hedgehog and TGFβ signaling pathways associated with EMT progression; Figure S4: Differential phosphokinase-array profiles of different kinases in GFP control 4 as well as KDM5C knockdown clones; Figure S5: Expression of CDH1, CDH2 and KDM5C in mouse xenografts after termination of the experiment; Figure S6: Uncropped Western blot from Figure 2A; Figure S7: Uncropped Western blot from Figure S1; Figure S8: Uncropped Western blot from Figure 3D; Figure S9: Uncropped Western blot from Figure 5J; Figure S10: Uncropped Western blot from Figure S3N.

Author Contributions: Conceptualization, J.K.; methodology, J.K., A.-L.L. and E.S.; validation, A.-L.L., E.S., H.P. and P.L.-K.; formal analysis, J.B.; investigation, A.-L.L., E.S., H.P., P.L.-K., N.K. and A.O.; resources, J.K.; data curation, A.-L.L. and J.K.; writing—original draft preparation, A.-L.L. and J.K.; writing—review and editing, A.-L.L., J.K., H.P., P.L.-K., V.S. and S.P.; visualization, A.-L.L.; supervision, J.K.; project administration, J.K.; funding acquisition, J.K. All authors have read and agreed to the published version of the manuscript.

Funding: This research was funded by the Deutsche Forschungsgemeinschaft (DFG), grant number KI672/6-1. The work was further supported by a grant of the Rudolf Becker Foundation (TO321/36080/2020/kg) to J.K. and S.P.

Institutional Review Board Statement: The study was conducted according to the guidelines of the Declaration of Helsinki, and approved by the Ethics Committee of the University of Luebeck (17-313). Animal experiments were performed by Charles River Discovery Research Services Germany according to a protocol approved by the authorized animal care committee.

Informed Consent Statement: Patient consent was waived since only anonymized clinico-pathological data were used retrospectively (approved from the Review Board of the University of Luebeck).

Data Availability Statement: All datasets generated and analyzed during the current study are available from the corresponding author on request.

Acknowledgments: We thank Maryam Rezaienia and Eva Dreyer for their excellent technical assistance.

Conflicts of Interest: The authors declare no conflict of interest. The funders had no role in the design of the study; in the collection, analyses, or interpretation of data; in the writing of the manuscript, or in the decision to publish the results.

References

1. Siegel, D.A.; O'Neil, M.E.; Richards, T.B.; Dowling, N.F.; Weir, H.K. Prostate Cancer Incidence and Survival, by Stage and Race/Ethnicity—United States, 2001–2017. *MMWR Morb. Mortal. Wkly. Rep.* **2020**, *69*, 1473–1480. [CrossRef]
2. Boutet, A.; De Frutos, C.A.; Maxwell, P.H.; Mayol, M.J.; Romero, J.; Nieto, M.A. Snail activation disrupts tissue homeostasis and induces fibrosis in the adult kidney. *Embo. J.* **2006**, *25*, 5603–5613. [CrossRef]
3. Berx, G.; Raspe, E.; Christofori, G.; Thiery, J.P.; Sleeman, J.P. Pre-EMTing metastasis? Recapitulation of morphogenetic processes in cancer. *Clin. Exp. Metastasis* **2007**, *24*, 587–597. [CrossRef] [PubMed]
4. McDonald, O.G.; Wu, H.; Timp, W.; Doi, A.; Feinberg, A.P. Genome-scale epigenetic reprogramming during epithelial-to-mesenchymal transition. *Nat. Struct. Mol. Biol.* **2011**, *18*, 867–874. [CrossRef] [PubMed]
5. Han, M.; Xu, W.; Cheng, P.; Jin, H.; Wang, X. Histone demethylase lysine demethylase 5B in development and cancer. *Oncotarget* **2017**, *8*, 8980–8991. [CrossRef]
6. Stein, J.; Majores, M.; Rohde, M.; Lim, S.; Schneider, S.; Krappe, E.; Ellinger, J.; Dietel, M.; Stephan, C.; Jung, K.; et al. KDM5C is overexpressed in prostate cancer and is a prognostic marker for prostate-specific antigen-relapse following radical prostatectomy. *Am. J. Pathol.* **2014**, *184*, 2430–2437. [CrossRef]
7. Xu, L.; Wu, W.; Cheng, G.; Qian, M.; Hu, K.; Yin, G.; Wang, S. Enhancement of proliferation and invasion of gastric cancer cell by KDM5C via decrease in p53 expression. *Technol. Cancer Res. Treat.* **2017**, *16*, 141–149. [CrossRef]
8. Ji, X.; Jin, S.; Qu, X.; Li, K.; Wang, H.; He, H.; Guo, F.; Dong, L. Lysine-specific demethylase 5C promotes hepatocellular carcinoma cell invasion through inhibition BMP7 expression. *BMC Cancer* **2015**, *15*, 801. [CrossRef]
9. Li, N.; Dhar, S.S.; Chen, T.Y.; Kan, P.Y.; Wei, Y.; Kim, J.H.; Chan, C.H.; Lin, H.K.; Hung, M.C.; Lee, M.G. JARID1D is a suppressor and prognostic marker of prostate cancer invasion and metastasis. *Cancer Res.* **2016**, *76*, 831–843. [CrossRef]
10. Shaikhibrahim, Z.; Offermann, A.; Braun, M.; Menon, R.; Syring, I.; Nowak, M.; Halbach, R.; Vogel, W.; Ruiz, C.; Zellweger, T.; et al. MED12 overexpression is a frequent event in castration-resistant prostate cancer. *Endocr-Relat Cancer* **2014**, *21*, 663–675. [CrossRef]
11. Sievers, E.; Trautmann, M.; Kindler, D.; Huss, S.; Gruenewald, I.; Dirksen, U.; Renner, M.; Mechtersheimer, G.; Pedeutour, F.; Aman, P.; et al. SRC inhibition represents a potential therapeutic strategy in liposarcoma. *Int. J. Cancer* **2015**, *137*, 2578–2588. [CrossRef] [PubMed]
12. Lim, S.; Janzer, A.; Becker, A.; Zimmer, A.; Schule, R.; Buettner, R.; Kirfel, J. Lysine-specific demethylase 1 (LSD1) is highly expressed in ER-negative breast cancers and a biomarker predicting aggressive biology. *Carcinogenesis* **2010**, *31*, 512–520. [CrossRef] [PubMed]
13. Schulte, J.H.; Lim, S.; Schramm, A.; Friedrichs, N.; Koster, J.; Versteeg, R.; Ora, I.; Pajtler, K.; Klein-Hitpass, L.; Kuhfittig-Kulle, S.; et al. Lysine-specific demethylase 1 is strongly expressed in poorly differentiated neuroblastoma: Implications for therapy. *Cancer Res.* **2009**, *69*, 2065–2071. [CrossRef] [PubMed]

14. Gandellini, P.; Folini, M.; Longoni, N.; Pennati, M.; Binda, M.; Colecchia, M.; Salvioni, R.; Supino, R.; Moretti, R.; Limonta, P.; et al. miR-205 exerts tumor-suppressive functions in human prostate through down-regulation of protein kinase Cepsilon. *Cancer Res.* **2009**, *69*, 2287–2295. [CrossRef] [PubMed]
15. Carvalho, F.L.; Simons, B.W.; Eberhart, C.G.; Berman, D.M. Notch signaling in prostate cancer: A moving target. *Prostate* **2014**, *74*, 933–945. [CrossRef] [PubMed]
16. Jordan, N.V.; Johnson, G.L.; Abell, A.N. Tracking the intermediate stages of epithelial-mesenchymal transition in epithelial stem cells and cancer. *Cell Cycle* **2011**, *10*, 2865–2873. [CrossRef] [PubMed]
17. Pastushenko, I.; Brisebarre, A.; Sifrim, A.; Fioramonti, M.; Revenco, T.; Boumahdi, S.; Van Keymeulen, A.; Brown, D.; Moers, V.; Lemaire, S.; et al. Identification of the tumour transition states occurring during EMT. *Nature* **2018**, *556*, 463–468. [CrossRef]
18. Simeonov, K.P.; Byrns, C.N.; Clark, M.L.; Norgard, R.J.; Martin, B.; Stanger, B.Z.; Shendure, J.; McKenna, A.; Lengner, C.J. Single-cell lineage tracing of metastatic cancer reveals selection of hybrid EMT states. *Cancer Cell* **2021**, *39*, 1150–1162.e9. [CrossRef]
19. Lamouille, S.; Xu, J.; Derynck, R. Molecular mechanisms of epithelial-mesenchymal transition. *Nat. Rev. Mol. Cell Biol.* **2014**, *15*, 178–196. [CrossRef]
20. Taciak, B.; Pruszynska, I.; Kiraga, L.; Bialasek, M.; Krol, M. Wnt signaling pathway in development and cancer. *J. Physiol Pharm.* **2018**, *69*, 185–196. [CrossRef]
21. Zaravinos, A. The Regulatory Role of MicroRNAs in EMT and Cancer. *J. Oncol.* **2015**, *2015*, 865816. [CrossRef] [PubMed]
22. Zhang, J.; Tian, X.J.; Xing, J. Signal transduction pathways of EMT induced by TGF-beta, SHH, and WNT and their crosstalks. *J. Clin. Med.* **2016**, *5*, 41. [CrossRef] [PubMed]
23. Sun, Y.; Schaar, A.; Sukumaran, P.; Dhasarathy, A.; Singh, B.B. TGFbeta-induced epithelial-to-mesenchymal transition in prostate cancer cells is mediated via TRPM7 expression. *Mol. Carcinog.* **2018**, *57*, 752–761. [CrossRef] [PubMed]
24. Bach, D.H.; Park, H.J.; Lee, S.K. The dual role of bone morphogenetic proteins in cancer. *Mol. Ther.-Oncolytics* **2018**, *8*, 1–13. [CrossRef]
25. Massague, J. How cells read TGF-beta signals. *Nat. Rev. Mol. Cell Biol.* **2000**, *1*, 169–178. [CrossRef]
26. Zeisberg, M.; Hanai, J.; Sugimoto, H.; Mammoto, T.; Charytan, D.; Strutz, F.; Kalluri, R. BMP-7 counteracts TGF-beta1-induced epithelial-to-mesenchymal transition and reverses chronic renal injury. *Nat. Med.* **2003**, *9*, 964–968. [CrossRef]
27. Yan, J.D.; Yang, S.; Zhang, J.; Zhu, T.H. BMP6 reverses TGF-beta1-induced changes in HK-2 cells: Implications for the treatment of renal fibrosis. *Acta Pharmacol. Sin.* **2009**, *30*, 994–1000. [CrossRef]
28. Buijs, J.T.; Rentsch, C.A.; van der Horst, G.; van Overveld, P.G.; Wetterwald, A.; Schwaninger, R.; Henriquez, N.V.; Ten Dijke, P.; Borovecki, F.; Markwalder, R.; et al. BMP7, a putat.tive regulator of epithelial homeostasis in the human prostate, is a potent inhibitor of prostate cancer bone metastasis in vivo. *Am. J. Pathol.* **2007**, *171*, 1047–1057. [CrossRef]
29. Nakao, A.; Afrakhte, M.; Moren, A.; Nakayama, T.; Christian, J.L.; Heuchel, R.; Itoh, S.; Kawabata, M.; Heldin, N.E.; Heldin, C.H.; et al. Identification of Smad7, a TGFbeta-inducible antagonist of TGF-beta signalling. *Nature* **1997**, *389*, 631–635. [CrossRef]
30. Villarroel, A.; Del Valle-Perez, B.; Fuertes, G.; Curto, J.; Ontiveros, N.; Garcia de Herreros, A.; Dunach, M. Src and Fyn define a new signaling cascade activated by canonical and non-canonical Wnt ligands and required for gene transcription and cell invasion. *Cell Mol. Life Sci.* **2020**, *77*, 919–935. [CrossRef]
31. Sandsmark, E.; Hansen, A.F.; Selnaes, K.M.; Bertilsson, H.; Bofin, A.M.; Wright, A.J.; Viset, T.; Richardsen, E.; Drablos, F.; Bathen, T.F.; et al. A novel non-canonical Wnt signature for prostate cancer aggressiveness. *Oncotarget* **2017**, *8*, 9572–9586. [CrossRef] [PubMed]
32. Asem, M.S.; Buechler, S.; Wates, R.B.; Miller, D.L.; Stack, M.S. Wnt5a signaling in cancer. *Cancers* **2016**, *8*, 79. [CrossRef] [PubMed]
33. Jho, E.H.; Zhang, T.; Domon, C.; Joo, C.K.; Freund, J.N.; Costantini, F. Wnt/beta-catenin/Tcf signaling induces the transcription of Axin2, a negative regulator of the signaling pathway. *Mol. Cell Biol.* **2002**, *22*, 1172–1183. [CrossRef] [PubMed]
34. Zhang, W.; Lu, W.; Ananthan, S.; Suto, M.J.; Li, Y. Discovery of novel frizzled-7 inhibitors by targeting the receptor's transmembrane domain. *Oncotarget* **2017**, *8*, 91459–91470. [CrossRef]
35. Xie, M.; Zhang, L.; He, C.S.; Xu, F.; Liu, J.L.; Hu, Z.H.; Zhao, L.P.; Tian, Y. Activation of Notch-1 enhances epithelial-mesenchymal transition in gefitinib-acquired resistant lung cancer cells. *J. Cell Biochem.* **2012**, *113*, 1501–1513. [CrossRef]
36. Bin Hafeez, B.; Adhami, V.M.; Asim, M.; Siddiqui, I.A.; Bhat, K.M.; Zhong, W.; Saleem, M.; Din, M.; Setaluri, V.; Mukhtar, H. Targeted knockdown of Notch1 inhibits invasion of human prostate cancer cells concomitant with inhibition of matrix metalloproteinase-9 and urokinase plasminogen activator. *Clin. Cancer Res.* **2009**, *15*, 452–459. [CrossRef]
37. Santagata, S.; Demichelis, F.; Riva, A.; Varambally, S.; Hofer, M.D.; Kutok, J.L.; Kim, R.; Tang, J.; Montie, J.E.; Chinnaiyan, A.M.; et al. JAGGED1 expression is associated with prostate cancer metastasis and recurrence. *Cancer Res.* **2004**, *64*, 6854–6857. [CrossRef]
38. Nanta, R.; Kumar, D.; Meeker, D.; Rodova, M.; Van Veldhuizen, P.J.; Shankar, S.; Srivastava, R.K. NVP-LDE-225 (Erismodegib) inhibits epithelial-mesenchymal transition and human prostate cancer stem cell growth in NOD/SCID IL2Rgamma null mice by regulating Bmi-1 and microRNA-128. *Oncogenesis* **2013**, *2*, e42. [CrossRef]
39. Ishii, A.; Shigemura, K.; Kitagawa, K.; Sung, S.Y.; Chen, K.C.; Yi-Te, C.; Liu, M.C.; Fujisawa, M. Anti-tumor Effect of Hedgehog Signaling Inhibitor, Vismodegib, on Castration-resistant Prostate Cancer. *Anticancer Res.* **2020**, *40*, 5107–5114. [CrossRef]

40. Yamamichi, F.; Shigemura, K.; Behnsawy, H.M.; Meligy, F.Y.; Huang, W.C.; Li, X.; Yamanaka, K.; Hanioka, K.; Miyake, H.; Tanaka, K.; et al. Sonic hedgehog and androgen signaling in tumor and stromal compartments drives epithelial-mesenchymal transition in prostate cancer. *Scand. J. Urol.* **2014**, *48*, 523–532. [CrossRef]
41. Dai, P.; Akimaru, H.; Tanaka, Y.; Maekawa, T.; Nakafuku, M.; Ishii, S. Sonic hedgehog-induced activation of the Gli1 promoter is mediated by GLI3. *J. Biol. Chem.* **1999**, *274*, 8143–8152. [CrossRef] [PubMed]
42. Sasaki, H.; Nishizaki, Y.; Hui, C.C.; Nakafuku, M.; Kondoh, H. Regulation of Gli2 and Gli3 activities by an amino-terminal repression domain: Implication of Gli2 and Gli3 as primary mediators of Shh signaling. *Development* **1999**, *126*, 3915–3924. [CrossRef]
43. Holtz, A.M.; Peterson, K.A.; Nishi, Y.; Morin, S.; Song, J.Y.; Charron, F.; McMahon, A.P.; Allen, B.L. Essential role for ligand-dependent feedback antagonism of vertebrate hedgehog signaling by PTCH1, PTCH2 and HHIP1 during neural patterning. *Development* **2013**, *140*, 3423–3434. [CrossRef] [PubMed]
44. Roshan, M.K.; Soltani, A.; Soleimani, A.; Kahkhaie, K.R.; Afshari, A.R.; Soukhtanloo, M. Role of AKT and mTOR signaling pathways in the induction of epithelial-mesenchymal transition (EMT) process. *Biochimie* **2019**, *165*, 229–234. [CrossRef] [PubMed]
45. Xu, W.; Yang, Z.; Lu, N. A new role for the PI3K/Akt signaling pathway in the epithelial-mesenchymal transition. *Cell Adh. Migr.* **2015**, *9*, 317–324. [CrossRef] [PubMed]
46. Chang, L.; Graham, P.H.; Hao, J.; Ni, J.; Bucci, J.; Cozzi, P.J.; Kearsley, J.H.; Li, Y. Acquisition of epithelial-mesenchymal transition and cancer stem cell phenotypes is associated with activation of the PI3K/Akt/mTOR pathway in prostate cancer radioresistance. *Cell Death Dis.* **2013**, *4*, e875. [CrossRef] [PubMed]
47. Chen, X.; Cheng, H.; Pan, T.; Liu, Y.; Su, Y.; Ren, C.; Huang, D.; Zha, X.; Liang, C. mTOR regulate EMT through RhoA and Rac1 pathway in prostate cancer. *Mol. Carcinog.* **2015**, *54*, 1086–1095. [CrossRef]
48. Garcia, G.E.; Nicole, A.; Bhaskaran, S.; Gupta, A.; Kyprianou, N.; Kumar, A.P. Akt-and CREB-mediated prostate cancer cell proliferation inhibition by Nexrutine, a Phellodendron amurense extract. *Neoplasia* **2006**, *8*, 523–533. [CrossRef]
49. Yin, X.; Yu, J.; Zhou, Y.; Wang, C.; Jiao, Z.; Qian, Z.; Sun, H.; Chen, B. Identification of CDK2 as a novel target in treatment of prostate cancer. *Future Oncol.* **2018**, *14*, 709–718. [CrossRef]
50. Arai, K.; Eguchi, T.; Rahman, M.M.; Sakamoto, R.; Masuda, N.; Nakatsura, T.; Calderwood, S.K.; Kozaki, K.; Itoh, M. A novel high-throughput 3D screening system for EMT inhibitors: A pilot screening discovered the EMT inhibitory activity of CDK2 inhibitor SU9516. *PLoS ONE* **2016**, *11*, e0162394. [CrossRef]
51. Hussain, S.S.; Huang, S.B.; Bedolla, R.G.; Rivas, P.; Basler, J.W.; Swanson, G.P.; Hui-Ming Huang, T.; Narayanasamy, G.; Papanikolaou, N.; Miyamoto, H.; et al. Suppression of ribosomal protein RPS6KB1 by Nexrutine increases sensitivity of prostate tumors to radiation. *Cancer Lett.* **2018**, *433*, 232–241. [CrossRef] [PubMed]
52. Mayr, B.; Montminy, M. Transcriptional regulation by the phosphorylation-dependent factor CREB. *Nat. Rev. Mol. Cell Biol.* **2001**, *2*, 599–609. [CrossRef] [PubMed]
53. Mazor, M.; Kawano, Y.; Zhu, H.; Waxman, J.; Kypta, R.M. Inhibition of glycogen synthase kinase-3 represses androgen receptor activity and prostate cancer cell growth. *Oncogene* **2004**, *23*, 7882–7892. [CrossRef] [PubMed]
54. Shepard, C.R.; Kassis, J.; Whaley, D.L.; Kim, H.G.; Wells, A. PLC gamma contributes to metastasis of in situ-occurring mammary and prostate tumors. *Oncogene* **2007**, *26*, 3020–3026. [CrossRef]
55. Yu, G.; Lee, Y.C.; Cheng, C.J.; Wu, C.F.; Song, J.H.; Gallick, G.E.; Yu-Lee, L.Y.; Kuang, J.; Lin, S.H. RSK promotes prostate cancer progression in bone through ING3, CKAP2, and PTK6-mediated cell survival. *Mol. Cancer Res.* **2015**, *13*, 348–357. [CrossRef]
56. Maffucci, T.; Raimondi, C.; Abu-Hayyeh, S.; Dominguez, V.; Sala, G.; Zachary, I.; Falasca, M. A phosphoinositide 3-kinase/phospholipase Cgamma1 pathway regulates fibroblast growth factor-induced capillary tube formation. *PLoS ONE* **2009**, *4*, e8285. [CrossRef]
57. Moritz, A.; Li, Y.; Guo, A.; Villen, J.; Wang, Y.; MacNeill, J.; Kornhauser, J.; Sprott, K.; Zhou, J.; Possemato, A.; et al. Akt-RSK-S6 kinase signaling networks activated by oncogenic receptor tyrosine kinases. *Sci. Signal.* **2010**, *3*, ra64. [CrossRef]
58. Peltier, J.; O'Neill, A.; Schaffer, D.V. PI3K/Akt and CREB regulate adult neural hippocampal progenitor proliferation and differentiation. *Dev. Neurobiol.* **2007**, *67*, 1348–1361. [CrossRef]
59. Wang, Y.; Wu, J.; Wang, Z. Akt binds to and phosphorylates phospholipase C-gamma1 in response to epidermal growth factor. *Mol. Biol. Cell* **2006**, *17*, 2267–2277. [CrossRef]
60. Zhang, C.; Su, L.; Huang, L.; Song, Z.Y. GSK3beta inhibits epithelial-mesenchymal transition via the Wnt/beta-catenin and PI3K/Akt pathways. *Int. J. Ophthalmol.* **2018**, *11*, 1120–1128. [CrossRef]
61. Puisieux, A.; Brabletz, T.; Caramel, J. Oncogenic roles of EMT-inducing transcription factors. *Nat. Cell Biol.* **2014**, *16*, 488–494. [CrossRef] [PubMed]
62. Emadi Baygi, M.; Soheili, Z.S.; Essmann, F.; Deezagi, A.; Engers, R.; Goering, W.; Schulz, W.A. Slug/SNAI2 regulates cell proliferation and invasiveness of metastatic prostate cancer cell lines. *Tumour. Biol.* **2010**, *31*, 297–307. [CrossRef] [PubMed]
63. Hanrahan, K.; O'Neill, A.; Prencipe, M.; Bugler, J.; Murphy, L.; Fabre, A.; Puhr, M.; Culig, Z.; Murphy, K.; Watson, R.W. The role of epithelial-mesenchymal transition drivers ZEB1 and ZEB2 in mediating docetaxel-resistant prostate cancer. *Mol. Oncol.* **2017**, *11*, 251–265. [CrossRef] [PubMed]
64. Yang, M.H.; Hsu, D.S.; Wang, H.W.; Wang, H.J.; Lan, H.Y.; Yang, W.H.; Huang, C.H.; Kao, S.Y.; Tzeng, C.H.; Tai, S.K.; et al. Bmi1 is essential in Twist1-induced epithelial-mesenchymal transition. *Nat. Cell Biol.* **2010**, *12*, 982–992. [CrossRef] [PubMed]

65. Shiota, M.; Itsumi, M.; Takeuchi, A.; Imada, K.; Yokomizo, A.; Kuruma, H.; Inokuchi, J.; Tatsugami, K.; Uchiumi, T.; Oda, Y.; et al. Crosstalk between epithelial-mesenchymal transition and castration resistance mediated by Twist1/AR signaling in prostate cancer. *Endocr. Relat. Cancer* **2015**, *22*, 889–900. [CrossRef] [PubMed]
66. Sanchez-Tillo, E.; de Barrios, O.; Siles, L.; Cuatrecasas, M.; Castells, A.; Postigo, A. beta-catenin/TCF4 complex induces the epithelial-to-mesenchymal transition (EMT)-activator ZEB1 to regulate tumor invasiveness. *Proc. Natl. Acad. Sci. USA* **2011**, *108*, 19204–19209. [CrossRef]
67. Lee, E.; Wang, J.; Yumoto, K.; Jung, Y.; Cackowski, F.C.; Decker, A.M.; Li, Y.; Franceschi, R.T.; Pienta, K.J.; Taichman, R.S. DNMT1 regulates epithelial-mesenchymal transition and cancer stem cells, which promotes prostate cancer metastasis. *Neoplasia* **2016**, *18*, 553–566. [CrossRef]
68. Wang, J.; He, C.; Gao, P.; Wang, S.; Lv, R.; Zhou, H.; Zhou, Q.; Zhang, K.; Sun, J.; Fan, C.; et al. HNF1B-mediated repression of SLUG is suppressed by EZH2 in aggressive prostate cancer. *Oncogene* **2020**, *39*, 1335–1346. [CrossRef]
69. Gregory, P.A.; Bracken, C.P.; Bert, A.G.; Goodall, G.J. MicroRNAs as regulators of epithelial-mesenchymal transition. *Cell Cycle* **2008**, *7*, 3112–3117. [CrossRef]
70. Nishikawa, R.; Goto, Y.; Kurozumi, A.; Matsushita, R.; Enokida, H.; Kojima, S.; Naya, Y.; Nakagawa, M.; Ichikawa, T.; Seki, N. MicroRNA-205 inhibits cancer cell migration and invasion via modulation of centromere protein F regulating pathways in prostate cancer. *Int. J. Urol.* **2015**, *22*, 867–877. [CrossRef]
71. Pastushenko, I.; Blanpain, C. EMT transition states during tumor progression and metastasis. *Trends Cell Biol.* **2019**, *29*, 212–226. [CrossRef] [PubMed]
72. Whiteside, T.L. The tumor microenvironment and its role in promoting tumor growth. *Oncogene* **2008**, *27*, 5904–5912. [CrossRef] [PubMed]

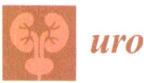 uro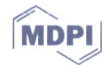

Review

The Prostate Cancer Immune Microenvironment, Biomarkers and Therapeutic Intervention

Yangyi Zhang [1,†], Bethany K. Campbell [1,2,†], Stanley S. Stylli [1,3], Niall M. Corcoran [1,2,4,5,6] and Christopher M. Hovens [1,2,4,6,*]

1. Department of Surgery, University of Melbourne, Parkville, VIC 3050, Australia; yangyiz@student.unimelb.edu.au (Y.Z.); bethany.campbell@unimelb.edu.au (B.K.C.); sstylli@unimelb.edu.au (S.S.S.); con@unimelb.edu.au (N.M.C.)
2. University of Melbourne Centre for Cancer Research, Victorian Comprehensive Cancer Centre, University of Melbourne, Parkville, VIC 3050, Australia
3. Department of Neurosurgery, The Royal Melbourne Hospital, Parkville, VIC 3050, Australia
4. Department of Urology, Royal Melbourne Hospital, Parkville, VIC 3050, Australia
5. Department of Urology, Western Health, Footscray, VIC 3011, Australia
6. University of Melbourne Centre for Cancer Research, Victorian Comprehensive Cancer Centre, Melbourne, VIC 3000, Australia
* Correspondence: chovens@unimelb.edu.au; Tel.: +61-3-9342-7294; Fax: 61-3-9342-8928
† These authors contributed equally to this work.

Simple Summary: Prostate cancer is the most commonly occurring internal malignancy in men. Immunotherapies are emerging as important cancer therapies, having been successfully applied to a range of solid tumour types. However, due to the highly immunosuppressive tumour microenvironment, these successes have not been replicated in prostate cancer. To aid in the selection of patients who would be responsive to immunotherapy, efforts are underway to identify biomarkers which may be indicative of a positive therapeutic response. This review provides an overview of the prostate tumour microenvironment, summarises the immunotherapy approaches being explored for use in prostate cancer, and examines the use of biomarkers for therapy selection.

Abstract: Advanced prostate cancers have a poor survival rate and a lack of effective treatment options. In order to broaden the available treatments, immunotherapies have been investigated. These include cancer vaccines, immune checkpoint inhibitors, chimeric antigen receptor T cells and bispecific antibodies. In addition, combinations of different immunotherapies and with standard therapy have been explored. Despite the success of the Sipuleucel-T vaccine in the metastatic, castrate-resistant prostate cancer setting, other immunotherapies have not shown the same efficacy in this population at large. Some individual patients, however, have shown remarkable responsiveness to these therapies. Therefore, work is underway to identify which populations will respond positively to therapy via the identification of predictive biomarkers. These include biomarkers of the immunologically active tumour microenvironment and biomarkers indicative of high neoantigen expression in the tumour. This review examines the constitution of the prostate tumour immune microenvironment, explores the effectiveness of immunotherapies, and finally investigates how therapy selection can be optimised by the use of biomarkers.

Keywords: prostate cancer; immunotherapy; predictive and prognostic biomarkers; tumour microenvironment; tumour immune microenvironment

1. Introduction

Prostate cancer is the second most frequently diagnosed cancer, and the fifth leading cause of cancer death among men in 2020 [1]. For instance, in 2018 in the U.S there were 3,245,430 men living with prostate cancer. In the U.S in 2021 there will be an estimated

248,530 new diagnoses of prostate cancer, and 34,130 deaths [2]. Due to this high prevalence, prostate cancer screening, consisting of prostate specific antigen (PSA) detection and digital rectal exam, generally commences in men in their 50s. Prostate cancer is a biologically heterogeneous disease that produces variable clinical outcomes. Low- and intermediate-risk localised prostate cancer is generally treated with curative attempts with ablative therapies such as surgery and radiotherapy. Of those patients treated for primary disease, up to 30–40% will eventually fail, and the disease will manifest through biochemical recurrence (BCR) [3,4]. Of these BCR patients who are treated with hormonal therapies approximately 10–20% will develop castrate-resistant cancer within 5 years [5]. Metastatic, castrate-resistant prostate cancer (mCRPC) is a highly aggressive stage of the disease, and has a prognosis of 9–13 months' survival [5]. Due to this poor survival rate of mCRPC, alternate avenues of treatment are being investigated.

Prostate cancer tissue is composed of tumour cells and host components such as immune cells, stromal matrix and soluble factors (e.g., cytokines) with the host components referred to as the Tumour Immune Microenvironment (TIME). Within the TIME, crosstalk occurs between the immune cells, stromal cells, the non-cellular components and the tumour cells, resulting not only in the evolution of the TIME, but also playing a role in tumour progression, tumour clearance or treatment response The TIME interacts with soluble factors secreted by the cancer cells, and in turn, also interacts with the tumour cells. Importantly, whilst providing structural support and contact with prostate cancer cells, the TIME also produce soluble factors, all of which combined can drive prostate cancer progression [6]. Traditionally, it is believed that tumour-intrinsic signalling pathways are oncogenic pathways, however, emerging evidence is showing that this signalling can also regulate the TIME and subsequently tumour immune escape [7,8]. In prostate cancer, this can include PI3K/PTEN/AKT signalling [9,10], TLR9 [11] and p53 loss of function [12], which drives the accumulation, expansion, infiltration and activation of MDSCs. However, immune cells within the prostate cancer TIME act as a double-edged sword, because across the various stages of the disease, the immune cells can also mediate their invasive capacity.

Immunotherapies have shown substantial benefit in other cancers, however, there have been challenges in overcoming the immunosuppressive tumour microenvironment of prostate cancer.

2. The Prostate Tumour Immune Microenvironment

Immune evasion is a hallmark of cancer and dysregulation of the immune microenvironment contributes to malignant progression in prostate cancer [13]. The prostate tumour microenvironment consists of three main compartments: the stroma, the tumour and the immune cells (Figure 1). Together, cellular populations, nutrients and signalling molecules generate a highly immunosuppressive tumour microenvironment.

2.1. The Stromal Compartment

The stromal compartment is inherently plastic and can rapidly respond to damage sustained by the adjacent epithelium. When responding to such damage, stromal cells are phenotypically and genotypically altered, and there is increased matrix remodelling and altered expression of repair-associated growth factors and cytokines. This state is known as reactive stroma [14,15]. In prostate cancer development, reactive stroma initiates during pre-malignant prostatic intraepithelial neoplasia, and co-evolves as the cancer develops [16]. Carcinoma-associated fibroblasts (CAFs) are the main type of cells present in reactive stroma and are central in mediating pro-survival signalling in cancer cells. In terms of the immune microenvironment, CAF proliferation has been shown to lead to the development of a fibrous stroma, which induces localized vasculature remodelling and a state of hypoxia and chronic inflammation [17]. Chronic inflammation is akin to a pre-cancerous state inducing re-modelling of the normal tissue environment, where NF-κB signalling pathways play a defining role. Here, NF-κB-controlled signalling networks modulate the expression of cascades of pro-inflammatory genes, particularly cytokines and chemokines, and also regulate inflammasome formation. In response, immunosuppressive cell populations are recruited to the microenvironment, while cytotoxic T-cell function and dendritic cell maturation are inhibited [18–21]. The transcription factor (HIF-1) which is regulated by oxygen, is also overexpressed in prostate cancer, and is correlated to the clinical stage of the disease [22,23]. Importantly, hypoxia can mediate prostatic adenocarcinoma cell plasticity with the acquisition of a mesenchymal phenotype in a process known as epithelial–mesenchymal transition (EMT). This process can also contribute to immune escape via a loss of cell–cell recognition, as observed with decreased e-cadherin modulating the T-cell synapse which is required for an efficient immune response [24]. In addition, mesenchymal cells exhibit decreased MHC1 expression levels which promotes differentiation/recruitment of T-regulatory lymphocytes (Tregs), immature DCs and ultimately tumour immunosuppression [24].

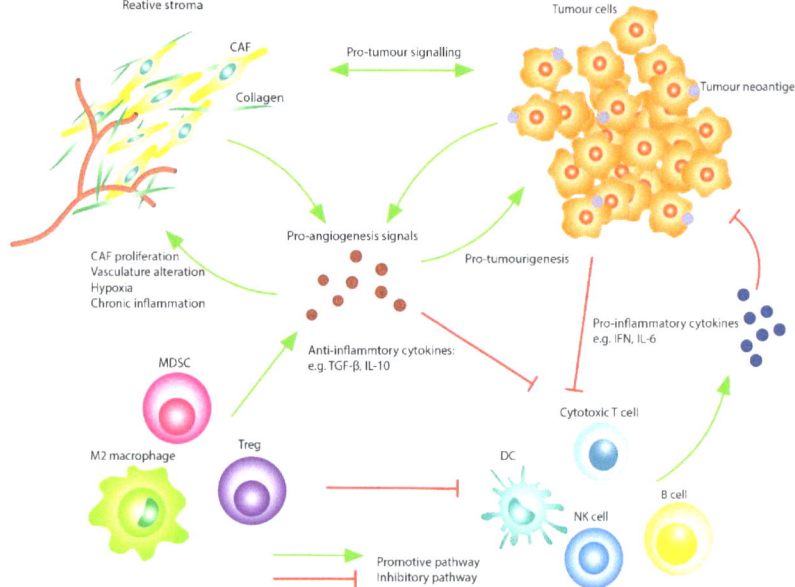

Figure 1. The tumour immune microenvironment of prostate cancer. The tumour microenvironment is composed of stroma, tumour cells and a variety of immune cells. The stromal components and tumour cells interact and promote a hypoxic and pro-tumour environment through cytokine production and pro-inflammatory signalling. As the immune cells infiltrate into the tumour microenvironment, immunosuppressive cells, such as regulatory T cells (Tregs), myeloid-derived suppressor cells (MDSCs) and M2 macrophages, suppress the anti-tumour activity of dendritic cells (DCs), cytotoxic T cells, natural killer (NK) and B cells, which together promote an immunosuppressive environment.

2.2. The Immune Cell Compartment

The prostate tumour microenvironment has altered levels of the various classes of immune cells compared to healthy prostate tissue. This includes tumour-associated macrophages (TAMs), T cells and neutrophils [25]. Interestingly, increased levels of inactive immune cells such as resting natural killer cells, naive B cells and resting dendritic cells are present, which may suggest that the prostate cancer microenvironment inhibits the activation of these cells [25].

The prostate cancer TIME is traditionally regarded as immunologically 'cold' due to its relatively low levels of infiltrating T lymphocytes [26]. This is in part due to the low tumour mutational burden observed in prostate tumours compared to tumours such as melanoma and renal cell carcinoma, thus reducing the presence of tumour neoantigens [25,27]. This, paired with the frequent loss or reduction in major histocompatibility complex (MHC) class I and II expression in antigen-presenting cells, means that the number of anti-tumour T cells being attracted to the tumour is minimal [28–31]. Further contributing to the immunosuppressive microenvironment is the lack of afferent lymphatics to the prostate and the immunosuppressive properties of seminal fluid [32].

In prostate cancer, T cells are the major class of tumour-infiltrating lymphocytes. Higher numbers of infiltrating T cells have been correlated with better clinical outcomes in a variety of solid tumours, including bladder cancer, colorectal cancer, ovarian cancer and melanoma [33–36]. In contrast, the prognostic value of tumour T-cell infiltration is controversial, with both very low and high levels being associated with worse clinical outcomes in prostatectomy specimens [37–40]. This suggests that in cases with low levels of T cells infiltrating, the immune system has failed to mount an effective anti-tumour response. On the other hand, cases with high levels of T-cell infiltration may suggest that the T cells being recruited are able to function effectively. Alternatively, there may be a defect in recruiting the appropriate T-cell subpopulations. For example, these patients might have high infiltration of Tregs. Tregs play an important role in downregulating the cytotoxic T-cell response, and high levels of FOXP3+ Treg infiltration is a negative predictor of overall survival in a range of cancers [41]. High levels of FOXP3+ Tregs have been identified in prostate cancer tumour samples and peripheral blood samples, and may in part explain the dysfunction observed in the cytotoxic CD8+ T cells [42,43].

CD8+ T cells have potent cytotoxic activity and play a key role in anti-tumour immunity. The prognostic value of CD8+ T-cell infiltration in prostate cancer is inconclusive. Several studies have suggested that high CD8+ T-cell infiltration in the tumour epithelium has been reported to be associated with improved overall survival or lower risk of disease relapse and progression in prostatectomy specimens [44,45]. Another study concluded that higher CD8+ and lower programmed death ligand 1 (PD-L1) expression was associated with lower risk of biochemical recurrence and metastasis development [46]. However, others have shown that high levels of CD8+ T cells are associated with worse prognosis [47,48]. One of these studies hypothesised that the failure of high levels of CD8+ T cells to reduce disease recurrence may be due to T-cell exhaustion, and associated expression of PD-1. Interestingly, another study demonstrated that low levels of PD-L1, an immune-suppression marker and ligand of PD-1, combined with high levels of CD8+ T cells, was associated with improved prognosis [46]. This suggests that T-cell exhaustion may play a role in this finding, given the importance of the PD-1/PD-L1 axis in T-cell activation.

Myeloid-derived suppressor cells (MDSCs) and TAMs are key inflammatory cells which also contribute to the immunosuppressive prostate cancer TIME. MDSCs are activated by Tregs and exert their immunosuppressive functions by depletion of arginine and tryptophan in the surrounding tissue. Ultimately, this leads to T-cell cell-cycle arrest and decreased expression of T-cell receptors [49,50]. TAMs can be stratified into two distinct subpopulations, however, the majority of TAMS present in prostate cancer are M2-like, which are associated with an anti-inflammatory phenotype [51]. The presence of M2-like TAMS in both epithelial and stromal compartments is associated with tumour aggressiveness and poorer patient outcomes [52,53].

2.3. Cytokines and Signalling Molecules

A plethora of cytokines are present in the TIME and play an important role in promoting tumorigenesis and regulating the immunosuppressive environment. One example is transforming growth factor-β (TGF-β). In healthy systems, TGF-β acts as a tumour suppressor, where it inhibits proliferation and induces apoptosis. However, when overexpressed in cancers, such as prostate cancer, TGF-β becomes a potent promoter of tumour invasiveness and metastasis [54,55]. One way it mediates this is through promotion of tumour immune evasion through suppression of proliferation and differentiation of lymphocytes, natural killer cells and macrophages [56,57]. On the other hand, anti-tumour cytokines, such as type I interferon (IFN), and their respective signalling pathways, are often suppressed in prostate cancer, especially in the metastatic state [58]. As IFN is important to the coordination of the immune response, the reactivation of the pathway with therapy may promote long-term anti-tumour immunity.

3. Immunotherapy Strategies in Prostate Cancer

Immunotherapy aims to enhance the adaptive immune response, either through enhancing specificity or promoting stronger activation against the tumour. This approach has found success in a range of cancers. However, the immunologically 'cold' nature of prostate cancer has made the development of effective immunotherapies more challenging. Clinical trials currently investigating the use of immunotherapies in prostate cancer patients are summarized in Supplementary Table S1.

3.1. Cancer Vaccines

One class of immunotherapies is cancer vaccines. Cancer vaccines prime the patient's immune system to recognise tumour-associated antigens (Figure 2A). Numerous types of cancer vaccines have been trialled in the prostate cancer setting, including autologous and allogeneic cellular vaccines to stimulate the function of antigen presenting cells, DNA and peptide vaccines which deliver engineered nucleic acids mimicking prostate tumour antigens, and oncolytic virus vaccines which cause direct lysis of tumour cells allowing for the release of a broad range of tumour antigens [59].

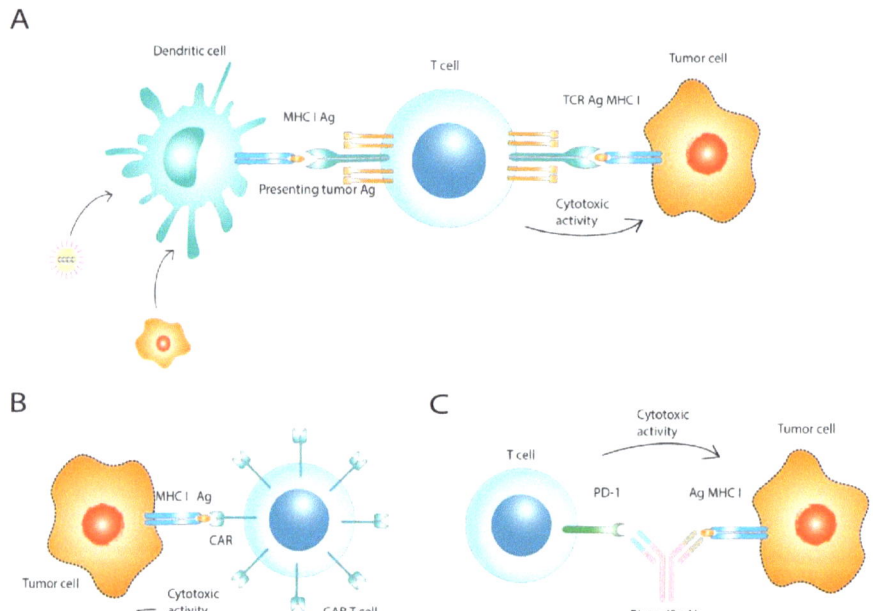

Figure 2. Immunotherapy Strategies in Prostate Cancer. Immunotherapy aims to enhance the adaptive immune response by enhancing specificity or promoting stronger activation against the tumour. (**A**) Cancer vaccines involve vaccination of the patient with tumour peptides, allogeneic whole tumour cells or autologous DCs as vehicles for delivery of the tumour antigen, priming the patient's immune system to recognize the tumour-associated antigens. (**B**) Chimeric Antigen Receptor T Cells (CAR-T) are genetically modified T cells which express a patient antigen-specific chimeric receptor combining both antibody specificity and T-cell effector and regulatory functions. (**C**) Bispecific antibodies (BiTEs) are designed to target the CD3 protein through an effector arm and a tumour antigen via a target arm, which promotes the interaction between tumour cells and CD8+ T cells, resulting in tumour cell death.

Sipuleucel-T is the only FDA-approved immunotherapy for mCRPC. Sipuleucel-T is an autologous cellular cancer vaccine which targets the immune system against prostatic acid phosphatase [60]. Sipuleucel-T treatment significantly increased median overall survival in mCRCP patients [61,62]. Of note, the greatest survival benefits were observed in patients with lower PSA [63]. This highlights that treatment may be more beneficial in the early disease stages, as newly activated cytotoxic T cells have more time to function [64,65]. The importance of an activated immune response is further highlighted by the fact that patients treated with Sipuleucel-T exhibited a 3-fold increase in the presence of activated effector T cells in the tumour microenvironment [64].

Additional vaccines which exhibit signs of efficacy in prostate cancer include PROST-VAC, GVAX and DCVAC/PCa. PROSTVAC is a virus-based vaccine which targets PSA and employs a triad of co-stimulatory molecules (TRICOM; CD-80, ICAM-1, LFA-3) which aid T-cell function, ultimately eliciting a robust immune response [66]. Despite promising initial results in mCRPC, other trials have failed to demonstrate its associated benefits as a monotherapy [67,68]. Similarly, despite promising results of improved patient survival in phase I and II trials, phase III trials with the allogenic GVAX in mCRPC demonstrated poor results and were terminated early [69–71].

3.2. Immune Checkpoint Inhibitors

In order to prevent autoimmunity, healthy cells display proteins known as immune checkpoint molecules. When a T cell binds these, an 'off' signal is sent to prevent T-cell-mediated destruction of the healthy cell. In cancer, however, these immune checkpoints are often upregulated and enhance immune evasion by the tumour. Immune checkpoint inhibitor (ICIs) monoclonal antibodies work by stopping this 'off' signal, and therefore allow the tumour to be targeted by the T cells (Figure 3) [72,73].

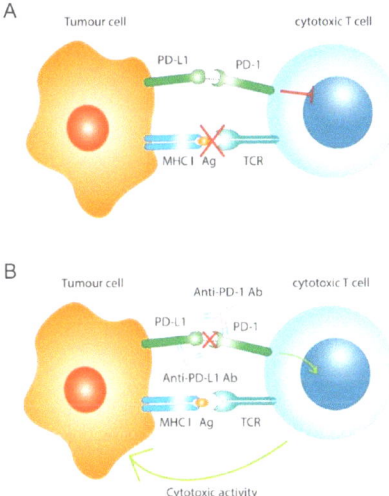

Figure 3. The PD-1 and PD-L1 interaction and its inhibition by immunotherapy. (**A**) PD-1 is expressed on cytotoxic T cells and PD-L1 is expressed on tumour cells. The T-cell receptor (TCR) binds to the tumour antigen (Ag) presented on the tumour cell surface by major histocompatibility complex class I (MHC I). When PD-L1 binds to PD-1, the activity of the cytotoxic T cell will be suppressed and the interaction between TCR and MHC I is blocked. The subsequent immune checkpoint activation can cause apoptosis of cytotoxic T cells. (**B**) Inhibition of PD-1 and PD-L1 activation by anti-PD-1/PD-L1 immunotherapy. Immune checkpoint inhibitors are antibodies that can specifically bind to the immune checkpoint molecules, such as PD-1 and its ligand PD-L1. This binding blocks the interaction between PD-1 and PD-L1 and promotes the anti-tumour activity of the cytotoxic T cell.

Ipilimumab is an ICI that targets CTLA-4, which has been trialled in mCRPC. In mCRPC patients who had failed docetaxel therapy, treatment with ipilimumab, alone or in combination with radiation therapy, resulted in increased median progression-free survival. However, no benefit to overall survival was observed [74]. The benefit was stronger in patients with favourable prognostic factors, especially the absence of visceral metastases. However, a follow-up study in asymptomatic or minimally symptomatic mCRPC patients without visceral metastases did not demonstrate any significant benefit to overall survival [75]. Similarly, anti-PD-1 and anti-PD-L1 agents, such as pembrolizumab, avelumab and nivolumab have been trialled in heavily pre-treated mCRPC. In a phase I trial of nivolumab, an objective response was not observed, while a phase 1 trial of aveulamab reported that 39% of patients had stable disease at >24 weeks [76]. In the same clinical settings, pembrolizmab treatment demonstrated an objective response rate of 17% [77].

3.3. Chimeric Antigen Receptor T Cells

Chimeric Antigen Receptor T Cells (CAR-T) are genetically enhanced T cells modified to engage with specific patient tumour antigens [78], (Figure 2B). This approach has found success in haematological cancers but has shown limited efficacy in the treatment of solid tumours. CAR-T cells targeting PSMA have been developed for the treatment of prostate cancer. This approach has had limited success in clearing tumours, but has demonstrated tumouristatic effects in some preliminary studies [79,80]. Newer generations of CAR-T therapy are integrating elements to counteract the immunosuppressive environment. One study looking at PSMA-directed/TGF-β-insensitive CAR-T cells has reported promising initial results [81,82].

3.4. Bispecific Antibodies

Bispecific antibodies consist of two monoclonal antibodies known as bispecific T-cell engagers (BiTEs) attached by a flexible linker (Figure 2C). These antibodies conjugate simultaneously with tumour antigens and the T cell to promote cytotoxic 4T-cell trafficking and function [83]. A phase I study using the BiTE Pasotuxizumab, which engages CD3 on T cells and PSMA, in androgen deprivation therapy (ADT) and chemotherapy-refractory mCRPC reported positive results, with 88% of patients exhibiting a PSA response in a dose-dependent manner. Interestingly, this resulted in a long-term response in 12.5% of the patients [84]. Another PMSA targeting BiTE, AMG 160, has resulted in a greater than 50% decline in PSA in about one-third of patients, with two patients showing a partial response and eight patients a stable disease (NCT03792841). Trispecific approaches are also being investigated, as demonstrated by the phase I study investigating the safety profile of HPN24 in mCRPC patients who have progressed in systemic therapy (NCT03577028). This is a CD3-PSMA-targeting monoclonal antibody with an albumin-binding domain for extending the half-life of the compound.

3.5. Combination Therapy Strategies

Given the lack of success in finding a single-agent immunotherapy for prostate cancer, the focus has shifted to identifying combination therapies. This includes combining with standard therapies as well as identifying useful dual-immunotherapy approaches.

As chemotherapy is one of the main treatments for cancer, there is strong interest in combining it with immunotherapies, and this approach has yielded early promise. A study of nivolumab plus docetaxel in chemotherapy-native mCRPC patients with ongoing ADT therapy reported an objective response rate of 40% and a median overall survival of 18 months following treatment [85]. Interim analysis from a second study of pembrolizumab and docetaxel and prednisone in mCRPC previously treated with ADT reported an objective response rate of 23.1% [86]. It has been suggested that chemotherapy releases neoantigens from the tumour upon cell death and these neoantigens promote the activation of CD8+ cells, thus promoting the efficacy of immunotherapies.

Like chemotherapy, poly-ADP ribose polymerase (PARP) inhibitors promote the necrotic release of tumour neoantigens. Additionally, like chemotherapy, their effectiveness as part of a combination therapy with immunotherapies has also been investigated. Most promisingly, treatment with durbalumab and PARP inhibitor, oliparib, in mCRPC patients who had progressed with androgen deprivation therapy reported that 53% of patients had a radiographic and/or PSA response [87]. An interim analysis of a second study reports a PSA response in 9%, and a partial response in 8% of those with measurable disease in mCRPC patients previously treated with docetaxel, following treatment with pembrolizumab and oliparib [88].

Another combination of interest is treatment with androgen-deprivation therapy and immunotherapies. It has been shown that ADT results in increased trafficking of anti-tumour immune cells, and as such, ADT may enhance the effectiveness of immunotherapies [89]. Across multiple studies, treatment with pembrolizumab in patients with mCRPC who had previously been treated with ADT reported a disease control rate of between 35 and 51%, however, one study did not show any benefit of therapy [90–92].

The combination of anti-angiogenic therapies with those of immunotherapies has also recently attracted interest. Here, it has been shown that tumour angiogenesis-targeted agents such as Sunitinib can induce a pro-immunogenic state in the tumour by inducing miR-221 expression. This is then thought to cause an induction of an interferon-related gene signature in the prostate cancer cells supported by miR-221 upregulation [93]. These data would suggest that the treatment combination of tumour kinase inhibitors (TKIs) and immune-based approaches might be a promising avenue to explore with TKIs treatment, inducing an immune responsive environment due to boosting miR-221 expression levels.

One of the main immunotherapy combination strategies under investigation is co-treatment with anti-PD-1 and anti-CTLA-4 agents. A study on asymptomatic or minimally symptomatic mCRPC patients not previously treated with ipilimumab and nivolumab showed an objective response rate of 26% at interim reporting, while in those who had progressed with chemotherapy, the objective response rate was 10% [94,95]. Ipilimumab and nivolumab have also been trialled in a subgroup of mCRPC patients positive for AR-V7. Outcomes tended to be better in a subset of patients, specifically in those with DNA damage repair mutations, however this was only significantly different in terms of progression-free survival [96]. This highlights the importance of biomarkers to enable selection of patients who will respond to therapy.

4. Immune Therapy Biomarkers

Metastatic prostate cancer presents a range of challenges to treatment with immunotherapy. Early studies on the use of these agents in prostate cancer have been characterised by a lack of response in a high percentage of patients. However, there is evidence that some subpopulations are highly responsive to immunotherapy. Therefore, it will likely be pertinent to identify improved molecular biomarkers that will allow for the selection of those patients that are most likely to benefit.

4.1. Immune Checkpoint Molecules as Biomarkers

ICI directly targets the immune checkpoint molecules; therefore, it follows that the expression of such molecules may be an important determinant of therapy response. PD-L1 levels have been shown to have varying degrees of association with therapy, with expression correlated with ICI response in melanoma but not in squamous cell carcinoma and non-small-cell lung cancer [97–99]. The expression of PD-L1 and PD-1 is low in healthy prostate tissue, present in around 0.5% and 1.5% of cases, respectively, and is increased in prostate cancer cases, with one study reporting positive staining in 13.2% and 7.7%, respectively [100]. Although dynamic expression is observed, high PD-L1 expression is associated with prostate cancer aggressiveness, with 61.7% of aggressive primary prostate tumours and 50% of CRPC expressing PD-L1 [101,102]. Despite this, PD-L1 expression does not strongly predict response to ICI in prostate cancer. A study examining pembrolizumab efficacy in PD-L1-positive versus PD-L1-negative cohorts of treatment-refractory mCRPC patients reported objective response rates of 5% and 3%, respectively [103]. This suggests that other factors contribute to the effectiveness of anti-PD-L1 therapy in these patients and that simple measurement of PD-L1 levels in tissue may not be an effective biomarker of treatment response.

4.2. Genetic Variations as Biomarkers

Genetic mutations present in a tumour can be a powerful predictor of therapy response. Prostate cancer has traditionally been difficult to target with immunotherapy due to its low number of mutations and therefore presence of fewer neoantigens, especially in relation to other highly mutated cancers such as melanoma and lung cancer [27].

Patients with high microsatellite instability (MSI-H) or mismatch-repair-deficient (MMRd) tumours have a high tumour mutational burden (TMB) and increased presence of tumour neoantigens, and are therefore strong candidates for immune checkpoint inhibitor immunotherapy [104,105]. The ICI pembrolizumab is FDA-approved for use in metastatic/unresectable MSI-H/MMRd tumours, however it is only effective in a subset of prostate cancer patients [106]. A retrospective study reported durable clinical benefit in 45.5% of MSI-H/MMRd prostate tumours treated with anti-PD1 or anti-PDL1 agents, either as monotherapy or combination therapy [107]. In addition, a second study observed increased overall survival in patients with higher-than-median TMB following ICI therapy [94].

Increased neoantigen expression and higher TMB is also associated with mutations in specific genes, particularly those involved in DNA damage repair such as BRCA1/2, ATM, MSH2, POLE and CDK12 [108–111]. A comprehensive analysis of POLE/POLD1 mutation in multiple cancer types reported that 1.8% of primary prostate tumours had mutations in one or both genes, correlating with a significantly higher TMB. Patients with POLE/POLD1 mutations have been shown to have longer overall survival following ICI treatment across all tumour types, with POLE/POLD1 reported as an independent risk factor for identifying prostate cancer patients who benefited from ICI [110].

CDK12 mutations are observed in 1.2% of primary prostate tumours, rising to 6.9% of mCRPC. A unique mutation signature was observed for CDK12-deficient tumours, differentiating it distinctly from MMRd prostate tumours [105]. PSA decline following ICI treatment has been observed in patients with CDK-12 mutations in a number of studies [105,111–113]. Interestingly, there was no difference observed between patients with mono- versus bi-allelic mutations in PSA decline, however, PSA-progression-free survival was marginally improved for those with biallelic mutations [113]. These retrospective studies indicate that prospective randomized trials incorporating genomic screening and selection of patients with MSI-H/MMRd prostate tumours with higher-than-median TMB or CDK12 mutations would be highly informative as to the usefulness of treating these patients with ICI-based therapies. At the present time, this combined strategy would appear to be the most promising of the genomic-based approaches to enhance ICI response rates in prostate cancer.

4.3. Peripheral Immune-Based Biomarkers

Traditionally, mutational status of tumours has been assessed via biopsy, however biopsy acquisition is an invasive procedure that is not always practical for cancer patients. In contrast, blood samples are relatively easy to obtain and are being investigated as a potentially rich source of biomarkers.

One such source of biomarkers is circulating tumour DNA (ctDNA). ctDNA-based assays are becoming increasingly popular as an alternative to biopsy for the detection of actionable genetic mutations. A case series reported the detection of MSI-H status in two prostate cancer patients via ctDNA samples. Importantly, they were able to monitor the response to treatment by using the frequency of variant alleles in blood samples as a readout, since it can be repeated for real-time monitoring of tumour clones [114]. This demonstrates the utility of such technologies as biomarkers of potential treatment efficacy and in monitoring response.

Cytokines are key regulators of the immune response; therefore, several studies have explored cytokine levels at baseline and their correlation with response to immunotherapy treatment, in particular treatment with cancer vaccines. One study suggests that higher baseline circulating interleukin-10 (IL-10) levels in CRPC patients may be negatively associated with response to treatment with a DNA vaccine encoding prostatic acid phosphatase [115]. A second study demonstrated that higher baseline levels of interleukin-6 (IL-6) was associated with shorter survival in patients treated with the personalized peptide vaccine [116].

The presence of various immune cell populations, such as T cells and MDSCs, have also been investigated for their merit as predictive biomarkers for clinical response to immunotherapy. Lower baseline levels of PD-1$^+$Tim-3^{NEG} CD4 effector memory cells and higher baseline PD-1^{NEG}Tim-3$^+$ CD8 and CTLA-4^{NEG} Tregs in mCRPC predicted improved survival following treatment with PROSTVAC and ipilimumab [117]. Similarly, higher baseline levels of CD4$^+$CTLA-4$^+$ T cells predicted improved survival when treated with GVAX and ipilimumab. In contrast, CRPC patients with higher CD14$^+$HLA-DR-monocytic MDSCs had worse survival following treatment [118]. There is also evidence that early changes in circulating immune cells can be used to monitor the response and adjust treatments accordingly, as a study reported that in mCRPC patients treated with DCVac and docetaxel an on-treatment decrease in MDSC independently predicted disease-specific survival [119].

5. Conclusions

As the second most commonly diagnosed cancer in males, prostate cancer is a major health concern. In particular, metastatic, castrate-resistant prostate cancer patients have poor survival rates. Immunotherapies have seen success in many other cancers; however, the treatment of prostate cancer through these methods suffers due to the immunosuppressive tumour microenvironment. Recent studies have helped elucidate many of the immune-suppressive mechanisms at play in prostate cancer. This knowledge, in combination with biomarkers, can help inform treatment selection and allow these mechanisms to be overcome through combination therapy strategies.

Supplementary Materials: The following supporting information can be downloaded at: https://www.mdpi.com/article/10.3390/uro2020010/s1, Table S1: Current immunotherapy clinical trials in prostate cancer [120–159].

Author Contributions: Writing—original draft preparation, Y.Z., B.K.C.; writing—review and editing, B.K.C., S.S.S., N.M.C., C.M.H.; supervision, N.M.C., C.M.H. All authors have read and agreed to the published version of the manuscript.

Funding: Support for this work was provided through the NHMRC project grant 1162514 to C.M.H. and the PRECEPT program grant, co-funded by Movember and the Australian Federal Government to N.M.C. N.M.C. was supported by a David Bickart Clinician Researcher Fellowship from the Faculty of Medicine, Dentistry and Health Sciences, University of Melbourne, and more recently by a Movember—Distinguished Gentleman's Ride Clinician Scientist Award through the Prostate Cancer Foundation of Australia's Research Program.

Institutional Review Board Statement: Not applicable.

Informed Consent Statement: Not applicable.

Data Availability Statement: Not applicable.

Conflicts of Interest: The authors declare no conflict of interest.

Abbreviations

ADT (Androgen-deprivation therapy); AKT (Ak strain transforming); ATM (ataxia telangiectasia mutated); BCR (biochemical recurrence); BRCA1 (Breast Cancer gene 1); BRAC2 (Breast Cancer Gene 2); CAFS (carcinoma-associated fibroblasts); CAR-T (Chimeric antigen receptor T cells); CD3 (cluster of differentiation 3); CD38 (cluster of differentiation 38); CD39 (cluster of differentiation 39); CD73 (cluster of differentiation 73); CDK12 (cyclin-dependent kinase 12); CRPC (castrate-resistant prostate cancer); CtDNA (circulating tumour DNA); (CTLA-4 cytotoxic T-lymphocyte-associated protein 4); DCs (dendritic cells); DLL3 (delta-like ligand 3); FDA (Food and Drug Administration); FOXP3 (Forkhead box P3); DNA (deoxyribonucleic acid); ICAM-1 (intercellular adhesion molecule-1); ICI (immune checkpoint inhibitor); IFN (interferon); IL-6 (interleukin 6); IL-8 (interleukin 8); IL-10 (interleukin 10); LFA-3 (Lymphocyte Function-Associated Antigen 3); mCRPC (metastatic, castrate-resistant prostate cancer); MDSCs (myeloid-derived suppressor cells); MHC (major histocompatibility complex); MMRd (mismatch repair deficient); MSH-I (high microsatellite instability); NK (natural killer cells); MSH2 (MutS homolog 2); PAP (prostatic acid phosphatase); PARP (poly-ADP ribose polymerase); (PD-1 (Programmed cell death protein 1); PD-L1 (Programmed death-ligand 1); PI3K (phosphoinositide 3-kinases); POLD1 (DNA Polymerase Delta 1); POLE (DNA polymerase epsilon); PSA (prostate-specific antigen); PSMA (Prostate Specific Membrane Antigen); PTEN (phosphatase and tensin homolog); STEAP1 (six-transmembrane epithelial antigen of prostate); TAMS (tumour-associated macrophages); TCR (T-cell receptor); TGF-β (transforming growth factor-β); TGF-β RII (transforming growth factor-β receptor II); TIME (tumour immune microenvironment); TKI (tyrosine kinase inhibitor); Tregs (regulatory T cells); Tumour mutational burden (TMB)

References

1. Sung, H.; Ferlay, J.; Siegel, R.L.; Laversanne, M.; Soerjomataram, I.; Jemal, A.; Bray, F. Global Cancer Statistics 2020: GLOBOCAN Estimates of Incidence and Mortality Worldwide for 36 Cancers in 185 Countries. *CA Cancer J. Clin.* **2021**, *71*, 209–249. [CrossRef] [PubMed]
2. Islami, F.; Ward, E.M.; Sung, H.; Cronin, K.A.; Tangka, F.K.L.; Sherman, R.L.; Zhao, J.; Anderson, R.N.; Henley, S.J.; Yabroff, K.R.; et al. Annual Report to the Nation on the Status of Cancer, Part 1: National Cancer Statistics. *JNCI J. Natl. Cancer Inst.* **2021**, *113*, 1648–1669. [CrossRef] [PubMed]
3. Freedland, S.J.; Humphreys, E.B.; Mangold, L.A.; Eisenberger, M.; Dorey, F.J.; Walsh, P.C.; Partin, A.W. Risk of prostate cancer-specific mortality following biochemical recurrence after radical prostatectomy. *J. Am. Med. Assoc.* **2005**, *294*, 433–439. [CrossRef] [PubMed]
4. Roehl, K.A.; Han, M.; Ramos, C.G.; Antenor, J.A.V.; Catalona, W.J. Cancer progression and survival rates following anatomical radical retropubic prostatectomy in 3,478 consecutive patients: Long-term results. *J. Urol.* **2004**, *172*, 910–914. [CrossRef]
5. Kirby, M.; Hirst, C.; Crawford, E.D. Characterising the castration-resistant prostate cancer population: A systematic review. *Int. J. Clin. Pract.* **2011**, *65*, 1180–1192. [CrossRef]
6. Keller, E.T.; Zhang, J.; Cooper, C.R.; Smith, P.C.; McCauley, L.K.; Pienta, K.J.; Taichman, R.S. Prostate carcinoma skeletal metastases: Cross-talk between tumor and bone. *Cancer Metastasis Rev.* **2001**, *20*, 333–349. [CrossRef]
7. Altorki, N.K.; Markowitz, G.J.; Gao, D.; Port, J.L.; Saxena, A.; Stiles, B.; McGraw, T.; Mittal, V. The lung microenvironment: An important regulator of tumour growth and metastasis. *Nat. Rev. Cancer* **2019**, *19*, 9–31. [CrossRef]
8. Spranger, S.; Gajewski, T.F. Tumor-intrinsic oncogene pathways mediating immune avoidance. *Oncoimmunology* **2016**, *5*, e1086862. [CrossRef]
9. Garcia, A.J.; Ruscetti, M.; Arenzana, T.L.; Tran, L.M.; Bianci-Frias, D.; Sybert, E.; Priceman, S.J.; Wu, L.; Nelson, P.S.; Smale, S.T.; et al. Pten null prostate epithelium promotes localized myeloid-derived suppressor cell expansion and immune suppression during tumor initiation and progression. *Mol. Cell. Biol.* **2014**, *34*, 2017–2028. [CrossRef]
10. Wang, G.; Lu, X.; Dey, P.; Deng, P.; Wu, C.C.; Jiang, S.; Fang, Z.; Zhao, K.; Konaparthi, R.; Hua, S.; et al. Targeting YAP-Dependent MDSC Infiltration Impairs Tumor Progression. *Cancer Discov.* **2016**, *6*, 80–95. [CrossRef]
11. Won, H.; Moreira, D.; Gao, C.; Duttagupta, P.; Zhao, X.; Manuel, E.; Diamond, D.; Yuan, Y.; Liu, Z.; Jones, J.; et al. TLR9 expression and secretion of LIF by prostate cancer cells stimulates accumulation and activity of polymorphonuclear MDSCs. *J. Leukoc. Biol.* **2017**, *102*, 423–436. [CrossRef] [PubMed]

12. Guo, G.; Marrero, L.; Rodriguez, P.; Del Valle, L.; Ochoa, A.; Cui, Y. Trp53 inactivation in the tumor microenvironment promotes tumor progression by expanding the immunosuppressive lymphoid-like stromal network. *Cancer Res.* **2013**, *73*, 1668–1675. [CrossRef] [PubMed]
13. Vinay, D.S.; Ryan, E.P.; Pawelec, G.; Talib, W.H.; Stagg, J.; Elkord, E.; Lichtor, T.; Decker, W.K.; Whelan, R.L.; Kumara, H.M.C.S.; et al. Immune evasion in cancer: Mechanistic basis and therapeutic strategies. *Semin. Cancer Biol.* **2015**, *35*, S185–S198. [CrossRef] [PubMed]
14. Rowley, D.R. What might a stromal response mean to prostate cancer progression? *Cancer Metastasis Rev.* **1998**, *17*, 411–419. [CrossRef] [PubMed]
15. Tuxhorn, J.A.; Ayala, G.E.; Smith, M.J.; Smith, V.C.; Dang, T.D.; Rowley, D.R. Reactive stroma in human prostate cancer: Induction of myofibroblast phenotype and extracellular matrix remodeling. *Clin. Cancer Res.* **2002**, *8*, 2912–2923. [PubMed]
16. Tuxhorn, J.A.; Ayala, G.E.; Rowley, D.R. Reactive stroma in prostate cancer progression. *J. Urol.* **2001**, *166*, 2472–2483. [CrossRef]
17. Ammirante, M.; Shalapour, S.; Kang, Y.; Jamieson, C.A.M.; Karin, M. Tissue injury and hypoxia promote malignant progression of prostate cancer by inducing CXCL13 expression in tumor myofibroblasts. *Proc. Natl. Acad. Sci. USA* **2014**, *111*, 14776–14781. [CrossRef]
18. Huang, Y.; Yuan, J.; Righi, E.; Kamoun, W.S.; Ancukiewicz, M.; Nezivar, J.; Santosuosso, M.; Martin, J.D.; Martin, M.R.; Vianello, F.; et al. Vascular normalizing doses of antiangiogenic treatment reprogram the immunosuppressive tumor microenvironment and enhance immunotherapy. *Proc. Natl. Acad. Sci. USA* **2012**, *109*, 17561–17566. [CrossRef]
19. Gabrilovich, D.; Ishida, T.; Oyama, T.; Ran, S.; Kravtsov, V.; Nadaf, S.; Carbone, D.P. Vascular endothelial growth factor inhibits the development of dendritic cells and dramatically affects the differentiation of multiple hematopoietic lineages in vivo. *Blood* **1998**, *92*, 4150–4166. [CrossRef]
20. Gabrilovich, D.I.; Chen, H.L.; Girgis, K.R.; Cunningham, H.T.; Meny, G.M.; Nadaf, S.; Kavanaugh, D.; Carbone, D.P. Production of vascular endothelial growth factor by human tumors inhibits the functional maturation of dendritic cells. *Nat. Med.* **1996**, *2*, 1096–1103. [CrossRef]
21. Voron, T.; Colussi, O.; Marcheteau, E.; Pernot, S.; Nizard, M.; Pointet, A.L.; Latreche, S.; Bergaya, S.; Benhamouda, N.; Tanchot, C.; et al. VEGF-A modulates expression of inhibitory checkpoints on CD8++ T cells in tumors. *J. Exp. Med.* **2015**, *212*, 139–148. [CrossRef] [PubMed]
22. Movsas, B.; Chapman, J.D.; Greenberg, R.E.; Hanlon, A.L.; Horwitz, E.M.; Pinover, W.H.; Stobbe, C.; Hanks, G.E. Increasing levels of hypoxia in prostate carcinoma correlate significantly with increasing clinical stage and patient age: An Eppendorf pO2 study. *Cancer* **2000**, *89*, 2018–2024. [CrossRef]
23. Turaka, A.; Buyyounouski, M.K.; Hanlon, A.L.; Horwitz, E.M.; Greenberg, R.E.; Movsas, B. Hypoxic prostate/muscle Po 2 ratio predicts for outcome in patients with localized prostate cancer: Long-term results. *Int. J. Radiat. Oncol. Biol. Phys.* **2012**, *82*, e433–e439. [CrossRef] [PubMed]
24. Terry, S.; Savagner, P.; Ortiz-Cuaran, S.; Mahjoubi, L.; Saintigny, P.; Thiery, J.P.; Chouaib, S. New insights into the role of EMT in tumor immune escape. *Mol. Oncol.* **2017**, *11*, 824–846. [CrossRef] [PubMed]
25. Wu, Z.; Chen, H.; Luo, W.; Zhang, H.; Li, G.; Zeng, F.; Deng, F. The Landscape of Immune Cells Infiltrating in Prostate Cancer. *Front. Oncol.* **2020**, *10*, 517637. [CrossRef]
26. Bonaventura, P.; Shekarian, T.; Alcazer, V.; Valladeau-Guilemond, J.; Valsesia-Wittmann, S.; Amigorena, S.; Caux, C.; Depil, S. Cold tumors: A therapeutic challenge for immunotherapy. *Front. Immunol.* **2019**, *10*, 168. [CrossRef]
27. Berger, M.F.; Lawrence, M.S.; Demichelis, F.; Drier, Y.; Cibulskis, K.; Sivachenko, A.Y.; Sboner, A.; Esgueva, R.; Pflueger, D.; Sougnez, C.; et al. The genomic complexity of primary human prostate cancer. *Nature* **2011**, *470*, 214–220. [CrossRef]
28. Sharpe, J.C.; Abel, P.D.; Gilbertston, J.A.; Brawn, P.; Foster, C.S. Modulated expression of human leucocyte antigen class I and class II determinants in hyperplastics and malignant human prostatic epithelium. *Br. J. Urol.* **1994**, *74*, 609–616. [CrossRef]
29. Blades, R.A.; Keating, P.J.; McWilliam, L.J.; George, N.J.R.; Stern, P.L. Loss of HLA class I expression in prostate cancer: Implications for immunotherapy. *Urology* **1995**, *46*, 681–687. [CrossRef]
30. Blumenfeld, W.; Ye, J.Q.; Dahiya, R.; Griffiss, J.M.; Narayan, P. HLA expression by benign and malignant prostatic epithelium: Augmentation by interferon-gamma. *J. Urol.* **1993**, *150*, 1289–1292. [CrossRef]
31. Bander, N.H.; Yao, D.; Liu, H.; Chen, Y.T.; Steiner, M.; Zuccaro, W.; Moy, P. MHC class I and II expression in prostate carcinoma and modulation by interferon-alpha and -gamma. *Prostate* **1997**, *33*, 233–239. [CrossRef]
32. McClinton, S.; Miller, I.D.; Eremin, O. An immunohistochemical characterisation of the inflammatory cell infiltrate in benign and malignant prostatic disease. *Br. J. Cancer* **1990**, *61*, 400–403. [CrossRef] [PubMed]
33. Bogunovic, D.; O'Neill, D.W.; Belitskaya-Levy, I.; Vacic, V.; Yu, Y.L.; Adams, S.; Darvishian, F.; Berman, R.; Shapiro, R.; Pavlick, A.C.; et al. Immune profile and mitotic index of metastatic melanoma lesions enhance clinical staging in predicting patient survival. *Proc. Natl. Acad. Sci. USA* **2009**, *106*, 20429–20434. [CrossRef]
34. Simpson, J.A.D.; Al-Attar, A.; Watson, N.F.S.; Scholefield, J.H.; Ilyas, M.; Durrant, L.G. Intratumoral T cell infiltration, MHC class I and STAT1 as biomarkers of good prognosis in colorectal cancer. *Gut* **2010**, *59*, 926–933. [CrossRef] [PubMed]
35. Oble, D.A.; Loewe, R.; Yu, P.; Mihm, M.C. Focus on TILs: Prognostic significance of tumor infiltrating lymphocytes in human melanoma. *Cancer Immun.* **2009**, *9*, 3. [PubMed]

36. Zhang, L.; Conejo-Garcia, J.R.; Katsaros, D.; Gimotty, P.A.; Massobrio, M.; Regnani, G.; Makrigiannakis, A.; Gray, H.; Schlienger, K.; Liebman, M.N.; et al. Intratumoral T Cells, Recurrence, and Survival in Epithelial Ovarian Cancer. *N. Engl. J. Med.* **2003**, *348*, 203–213. [CrossRef] [PubMed]
37. Flammiger, A.; Bayer, F.; Cirugeda-Kühnert, A.; Huland, H.; Tennstedt, P.; Simon, R.; Minner, S.; Bokemeyer, C.; Sauter, G.; Schlomm, T.; et al. Intratumoral T but not B lymphocytes are related to clinical outcome in prostate cancer. *APMIS* **2012**, *120*, 901–908. [CrossRef]
38. Kärjä, V.; Aaltomaa, S.; Lipponen, P.; Isotalo, T.; Talja, M.; Mokka, R. Tumour-infiltrating lymphocytes: A prognostic factor of psa-free survival in patients with local prostate carcinoma treated by radical prostatectomy. *Anticancer Res.* **2005**, *25*, 4435–4438.
39. Vesalainen, S.; Lipponen, P.; Talja, M.; Syrjänen, K. Histological grade, perineural infiltration, tumour-infiltrating lymphocytes and apoptosis as determinants of long-term prognosis in prostatic adenocarcinoma. *Eur. J. Cancer* **1994**, *30*, 1797–1803. [CrossRef]
40. Irani, J.; Goujon, J.M.; Ragni, E.; Peyrat, L.; Hubert, J.; Saint, F.; Mottet, N. High-grade inflammation in prostate cancer as a prognostic factor for biochemical recurrence after radical prostatectomy. *Urology* **1999**, *54*, 467–472. [CrossRef]
41. Saleh, R.; Elkord, E. FoxP3+ T regulatory cells in cancer: Prognostic biomarkers and therapeutic targets. *Cancer Lett.* **2020**, *490*, 174–185. [CrossRef] [PubMed]
42. Miller, A.M.; Lundberg, K.; Özenci, V.; Banham, A.H.; Hellström, M.; Egevad, L.; Pisa, P. CD4 + CD25 high T Cells Are Enriched in the Tumor and Peripheral Blood of Prostate Cancer Patients. *J. Immunol.* **2006**, *177*, 7398–7405. [CrossRef] [PubMed]
43. Kiniwa, Y.; Miyahara, Y.; Wang, H.Y.; Peng, W.; Peng, G.; Wheeler, T.M.; Thompson, T.C.; Old, L.J.; Wang, R.F. CD8+ Foxp3+ regulatory T cells mediate immunosuppression in prostate cancer. *Clin. Cancer Res.* **2007**, *13*, 6947–6958. [CrossRef] [PubMed]
44. Yang, Y.; Attwood, K.; Bshara, W.; Mohler, J.L.; Guru, K.; Xu, B.; Kalinski, P.; Chatta, G. High intratumoral CD8+ T-cell infiltration is associated with improved survival in prostate cancer patients undergoing radical prostatectomy. *Prostate* **2021**, *81*, 20–28. [CrossRef]
45. Sorrentino, C.; Musiani, P.; Pompa, P.; Cipollone, G.; Di Carlo, E. Androgen deprivation boosts prostatic infiltration of cytotoxic and regulatory T lymphocytes and has no effect on disease-free survival in prostate cancer patients. *Clin. Cancer Res.* **2011**, *17*, 1571–1581. [CrossRef]
46. Vicier, C.; Ravi, P.; Kwak, L.; Werner, L.; Huang, Y.; Evan, C.; Loda, M.; Hamid, A.A.; Sweeney, C.J. Association between CD8 and PD-L1 expression and outcomes after radical prostatectomy for localized prostate cancer. *Prostate* **2021**, *81*, 50–57. [CrossRef]
47. Ness, N.; Andersen, S.; Valkov, A.; Nordby, Y.; Donnem, T.; Al-Saad, S.; Busund, L.T.; Bremnes, R.M.; Richardsen, E. Infiltration of CD8+ lymphocytes is an independent prognostic factor of biochemical failure-free survival in prostate cancer. *Prostate* **2014**, *74*, 1452–1461. [CrossRef]
48. Zhao, S.G.; Lehrer, J.; Chang, S.L.; Das, R.; Erho, N.; Liu, Y.; Sjöström, M.; Den, R.B.; Freedland, S.J.; Klein, E.A.; et al. The immune landscape of prostate cancer and nomination of PD-L2 as a potential therapeutic target. *J. Natl. Cancer Inst.* **2019**, *111*, 301–310. [CrossRef]
49. Rodriguez, P.C.; Quiceno, D.G.; Zabaleta, J.; Ortiz, B.; Zea, A.H.; Piazuelo, M.B.; Delgado, A.; Correa, P.; Brayer, J.; Sotomayor, E.M.; et al. Arginase I production in the tumor microenvironment by mature myeloid cells inhibits T-cell receptor expression and antigen-specific T-cell responses. *Cancer Res.* **2004**, *64*, 5839–5849. [CrossRef]
50. Rodriguez, P.C.; Quiceno, D.G.; Ochoa, A.C. L-arginine availability regulates T-lymphocyte cell-cycle progression. *Blood* **2007**, *109*, 1568–1573. [CrossRef]
51. Lundholm, M.; Hägglöf, C.; Wikberg, M.L.; Stattin, P.; Egevad, L.; Bergh, A.; Wikström, P.; Palmqvist, R.; Edin, S. Secreted factors from colorectal and prostate cancer cells skew the immune response in opposite directions. *Sci. Rep.* **2015**, *5*, 15651. [CrossRef]
52. Lanciotti, M.; Masieri, L.; Raspollini, M.R.; Minervini, A.; Mari, A.; Comito, G.; Giannoni, E.; Carini, M.; Chiarugi, P.; Serni, S. The Role of M1 and M2 Macrophages in Prostate Cancer in relation to Extracapsular Tumor Extension and Biochemical Recurrence after Radical Prostatectomy. *BioMed Res. Int.* **2014**, *2014*, 486798. [CrossRef] [PubMed]
53. Erlandsson, A.; Carlsson, J.; Lundholm, M.; Fält, A.; Andersson, S.O.; Andrén, O.; Davidsson, S. M2 macrophages and regulatory T cells in lethal prostate cancer. *Prostate* **2019**, *79*, 363–369. [CrossRef]
54. Cao, Z.; Kyprianou, N. Mechanisms navigating the TGF-β pathway in prostate cancer. *Asian J. Urol.* **2015**, *2*, 11–18. [CrossRef] [PubMed]
55. Haas, C.; Krinner, E.; Brischwein, K.; Hoffmann, P.; Lutterbüse, R.; Schlereth, B.; Kufer, P.; Baeuerle, P.A. Mode of cytotoxic action of T cell-engaging BiTE antibody MT110. *Immunobiology* **2009**, *214*, 441–453. [CrossRef] [PubMed]
56. Donkor, M.K.; Sarkar, A.; Savage, P.A.; Franklin, R.A.; Johnson, L.K.; Jungbluth, A.A.; Allison, J.P.; Li, M.O. T cell surveillance of oncogene-induced prostate cancer is impeded by T cell-derived TGF-β1 cytokine. *Immunity* **2011**, *35*, 123–134. [CrossRef]
57. Li, M.O.; Wan, Y.Y.; Sanjabi, S.; Robertson, A.K.L.; Flavell, R.A. Transforming growth factor-β regulation of immune responses. *Annu. Rev. Immunol.* **2006**, *24*, 99–146. [CrossRef]
58. Owen, K.L.; Gearing, L.J.; Zanker, D.J.; Brockwell, N.K.; Khoo, W.H.; Roden, D.L.; Cmero, M.; Mangiola, S.; Hong, M.K.; Spurling, A.J.; et al. Prostate cancer cell-intrinsic interferon signaling regulates dormancy and metastatic outgrowth in bone. *EMBO Rep.* **2020**, *21*, e50162. [CrossRef]
59. Paston, S.J.; Brentville, V.A.; Symonds, P.; Durrant, L.G. Cancer Vaccines, Adjuvants, and Delivery Systems. *Front. Immunol.* **2021**, *12*, 627932. [CrossRef]
60. Thara, E.; Dorff, T.B.; Pinski, J.K.; Quinn, D.I. Vaccine therapy with sipuleucel-T (Provenge) for prostate cancer. *Maturitas* **2011**, *69*, 296–303. [CrossRef]

61. Small, E.J.; Schellhammer, P.F.; Higano, C.S.; Redfern, C.H.; Nemunaitis, J.J.; Valone, F.H.; Verjee, S.S.; Jones, L.A.; Hershberg, R.M. Placebo-controlled phase III trial of immunologic therapy with Sipuleucel-T (APC8015) in patients with metastatic, asymptomatic hormone refractory prostate cancer. *J. Clin. Oncol.* **2006**, *24*, 3089–3094. [CrossRef] [PubMed]
62. Kawalec, P.; Paszulewicz, A.; Holko, P.; Pilc, A. Sipuleucel-T immunotherapy for castration-resistant prostate cancer. A systematic review and meta-analysis. *Arch. Med. Sci.* **2012**, *8*, 767–775. [CrossRef] [PubMed]
63. Schellhammer, P.F.; Chodak, G.; Whitmore, J.B.; Sims, R.; Frohlich, M.W.; Kantoff, P.W. Lower baseline prostate-specific antigen is associated with a greater overall survival benefit from sipuleucel-T in the immunotherapy for prostate adenocarcinoma treatment (IMPACT) trial. *Urology* **2013**, *81*, 1297–1302. [CrossRef] [PubMed]
64. Fong, L.; Carroll, P.; Weinberg, V.; Chan, S.; Lewis, J.; Corman, J.; Amling, C.L.; Stephenson, R.A.; Simko, J.; Sheikh, N.A.; et al. Activated lymphocyte recruitment into the tumor microenvironment following preoperative sipuleucel-T for localized prostate cancer. *J. Natl. Cancer Inst.* **2014**, *106*, dju268. [CrossRef] [PubMed]
65. Hagihara, K.; Chan, S.; Zhang, L.; Oh, D.Y.; Wei, X.X.; Simko, J.; Fong, L. Neoadjuvant sipuleucel-T induces both Th1 activation and immune regulation in localized prostate cancer. *Oncoimmunology* **2019**, *8*, e1486953. [CrossRef] [PubMed]
66. Gulley, J.L.; Madan, R.A.; Tsang, K.Y.; Jochems, C.; Marté, J.L.; Farsaci, B.; Tucker, J.A.; Hodge, J.W.; Liewehr, D.J.; Steinberg, S.M.; et al. Immune impact induced by PROSTVAC (PSA-TRICOM), a therapeutic vaccine for prostate cancer. *Cancer Immunol. Res.* **2014**, *2*, 133–141. [CrossRef]
67. Kantoff, P.W.; Schuetz, T.J.; Blumenstein, B.A.; Michael Glode, L.; Bilhartz, D.L.; Wyand, M.; Manson, K.; Panicali, D.L.; Laus, R.; Schlom, J.; et al. Overall survival analysis of a phase II randomized controlled trial of a poxviral-based PSA-targeted immunotherapy in metastatic castration-resistant prostate cancer. *J. Clin. Oncol.* **2010**, *28*, 1099–1105. [CrossRef]
68. Gulley, J.L.; Borre, M.; Vogelzang, N.J.; Ng, S.; Agarwal, N.; Parker, C.C.; Pook, D.W.; Rathenborg, P.; Flaig, T.W.; Carles, J.; et al. Phase III Trial of PROSTVAC in asymptomatic or minimally symptomatic metastatic castration-resistant prostate cancer. *J. Clin. Oncol.* **2019**, *37*, 1051–1061. [CrossRef]
69. Higano, C.S.; Corman, J.M.; Smith, D.C.; Centeno, A.S.; Steidle, C.P.; Gittleman, M.; Simons, J.W.; Sacks, N.; Aimi, J.; Small, E.J. Phase 1/2 dose-escalation study of a GM-CSF-secreting, allogeneic, cellular immunotherapy for metastatic hormone-refractory prostate cancer. *Cancer* **2008**, *113*, 975–984. [CrossRef]
70. Small, E.J.; Sacks, N.; Nemunaitis, J.; Urba, W.J.; Dula, E.; Centeno, A.S.; Nelson, W.G.; Ando, D.; Howard, C.; Borellini, F.; et al. Granulocyte macrophage colony-stimulating factor-secreting allogeneic cellular immunotherapy for hormone-refractory prostate cancer. *Clin. Cancer Res.* **2007**, *13*, 3883–3891. [CrossRef]
71. Higano, C.; Saad, F.; Somer, B.; Curti, B.; Petrylak, D.; Drake, C.G.; Schnell, F.; Redfern, C.H.; Schrijvers, D.; Sacks, N. A phase III trial of GVAX immunotherapy for prostate cancer versus docetaxel plus prednisone in asymptomatic, castration-resistant prostate cancer (CRPC). In Proceedings of the 2009 Genitourinary Cancers Symposium, Orlando, FL, USA, 26–28 February 2009; p. LBA150.
72. He, X.; Xu, C. Immune checkpoint signaling and cancer immunotherapy. *Cell Res.* **2020**, *30*, 660–669. [CrossRef] [PubMed]
73. Ribas, A.; Wolchok, J.D. Cancer immunotherapy using checkpoint blockade. *Science* **2018**, *359*, 1350–1355. [CrossRef] [PubMed]
74. Kwon, E.D.; Drake, C.G.; Scher, H.I.; Fizazi, K.; Bossi, A.; Van den Eertwegh, A.J.M.; Krainer, M.; Houede, N.; Santos, R.; Mahammedi, H.; et al. Ipilimumab versus placebo after radiotherapy in patients with metastatic castration-resistant prostate cancer that had progressed after docetaxel chemotherapy (CA184-043): A multicentre, randomised, double-blind, phase 3 trial. *Lancet Oncol.* **2014**, *15*, 700–712. [CrossRef]
75. Beer, T.M.; Kwon, E.D.; Drake, C.G.; Fizazi, K.; Logothetis, C.; Gravis, G.; Ganju, V.; Polikoff, J.; Saad, F.; Humanski, P.; et al. Randomized, double-blind, phase III trial of ipilimumab versus placebo in asymptomatic or minimally symptomatic patients with metastatic chemotherapy-naive castration-resistant prostate cancer. *J. Clin. Oncol.* **2017**, *35*, 40–47. [CrossRef] [PubMed]
76. Topalian, S.L.; Hodi, F.S.; Brahmer, J.R.; Gettinger, S.N.; Smith, D.C.; McDermott, D.F.; Powderly, J.D.; Carvajal, R.D.; Sosman, J.A.; Atkins, M.B.; et al. Safety, Activity, and Immune Correlates of Anti–PD-1 Antibody in Cancer. *N. Engl. J. Med.* **2012**, *366*, 2443–2454. [CrossRef]
77. Hansen, A.R.; Massard, C.; Ott, P.A.; Haas, N.B.; Lopez, J.S.; Ejadi, S.; Wallmark, J.M.; Keam, B.; Delord, J.P.; Aggarwal, R.; et al. Pembrolizumab for advanced prostate adenocarcinoma: Findings of the KEYNOTE-028 study. *Ann. Oncol.* **2018**, *29*, 1807–1813. [CrossRef] [PubMed]
78. Ramos, C.A.; Dotti, G. Chimeric antigen receptor (CAR)-engineered lymphocytes for cancer therapy. *Expert Opin. Biol. Ther.* **2011**, *11*, 855–873. [CrossRef]
79. Junghans, R.P.; Ma, Q.; Rathore, R.; Gomes, E.M.; Bais, A.J.; Lo, A.S.Y.; Abedi, M.; Davies, R.A.; Cabral, H.J.; Al-Homsi, A.S.; et al. Phase I Trial of Anti-PSMA Designer CAR-T Cells in Prostate Cancer: Possible Role for Interacting Interleukin 2-T Cell Pharmacodynamics as a Determinant of Clinical Response. *Prostate* **2016**, *76*, 1257–1270. [CrossRef]
80. Slovin, S.F.; Wang, X.; Hullings, M.; Arauz, G.; Bartido, S.; Lewis, J.S.; Schöder, H.; Zanzonico, P.; Scher, H.I.; Sadelain, M.; et al. Chimeric antigen receptor (CAR +) modified T cells targeting prostate-specific membrane antigen (PSMA) in patients (pts) with castrate metastatic prostate cancer (CMPC). *J. Clin. Oncol.* **2013**, *31*, 72. [CrossRef]
81. Kloss, C.C.; Lee, J.; Zhang, A.; Chen, F.; Melenhorst, J.J.; Lacey, S.F.; Maus, M.V.; Fraietta, J.A.; Zhao, Y.; June, C.H. Dominant-Negative TGF-β Receptor Enhances PSMA-Targeted Human CAR T Cell Proliferation And Augments Prostate Cancer Eradication. *Mol. Ther.* **2018**, *26*, 1855–1866. [CrossRef]

82. Narayan, V.; Barber-Rotenberg, J.; Fraietta, J.; Hwang, W.-T.; Lacey, S.F.; Plesa, G.; Carpenter, E.L.; Maude, S.L.; Lal, P.; Vapiwala, N.; et al. A phase I clinical trial of PSMA-directed/TGFβ-insensitive CAR-T cells in metastatic castration-resistant prostate cancer. *J. Clin. Oncol.* **2021**, *39*, 125. [CrossRef]
83. Hummel, H.D.; Kufer, P.; Grüllich, C.; Seggewiss-Bernhardt, R.; Deschler-Baier, B.; Chatterjee, M.; Goebeler, M.E.; Miller, K.; De Santis, M.; Loidl, W.; et al. Pasotuxizumab, a BiTE® therapy for castration-resistant prostate cancer: Phase I, dose-escalation study findings. *Immunotherapy* **2021**, *13*, 125–141. [CrossRef] [PubMed]
84. Hummel, H.-D.; Kufer, P.; Grüllich, C.; Deschler-Baier, B.; Chatterjee, M.; Goebeler, M.-E.; Miller, K.; De Santis, M.; Loidl, W.C.; Buck, A.; et al. Phase 1 study of pasotuxizumab (BAY 2010112), a PSMA-targeting Bispecific T cell Engager (BiTE) immunotherapy for metastatic castration-resistant prostate cancer (mCRPC). *J. Clin. Oncol.* **2019**, *37*, 5034. [CrossRef]
85. Fizazi, K.; González Mella, P.; Castellano, D.; Minatta, J.N.; Rezazadeh, A.; Shaffer, D.R.; Vazquez Limon, J.C.; Sánchez López, H.M.; Armstrong, A.J.; Horvath, L.; et al. CheckMate 9KD Arm B final analysis: Efficacy and safety of nivolumab plus docetaxel for chemotherapy-naïve metastatic castration-resistant prostate cancer. *J. Clin. Oncol.* **2021**, *39*, 12. [CrossRef]
86. Appleman, L.J.; Kolinsky, M.P.; Berry, W.R.; Retz, M.; Mourey, L.; Piulats, J.M.; Romano, E.; Gravis, G.; Gurney, H.; De Bono, J.S.; et al. KEYNOTE-365 cohort B: Pembrolizumab (pembro) plus docetaxel and prednisone in abiraterone (abi) or enzalutamide (enza)–pretreated patients with metastatic castration-resistant prostate cancer (mCRPC)—New data after an additional 1 year of follow-up. *J. Clin. Oncol.* **2021**, *39*, 10. [CrossRef]
87. Karzai, F.; Madan, R.A.; Owens, H.; Couvillon, A.; Hankin, A.; Williams, M.; Bilusic, M.; Cordes, L.M.; Trepel, J.B.; Killian, K.; et al. A phase 2 study of olaparib and durvalumab in metastatic castrate-resistant prostate cancer (mCRPC) in an unselected population. *J. Clin. Oncol.* **2018**, *36*, 163. [CrossRef]
88. Yu, E.Y.; Piulats, J.M.; Gravis, G.; Laguerre, B.; Arranz Arija, J.A.; Oudard, S.; Fong, P.C.C.; Kolinsky, M.P.; Augustin, M.; Feyerabend, S.; et al. KEYNOTE-365 cohort A updated results: Pembrolizumab (pembro) plus olaparib in docetaxel-pretreated patients (pts) with metastatic castration-resistant prostate cancer (mCRPC). *J. Clin. Oncol.* **2020**, *38*, 100. [CrossRef]
89. Long, X.; Hou, H.; Wang, X.; Liu, S.; Diao, T.; Lai, S.; Hu, M.; Zhang, S.; Liu, M.; Zhang, H. Immune signature driven by ADT-induced immune microenvironment remodeling in prostate cancer is correlated with recurrence-free survival and immune infiltration. *Cell Death Dis.* **2020**, *11*, 779. [CrossRef]
90. Graff, J.N.; Antonarakis, E.S.; Hoimes, C.J.; Tagawa, S.T.; Hwang, C.; Kilari, D.; Ten Tije, A.; Omlin, A.G.; McDermott, R.S.; Vaishampayan, U.N.; et al. Pembrolizumab (pembro) plus enzalutamide (enza) for enza-resistant metastatic castration-resistant prostate cancer (mCRPC): KEYNOTE-199 cohorts 4-5. *J. Clin. Oncol.* **2020**, *38*, 15. [CrossRef]
91. Yu*, E.Y.; Fong, P.; Piulats, J.M.; Appleman, L.; Conter, H.; Feyerabend, S.; Shore, N.; Gravis, G.; Laguerre, B.; Gurney, H.; et al. PD16-12 pembrolizumab plus enzalutamide in abiraterone-pretreated patients with metastatic castration-resistant prostate cancer: Updated results from KEYNOTE-365 cohort C. *J. Urol.* **2020**, *203*, e368. [CrossRef]
92. Powles, T.; Fizazi, K.; Gillessen, S.; Drake, C.G.; Rathkopf, D.E.; Narayanan, S.; Green, M.C.; Mecke, A.; Schiff, C.; Sweeney, C. A phase III trial comparing atezolizumab with enzalutamide vs enzalutamide alone in patients with metastatic castration-resistant prostate cancer (mCRPC). *J. Clin. Oncol.* **2017**, *35*, TPS5090. [CrossRef]
93. Krebs, M.; Solimando, A.G.; Kalogirou, C.; Marquardt, A.; Frank, T.; Sokolakis, I.; Hatzichristodoulou, G.; Kneitz, S.; Bargou, R.; Kübler, H.; et al. miR-221-3p Regulates VEGFR2 Expression in High-Risk Prostate Cancer and Represents an Escape Mechanism from Sunitinib In Vitro. *J. Clin. Med.* **2020**, *9*, 670. [CrossRef] [PubMed]
94. Sharma, P.; Pachynski, R.K.; Narayan, V.; Fléchon, A.; Gravis, G.; Galsky, M.D.; Mahammedi, H.; Patnaik, A.; Subudhi, S.K.; Ciprotti, M.; et al. Nivolumab Plus Ipilimumab for Metastatic Castration-Resistant Prostate Cancer: Preliminary Analysis of Patients in the CheckMate 650 Trial. *Cancer Cell* **2020**, *38*, 489–499.e3. [CrossRef] [PubMed]
95. Sharma, P.; Pachynski, R.K.; Narayan, V.; Flechon, A.; Gravis, G.; Galsky, M.D.; Mahammedi, H.; Patnaik, A.; Subudhi, S.K.; Ciprotti, M.; et al. Initial results from a phase II study of nivolumab (NIVO) plus ipilimumab (IPI) for the treatment of metastatic castration-resistant prostate cancer (mCRPC.; CheckMate 650). *J. Clin. Oncol.* **2019**, *37*, 142. [CrossRef]
96. Boudadi, K.; Suzman, D.L.; Anagnostou, V.; Fu, W.; Luber, B.; Wang, H.; Niknafs, N.; White, J.R.; Silberstein, J.L.; Sullivan, R.; et al. Ipilimumab plus nivolumab and DNA-repair defects in AR-V7-expressing metastatic prostate cancer. *Oncotarget* **2018**, *9*, 28561–28571. [CrossRef]
97. Larkin, J.; Chiarion-Sileni, V.; Gonzalez, R.; Grob, J.J.; Cowey, C.L.; Lao, C.D.; Schadendorf, D.; Dummer, R.; Smylie, M.; Rutkowski, P.; et al. Combined Nivolumab and Ipilimumab or Monotherapy in Untreated Melanoma. *N. Engl. J. Med.* **2015**, *373*, 23–34. [CrossRef]
98. Ferris, R.L.; Blumenschein, G.; Fayette, J.; Guigay, J.; Colevas, A.D.; Licitra, L.; Harrington, K.; Kasper, S.; Vokes, E.E.; Even, C.; et al. Nivolumab for Recurrent Squamous-Cell Carcinoma of the Head and Neck. *N. Engl. J. Med.* **2016**, *375*, 1856–1867. [CrossRef]
99. Brahmer, J.; Reckamp, K.L.; Baas, P.; Crinò, L.; Eberhardt, W.E.E.; Poddubskaya, E.; Antonia, S.; Pluzanski, A.; Vokes, E.E.; Holgado, E.; et al. Nivolumab versus Docetaxel in Advanced Squamous-Cell Non–Small-Cell Lung Cancer. *N. Engl. J. Med.* **2015**, *373*, 123–135. [CrossRef]
100. Sharma, M.; Yang, Z.; Miyamoto, H.; Lucarelli, G. Immunohistochemistry of immune checkpoint markers PD-1 and PD-L1 in prostate cancer. *Medicine* **2019**, *98*, e17257. [CrossRef]

101. Gevensleben, H.; Dietrich, D.; Golletz, C.; Steiner, S.; Jung, M.; Thiesler, T.; Majores, M.; Stein, J.; Uhl, B.; Müller, S.; et al. The immune checkpoint regulator PD-L1 is highly expressed in aggressive primary prostate cancer. *Clin. Cancer Res.* **2016**, *22*, 1969–1977. [CrossRef]
102. Massari, F.; Ciccarese, C.; Caliò, A.; Munari, E.; Cima, L.; Porcaro, A.B.; Novella, G.; Artibani, W.; Sava, T.; Eccher, A.; et al. Magnitude of PD-1, PD-L1 and T Lymphocyte Expression on Tissue from Castration-Resistant Prostate Adenocarcinoma: An Exploratory Analysis. *Target. Oncol.* **2016**, *11*, 345–351. [CrossRef]
103. Antonarakis, E.S.; Piulats, J.M.; Gross-Goupil, M.; Goh, J.; Ojamaa, K.; Hoimes, C.J.; Vaishampayan, U.; Berger, R.; Sezer, A.; Alanko, T.; et al. Pembrolizumab for treatment-refractory metastatic castration-resistant prostate cancer: Multicohort, open-label phase II KEYNOTE-199 study. *J. Clin. Oncol.* **2020**, *38*, 395–405. [CrossRef] [PubMed]
104. Alexandrov, L.B.; Nik-Zainal, S.; Wedge, D.C.; Aparicio, S.A.J.R.; Behjati, S.; Biankin, A.V.; Bignell, G.R.; Bolli, N.; Borg, A.; Børresen-Dale, A.L.; et al. Signatures of mutational processes in human cancer. *Nature* **2013**, *500*, 415–421. [CrossRef] [PubMed]
105. Wu, Y.M.; Cieślik, M.; Lonigro, R.J.; Vats, P.; Reimers, M.A.; Cao, X.; Ning, Y.; Wang, L.; Kunju, L.P.; de Sarkar, N.; et al. Inactivation of CDK12 Delineates a Distinct Immunogenic Class of Advanced Prostate Cancer. *Cell* **2018**, *173*, 1770–1782.e14. [CrossRef] [PubMed]
106. Marcus, L.; Lemery, S.J.; Keegan, P.; Pazdur, R. FDA approval summary: Pembrolizumab for the treatment of microsatellite instability-high solid tumors. *Clin. Cancer Res.* **2019**, *25*, 3753–3758. [CrossRef]
107. Abida, W.; Cheng, M.L.; Armenia, J.; Middha, S.; Autio, K.A.; Vargas, H.A.; Rathkopf, D.; Morris, M.J.; Danila, D.C.; Slovin, S.F.; et al. Analysis of the Prevalence of Microsatellite Instability in Prostate Cancer and Response to Immune Checkpoint Blockade. *JAMA Oncol.* **2019**, *5*, 471–478. [CrossRef] [PubMed]
108. Pritchard, C.C.; Morrissey, C.; Kumar, A.; Zhang, X.; Smith, C.; Coleman, I.; Salipante, S.J.; Milbank, J.; Yu, M.; Grady, W.M.; et al. Complex MSH2 and MSH6 mutations in hypermutated microsatellite unstable advanced prostate cancer. *Nat. Commun.* **2014**, *5*, 4988. [CrossRef]
109. Strickland, K.C.; Howitt, B.E.; Shukla, S.A.; Rodig, S.; Ritterhouse, L.L.; Liu, J.F.; Garber, J.E.; Chowdhury, D.; Wu, C.J.; D'Andrea, A.D.; et al. Association and prognostic significance of BRCA1/2-mutation status with neoantigen load, number of tumor-infiltrating lymphocytes and expression of PD-1/PD-L1 in high grade serous ovarian cancer. *Oncotarget* **2016**, *7*, 13587–13598. [CrossRef]
110. Wang, F.; Zhao, Q.; Wang, Y.N.; Jin, Y.; He, M.M.; Liu, Z.X.; Xu, R.H. Evaluation of POLE and POLD1 Mutations as Biomarkers for Immunotherapy Outcomes Across Multiple Cancer Types. *JAMA Oncol.* **2019**, *5*, 1504–1506. [CrossRef]
111. Antonarakis, E.S. Cyclin-Dependent Kinase 12, Immunity, and Prostate Cancer. *N. Engl. J. Med.* **2018**, *379*, 1087–1089. [CrossRef]
112. Antonarakis, E.S.; Isaacsson Velho, P.; Fu, W.; Wang, H.; Agarwal, N.; Santos, V.S.; Maughan, B.L.; Pili, R.; Adra, N.; Sternberg, C.N.; et al. CDK12 -Altered Prostate Cancer: Clinical Features and Therapeutic Outcomes to Standard Systemic Therapies, Poly (ADP-Ribose) Polymerase Inhibitors, and PD-1 Inhibitors. *JCO Precis. Oncol.* **2020**, *4*, 370–381. [CrossRef] [PubMed]
113. Schweizer, M.T.; Ha, G.; Gulati, R.; Brown, L.C.; McKay, R.R.; Dorff, T.; Hoge, A.C.H.; Reichel, J.; Vats, P.; Kilari, D.; et al. CDK12 -Mutated Prostate Cancer: Clinical Outcomes With Standard Therapies and Immune Checkpoint Blockade. *JCO Precis. Oncol.* **2020**, *4*, 382–392. [CrossRef] [PubMed]
114. Ravindranathan, D.; Russler, G.A.; Yantorni, L.; Drubosky, L.M.; Bilen, M.A. Detection of Microsatellite Instability via Circulating Tumor DNA and Response to Immunotherapy in Metastatic Castration-Resistant Prostate Cancer: A Case Series. *Case Rep. Oncol.* **2021**, *14*, 190–196. [CrossRef] [PubMed]
115. Johnson, L.E.; Olson, B.M.; McNeel, D.G. Pretreatment antigen-specific immunity and regulation—association with subsequent immune response to anti-tumor DNA vaccination. *J. Immunother. Cancer* **2017**, *5*, 56. [CrossRef] [PubMed]
116. Komatsu, N.; Matsueda, S.; Tashiro, K.; Ioji, T.; Shichijo, S.; Noguchi, M.; Yamada, A.; Doi, A.; Suekane, S.; Moriya, F.; et al. Gene expression profiles in peripheral blood as a biomarker in cancer patients receiving peptide vaccination. *Cancer* **2012**, *118*, 3208–3221. [CrossRef]
117. Jochems, C.; Tucker, J.A.; Tsang, K.Y.; Madan, R.A.; Dahut, W.L.; Liewehr, D.J.; Steinberg, S.M.; Gulley, J.L.; Schlom, J. A combination trial of vaccine plus ipilimumab in metastatic castration-resistant prostate cancer patients: Immune correlates. *Cancer Immunol. Immunother.* **2014**, *63*, 407–418. [CrossRef]
118. Santegoets, S.J.A.M.; Stam, A.G.M.; Lougheed, S.M.; Gall, H.; Scholten, P.E.T.; Reijm, M.; Jooss, K.; Sacks, N.; Hege, K.; Lowy, I.; et al. T cell profiling reveals high CD4+CTLA-4+ T cell frequency as dominant predictor for survival after Prostate GVAX/ipilimumab treatment. *Cancer Immunol. Immunother.* **2013**, *62*, 245–256. [CrossRef] [PubMed]
119. Kongsted, P.; Borch, T.H.; Ellebaek, E.; Iversen, T.Z.; Andersen, R.; Met, Ö.; Hansen, M.; Lindberg, H.; Sengeløv, L.; Svane, I.M. Dendritic cell vaccination in combination with docetaxel for patients with metastatic castration-resistant prostate cancer: A randomized phase II study. *Cytotherapy* **2017**, *19*, 500–513. [CrossRef]
120. Ross, A.; Armstrong, A.J.; Pieczonka, C.M.; Bailen, J.L.; Tutrone, R.F.; Cooperberg, M.R.; Pavlovich, C.P.; Renzulli, J.F.; Haynes, H.; Sheikh, N.A.; et al. A comparison of sipuleucel-T (sip-T) product parameters from two phase III studies: PROVENT in active surveillance prostate cancer and IMPACT in metastatic castrate-resistant prostate cancer (mCRPC). *J. Clin. Oncol.* **2020**, *38*, 321. [CrossRef]

121. Madan, R.A.; Slovin, S.; Harshman, L.C.; Wei, X.X.; Bilusic, M.; Karzai, F.H.; Donahue, R.N.; Toney, N.J.; Strauss, J.; Cordes, L.; et al. 681P Clinical and immune responses to immunotherapy in biochemically recurrent (non-metastatic castration sensitive) prostate cancer (BCRpc). *Ann. Oncol.* **2020**, *31*, S542. [CrossRef]
122. Tran, B.; Horvath, L.; Dorff, T.B.; Greil, R.; Machiels, J.-P.H.; Roncolato, F.; Autio, K.A.; Rettig, M.; Fizazi, K.; Lolkema, M.P.; et al. Phase I study of AMG 160, a half-life extended bispecific T-cell engager (HLE BiTE) immune therapy targeting prostate-specific membrane antigen (PSMA), in patients with metastatic castration-resistant prostate cancer (mCRPC). *J. Clin. Oncol.* **2020**, *38*, TPS261. [CrossRef]
123. Kelly, W.K.; Pook, D.W.; Appleman, L.J.; Waterhouse, D.M.; Horvath, L.; Edenfield, W.J.; Matsubara, N.; Danila, D.C.; Aggarwal, R.R.; Petrylak, D.P.; et al. Phase I study of AMG 509, a STEAP1 x CD3 T-cell recruiting XmAb 2+1 immune therapy, in patients with metastatic castration-resistant prostate cancer (mCRPC). *J. Clin. Oncol.* **2021**, *39*, TPS183. [CrossRef]
124. Markowski, M.C.; Kilari, D.; Eisenberger, M.A.; McKay, R.R.; Dreicer, R.; Trikha, M.; Heath, E.I.; Li, J.; Garzone, P.D.; Young, T.S. Phase I study of CCW702, a bispecific small molecule-antibody conjugate targeting PSMA and CD3 in patients with metastatic castration-resistant prostate cancer (mCRPC). *J. Clin. Oncol.* **2021**, *39*, TPS5094. [CrossRef]
125. Chang Lee, S.; Ma, J.S.Y.; Kim, M.S.; Laborda, E.; Choi, S.H.; Hampton, E.N.; Yun, H.; Nunez, V.; Muldong, M.T.; Wu, C.N.; et al. A PSMA-targeted bispecific antibody for prostate cancer driven by a small-molecule targeting ligand. *Sci. Adv.* **2021**, *7*, eabi8193. [CrossRef]
126. Aggarwal, R.R.; Aparicio, A.; Heidenreich, A.; Sandhu, S.K.; Zhang, Y.; Salvati, M.; Shetty, A.; Hashemi Sadraei, N. Phase 1b study of AMG 757, a half-life extended bispecific T-cell engager (HLE BiTEimmune-oncology therapy) targeting DLL3, in de novo or treatment emergent neuroendocrine prostate cancer (NEPC). *J. Clin. Oncol.* **2021**, *39*, TPS5100. [CrossRef]
127. Tsimberidou, A.M.; Drakaki, A.; Khalil, D.; Kummar, S.; Hodi, F.S.; Oh, D.Y.; Cabanski, C.R.; Tezlaff, M.; LaVallee, T.; Spasic, M.; et al. An exploratory study of nivolumab (nivo) with or without ipilimumab (ipi) according to the percentage of tumoral CD8 cells in advanced metastatic cancer. *J. Clin. Oncol.* **2021**, *39*, 2573. [CrossRef]
128. Reimers, M.A.; Abida, W.; Chou, J.; George, D.J.; Heath, E.I.; McKay, R.R.; Pachynski, R.K.; Zhang, J.; Choi, J.E.; Feng, F.Y.; et al. IMPACT: Immunotherapy in patients with metastatic cancers and CDK12 mutations. *J. Clin. Oncol.* **2019**, *37*, TPS5091. [CrossRef]
129. Wong, Y.N.S.; Sankey, P.; Josephs, D.H.; Jones, R.J.; Crabb, S.J.; Beare, S.; Duggan, M.; White, L.; Charlaftis, N.; Wheeler, G.; et al. Nivolumab and ipilimumab treatment in prostate cancer with an immunogenic signature (NEPTUNES). *J. Clin. Oncol.* **2019**, *37*, TPS5090. [CrossRef]
130. Mehra, N.; Kloots, I.; Slootbeek, P.; den Brok, M.; Adema, G.; Kerkmeijer, L.; Smeenk, R.J.; Westdorp, H.; Bloemendal, H.; Schalken, J.; et al. 642TiP Phase II CA184-585 (INSPIRE) trial of ipilimumab with nivolumab for molecular-selected patients with castration-resistant prostate cancer. *Ann. Oncol.* **2021**, *32*, S671. [CrossRef]
131. Bansal, D.; Beck, R.; Arora, V.; Knoche, E.M.; Picus, J.; Reimers, M.A.; Roth, B.J.; Gulley, J.L.; Schreiber, R.; Pachynski, R.K. A pilot trial of neoantigen DNA vaccine in combination with nivolumab/ipilimumab and prostvac in metastatic hormone-sensitive prostate cancer (mHSPC). *J. Clin. Oncol.* **2021**, *39*, TPS192. [CrossRef]
132. Redman, J.M.; Steinberg, S.M.; Gulley, J.L. Quick efficacy seeking trial (QuEST1): A novel combination immunotherapy study designed for rapid clinical signal assessment metastatic castration-resistant prostate cancer 11 Medical and Health Sciences 1107 Immunology. *J. Immunother. Cancer* **2018**, *6*, 91. [CrossRef] [PubMed]
133. Autio, K.A.; Eastham, J.A.; Danila, D.C.; Slovin, S.F.; Morris, M.J.; Abida, W.; Laudone, V.P.; Touijer, K.A.; Gopalan, A.; Wong, P.; et al. A phase II study combining ipilimumab and degarelix with or without radical prostatectomy (RP) in men with newly diagnosed metastatic noncastration prostate cancer (mNCPC) or biochemically recurrent (BR) NCPC. *J. Clin. Oncol.* **2017**, *35*, 203. [CrossRef]
134. Gratzke, C.; Burgents, J.E.; Niu, C.; Poehlein, C.H.; Drake, C.G. Phase III study of pembrolizumab (pembro) plus enzalutamide (enza) and androgen deprivation therapy (ADT) for patients (pts) with metastatic hormone-sensitive prostate cancer (mHSPC): KEYNOTE-991. *J. Clin. Oncol.* **2020**, *38*, TPS5595. [CrossRef]
135. Fizazi, K.; González Mella, P.; Castellano, D.; Minatta, J.N.; Rezazadeh Kalebasty, A.; Shaffer, D.; Vázquez Limón, J.C.; Sánchez López, H.M.; Armstrong, A.J.; Horvath, L.; et al. Nivolumab plus docetaxel in patients with chemotherapy-naïve metastatic castration-resistant prostate cancer: Results from the phase II CheckMate 9KD trial. *Eur. J. Cancer* **2022**, *160*, 61–71. [CrossRef] [PubMed]
136. Drake, C.G.; Saad, F.; Clark, W.R.; Ciprotti, M.; Sharkey, B.; Subudhi, S.K.; Fizazi, K. 690TiP A phase III, randomized, double-blind trial of nivolumab or placebo combined with docetaxel for metastatic castration-resistant prostate cancer (mCRPC; CheckMate 7DX). *Ann. Oncol.* **2020**, *31*, S546. [CrossRef]
137. Graff, J.N.; Liang, L.W.; Kim, J.; Stenzl, A. KEYNOTE-641: A Phase III study of pembrolizumab plus enzalutamide for metastatic castration-resistant prostate cancer. *Futur. Oncol.* **2021**, *17*, 3017–3026. [CrossRef] [PubMed]
138. Piulats, J.; Ferrario, C.; Linch, M.; Stoeckle, M.; Laguerre, B.; Arranz, J.; Todenhoefer, T.; Fong, P.; Berry, W.; Emmenegger, U.; et al. 351 KEYNOTE-365 cohort D: Pembrolizumab plus abiraterone acetate and prednisone in patients with chemotherapy-naive metastatic castration-resistant prostate cancer (mCRPC). *J. Immunother. Cancer* **2021**, *9*, A378. [CrossRef]
139. Berry, W.R.; Fong, P.C.C.; Piulats, J.M.; Appleman, L.J.; Conter, H.J.; Feyerabend, S.; Shore, N.D.; Gravis, G.; Laguerre, B.; Gurney, H.; et al. KEYNOTE-365 cohort C updated results: Pembrolizumab (pembro) plus enzalutamide (enza) in abiraterone (abi)-pretreated patients (pts) with metastatic castrate-resistant prostate cancer (mCRPC). *J. Clin. Oncol.* **2020**, *38*, 102. [CrossRef]

140. Kolinsky, M.P.; Gravis, G.; Mourey, L.; Piulats, J.M.; Sridhar, S.S.; Romano, E.; Berry, W.R.; Gurney, H.; Retz, M.; Appleman, L.J.; et al. KEYNOTE-365 cohort B updated results: Pembrolizumab (pembro) plus docetaxel and prednisone in abiraterone (abi) or enzalutamide (enza)-pretreated patients (pts) with metastatic castrate-resistant prostate cancer (mCRPC). *J. Clin. Oncol.* **2020**, *38*, 103. [CrossRef]
141. Danila, D.C.; Kuzel, T.; Cetnar, J.P.; Rathkopf, D.E.; Morris, M.J.; Alumkal, J.J.; Butler, A.; Curley, T.; Hullings, M.; Buddle, J.R.; et al. A phase 1/2 study combining ipilimumab with abiraterone acetate plus prednisone in chemotherapy- and immunotherapy-naïve patients with progressive metastatic castration resistant prostate cancer (mCRPC). *J. Clin. Oncol.* **2016**, *34*, e16507. [CrossRef]
142. Gandhy, S.U.; Karzai, F.; Marte, J.L.; Bilusic, M.; McMahon, S.; Strauss, J.; Couvillon, A.; Williams, M.; Hankin, A.; Steinberg, S.M.; et al. PSA progression compared to radiographic or clinical progression in metastatic castration-resistant prostate cancer patients treated with enzalutamide. *J. Clin. Oncol.* **2020**, *38*, 105. [CrossRef]
143. Gandhy, S.; Gonzales, E.M.; Karzai, F.; Marte, J.; Bilusic, M.; McMahon, S.; Strauss, J.; Steinberg, S.; Gill, A.; Tubbs, A.; et al. 643P Evaluating biomarkers in metastatic castration resistant prostate cancer (mCRPC) patients (Pts) treated with enzalutamide (Enza): PSA, circulating tumor cell (CTC) counts, AR-V7 status, PET imaging vs. CT & Tc99 scans. *Ann. Oncol.* **2020**, *31*, S527–S528. [CrossRef]
144. Petrylak, D.P.; Ratta, R.; Gafanov, R.; Facchini, G.; Piulats, J.M.; Kramer, G.; Flaig, T.W.; Chandana, S.R.; Li, B.; Burgents, J.; et al. KEYNOTE-921: Phase III study of pembrolizumab plus docetaxel for metastatic castration-resistant prostate cancer. *Futur. Oncol.* **2021**, *17*, 3291–3299. [CrossRef] [PubMed]
145. Agarwal, N.; Azad, A.; Carles, J.; Chowdhury, S.; McGregor, B.A.; Merseburger, A.S.; Oudard, S.; Saad, F.; Soares, A.; Panneerselvam, A.; et al. A phase III, randomized, open-label, study (CONTACT-02) of cabozantinib plus atezolizumab versus second novel hormone therapy (NHT) in patients (pts) with metastatic, castration-resistant prostate cancer (mCRPC). *J. Clin. Oncol.* **2021**, *39*, TPS190. [CrossRef]
146. Atiq, M.O.; Gandhy, S.; Karzai, F.; Bilusic, M.; Cordes, L.M.; Owens, H.; Couvillon, A.; Hankin, A.; Williams, M.; Figg, W.D.; et al. Patients with undetectable PSA 2 years after docetaxel for metastatic castration sensitive prostate cancer (mCSPC). *J. Clin. Oncol.* **2021**, *39*, e17044. [CrossRef]
147. Chandran, E.B.A.; Atiq, M.O.; Donahue, R.N.; Karzai, F.; Bilusic, M.; Marte, J.L.; Arlen, P.M.; Cordes, L.M.; Owens, H.; Hankin, A.; et al. Evaluating the optimal sequence of immunotherapy and docetaxel in men with metastatic castration-sensitive prostate cancer. *J. Clin. Oncol.* **2022**, *40*, 130. [CrossRef]
148. Sokolova, A.; Gulati, R.; Cheng, H.H.; Beer, T.M.; Graff, J.N.; Amador, M.; Toulouse, A.; Taylor, K.; Bailey, S.; Smith, S.; et al. Trial in progress: Durvalumab and olaparib for the treatment of prostate cancer in men predicted to have a high neoantigen load. *J. Clin. Oncol.* **2022**, *40*, TPS202. [CrossRef]
149. Pachynski, R.K.; Retz, M.; Goh, J.C.; Burotto, M.; Gravis, G.; Castellano, D.; Flechon, A.; Zschaebitz, S.; Shaffer, D.R.; Vazquez Limon, J.C.; et al. CheckMate 9KD cohort A1 final analysis: Nivolumab (NIVO) + rucaparib for post-chemotherapy (CT) metastatic castration-resistant prostate cancer (mCRPC). *J. Clin. Oncol.* **2021**, *39*, 5044. [CrossRef]
150. Petrylak, D.P.; Perez-Gracia, J.L.; Lacombe, L.; Bastos, D.A.; Mahammedi, H.; Kwan, E.M.; Zschäbitz, S.; Armstrong, A.J.; Pachynski, R.K.; Goh, J.C.; et al. 579MO CheckMate 9KD cohort A2 final analysis: Nivolumab (NIVO) + rucaparib for chemotherapy (CT)-naïve metastatic castration-resistant prostate cancer (mCRPC). *Ann. Oncol.* **2021**, *32*, S629–S630. [CrossRef]
151. Subudhi, S.K.; Aparicio, A.; Zurita, A.J.; Doger, B.; Kelly, W.K.; Peer, A.; Rathkopf, D.E.; Karsh, L.I.; Tryon, J.J.; Kothari, N.; et al. A phase Ib/II study of niraparib combination therapies for the treatment of metastatic castration-resistant prostate cancer (NCT03431350). *J. Clin. Oncol.* **2019**, *37*, TPS5087. [CrossRef]
152. Yu, E.Y.; Park, S.H.; Huang, Y.-H.; Bennamoun, M.; Xu, L.; Kim, J.; Antonarakis, E.S. Phase III study of pembrolizumab (pembro) plus olaparib versus enzalutamide (enza) or abiraterone acetate (abi) in patients (pts) with metastatic castration-resistant prostate cancer (mCRPC) who progressed on chemotherapy: KEYLYNK-010. *J. Clin. Oncol.* **2020**, *38*, TPS256. [CrossRef]
153. Supiot, S.; Libois, V.; Guimas, V.; Rio, E.; Rolland, F.; Bompas, E.; Vansteene, D.; Tigreat, M.; Lisbona, A.; Colliaux, J.; et al. Prostate cancer with oligometastatic relapse: Combining stereotactic ablative radiotherapy and durvalumab, a randomized phase II trial (POSTCARD—GETUG-P13). *J. Clin. Oncol.* **2019**, *37*, TPS5088. [CrossRef]
154. Aggarwal, R.R.; Luch Sam, S.; Koshkin, V.S.; Small, E.J.; Feng, F.Y.; de Kouchkovsky, I.; Kwon, D.H.; Friedlander, T.W.; Borno, H.; Bose, R.; et al. Immunogenic priming with 177 Lu-PSMA-617 plus pembrolizumab in metastatic castration resistant prostate cancer (mCRPC): A phase 1b study. *J. Clin. Oncol.* **2021**, *39*, 5053. [CrossRef]
155. Sandhu, S.K.; Joshua, A.M.; Emmett, L.; Spain, L.; Horvath, L.G.; Crumbaker, M.; Anton, A.; Wallace, R.; Pasam, A.; Bressel, M.; et al. 577O PRINCE: Interim analysis of the phase Ib study of 177Lu-PSMA-617 in combination with pembrolizumab for metastatic castration resistant prostate cancer (mCRPC). *Ann. Oncol.* **2021**, *32*, S626. [CrossRef]
156. Dohopolski, M.; Watumull, L.; Mathews, D.; Gao, A.; Garant, A.; Choy, H.; Ahn, C.; Timmerman, R.D.; Courtney, K.; Hannan, R. Phase II Trial of Sipuleucel-T and Stereotactic Ablative Radiation therapy (SAbR) for Patients with Metastatic Castrate-Resistant Prostate Cancer (mCRPC). *Int. J. Radiat. Oncol.* **2020**, *108*, e879. [CrossRef]
157. Reimers, M.A.; Visconti, J.L.; Cittolin Santos, G.F.; Pachynski, R.K. A phase 1b clinical trial of cabozantinib (CABO) and abiraterone (ABI) with checkpoint inhibitor immunotherapy (CPI) in metastatic hormone-sensitive prostate cancer (mHSPC) (CABIOS Trial). *J. Clin. Oncol.* **2022**, *40*, TPS214. [CrossRef]

158. Yuan, Z.; Fernandez, D.; Dhillon, J.; Abraham-Miranda, J.; Awasthi, S.; Kim, Y.; Zhang, J.; Jain, R.; Serna, A.; Pow-Sang, J.M.; et al. Proof-of-principle Phase I results of combining nivolumab with brachytherapy and external beam radiation therapy for Grade Group 5 prostate cancer: Safety, feasibility, and exploratory analysis. *Prostate Cancer Prostatic Dis.* **2021**, *24*, 140–149. [CrossRef]
159. Tagawa, S.T.; Osborne, J.; Dallos, M.; Nauseef, J.; Sternberg, C.N.; Gregos, P.; Patel, A.; Tan, A.; Singh, S.; Bissassar, M.; et al. Phase I/II trial of pembrolizumab and AR signaling inhibitor +/- 225Ac-J591 for chemo-naive metastatic castration-resistant prostate cancer (mCRPC). *J. Clin. Oncol.* **2022**, *40*, TPS216. [CrossRef]

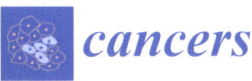

Article

Application of Proteogenomics to Urine Analysis towards the Identification of Novel Biomarkers of Prostate Cancer: An Exploratory Study

Tânia Lima [1,2], António S. Barros [3], Fábio Trindade [3], Rita Ferreira [4], Adelino Leite-Moreira [3], Daniela Barros-Silva [2], Carmen Jerónimo [2,5,6], Luís Araújo [7], Rui Henrique [2,5,6], Rui Vitorino [1,3,4,†] and Margarida Fardilha [1,*,†]

1. Department of Medical Sciences, Institute of Biomedicine-iBiMED, University of Aveiro, 3810-193 Aveiro, Portugal; tanialima@ua.pt (T.L.); rvitorino@ua.pt (R.V.)
2. Cancer Biology and Epigenetics Group, Research Center of Portuguese Oncology Institute of Porto (GEBC CI-IPOP) & Porto Comprehensive Cancer Center (P.CCC), 4200-072 Porto, Portugal; daniela.silva@ipoporto.min-saude.pt (D.B.-S.); carmenjeronimo@ipoporto.min-saude.pt (C.J.); henrique@ipoporto.min-saude.pt (R.H.)
3. UnIC@RISE, Department of Surgery and Physiology, Faculty of Medicine of the University of Porto, 4200-319 Porto, Portugal; asbarros@med.up.pt (A.S.B.); ftrindade@med.up.pt (F.T.); amoreira@med.up.pt (A.L.-M.)
4. LAQV/REQUIMTE, Department of Chemistry, University of Aveiro, 3810-193 Aveiro, Portugal; ritaferreira@ua.pt
5. Department of Pathology, Portuguese Oncology Institute of Porto (IPO Porto) & Porto Comprehensive Cancer Center (P.CCC), 4200-072 Porto, Portugal
6. Department of Pathology and Molecular Immunology, Institute of Biomedical Sciences Abel Salazar, University of Porto (ICBAS-UP), 4050-513 Porto, Portugal
7. Department of Clinical Pathology, Portuguese Oncology Institute of Porto (IPO Porto) & Porto Comprehensive Cancer Center (P.CCC), 4200-072 Porto, Portugal; laraujo@ipoporto.min-saude.pt
* Correspondence: mfardilha@ua.pt; Tel.: +351-234-247240; Fax: +351-234-377220
† These authors contributed equally to this work.

Simple Summary: Prostate cancer (PCa) is one of the most common cancers. Due to the limited and invasive approaches for PCa diagnosis, it is crucial to identify more accurate and non-invasive biomarkers for its detection. The aim of our study was to non-invasively uncover new protein targets for detecting PCa using a proteomics and proteogenomics approach. This work identified several dysregulated mutant protein isoforms in urine from PCa patients, some of them predicted to have a protective or an adverse role in these patients. These results are promising given urine's non-invasive nature and offers an auspicious opportunity for research and development of PCa biomarkers.

Abstract: To identify new protein targets for PCa detection, first, a shotgun discovery experiment was performed to characterize the urinary proteome of PCa patients. This revealed 18 differentially abundant urinary proteins in PCa patients. Second, selected targets were clinically tested by immunoblot, and the soluble E-cadherin fragment was detected for the first time in the urine of PCa patients. Third, the proteogenome landscape of these PCa patients was characterized, revealing 1665 mutant protein isoforms. Statistical analysis revealed 6 differentially abundant mutant protein isoforms in PCa patients. Analysis of the likely effects of mutations on protein function and PPIs involving the dysregulated mutant protein isoforms suggests a protective role of mutations HSPG2*Q1062H and VASN*R161Q and an adverse role of AMBP*A286G and CD55*S162L in PCa patients. This work originally characterized the urinary proteome, focusing on the proteogenome profile of PCa patients, which is usually overlooked in the analysis of PCa and body fluids. Combined analysis of mass spectrometry data using two different software packages was performed for the first time in the context of PCa, which increased the robustness of the data analysis. The application of proteogenomics to urine proteomic analysis can be very enriching in mutation-related diseases such as cancer.

Citation: Lima, T.; Barros, A.S.; Trindade, F.; Ferreira, R.; Leite-Moreira, A.; Barros-Silva, D.; Jerónimo, C.; Araújo, L.; Henrique, R.; Vitorino, R.; et al. Application of Proteogenomics to Urine Analysis towards the Identification of Novel Biomarkers of Prostate Cancer: An Exploratory Study. *Cancers* 2022, 14, 2001. https://doi.org/10.3390/cancers14082001

Academic Editor: Anne Chauchereau

Received: 22 February 2022
Accepted: 13 April 2022
Published: 15 April 2022

Publisher's Note: MDPI stays neutral with regard to jurisdictional claims in published maps and institutional affiliations.

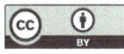

Copyright: © 2022 by the authors. Licensee MDPI, Basel, Switzerland. This article is an open access article distributed under the terms and conditions of the Creative Commons Attribution (CC BY) license (https://creativecommons.org/licenses/by/4.0/).

Keywords: prostate cancer; urine; human; biomarker; proteome; proteogenome; label-free quantitation; immunoblot

1. Introduction

Prostate cancer (PCa) is one of the most prevalent cancers among men and the fifth leading cause of cancer-related death [1]. When detected at early stages, PCa can be treated. However, PCa diagnosis is challenging, largely due to the low specificity of PSA tests, particularly in the diagnostic window of 4–10 ng/mL [2], which underscores the need to identify new and more accurate biomarkers.

An ideal biomarker for PCa should be non-invasively assessed, inexpensive, highly sensitive, and specific [3]. For anatomical reasons, urine is enriched in prostatic secretions and better reflects the molecular changes associated with the prostate than blood, which contains markers and confounding factors from the whole body. Urine can be serially collected, requiring minimal processing steps, and presents a simpler matrix with more stability than blood [4].

The phenotype role of proteins combined with the variety of techniques available for proteome analysis makes the search for protein markers in cancer a very attractive strategy [5]. Some promising single-protein biomarkers have been reported, such as AMBP [6] and zinc-alpha-2-glycoprotein (AZGP1) [7,8]. AMBP discriminated PCa and benign prostatic hyperplasia (BPH) patients with a highest accuracy than that estimated for PSA [9], using 2D-DIGE MALDI-TOF/TOF and immunoturbidimetry as discovery and validation approaches, respectively. AZGP1 significantly improved the prediction of PCa in a cohort of candidates for a prostatic biopsy, using isobaric stable isotope labeling and 2D-LC-MS/MS as the discovery method and Western Blot as the validation approach. Multi-marker panels have been shown to improve performance because they better reflect the cancer complexity and heterogeneity, addressing the limitations of single biomarkers. Although promising, no urine protein panel is available for clinical practice due partly to failure in clinical validation, reflecting the need to discover new biomarkers and/or new combinations of biomarkers [7,8]. Interestingly, and to the best of our knowledge, only one assay (Promark®) that quantifies a protein panel in prostate tissue by Mass Spectrometry (MS) is commercially available [10] and, to date, only four mRNA-based urine tests—PCA3 [11], SelectMDX [12], ExoDx Prostate(IntelliScore) [13], and MyProstateScore [14]—have been commercialized.

Cancer is driven by accumulated mutations and other genomic alterations [15]. Mutations on proteins can affect their structure, function, and stability, which may increase their susceptibility to being degraded [16]. As in other types of cancer, in PCa, a weak correlation between RNA and proteins expression is observed. Therefore, the effect of mutations should also be directly investigated at the protein level [17]. To address this inference problem, integration of genome and proteome data (proteogenome) analyses has been performed to identify mutant protein isoforms. Integrated proteogenome analysis can provide new insights into PCa pathophysiology and unveil powerful clinically applicable biomarkers. A shotgun proteomics approach combined with a mutation database has been used to detect mutated peptides related to various types of cancer, such as breast [18], colon [19], and rectal cancer [20]. Still, in PCa, it is mostly unexplored. In 2018, Kwon et al. first applied a proteogenome approach to identify six mutated peptides in the conditioned media from human PCa cell lines related to androgen-independent PCa, which are specific markers for PCa and for metastasis sites [21]. More recently, the same team identified seventy mutant peptides in PCa cell lines, of which seven were differentially expressed in PCa compared to normal tissues [22].

To identify a panel of putative protein markers to be evaluated in a non-invasively collected body fluid for PCa screening, the urine proteome and proteogenome of PCa patients were characterized by an MS-based approach. The integration of results was used to select candidate targets for small-scale clinical testing. MS is widely used to discover urinary protein biomarkers for cancer, including PCa [23]. Usually, biomarker discovery relies on a shotgun proteomics approach, followed by a validation phase using antibody-based techniques or targeted MS. Considering the complex mixture of proteins in urine, separation methodologies are important to increase sensitivity. Thus, a combination of gel-based and gel-free methods, such as GeLC-MS/MS, appears to be a robust and reproducible method for proteome analysis [24], warranting its application in the present work.

This work aims to improve the diagnosis of PCa by investigating the effect of new mutations in proteins that can be detected in urine, a non-invasively collected fluid. Additipnally, it overcomes the limitations of prior studies by using a combination of two software packages for MS data analysis, a proteogenome approach, and a detailed revision and integration of other exploratory proteome analyses to select protein targets.

2. Materials and Methods

2.1. Urine Proteome Profile of PCa Patients and Cancer-Free Subjects

2.1.1. Patients and Sample Collection

Urine samples were collected, without a prior prostate massage, from patients diagnosed with PCa at the Portuguese Oncology Institute of Porto (IPO Porto, Porto, Portugal), before surgery or therapy. Patients with other types of cancer, obesity, or autoimmune diseases were excluded, and cancer-free subjects had no clinically apparent prostatic disease. All available clinical data of the subjects enrolled in this study (discovery (d) and testing cohorts) is depicted in Tables S1 and S2. The discovery cohort comprised five PCa patients and five cancer-free subjects (controls). The testing cohort comprised thirty patients and thirty cancer-free subjects, not considering benign prostate diseases, such as BPH, due to the unavailability of samples.

2.1.2. Urine Sample Preparation

Urine samples were kept at 4 °C and centrifuged at $4000 \times g$ for 20 min at 4 °C. The supernatant (4.5 mL per sample) was collected and stored at −80 °C until laboratory analysis. Each urine sample was concentrated using a filter device (10 kDa cut-off, Vivaspin 500 Sartorius Biotech) by sequential centrifugations at $10,000 \times g$ for 10 min at 10 °C. Afterward, the retentate was resuspended in 0.5 M Tris pH 6.8 and 4% SDS and protein concentration were assessed by DC™ kit (Bio-Rad, Hercules, CA, USA).

2.1.3. SDS-PAGE

The volume equivalent to 50 µg of protein was precipitated overnight with cold acetone (−20 °C) and centrifuged at $14,000 \times g$ for 30 min at 4 °C. Then, the precipitated protein was mixed 1:1 with sample Laemmli loading buffer (0.5 M Tris-HCl pH 6.8, 15% glycerol, 4% SDS, 20% 2-mercaptoethanol, bromophenol blue), heated to 100 °C for 5 min, and separated on 12% Tris-Glycine gels. Following electrophoretic separation, gels were fixed in methanol:acetic acid:water (4:1:5; for 30 min) and stained with Colloidal Coomassie Blue G250 (overnight). Gels were distained with 20% methanol until optimal contrast was achieved.

2.1.4. Liquid Chromatography Tandem-Mass-Spectrometry (LC-MS/MS)

Tryptic digestion was performed according to Shevchenko et al. [25], with a few modifications. All protein bands were manually excised from the gels and sliced into ten sections. The gel pieces were washed with ammonium bicarbonate (NH_4HCO_3) (25 mM) and ACN (acetonitrile). Proteins were reduced with dithiothreitol (10 mM, 30 min, 60 °C) and alkylated in the dark with iodoacetamide (55 mM, 30 min, 25 °C). The gel pieces were washed with 100 mM NH_4HCO_3 and then with ACN. Gel pieces were vacuum-dried (SpeedVac, Thermo Savant) and proteins digested with trypsin (Thermo Scientific™, Waltham, MA, USA. Pierce™ Trypsin Protease, MS Grade) in 50 mM NH_4HCO_3 to a final protease: protein ratio of 1:25 (w/w). After 30 min on ice, 50 µL of 50 mM NH_4HCO_3 was added, and the samples were incubated for 16 h at 37 °C. The extraction of tryptic peptides was performed by the serial addition of 10% formic acid (FA), 10% FA:ACN (1:1) twice, and 90% ACN. Tryptic peptides were lyophilized and resuspended in 1% FA upon HPLC injection. The samples were analyzed with an Orbitrap Q Exactive (Thermo Fisher Scientific, Bremen, Germany) through the EASY-spray nano ESI source (Thermo Fisher Scientific, Bremen) that was coupled to an Ultimate 3000 (Dionex, Sunnyvale, CA, USA) HPLC system. The trap (5 mm × 300 μm inner diameter) and the EASY-spray analytical (150 mm × 75 μm) columns used were C18 Pepmap100 (Dionex, LC Packings, Sunnyvale, CA, USA), having a particle size of 3 μm. One analytical replicate was performed for each sample and blank runs were acquired between samples. For quality control of the performance of the nano-LC system, the acquisition of cytochrome C digest (1 pmol/μL) (cytochrome c digest lyophilized P/N 161089-thermo scientific) was routinely performed. Peptides were trapped at 30 μL/min in 96% of solvent A (0.1% FA). Elution was achieved with the solvent B (0.1% FA/80% acetonitrile v/v) at 300 nL/min. The 92 min gradient used was as follows: 0–3 min, 4 solvent B; 3–70 min, 4–25% solvent B; 70–90 min, 25–40% solvent B; 90–92 min, 40–90% solvent B; 92–100 min, 90% solvent B; 100–101 min, 90–4% solvent B; 101–120 min, 4% solvent B. The mass spectrometer was operated at 2.2 kV in the data-dependent acquisition mode. An MS2 method was used with an FT survey scan from 400 to 1600 m/z (resolution 70,000; auto-gain control target 1×10^6). The 10 most intense peaks were subjected to high collision dissociation fragmentation (resolution 17,500; auto-gain control target 5×10^4, normalized collision energy 28%, max. injection time 100 ms, dynamic exclusion 35 s).

2.1.5. Protein Identification and Quantification

The MaxQuant (version 1.6.5.0, Thermo software) and Proteome Discoverer (version 2.2, Thermo Fisher Scientific) software packages were used for peptide identification and label-free quantification. In MaxQuant, the Andromeda, and Proteome Discoverer, the MS Amanda, and Sequest HT search engines were used to search the MS/MS spectra against the Uniprot (TrEMBL and Swiss-Prot) protein sequence database under Homo Sapiens (version December 2018). Both database search parameters were as follows: methionine oxidation, protein N-term acetylation and phosphorylation, as variable modifications, and cysteine carbamidomethylation as a fixed modification. The mass tolerance of precursor mass was 20 ppm for MaxQuant and 10 ppm for Proteome Discoverer, and fragment ion mass tolerance was 0.15 Da (MaxQuant) and 0.02 Da (Proteome Discoverer). Minimal peptide length was set to 7 amino acids and, at most, 2 missed cleavages were allowed for both software. The false discovery rate (FDR) for identification was set to 1% at peptide and protein levels. Only the top-ranking protein of each group (master proteins), identified with at least two peptides, were considered. Exclusion of contaminants relied on those identified by the MaxQuant software and the cRAP protein sequences—THE GPM (https://www.thegpm.org/crap/) (accessed on 2 April 2019).

The MS proteome data have been deposited on the ProteomeXchange Consortium via the PRIDE [26] partner repository with the data set identifier PXD017902.

2.1.6. Exploratory Analysis of Urine Proteome Data

The protein abundances in Proteome Discoverer (normalized to the respective median) and normalized LFQ intensities in MaxQuant were log 2-transformed. In an exploratory analysis of proteome data, the proteins identified in all individuals were used as variables to perform Principal Component Analysis (PCA) and Heatmap analyses. These analyses were performed on MetaboAnalyst 5.0 [27]. To identify dysregulated proteins in PCa patients, the fold-change in protein abundance between PCa patients and cancer-free subjects was then calculated from the average log2 difference of protein intensities. Student's t-test assessed the statistical significance of this difference.

2.1.7. Comparison with a Previous Bioinformatic Analysis of Putative Urinary Markers of PCa and Selection of Candidate Protein Targets for the Testing Phase

Dysregulated proteins were compared with the results of a bioinformatic analysis focused on comparing and mining the proteome profile of tumor prostate tissue and urine from PCa patients reported by several MS studies [28]. The bioinformatic analysis reported 2641 and 616 dysregulated proteins in tumor prostate tissue and urine from PCa patients, respectively. To place urine proteome as a reflection of events taking place in prostate tissue and to identify specific urinary protein targets for PCa, the dysregulated proteins identified in tumor prostate tissue and urine from PCa patients were compared, resulting in 339 overlapping proteins. In this sense, the dysregulated proteins identified by MS in the present work, common to the 2641 dysregulated proteins expressed in tumor prostate tissue or to the 339 urinary proteins with prostate expression, correspond to the selection criteria of candidate proteins to be tested. Then, the selected proteins were compared with the normal human urinary proteome [29].

2.1.8. Measurement of Candidate Protein Targets in Urine Using Immunoblot

The selected protein targets from the discovery phase were tested by slot blot or Western blot immunoassays. In slot blot analysis, performed according to Caseiro et al. [30], the urine protein concentrated fraction was diluted in TBS to a final protein concentration of 0.01 µg/µL and slot-blotted onto a nitrocellulose membrane (Amersham Protran NC 0.45; Amersham Pharmacia Biotech, Buckinghamshire, UK). Antibodies specificity, selectivity, and sensitivity were assessed previously through Western blot by the bands appearing at the expected molecular weights without evidence of non-specific binding of the antibodies. The blocking and incubation conditions were optimized as follows: EFEMP1 (GTX111657: 1:1000, 1 h; GE Amersham-NA934: HRP-linked donkey anti-rabbit 1:10,000); AMBP (sc-81948: 1:1000, 1 h; GE Amersham-NA931: HRP-linked sheep anti-mouse 1:5000); LMAN2 (sc-130026, 1 h; GE Amersham-NA931: HRP-linked sheep anti-mouse 1:5000). Regarding Western blot, 20 µg of protein from each sample was separated on a 12% SDS-PAGE gel and transferred onto nitrocellulose membranes. In both immunoblot experiments, Ponceau S staining was used to normalize the antibody signal to total protein levels. In any case, the membranes were washed with TBS-T (TBS 25 Mm Tris–HCl, pH 7.4, 150 Mm NaCl, 0.1% Tween 20) and imaged in a ChemiDocTM Touch imaging system (Bio-Rad) using the Enhanced Chemiluminescence kit (ECL Select Western Blotting Detection Reagent, RPN2235, Amersham). Optical density was assessed with Image Lab Software (Bio-Rad) and normalized to a loading control sample. Western blot conditions were: CDH1 (GTX629691: 1:1000, 1 h; GE Amersham-NA931: HRP-linked sheep anti-mouse 1:5000); TTR (GTX100577: 1:500, 1 h; GE Amersham-NA934: HRP-linked donkey anti-rabbit 1:10,000).

2.1.9. Measurement of Urinary PSA Levels

Urinary PSA levels were determined using the same method (Elecsys total PSA, 08791732500) used to determine serum PSA levels. This electrochemiluminescence assay is used in the clinical routine of IPO Porto. It quantifies total PSA (free + complexed PSA) using a Cobas e 801 module, a member of Roche Cobas 8000 Modular Analyzer (Roche, Woerden, The Netherlands).

2.2. Urine Proteogenome Profile of PCa Patients and Cancer-Free Subjects

2.2.1. Identification of Cancer-Associated Mutations

Considering the high impact of mutations on cancer progression, the proteogenome profile of urine from PCa patients was explored. For this, mass spectra resulting from the MS analysis were searched against a database built into the Pinnacle software (https://rimuhc.ca/-/protein-quantification-software-pinnacle?redirect=%2Fproteomics-software, accessed on 5 January 2022). This type of analysis aimed to investigate the existence of cancer-associated mutations that were translated in proteins present in the urine from PCa patients. To select high-confidence urinary proteins with a very likely origin in the prostate, only mutations on proteins present in all samples and with known prostate expression were considered. The prostate proteome was searched in the HPA database and in the above-mentioned bioinformatic analysis [28]. The prostate proteome in the HPA consisted of proteins with evidence at the protein level and its last access was on 8 November 2021.

2.2.2. Exploratory Analysis of Urine Proteogenome Data

The abundances of proteins with known prostate expression in Pinnacle were log 2-transformed. In an exploratory analysis of proteogenome data, the levels of mutant protein isoforms identified in all individuals were used as variables to perform Principal Component Analysis (PCA) and Heatmap analyses. These analyses were performed on MetaboAnalyst 5.0 [27]. To identify dysregulated proteins with mutations in PCa patients, the fold-change in protein abundance between PCa patients and cancer-free subjects was then calculated from the average log2 difference of protein intensities. Student's t-test assessed the statistical significance of this difference.

2.2.3. Integration with the Cancer Genome Atlas (TCGA), DisGeNET and Literature Data

To investigate whether mutations identified in proteins with known prostate expression were already described in PCa, TCGA, DisGeNET (v7.0), and literature data were searched.

TCGA is a cancer genomics consortium that generates data (https://www.cancer.gov/tcga, accessed on 12 January 2022) encompassing the profiling of over 20,000 primary tumors and matched non-tumoral samples related to various human cancers, including PCa. The characterization of PCa samples disclosed 20,237 mutated genes and 33,334 mutations. DisGeNET is one of the largest repositories of Gene-Disease (GDA) and Variant-Disease (VDA) Associations [31]. The latest version of DisGeNET contains 1,134,942 GDAs and 369,554 VDAs. In the present work, variants associated with PCa were extracted from the Prostate Carcinoma C0600139 (January 2022).

2.2.4. Comparison of the Levels of Native and Mutant Forms of Proteins in the Urine from PCa Patients

To investigate the influence of mutations on the abundance of proteins with known expression in the prostate, the levels of their native and mutant forms were compared.

2.2.5. Prediction of the Likely Impact of Single-Residue Substitutions in Proteins

The PolyPhen-2 (Polymorphism Phenotyping v2) web tool was used to predict the likely impact of each amino acid substitution on the structure and function of the proteins with known prostate expression [32]. Each mutation is assigned a score, which is the probability of the substitution being damaging, in addition to a sensitivity and specificity value of the prediction confidence. According to the PolyPhen-2 tool, single-residue substitutions in the protein sequence can be classified as benign (score: 0–0.4), possibly damaging (score: 0.4–0.9), or probably damaging (score: 0.9–1) [33].

2.2.6. Protein–Protein Interaction Analysis

Due to the pivotal role of Protein–Protein interactions (PPIs) in cancer and the possible effect of mutations on its dynamics, the interactions between proteins in which point mutations has been identified were explored. For this, the STRING database v 11.5 was sourced on 12 January 2022, and only protein interactions with a confidence score of ≥ 0.4 were considered [34]. However, we must be cautious when extrapolating the significance of these PPIs to biological fluids such as urine, as most PPIs are identified or predicted from studies in cells and tissues.

2.2.7. Prediction of the Likely Impact of Single-Residue Substitutions in Protein–Protein Affinity

Considering the impact of mutations on PPIs, the SAAMBE-SEQ Web Server was used to predict the effect of point mutations detected in this work on protein binding affinity [35].

2.3. Statistical Data Analysis

Statistical analyses were carried out in R software for Windows version 3.6.2 and GraphPad Prism version 6.0 (GraphPad Software, Inc.; San Diego, CA, USA). The Shapiro normality test and visual inspection of the histograms were used to assess the data distribution. To evaluate the effect size of the dysregulated proteins when comparing the tested groups, Cohen's d was determined. Differences were considered statistically significant if p-value was ≤ 0.05. The clinical parameters and protein levels are expressed as mean $\pm$ standard deviation (SD).

3. Results

3.1. Urine Proteome Profile of PCa Patients and Cancer-Free Subjects

To identify potential protein targets for PCa prediction, shotgun proteomics was performed in urine collected from PCa patients and cancer-free subjects. To boost MS data analysis, a combination of two different software packages, MaxQuant and Proteome Discover, sourcing three databases (Andromeda, Amanda, and Sequest HT) in total, was used.

Considering only the top-ranking protein of each group identified with at least two peptides and filtering out identifications from reversed sequences and contaminants, 605 and 592 urinary proteins were identified by MaxQuant and Proteome Discoverer, respectively. In total, 732 proteins were identified, excluding those common to both software.

3.1.1. Exploratory Analysis of Urine Proteome Data

Aiming to select and identify proteins of interest for PCa monitoring, only proteins present in all samples analyzed by MaxQuant (82 proteins) and by Proteome Discoverer (84 proteins) were considered for further analysis. These high-confidence proteins were separately used for Principal Component Analysis (PCA) (Figures 1A and 2A) and Heatmap analyses (Figures 1B and 2B). In both software, no separation of groups was observed in the PCa analysis. However, the proteins identified by the MaxQuant software alone seem to provide a discrimination between PCa patients and non-cancer subjects based on two protein clusters, depicted in the heatmap: AZGP1(zinc-alpha-2-glycoprotein)-SPP1 (Osteopontin); CD14 (Monocyte differentiation antigen CD14)-MASP2 (Mannan-binding lectin serine protease 2) (Figure 1B). In the first cluster, proteins are mostly upregulated in PCa patients compared to non-cancer subjects, while in the second cluster proteins are predominantly downregulated in PCa patients.

Then, differential protein analysis revealed 18 dysregulated proteins in PCa, with 4 proteins (p-value ≤ 0.05) identified only by Proteome Discoverer, 9 proteins only by MaxQuant analysis, and 5 proteins (Cadherin-1 (CDH1), EGF-containing fibulin-like extracellular matrix protein 1 (EFEMP1), Prostate-specific antigen (PSA) (KLK3), Secreted and transmembrane protein 1 (SECTM1), and Transthyretin (TTR)) discovered by both software. Altogether, 11 proteins were significantly downregulated (fold change less than 1), and 7 proteins were significantly upregulated (fold change greater than 1) in PCa patients (Tables 1 and 2). Reassuringly, the most widely used biomarker for PCa diagnosis, PSA, was one of the dysregulated proteins in common in the analysis by both software packages. When the tested groups were compared, proteins showing significant differences (p-value ≤ 0.05) and revealed a "large" effect-size (|Cohen's d|) > 0.8 (Tables 1 and 2). Besides a large effect-size, dysregulated proteins identified by both software presented a consistent direction of dysregulation. It is noteworthy that in the heatmap of MaxQuant data, seven proteins (TTR, KLK3, SECTM1, CDH13, AMY2A, EFEMP1, ITIH4, HSPG2, PTGDS, CDH1, and LMAN2) responsible for the separation of groups were also found dysregulated in PCa patients. It was observed that the decreased levels of SECTM1, CDH13, AMY2A, EFEMP1, ITIH4, HSPG2, PTGDS, CDH1, and LMAN2 and increased levels of TTR and KLK3 characterized the urine proteome of PCa patients.

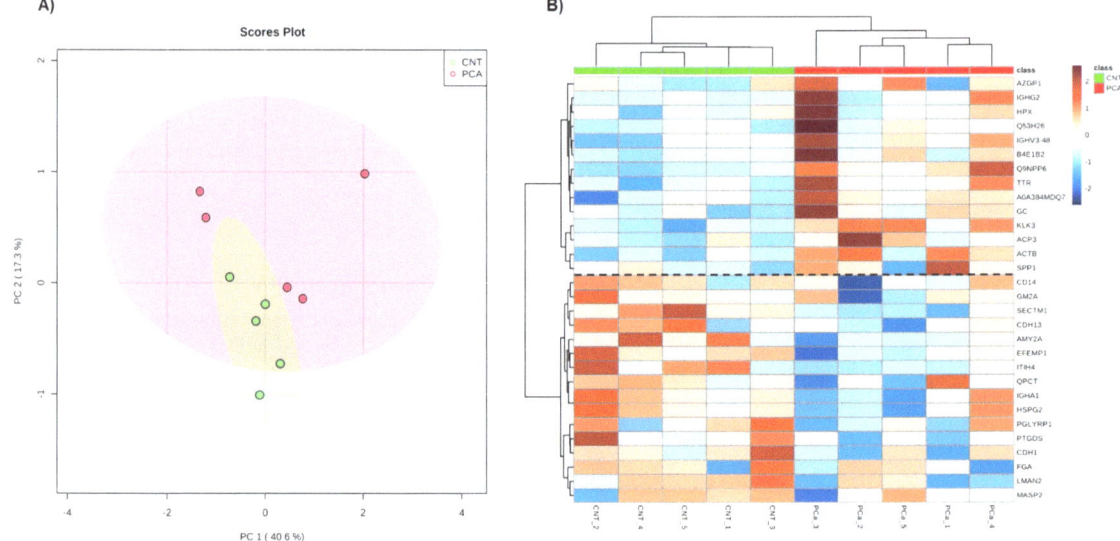

Figure 1. Exploratory analysis of proteome data from MaxQuant. (**A**) Principal Component Analysis of the urine proteome of the two groups. (**B**) The heatmap of proteins identified in all individuals. Samples are represented in columns and proteins in rows. Proteins whose gene name is not available are indicated by their UniProt accession number. The dashed line on the heatmap indicates the two clusters of proteins.

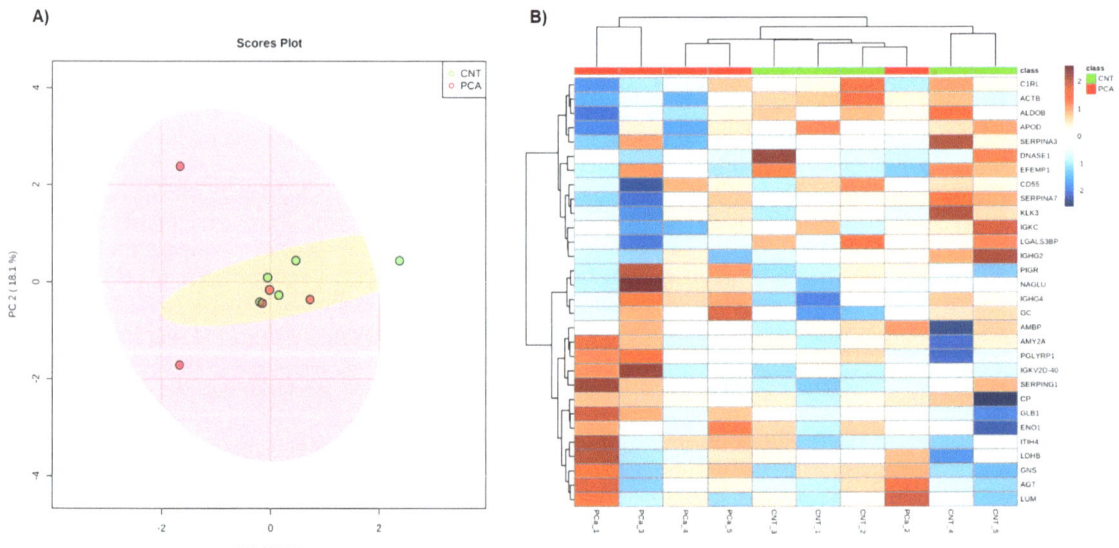

Figure 2. Exploratory analysis of proteome data from Proteome discoverer. (**A**) Principal Component Analysis of the urine proteome of the two groups. (**B**) The heatmap of proteins identified in all individuals. Samples are represented in columns and proteins in rows.

Table 1. Dysregulated proteins between PCa patients and cancer-free subjects (Proteome Discoverer).

Uniprot ID	Protein Name	Gene Name	p-Value	Cohen's d [Lower; Upper 95% CI]
P07288	Prostate-specific antigen	KLK3	0.00	4.21 (3.50; 4.91)
Q8WVN6	Secreted and transmembrane protein 1	SECTM1	0.01	−2.16 (−2.39; −1.93)
P12830	Cadherin-1	CDH1	0.03	−1.73 (−2.05; −1.41)
P0DOX5	Immunoglobulin gamma-1 heavy chain	N/A	0.03	1.73 (1.39; 2.07)
Q12805	EGF-containing fibulin-like extracellular matrix protein 1	EFEMP1	0.03	−1.68 (−2.25; −1.12)
P02766	Transthyretin	TTR	0.03	1.66 (0.86; 2.46)
P01861	Immunoglobulin heavy constant gamma 4	IGHG4	0.04	1.52 (0.90; 2.15)
P01034	Cystatin-C	CST3	0.05	1.50 (0.91; 2.08)
Q01459	Di-N-acetylchitobiase	CTBS	0.05	−1.44 (−1.86; −1.02)

The protein identification and label-free quantification performed by the Proteome Discoverer software revealed nine dysregulated proteins (p-value ≤ 0.05) between the tested groups. These proteins are shown in this table along with their p-value and effect size. The Cohen's d for individual proteins is presented together with the lower and upper 95% confidence interval (CI). Abbreviation: Confidence interval (CI).

Table 2. Dysregulated proteins between PCa patients and cancer-free subjects (MaxQuant).

Uniprot ID	Protein Name	Gene Name	p-Value	Cohen's d [Lower; Upper 95% CI]
Q8WVN6	Secreted and transmembrane protein 1	SECTM1	0.01	−2.10 (−2.48; −1.73)
P07288	Prostate-specific antigen	KLK3	0.01	2.01 (1.08; 2.95)
P41222	Prostaglandin-H2 D-isomerase	PTGDS	0.01	−1.97 (−2.44; −1.49)
Q14624	Inter-alpha-trypsin inhibitor heavy chain H4	ITIH4	0.01	−1.96 (−2.32; −1.60)
Q12805	EGF-containing fibulin-like extracellular matrix protein 1	EFEMP1	0.01	−1.84 (−2.33; −1.35)
P55290	Cadherin-13	CDH13	0.02	−1.75 (−2.11; −1.40)
P98160	Basement membrane-specific heparan sulfate proteoglycan core protein	HSPG2	0.03	−1.63 (−2.07; −1.19)
P04746	Pancreatic alpha -amylase	AMY2A	0.03	−1.57 (−1.95; −1.19)
P01876	Immunoglobulin heavy constant alpha 1	IGHA1	0.04	1.55 (1.32; 1.78)
P02760	Protein AMBP	AMBP	0.04	−1.51 (−1.88; −1.13)
P12830	Cadherin-1	CDH1	0.05	−1.48 (−1.90; −1.07)
Q12907	Vesicular integral-membrane protein VIP36	LMAN2	0.05	−1.46 (−2.10; −0.83)
Q9NPP6	Immunoglobulin heavy chain variant	N/A	0.04	1.58 (1.22; 1.93)
P02766	Transthyretin	TTR	0.05	1.42 (0.97; 1.87)

The protein identification and label-free quantification performed by the MaxQuant software revealed fourteen dysregulated proteins (p-value ≤ 0.05) between the tested groups. These proteins are shown in this table along with their p-value and effect size. The Cohen's d fof individual proteins is presented together with the lower and upper 95% confidence interval (CI). Abbreviation: Confidence interval (CI).

3.1.2. Comparison with a Previous Bioinformatic Analysis of Putative Urinary Markers of PCa and Selection of Candidate Protein Targets for the Testing Phase

To select the most promising proteins for further analysis, dysregulated proteins revealed by MS analysis were compared with proteins resulting from a bioinformatic analysis integrating urine and tumor tissue proteomes of PCa from several MS studies [28]. From this comparison, some common proteins emerged, such as AMBP, CDH1, EFEMP1, KLK3, SECTM1, LMAN2, and TTR.

From the previous study of our group, the dysregulated proteins AMBP, KLK3, LMAN2, and TTR were found dysregulated in urine and tumor tissue from PCa patients, while SECTM1 was only found in urine from PCa patients, and CDH1 and EFEMP1 were only in PCa tissue.

Taken together, and keeping in mind that candidate targets should be urinary proteins with prostate expression, AMBP, CDH1, EFEMP1, KLK3, LMAN2, and TTR were selected for testing in an independent cohort. The presence of these proteins in the urine was already expected, because they are characteristic of the normal human urine proteome [29].

3.1.3. Measurement of Candidate Protein Targets in Urine

Five protein targets, AMBP, CDH1, EFEMP1, LMAN2, and TTR were selected for immunoblot-based testing in a larger and independent cohort (testing group). However, none of the MS findings could be reproduced (Table S3, Figure S1). Measurement of urinary PSA levels in the testing cohort did not agree with the MS findings ($p = 0.29$, Mann–Whiney test). The results are shown in Figure 3.

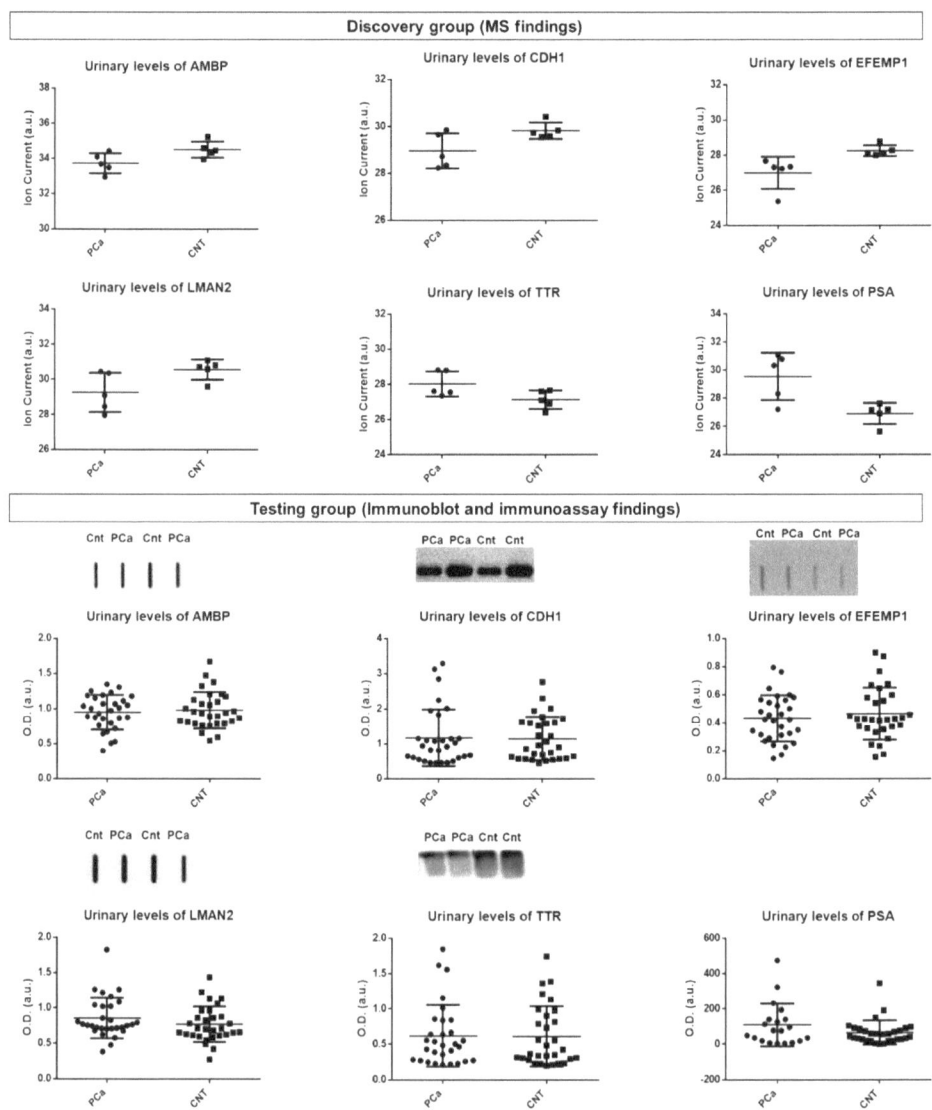

Figure 3. Urinary protein levels of the candidate targets for PCa in the discovery group (using MS) and in the testing group (using immunoblot and immunoassay). MS: mass spectrometry.

3.2. Urine Proteogenome Profile of PCa Patients and Cancer-Free Subjects

3.2.1. Identification of Cancer-Associated Mutations

To characterize the proteogenome landscape of urine from PCa patients, MS/MS spectra were searched against a repository of information from a wide variety of databases encompassing somatic mutations. This search resulted in identifying 6418 mutated peptides corresponding to 1665 mutant protein isoforms. Of these, 609 mutated peptides, which correspond to 417 mutant protein isoforms, were associated with cancer. Only mutant protein isoforms that occurred in all urine samples (322 proteins) were selected for further analysis. Immunoglobulins and highly abundant urinary proteins (serum albumin, uromodulin, serotransferrin) were excluded due to their high abundance in biological samples and the lack of specificity for cancer, resulting in 170 proteins. These 170 proteins corresponded to 122 proteins after filtering out duplicates. As our focus was high confidence proteins with mutations whose origin was very likely the prostate, these data were integrated with the prostate proteome searched in the HPA database and in a bioinformatic analysis [28], resulting in 86 proteins with known expression in the prostate (Table S4). Among these proteins are some of known relevance for PCa, namely Acid ceramidase (ASAH1), Extracellular superoxide dismutase [Cu-Zn] (SOD3), Glutathione S-transferase P (GSTP1), Osteopontin (SPP1), Prostatic acid phosphatase (PAP), and Zinc-alpha-2-glycoprotein (ZAG).

3.2.2. Exploratory Analysis of Urine Proteogenome Data

The levels of the mutant protein isoforms were used for PCA (Principal Component Analysis) (Figure 4A) and Heatmap analyses (Figure 4B). No group separation was observed in the PCA of the proteogenome profile of PCa patients. However, the heatmap indicates a discrimination between PCa patients and non-cancer subjects based on two protein clusters: ITIH4*G893S (Inter-alpha-trypsin inhibitor heavy chain H4)-LMAN2*D222N (Vesicular integral-membrane protein VIP36); KLK3*C209Y (PSA)-MVB12B*T198M (Multivesicular body subunit 12B) (Figure 4B). In the first cluster, mutant forms of proteins are mostly downregulated in PCa patients compared to non-cancer subjects, while in the second cluster mutant forms of proteins are upregulated predominantly in PCa patients.

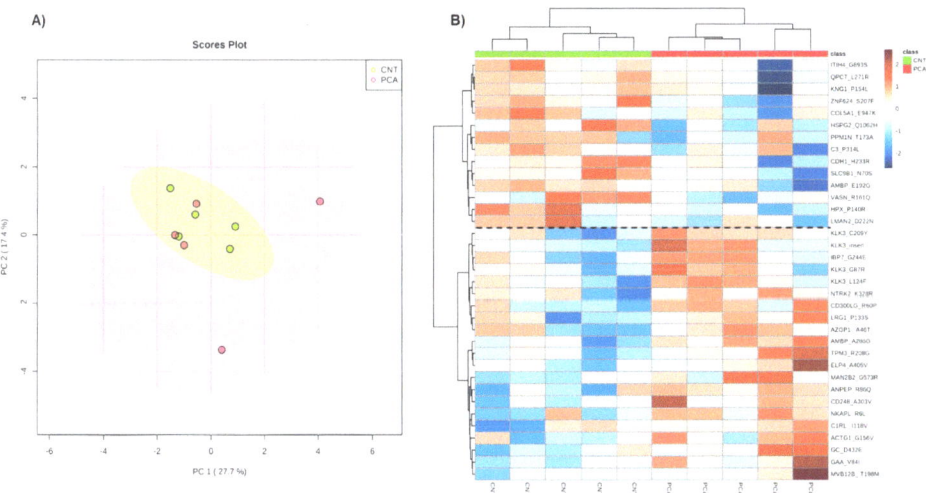

Figure 4. Exploratory analysis of proteogenome data from Pinnacle. (**A**) Principal Component Analysis of the urine proteogenome of the two groups. (**B**) The heatmap of mutant proteins identified in all individuals. Samples are represented in columns and proteins in rows. Proteins are identified by their gene name, and the mutation identified. The dashed line on the heatmap indicates the two clusters of proteins.

3.2.3. Integration with the Cancer Genome Atlas (TCGA), DisGeNET and Literature Data

According to TCGA, DisGeNET, and the literature, only three of the mutations identified in the 86 proteins with known prostate expression have already been described. These mutations (rs17632542, rs1695, rs7041) were mapped on KLK3 (PSA) [36], GSTP1 (Glutathione S-transferase P) [37,38], and GC (Vitamin D-binding protein) [39], respectively. To the best of our knowledge, there is no association of the remaining mutant protein isoforms with PCa. Especially notable are the proteins SPP1, VASN, ASAH1, RBP4, and ASS1, which, until now, have had no mutation related to PCa described in the literature.

3.2.4. Comparison of the Levels of Native and Mutant Forms of Proteins in the Urine from PCa Patients

The analysis of proteogenome data revealed 6 differentially abundant mutant protein isoforms in PCa patients compared with cancer-free individuals, namely Protein AMBP (AMBP*A286G), Sodium/hydrogen exchanger 9B1 (SLC9B1*N70S), Basement membrane-specific heparan sulfate proteoglycan core protein (HSPG2*Q1062H), Zinc finger protein 624 (ZNF624*S207F), Vasorin (VASN*R161Q), and Complement decay-accelerating factor (CD55*S162L) (Table S4, Figure S2). Mutant AMBP isoform was upregulated in PCa patients, while the remaining 5 differentially abundant mutant protein isoforms were downregulated.

Comparing the proteome profile analysis of MaxQuant and Proteome Discoverer with the proteogenome profile of PCa patients resulted in 30 and 31 common proteins, respectively. Of these common proteins, AMBP, CDH1, EFEMP1, HSPG2, ITIH4, KLK3, LMAN2, PTGDS, VASN, and CD55 proteins stood out. The native form of AMBP, CDH1, EFEMP1, HSPG2, ITIH4, KLK3, LMAN2, and PTGDS proteins was found dysregulated in urine from PCa patients, but only the mutant protein isoforms (AMBP*A286G; HSPG2*Q1062H) were found dysregulated (Figure S2). In the remaining common proteins, the presence of mutations did not affect their abundance in urine. The native form of VASN and CD55 proteins was not found dysregulated in the urine from PCa patients, but their mutant protein isoforms (VASN*R161Q; CD55*S162L) were.

The mutations identified in these proteins and in those with recognized relevance to PCa are summarized in Table 3.

Table 3. List of mutations mapped on some proteins and respective mutant peptides identified in urine from PCa patients.

Uniprot ID	Protein Name	Gene Name	Mutation Description	Mutation Type	Protein Role in PCa or Other Types of Cancer
P02760	Protein AMBP	AMBP	G238S; E192G; V69M; A286G; P197S; R185Q; G338S; G341A; I198T; V313I; G186R; R185Q	missense	AMBP is an inflammation-regulating protein, associated with human cancers [40,41], including PCa [42,43]. Increased urinary levels [6,42,44,45] but diminished levels in tumor prostate tissue have been reported in PCa patients [46–48].
P12830	Cadherin-1	CDH1	H233R; A408E	missense	CDH1 is a protein implicated in cell adhesion, migration, and epithelial-mesenchymal transition [49,50] and its downregulation is correlated with a poor prognosis in PCa patients [51].
Q12805	EGF-containing fibulin-like extracellular matrix protein 1	EFEMP1	V463M	missense	EFMP1 plays a role in cell adhesion and migration, acting as a tumor suppressor in PCa. Diminished EFEMP1 mRNA and protein levels [52] and EFEMP1 promoter hypermethylation were observed in PCa patients [53,54].

Table 3. Cont.

Uniprot ID	Protein Name	Gene Name	Mutation Description	Mutation Type	Protein Role in PCa or Other Types of Cancer
P98160	Basement membrane-specific heparan sulfate proteoglycan core protein	HSPG2	V4332I; A1503V; S970F; M638V; Q1062H	missense	HSPG2, found predominantly in the ECM and bone marrow, modulates tumor angiogenesis, proliferation, and differentiation. It is overexpressed in PCa tissues compared to non-malignant tissues, correlating with high GS and PCa cell proliferation and viability [55–57].
Q14624	Inter-alpha-trypsin inhibitor heavy chain H4	ITIH4	R866C; G893S	missense	ITIH4 is an acute-phase response protein whose function remains unclear [58]. Research points to a tumor suppressor activity of ITIH4 in human cancers and dysregulation in PCa [43,59].
P07288	Prostate-specific antigen (PSA)	KLK3	C209Y; V55M; G156V; AVCG (47–50); S117P; G87R; L124F; A154T; I179T	Missense; inframe_insertion	PSA is widely used as serum biomarker for PCa. It was approved by the US Food and Drug Administration (FDA) in 1994 [60].
Q12907	Vesicular integral-membrane protein VIP36	LMAN2	G250S; D229N	missense	LMAN2 protein is involved in endoplasmic reticulum to Golgi trafficking of some glycoproteins [61]. Dysregulation of the LMAN2 gene has been indicated in some cancers [62–64], while the role in PCa remains obscure. However, raised LMAN2 urinary levels were detected in PCa patients [44].
P41222	Prostaglandin-H2 D-isomerase	PTGDS	L130M	missense	PTGDS is involved in prostaglandins metabolism and lipid transport. The PTGDS gene is downregulated in malignant prostate tissues compared to non-malignant tissues and integrates a signature that predicts relapse after prostatectomy. In vitro, its overexpression increased death and suppressed the growth of PCa cells [65,66].
Q13510	Acid ceramidase	ASAH1	V246A	missense	ASAH1 hydrolyzes ceramide to sphingosine and fatty acid [67] and its protein levels are elevated in tumor prostate tissue [68]. Its increased levels have been suggested as a therapeutic target in PCa as they have been correlated with metastasis establishment and resistance to chemotherapy [69,70].
P08294	Extracellular superoxide dismutase [Cu-Zn]	SOD3	A58T	missense	SOD3 is a known tumor suppressor gene in PCa. It is an antioxidant enzyme that catalyzes the dismutation of the superoxide radical anion [71]. SOD3-reduced levels were reported in PCa patients, and its overexpression in PCa cells prevented cell proliferation, migration, and invasion, suggesting a role as a therapeutic target and predictive marker [72,73].
P09211	Glutathione S-transferase P	GSTP1	I105V	missense	GSTP1 is a known tumor suppressor gene in PCa and is responsible for cellular detoxification through glutathione conjugation [74]. PCa is characterized by loss of GSTP1 function, mostly due to hypermethylation of its regulatory CpG island [75], and it is purported to occur early in prostatic carcinogenesis [76,77].

Table 3. Cont.

Uniprot ID	Protein Name	Gene Name	Mutation Description	Mutation Type	Protein Role in PCa or Other Types of Cancer
P10451	Osteopontin	SPP1	A22G	missense	SPP1 is a bone matrix protein involved in bone remodeling, modulation of inflammation, cell adhesion, and migration and angiogenesis [78]. In PCa, SPP1 is associated with metastasis and proliferation [79], lower overall survival and biochemical relapse-free survival, and high GS [80]. Higher SPP1 levels were reported in PCa patients [80–82].
P15309	Prostatic acid phosphatase	PAP	G68D	missense	PAP is one of the main secreted proteins by the prostate cells and was the first serum screening marker for PCa. PAP was later replaced by PSA [83,84].
P25311	Zinc-alpha-2-glycoprotein	ZAG	P187L; A46T	missense	ZAG promotes adipocyte lipolysis, resulting in cancer cachexia [85]. Elevated levels of this protein have been proposed as a serum marker for PCa [86,87], and a significant predictive ability was found for urinary ZAG [8].
Q4ZJI4	Sodium/hydrogen exchanger 9B1	SLC9B1	N70S	missense	SLC9B1 is a Na^+/H^+ transporter responsible for preserving cellular homeostasis [88], but this transporter has not yet been correlated with any type of cancer.
Q9P2J8	Zinc finger protein 624	ZNF624	S207F	missense	ZNF624 has not been well studied yet, but in breast cancer was one of the target genes of a microRNA found to be significantly and independently correlated with patient prognosis [89].
Q6EMK4	Vasorin	VASN	R161Q	missense	VASN, an inhibitor of TGF-beta signaling, is upregulated in PCa tissues and stimulates PCa proliferation [90].
P08174	Complement decay-accelerating factor	CD55	S162L	missense	CD55 inhibits the complement system [91]. In PCa, CD55 mediates tumor cells survival and growth [92].

This table shows the UniProt IDs, protein and gene names, mutation site/description and type, and the role of proteins in PCa.

3.2.5. Prediction of the Likely Impact of Single-Residue Substitutions in Proteins

With the purpose of determining the potential impact of point mutations on protein function, PolyPhen-2 tool was used. It is worthy of mention that AMBP*A286G and CD55*S162L mutant protein isoforms were predicted to be probably damaging, while SLC9B1*N70S, ZNF624*S207F, VASN*R161Q, and HSPG2*Q1062H were predicted to be benign. Most point mutations were predicted to be possibly or probably damaging. The results are presented in Tables 4 and S5.

Table 4. Results of Polyphen-2 score and prediction for the mapped mutations.

Gene Name	Mutation	Prediction	Score	Sensitivity	Specificity
AMBP	G238S	Probably damaging	1.000	0.00	1.00
AMBP	E192G	Probably damaging	0.75	0.981	0.96
AMBP	V69M	Possibly damaging	0.758	0.85	0.92
AMBP	A286G	Probably damaging	1.000	0.00	1.00
AMBP	P197S	Benign	0.051	0.94	0.83
AMBP	G338S	Probably damaging	0.994	0.69	0.97
AMBP	G341A	Probably damaging	0.958	0.78	0.95
AMBP	V313I	Benign	0.025	0.95	0.81
AMBP	G186R	Probably damaging	1.000	0.00	1.00
AMBP	R185Q	Probably damaging	0.992	0.70	0.97
CDH1	H233R	Possibly damaging	0.831	0.84	0.93
CDH1	A408E	Possibly damaging	0.798	0.84	0.93
EFEMP1	V463M	Probably damaging	0.999	0.14	0.99
HSPG2	V4332I	Benign	0.001	0.99	0.15
HSPG2	A1503V	Probably damaging	1.00	0.00	1.00
HSPG2	S970F	Possibly damaging	0.498	0.88	0.90
HSPG2	M638V	Benign	0.00	1.00	0.00
HSPG2	Q1062H	Benign	0.00	1.00	0.00
ITIH4	R866C	Probably damaging	1	0.00	1.00
ITIH4	G893S	Benign	0.00	1.00	0.00
KLK3	C209Y	Probably damaging	1.000	0.00	1.00
KLK3	G156V	Probably damaging	1.000	0.00	1.00
KLK3	V55M	Probably damaging	0.972	0.77	0.96
KLK3	S117P	Possibly damaging	0.621	0.87	0.91
KLK3	G87R	Benign	0.128	0.93	0.86
KLK3	L124F	Probably damaging	1.000	0.00	1.00
KLK3	A154T	Possibly damaging	0.657	0.86	0.91
KLK3	I179T	Possibly damaging	0.800	0.84	0.93
LMAN2	G250S	Probably damaging	1.00	0.00	1.00
LMAN2	D229N	Probably damaging	0.983	0.74	0.96
PTGDS	L130M	Probably damaging	1.00	0.00	1.00
ASAH1	V246A	Benign	0.00	1.00	0.00
SOD3	A58T	Benign	0.188	0.92	0.87
GSTP1	I105V	Benign	0.00	1.00	0.00
SPP1	A22G	Possibly damaging	0.611	0.87	0.91
ACP3	G68D	Probably damaging	1.00	0.00	1.00
AZGP1	P187L	Probably damaging	0.94	0.69	0.97
AZGP1	A46T	Benign	0.002	0.99	0.30
SLC9B1	N70S	Benign	0.036	0.94	0.82
ZNF624	S207F	Benign	0.214	0.92	0.88
VASN	R161Q	Benign	0.019	0.95	0.80
CD55	S162L	Probably damaging	0.990	0.72	0.97

3.2.6. Protein–Protein Interaction Analysis

In addition to impacting the function of proteins, mutations can also affect interactions between proteins and, consequently, important biological processes and signaling pathways. To predict interactions between the proteins in which point mutations were identified, the STRING search tool was used. As shown in Figure 5, the network consisted of 86 connected proteins (nodes) through 214 edges with different confidence levels. The protein–protein interaction enrichment p-value was $<1.0 \times 10^{-16}$. Reactome enrichment analysis showed 12 pathways enriched in this network (Table S6). Regulation of Insulin-like Growth Factor (IGF) transport and uptake by Insulin-like Growth Factor Binding Proteins (IGFBPs) was the third most important pathway in this network, while Extracellular matrix (ECM) organization was the tenth. This network shows predicted interactions between most of the proteins.

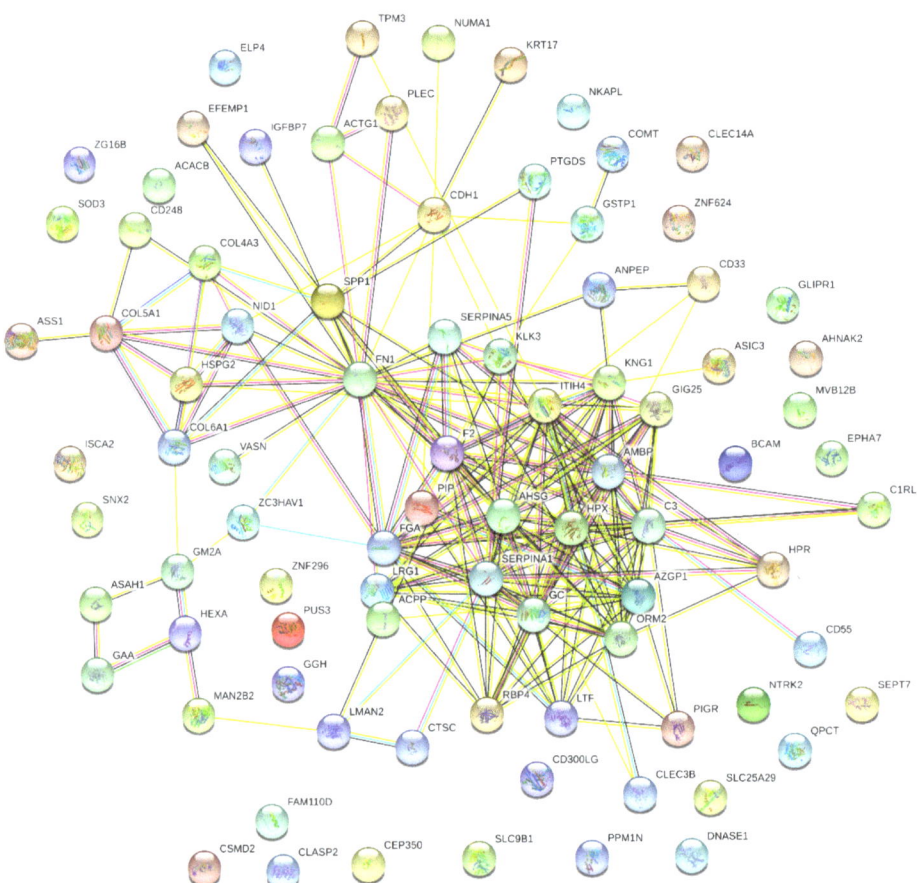

Figure 5. PPI network of 86 mutated proteins with known expression in the prostate.

3.2.7. Prediction of the Likely Impact of Single-Residue Substitutions in Protein–Protein Affinity

To predict the impact of point mutations on PPIs, the SAAMBE-SEQ tool was used. The likely effect of AMBP*A286G, HSPG2*Q1062H, VASN*R161Q, and CD55*S162L point mutations on protein–protein interactions was scrutinized. Point mutations detected on SLC9B1 and ZNF624 were not examined as these proteins do not interact with any proteins in the network. Additionally, the impact of point mutations on proteins involved in the

IGF pathway was also explored. This analysis revealed that the likely effect of these point mutations is destabilizing for PPIs (Table S7).

4. Discussion

The limitations and the invasive nature of serum PCa screening have driven the discovery of new candidate urinary biomarkers, especially protein markers. However, so far, none has translated into clinically useful tools, reflecting the need to discover novel biomarkers and/or new combinations of biomarkers. Thus, this study aimed to take advantage of a non-invasively collected biofluid, urine, and a high throughput approach, proteomics, to identify new protein targets for predicting the risk of developing PCa. This work was divided into three stages: characterization of the urine proteome profile and selection of protein targets; testing of shortlisted protein targets in a larger, independent cohort; and characterization of the urine proteogenome profile. The urine proteome profile of PCa and cancer-free subjects was analyzed by two software packages and 18 dysregulated proteins, of which 5 (TTR, EFEMP1, CDH1, SECTM1, KLK3) common to both software, were found. The integration of the urine proteome profile of PCa patients with proteome data from other studies reviewed by us [28] supported the selection of potential discriminatory protein targets. As a result, AMBP, CDH1, EFEMP1, LMAN2, and TTR stood out as potential targets and were tested in an independent cohort of patients. In this testing phase, incubation with anti-E-cadherin did not result in a band around 120 kDa (full-length protein), but rather a band about 80 kDa. We realized that this 80 kDa fragment corresponded to soluble E-cadherin (sE-cadherin) and has been previously identified in tissue and serum from PCa patients [93,94] and in urine from patients with other cancers [95,96], using antibody-based techniques. Concerning PCa, as far as we know, here we present the first report of the detection of sE-cadherin fragment in the urine. Kuefer et al. [93] suggested that the 80 kDa fragment is originated from the extracellular domain of full-length E-cadherin. Increased levels of sE-cadherin have been reported in serum and tumor prostate tissue from PCa patients and are correlated with disease stage [94,97,98]. Differential abundances of these MS-detected proteins were tested in an independent cohort using immunoblot, but different variations were observed. Additionally, urinary PSA levels were also assessed in this independent cohort, but did not distinguish PCa patients from controls, which agrees with other studies [99].

The proteogenome landscape of urine from PCa patients was then characterized and 1665 mutant protein isoforms were disclosed, of which 417 were cancer-related mutations. After considering only mutations present in all urine samples and proteins with known prostate expression, 86 mutant protein isoforms emerged. Among these proteins are some of known relevance for PCa, namely Acid ceramidase (ASAH1), Extracellular superoxide dismutase [Cu-Zn] (SOD3), Glutathione S-transferase P (GSTP1), Osteopontin (SPP1), Prostatic Acid Phosphatase (PAP), and Zinc-Alpha-2-Glycoprotein (ZAG). PAP is gaining renewed interest due to its superior predictive role of cause-specific survival and GS compared to serum PSA in men with high risk PCa [100,101]. Remarkably, it was recently suggested that a form of PAP (PLPAcP) associates with early PCa [102]. Identifying a new mutation in this protein in a non-invasive biological fluid, adding to the prediction of PAP mutation to be probably damaging, strengthens the renewed interest in its study in PCa. Mutations found on the 86 proteins were searched for in databases and the literature and, to the best of our knowledge, only rs17632542 [36,103–105], rs1695 [37,38,106,107], and rs7041 [39] mutations mapped on PSA, GSTP1, and GC proteins have been described in the PCa context. In that vein, these results validate the proteogenome analysis performed in the present study.

The analysis of the urine proteogenome profile of PCa patients revealed 6 differentially abundant mutant protein isoforms, namely AMBP*A286G, SLC9B1*N70S, HSPG2*Q1062H, ZNF624*S207F, VASN*R161Q, and CD55*S162L. From the comparison of the proteome and proteogenome profile of PCa patients, AMBP, CDH1, EFEMP1, KLK3, and LMAN2 proteins stood out. Their native form was found dysregulated in urine from PCa patients, but the same was not observed with their mutant form, with the exception of AMBP*A286G and HSPG2*Q1062H. These results may explain the differences between MS and immunoblot data, because the antibodies either do not recognize the mutated peptides or do not specifically recognize them.

PPIs play a pivotal role in most biological processes. Dysregulation of these protein interactions may result in pathological conditions, such as cancer, being involved in tumor progression, invasion, and metastasis [108,109]. In this sense, PPIs have been claimed as promising therapeutic targets for numerous types of cancer, including for PCa. For this type of cancer, 28 small molecules and 14 peptides have been proposed to disrupt PPIs with relevance to PCa progression [110]. To explore PPIs between proteins with known prostate expression and the pathways in which these interactions were involved, the STRING tool was used. In this analysis, the IGF transport and uptake by IGFBPs proved to be the third most important pathway in the network. The IGF axis is a network of ligands (GF1, IGF2, insulin) and IGFBP receptors (IGF1R, IGF2R, INSR), the latter being responsible for mediating the activity of IGFs [111]. IGFs are oncogenic regulators, promoting prostate tumor growth, survival, and proliferation, and the role of IGF axis has been well documented in PCa. For instance, IGFBP-2 enhanced proliferation of androgen-independent prostate cancer cells [112] and IGF-I levels were found raised in serum and prostate tissue from PCa patients, being a predictor of risk for this type of cancer [113,114]. In accordance with this, IGF1R and INSR act as oncogenes in PCa, enhancing tumor growth, proliferation, invasion, and angiogenesis [115]. Considering the relevance of the IGF pathway in PCa, the impact of mutations on the interaction of proteins involved in this pathway was predicted. According to SAAMBE-SEQ, the mutations were predicted to destabilize all PPIs involved in the IGF pathway, which naturally could affect this pathway and consequently the progression of PCa.

To investigate the likely impact of each amino acid substitution on protein function and PPIs involving the dysregulated mutant protein isoforms (AMBP*A286G, SLC9B1*N70S, HSPG2*Q1062H, ZNF624*S207F, VASN*R161Q, and CD55*S162L), the PolyPhen-2 and SAAMBE-SEQ prediction tools were used. The role of the SLC9B1 and ZNF624 proteins on cancer is completely unknown, so the downregulation of their mutant protein isoforms and the prediction of their benign impact do not allow conclusions to be drawn. HSPG2, in its intact form, is a well-described pro-angiogenic molecule, being correlated with GS and increased cell proliferation and viability [55,56,116]. The intact form of this protein was found increased in tumor prostate tissue, but in sera from PCa patients raised levels of HSPG2-derived fragments resulting from matrix metalloproteinase 7 (MMP7) degradation were observed. These fragments were mostly originated from domain IV and were not present in sera from non-cancer subjects, suggesting that HSPG2 cleavage occurs during metastasis and before the protein enters the bloodstream. Using an in silico analysis, Grindel et al. predicted that domains III and V of HSPG2 are the most prone to cleavage by MMP-7 and generate new peptides for other extracellular proteases to digest [55]. Curiously, in this work, the mutated peptide identified in the mutant HSPG2 isoform is located on domain III. The cleavage of HSPG2 and other components of basement membrane occurs during PCa cell invasion and is orchestrated by proteases such as MMPs, cathepsin L, and BMP1/Tolloid-like proteases. Both Cathepsin L and BMP1/Tolloid-like proteases cleave HSPG2 in domain V, originating the Endorepellin [117] and LG3 [118] peptides, respectively. Unlike the intact form, cleaved Endorepellin and LG3 peptides behave as powerful anti-angiogenic factors, being claimed as potential therapeutic targets for cancer [118]. In fact, the administration of endorepellin to mice with squamous cell carcinomas and lung carcinomas resulted in mitigation of tumor growth, angiogenesis and metabolism and promotion of tumor hypoxia [119]. Accordingly, LG3-diminished levels were noticed in breast cancer cells and in plasma from breast cancer patients [120]. Only the LG3 peptide has been detected in urine [121,122]. In PCa, both the existence and the role of these peptides are unknown, and the only recognized HSPG2 protease is MMP7. A complex network between HSPG2 and other basement membrane components, such as collagens, laminin, and nidogen is responsible for ECM integrity. When this integrity is disturbed, the metastatic process is compromised [123]. In the present work, mutations were identified in HSPG2, collagens, nidogen, and in other proteins involved in ECM organization. When the impact of these mutations on PPIs was predicted, they all proved to be destabilizing, which eventually affects ECM dynamics and tumor progression. All these results, together with the fact that the HSPG2*Q1062H point mutation was predicted to be benign and the mutant peptide was downregulated in PCa patients, suggest that this mutant peptide may have beneficial effects in patients with PCa and opens doors for its study in PCa treatment. Concerning the AMBP protein, it is cleaved into three chains, namely Alpha-1-microglobulin, Bikunin, and Trypstatin. The function of the AMBP protein in cancer remains undisclosed. However, it has been claimed that the AMBP-derived product bikunin is underexpressed in oral squamous cell carcinoma and plays an antitumor role [40]. In line with this, there is evidence that bikunin significantly prevented tumor invasion and metastasis in Lewis lung carcinoma and ovarian carcinoma cells [124,125]. Curiously, in this work, the mutant peptide identified in the AMBP isoform is located on the bikunin fragment. The mutation identified in AMBP was predicted to be probably damaging, destabilized all PPIs in which AMBP was involved, and resulted in an upregulation of mutant AMBP isoform in PCa patients. This may suggest a detrimental role of this mutation on PCa patients. Regarding CD55, it blocks complement response by accelerating the decay of C3 and C5 convertases [126] and is involved in PCa cell survival and metastasis [92]. This interplay between CD55 and C3 is visible by their interaction in the STRING network. The mutation detected on the CD55 protein was predicted to be probably damaging and destabilizing for CD55-C3 interaction. With these findings, it seems reasonable to suspect the detrimental role of this mutation on PCa patients. Regarding VASN, it is a known inhibitor of TGF-β signaling [127]. The TGF-β pathway has a dual role in cancer, because it prevents cell proliferation in early stages and in advanced stages stimulates proliferation, epithelial-to-mesenchymal transition (EMT) and evasion of immune surveillance, and attenuates apoptosis [128]. The mechanism involved in this inhibitory action of VASN on TGF-beta was revealed in breast cancer cell lines. It was demonstrated that a soluble form of VASN resulting from the proteolytic shedding of its extracellular domain by Metalloprotease domain 17 (ADAM17) is responsible for controlling the TGFβ pathway [129]. In PCa, the role of VASN is largely unexplored, including the interplay between the VASN and TGFβ pathways. However, overexpression of VASN in prostate tumor tissue and in serum from PCa patients and the subsequent promotion of cell proliferation and PCa progression have already been reported, in agreement with other types of cancer [90]. Interestingly, in this work, the mutated peptide identified in the VASN protein is located on the extracellular domain of the protein, the domain cleaved by ADAM17. The mutation identified in VASN resulted in a downregulation of this mutant protein isoform in PCa patients and was predicted to be benign, which may suggest a protective role of this mutation on PCa patients.

These findings indicate that, in mutational diseases such as cancer and in biofluids with high proteolytic activity, such as urine, the application of proteogenomics to urine analysis and the study of peptides can be very enriching because point mutations can go unnoticed at the protein level but are detected at the peptide level. This may sharpen or renew interest in underexplored targets, as observed in this work. We hope to address some of these questions in future work. Furthermore, it would be interesting to test these mutant peptides by an MS-targeted approach such as MRM, but this is beyond the scope of this work. This work's novelty lies in the proteogenome characterization of urine from PCa patients and the combined analysis of MS data using two different software packages, increasing certainty in the identification of urinary proteins modulated by PCa.

5. Conclusions

The majority of mutations identified in this work have never been associated with PCa, and some are predicted to be damaging, which offers an auspicious opportunity for research and development of PCa biomarkers, especially in the HSPG2 context. Additionally, the discovery of cancer-associated mutations in PCa-related proteins in urine is promising given this biofluid's non-invasive and dynamic nature.

Supplementary Materials: The following supporting information can be downloaded at: https://www.mdpi.com/article/10.3390/cancers14082001/s1: Table S1, Clinical data of subjects included in the discovery cohort group; Table S2, Clinical data of subjects included in the testing cohort group; Table S3, Summary of statistical analysis results of shortlisted proteins evaluated in the testing group; Table S4, List of mutant protein isoforms identified in the 86 proteins with known prostate expression; Table S5, Prediction of likely impact of point mutations on protein function using PolyPhen-2 tool; Table S6, Reactome pathway enrichment analysis of the network; Table S7, Prediction of likely impact of point mutations on protein–protein interactions using SAAMBE-SEQ tool; Figure S1, Original Western blots figures; Figure S2, Levels of AMBP*A286G, SLC9B1*N70S, HSPG2*Q1062H, ZNF624*S207F, VASN*R161Q, and CD55*S162L mutant protein isoforms and respective levels of native form (when applicable) in the urine from PCa patients.

Author Contributions: Conceptualization, T.L., R.H., R.V. and M.F.; methodology, T.L., R.H., R.V. and M.F.; validation, T.L., R.H., R.V. and M.F.; formal analysis, T.L., A.S.B., F.T., R.F., C.J., A.L.-M., R.H., R.V. and M.F.; investigation, T.L.; resources, D.B.-S., C.J., L.A., A.L.-M., R.H., R.V. and M.F.; data curation, A.S.B., F.T. and R.F.; writing—original draft preparation, T.L.; writing—review and Editing, T.L., A.S.B., F.T., R.F., A.L.-M., D.B.-S., L.A., C.J., R.H., R.V. and M.F.; visualization, T.L., R.H., R.V. and M.F.; supervision, R.H., R.V. and M.F.; project administration, T.L.; funding acquisition, T.L., R.H., R.V. and M.F. All authors have read and agreed to the published version of the manuscript.

Funding: This work was supported by the Portuguese Foundation for Science and Technology (FCT), European Union, QREN, FEDER, and COMPETE for the Unidade de Investigação Cardiovascular (UIDB/IC/00051/2020 and UIDP/00051/2020), Institute of Biomedicine (iBiMED) (UIDB/04501/2020, POCI-01-0145-FEDER-007628), and FCT QOPNA ((FCT UID/QUI/00062/2019) and LAQV/REQUIMTE (UIDB/50006/2020) research units and the DOCnet (NORTE-01-0145-FEDER-000003), by Norte Portugal Regional Operational Programme (NORTE 2020), under the PORTUGAL 2020 Partnership Agreement, through the European Regional Development Fund (ERDF). T.L. is supported by an individual scholarship (SFRH/BD/136904/2018), F.T. by a post-doctoral research grant by UnIC (UIDP/00051/2020), and R.V. by individual fellowship grant (IF/00286/2015).

Institutional Review Board Statement: The study was conducted according to the guidelines of the Declaration of Helsinki and approved by the IPO-Porto Ethics Committee (Comissão de Ética para a Saúde, Reference 282R/2017).

Informed Consent Statement: Informed consent was obtained from all subjects involved in the study.

Data Availability Statement: Data generated during Mass Spectrometry analysis is available in the ProteomeXchange Consortium via the PRIDE partner repository with the data set identifier PXD017902.

Conflicts of Interest: The authors declare no conflict of interest.

References

1. Sung, H.; Ferlay, J.; Siegel, R.L.; Laversanne, M.; Soerjomataram, I.; Jemal, A.; Bray, F. Global cancer statistics 2020: GLOBOCAN estimates of incidence and mortality worldwide for 36 cancers in 185 countries. *CA Cancer J. Clin.* **2021**, *71*, 209–249. [CrossRef] [PubMed]
2. Saini, S. PSA and beyond: Alternative prostate cancer biomarkers. *Cell. Oncol.* **2016**, *39*, 97–106. [CrossRef] [PubMed]
3. Jakobsen, N.A.; Hamdy, F.C.; Bryant, R.J. Novel biomarkers for the detection of prostate cancer. *J. Clin. Urol.* **2016**, *9*, 3–10. [CrossRef] [PubMed]
4. Eskra, J.N.; Daniel, R.; Pavlovich, C.P.; Catalona, W.J.; Luo, J. Approaches to urinary detection of prostate cancer. *Prostate Cancer Prostatic Dis.* **2019**, *22*, 362–381. [CrossRef]
5. Van der Burgt, Y.E.M. Protein biomarker discovery is still relevant and has entered a new phase. *eBioMedicine* **2019**, *43*, 15. [CrossRef]

6. Davalieva, K.; Kiprijanovska, S.; Komina, S.; Petrusevska, G.; Zografska, C.C.; Polenakovic, M. Proteomics analysis of urine reveals acute phase response proteins as candidate diagnostic biomarkers for prostate cancer. *Proteome Sci.* **2015**, *13*, 2. [CrossRef]
7. Garbis, S.D.; Tyritzis, S.I.; Roumeliotis, T.; Zerefos, P.; Giannopoulou, E.G.; Vlahou, A.; Kossida, S.; Diaz, J.; Vourekas, S.; Tamvakopoulos, C.; et al. Search for potential markers for prostate cancer diagnosis, prognosis and treatment in clinical tissue specimens using amine-specific isobaric tagging (iTRAQ) with two-dimensional liquid chromatography and tandem mass spectrometry. *J. Proteome Res.* **2008**, *7*, 3146–3158. [CrossRef]
8. Katafigiotis, I.; Tyritzis, S.I.; Stravodimos, K.G.; Alamanis, C.; Pavlakis, K.; Vlahou, A.; Makridakis, M.; Katafigioti, A.; Garbis, S.D.; Constantinides, C.A. Zinc α2-glycoprotein as a potential novel urine biomarker for the early diagnosis of prostate cancer. *BJU Int.* **2012**, *110*, E688–E693. [CrossRef]
9. Louie, K.S.; Seigneurin, A.; Cathcart, P.; Sasieni, P. Do prostate cancer risk models improve the predictive accuracy of PSA screening? A meta-analysis. *Ann. Oncol.* **2015**, *26*, 848–864. [CrossRef]
10. Blume-Jensen, P.; Berman, D.M.; Rimm, D.L.; Shipitsin, M.; Putzi, M.; Nifong, T.P.; Small, C.; Choudhury, S.; Capela, T.; Coupal, L.; et al. Biology of human tumors development and clinical validation of an in situ biopsy-based multimarker assay for risk stratification in prostate cancer. *Clin. Cancer Res.* **2015**, *17*, 372–381. [CrossRef]
11. Deras, I.L.; Aubin, S.M.J.; Blase, A.; Day, J.R.; Koo, S.; Partin, A.W.; Ellis, W.J.; Marks, L.S.; Fradet, Y.; Rittenhouse, H.; et al. PCA3: A molecular urine assay for predicting prostate biopsy outcome. *J. Urol.* **2008**, *179*, 1587–1592. [CrossRef] [PubMed]
12. Van Neste, L.; Hendriks, R.J.; Dijkstra, S.; Trooskens, G.; Cornel, E.B.; Jannink, S.A.; de Jong, H.; Hessels, D.; Smit, F.P.; Melchers, W.J.G.; et al. Detection of high-grade prostate cancer using a urinary molecular biomarker—Based risk score. *Eur. Urol.* **2016**, *70*, 740–748. [CrossRef] [PubMed]
13. McKiernan, J.; Donovan, M.J.; O'Neill, V.; Bentink, S.; Noerholm, M.; Belzer, S.; Skog, J.; Kattan, M.W.; Partin, A.; Andriole, G.; et al. A novel urine exosome gene expression assay to predict high-grade prostate cancer at initial biopsy. *JAMA Oncol.* **2016**, *2*, 882–889. [CrossRef] [PubMed]
14. Tosoian, J.J.; Dunn, R.L.; Niknafs, Y.S.; Saha, A.; Vince, R.A.; St. Sauver, J.L.; Jacobson, D.J.; McGree, M.E.; Siddiqui, J.; Groskopf, J.; et al. Association of urinary myprostatescore, age, and prostate volume in a longitudinal cohort of healthy men: Long-term findings from the olmsted county study. *Eur. Urol. Open Sci.* **2021**, *29*, 30–35. [CrossRef]
15. Lin, T.; Zhang, T.; Kitata, R.B.; Liu, T.; Smith, R.D.; Qian, W.; Shi, T. Mass spectrometry-based targeted proteomics for analysis of protein mutations. *Mass Spectrom. Rev.* **2021**, e21741. [CrossRef]
16. Reva, B.; Antipin, Y.; Sander, C. Predicting the functional impact of protein mutations: Application to cancer genomics. *Nucleic Acids Res.* **2011**, *39*, e118. [CrossRef]
17. Sinha, A.; Huang, V.; Livingstone, J.; Wang, J.; Fox, N.S.; Kurganovs, N.; Ignatchenko, V.; Fritsch, K.; Donmez, N.; Heisler, L.E.; et al. The proteogenomic landscape of curable prostate cancer. *Cancer Cell* **2019**, *35*, 414–427.e6. [CrossRef]
18. Lazar, I.M.; Karcini, A.; Ahuja, S.; Estrada-Palma, C. Proteogenomic analysis of protein sequence alterations in breast cancer cells. *Sci. Rep.* **2019**, *9*, 10381. [CrossRef]
19. Mathivanan, S.; Ji, H.; Tauro, B.J.; Chen, Y.S.; Simpson, R.J. Identifying mutated proteins secreted by colon cancer cell lines using mass spectrometry. *J. Proteom.* **2012**, *76*, 141–149. [CrossRef]
20. Zhang, B.; Wang, J.; Wang, X.; Zhu, J.; Liu, Q.; Shi, Z.; Chambers, M.C.; Zimmerman, L.J.; Shaddox, K.F.; Kim, S.; et al. Proteogenomic characterization of human colon and rectal cancer. *Nature* **2014**, *513*, 382–387. [CrossRef]
21. Kwon, O.K.; Jeon, J.M.I.; Sung, E.; Na, A.Y.; Kim, S.J.; Lee, S. Comparative secretome profiling and mutant protein identification in metastatic prostate cancer cells by quantitative mass spectrometry-based proteomics. *Cancer Genom. Proteom.* **2018**, *15*, 279–290. [CrossRef] [PubMed]
22. Kwon, O.K.; Ha, Y.-S.; Lee, J.N.; Kim, S.; Lee, H.; Chun, S.Y.; Kwon, T.G.; Lee, S. Comparative proteome profiling and mutant protein identification in metastatic prostate cancer cells by quantitative mass spectrometry-based proteogenomics. *Cancer Genom. Proteom.* **2019**, *16*, 273–286. [CrossRef] [PubMed]
23. Yang, J.; Roy, R.; Jedinak, A.; Moses, M.A. Mining the human urinary proteome biomarker discovery for human cancer and its metastases. *Cancer J.* **2015**, *21*, 327–336. [CrossRef] [PubMed]
24. Dzieciatkowska, M.; Hill, R.C.; Hansen, K. GeLC-MS/MS analysis of complex protein mixtures. *Methods Mol. Biol.* **2014**, *1156*, 53–66. [CrossRef]
25. Shevchenko, A.; Tomas, H.; Havliš, J.; Olsen, J.V.; Mann, M. In-gel digestion for mass spectrometric characterization of proteins and proteomes. *Nat. Protoc.* **2007**, *1*, 2856–2860. [CrossRef]
26. Perez-Riverol, Y.; Csordas, A.; Bai, J.; Bernal-Llinares, M.; Hewapathirana, S.; Kundu, D.J.; Inuganti, A.; Griss, J.; Mayer, G.; Eisenacher, M.; et al. The PRIDE database and related tools and resources in 2019: Improving support for quantification data. *Nucleic Acids Res.* **2019**, *47*, D442–D450. [CrossRef]
27. Pang, Z.; Chong, J.; Zhou, G.; de Lima Morais, D.A.; Chang, L.; Barrette, M.; Gauthier, C.; Jacques, P.É.; Li, S.; Xia, J. MetaboAnalyst 5.0: Narrowing the gap between raw spectra and functional insights. *Nucleic Acids Res.* **2021**, *49*, W388–W396. [CrossRef]
28. Lima, T.; Henrique, R.; Vitorino, R.; Fardilha, M. Bioinformatic analysis of dysregulated proteins in prostate cancer patients reveals putative urinary biomarkers and key biological pathways. *Med. Oncol.* **2021**, *38*, 10381. [CrossRef]
29. Zhao, M.; Li, M.; Yang, Y.; Guo, Z.; Sun, Y.; Shao, C.; Li, M.; Sun, W.; Gao, Y. A comprehensive analysis and annotation of human normal urinary proteome. *Sci. Rep.* **2017**, *7*, 3024. [CrossRef]

30. Caseiro, A.; Barros, A.; Ferreira, R.; Padrão, A.; Aroso, M.; Quintaneiro, C.; Pereira, A.; Marinheiro, R.; Vitorino, R.; Amado, F. Pursuing type 1 diabetes mellitus and related complications through urinary proteomics. *Transl. Res.* **2014**, *163*, 188–199. [CrossRef]
31. Piñero, J.; Ramírez-Anguita, J.M.; Saüch-Pitarch, J.; Ronzano, F.; Centeno, E.; Sanz, F.; Furlong, L.I. The DisGeNET knowledge platform for disease genomics: 2019 update. *Nucleic Acids Res.* **2020**, *48*, D845–D855. [CrossRef]
32. Adzhubei, I.A.; Schmidt, S.; Peshkin, L.; Ramensky, V.E.; Gerasimova, A.; Bork, P.; Kondrashov, A.S.; Sunyaev, S.R. A method and server for predicting damaging missense mutations. *Nat. Methods* **2010**, *7*, 248–249. [CrossRef]
33. Adzhubei, I.; Jordan, D.M.; Sunyaev, S.R. Predicting functional effect of human missense mutations using PolyPhen-2. *Curr. Protoc. Hum. Genet.* **2013**, *76*, 7–20. [CrossRef]
34. Szklarczyk, D.; Gable, A.L.; Nastou, K.C.; Lyon, D.; Kirsch, R.; Pyysalo, S.; Doncheva, N.T.; Legeay, M.; Fang, T.; Bork, P.; et al. The STRING database in 2021: Customizable protein-protein networks, and functional characterization of user-uploaded gene/measurement sets. *Nucleic Acids Res.* **2021**, *49*, D605–D612. [CrossRef]
35. Li, G.; Pahari, S.; Murthy, A.K.; Liang, S.; Fragoza, R.; Yu, H.; Alexov, E. SAAMBE-SEQ: A sequence-based method for predicting mutation effect on protein-protein binding affinity. *Bioinformatics* **2021**, *37*, 992–999. [CrossRef]
36. Otto, J.J.; Correll, V.L.; Engstroem, H.A.; Hitefield, N.L.; Main, B.P.; Albracht, B.; Johnson-Pais, T.; Yang, L.F.; Liss, M.; Boutros, P.C.; et al. Targeted mass spectrometry of a clinically relevant psa variant from post-DRE urines for quantitation and genotype determination. *Proteom. Clin. Appl.* **2020**, *14*, e2000012. [CrossRef]
37. Santric, V.; Djokic, M.; Suvakov, S.; Pljesa-Ercegovac, M.; Nikitovic, M.; Radic, T.; Acimovic, M.; Stankovic, V.; Bumbasirevic, U.; Milojevic, B.; et al. GSTP1 rs1138272 polymorphism affects prostate cancer risk. *Medicina* **2020**, *56*, 128. [CrossRef]
38. Zhang, Y.; Yuan, Y.; Chen, Y.; Wang, Z.; Li, F.; Zhao, Q. Association between GSTP1 Ile105Val polymorphism and urinary system cancer risk: Evidence from 51 studies. *Onco. Targets. Ther.* **2016**, *9*, 3565–3569. [CrossRef]
39. Gilbert, R.; Bonilla, C.; Metcalfe, C.; Lewis, S.; Evans, D.M.; Fraser, W.D.; Kemp, J.P.; Donovan, J.L.; Hamdy, F.C.; Neal, D.E.; et al. Associations of vitamin D pathway genes with circulating 25-hydroxivitamin-D, 1, 25-dihydroxyvitamin-D, and prostate cancer: A nested case–control study. *Cancer Causes Control.* **2015**, *26*, 205–218. [CrossRef]
40. Sekikawa, S.; Onda, T.; Miura, N.; Nomura, T.; Takano, N.; Shibahara, T.; Honda, K. Underexpression of α-1-microglobulin/bikunin precursor predicts a poor prognosis in oral squamous cell carcinoma. *Int. J. Oncol.* **2018**, *53*, 2605–2614. [CrossRef]
41. Huang, M.; Han, Y.; Gao, J.; Feng, J.; Zhu, L.; Qu, L.; Shen, L.; Shou, C. High level of serum AMBP is associated with poor response to paclitaxel-capecitabine chemotherapy in advanced gastric cancer patients. *Med. Oncol.* **2013**, *30*, 748. [CrossRef]
42. Fujita, K.; Kume, H.; Matsuzaki, K.; Kawashima, A.; Ujike, T. Proteomic analysis of urinary extracellular vesicles from high Gleason score prostate cancer. *Sci. Rep.* **2017**, *7*, 42961. [CrossRef]
43. Hamm, A.; Veeck, J.; Bektas, N.; Wild, P.J.; Hartmann, A.; Heindrichs, U.; Kristiansen, G.; Werbowetski-Ogilvie, T.; Del Maestro, R.; Knuechel, R.; et al. Frequent expression loss of Inter-alpha-trypsin inhibitor heavy chain (ITIH) genes in multiple human solid tumors: A systematic expression analysis. *BMC Cancer* **2008**, *8*, 25. [CrossRef]
44. Davalieva, K.; Kiprijanovska, S.; Kostovska, I.M.; Stavridis, S.; Stankov, O.; Komina, S.; Petrusevska, G.; Polenakovic, M. Comparative proteomics analysis of urine reveals down-regulation of acute phase response signaling and LXR/RXR activation pathways in prostate cancer. *Proteomes* **2017**, *6*, 1. [CrossRef]
45. Zhao, H.; Zhao, X.; Lei, T.; Zhang, M. Screening, identification of prostate cancer urinary biomarkers and verification of important spots. *Invest. New Drugs* **2019**, *37*, 935–947. [CrossRef]
46. Rodríguez-Blanco, G.; Zeneyedpour, L.; Duijvesz, D.; Marije Hoogland, A.; Verhoef, E.I.; Kweldam, C.F.; Burgers, P.C.; Smitt, P.S.; Bangma, C.H.; Jenster, G.; et al. Tissue proteomics outlines AGR2 AND LOX5 as markers for biochemical recurrence of prostate cancer. *Oncotarget* **2018**, *9*, 36444–36456. [CrossRef]
47. Quanico, J.; Franck, J.; Gimeno, J.-P.; Sabbagh, R.; Salzet, M.; Day, R.; Fournier, I. Parafilm-assisted microdissection: A sampling method for mass spectrometry-based identification of differentially expressed prostate cancer protein biomarkers. *Chem. Commun.* **2015**, *51*, 4564–4567. [CrossRef]
48. Khan, A.P.; Poisson, L.M.; Bhat, V.B.; Fermin, D.; Zhao, R.; Kalyana-Sundaram, S.; Michailidis, G.; Nesvizhskii, A.I.; Omenn, G.S.; Chinnaiyan, A.M.; et al. Quantitative proteomic profiling of prostate cancer reveals a role for miR-128 in prostate cancer. *Mol. Cell. Proteom.* **2010**, *9*, 298–312. [CrossRef]
49. Debelec-Butuner, B.; Alapinar, C.; Ertunc, N.; Gonen-Korkmaz, C.; Yörükoğlu, K.; Korkmaz, K.S. TNFα-mediated loss of β-catenin/E-cadherin and subsequent increase in cell migration is partially restored by NKX3.1 expression in prostate cells. *PLoS ONE* **2014**, *9*, e109868. [CrossRef]
50. Tsui, K.-H.; Lin, Y.-H.; Chung, L.-C.; Chuang, S.-T.; Feng, T.-H.; Chiang, K.-C.; Chang, P.-L.; Yehg, C.-J.; Juang, H.H. Prostate-derived ets factor represses tumorigenesis and modulates epithelial-to-mesenchymal transition in bladder carcinoma cells. *Cancer Lett.* **2016**, *375*, 142–151. [CrossRef]
51. Li, F.; Pascal, L.E.; Stolz, D.B.; Wang, K.; Zhou, Y.; Chen, W.; Xu, Y.; Chen, Y.; Dhir, R.; Parwani, A.V.; et al. E-cadherin is down-regulated in benign prostate hyperplasia and required for tight junction formation and permeability barrier in prostatic epithelial cell monolayer. *Prostate* **2020**, *79*, 1226–1237. [CrossRef] [PubMed]
52. Shen, H.; Zhang, L.; Zhou, J.; Chen, Z.; Yang, G.; Liao, Y.; Zhu, M. Epidermal growth factor-containing fibulin-like extracellular matrix protein 1 (EFEMP1) acts as a potential diagnostic biomarker for prostate cancer. *Med. Sci. Monit.* **2017**, *23*, 216–222. [CrossRef] [PubMed]

53. Kim, Y.J.; Yoon, H.Y.; Kim, S.K.; Kim, Y.W.; Kim, E.J.; Kim, I.Y.; Kim, W.J. EFEMP1 as a novel DNA methylation marker for prostate cancer: Array-based DNA methylation and expression profiling. *Clin. Cancer Res.* **2011**, *17*, 4523–4530. [CrossRef] [PubMed]
54. Almeida, M.; Costa, V.L.; Costa, N.R.; Ramalho-Carvalho, J.; Baptista, T.; Ribeiro, F.R.; Paulo, P.; Teixeira, M.R.; Oliveira, J.; Lothe, R.A.; et al. Epigenetic regulation of EFEMP1 in prostate cancer: Biological relevance and clinical potential. *J. Cell. Mol. Med.* **2014**, *18*, 2287–2297. [CrossRef] [PubMed]
55. Grindel, B.; Li, Q.; Arnold, R.; Petros, J.; Zayzafoon, M.; Muldoon, M.; Stave, J.; Chung, L.W.K.; Farach-Carson, M.C. Perlecan/HSPG2 and matrilysin/MMP-7 as indices of tissue invasion: Tissue localization and circulating perlecan fragments in a cohort of 288 radical prostatectomy patients. *Oncotarget* **2016**, *7*, 10433–10447. [CrossRef]
56. Savorè, C.; Zhang, C.; Muir, C.; Liu, R.; Wyrwa, J.; Shu, J.; Zhau, H.E.; Chung, L.W.K.; Carson, D.D.; Farach-Carson, M.C. Perlecan knockdown in metastatic prostate cancer cells reduces heparin-binding growth factor responses in vitro and tumor growth in vivo. *Clin. Exp. Metastasis* **2005**, *22*, 377–390. [CrossRef]
57. Whitelock, J.; Melrose, J.; Iozzo, R.V. Diverse cell signaling events modulated by perlecan. *Biochemistry* **2008**, *47*, 11174–11183. [CrossRef]
58. Piñeiro, M.; Andrés, M.; Iturralde, M.; Carmona, S.; Hirvonen, J.; Pyörälä, S.; Heegaard, P.M.H.; Tjørnehøj, K.; Lampreave, F.; Piñeiro, A.; et al. ITIH4 (inter-alpha-trypsin inhibitor heavy chain 4) is a new acute-phase protein isolated from cattle during experimental infection. *Infect. Immun.* **2004**, *72*, 3777–3782. [CrossRef]
59. Huang, M.; Zhang, W.; Zhao, B.; Li, L. Relationship between inter-α-trypsin inhibitor heavy chain 4 and ovarian cancer. *Chin. J. Cancer Res.* **2019**, *31*, 955–964. [CrossRef]
60. Duffy, M.J. Biomarkers for prostate cancer: Prostate-specific antigen and beyond. *Clin. Chem. Lab. Med.* **2020**, *58*, 326–339. [CrossRef]
61. Söllner, T. Adaptor protein CD2AP and L-type lectin LMAN2 regulate exosome cargo protein trafficking through the golgi. *J. Biol. Chem.* **2016**, *291*, 25462–25475. [CrossRef]
62. The L-Type Lectin LMAN2 Is Over-Expressed in Brain Metastatic Breast Cancer. Available online: https://www.sciencegate.app/app/document/full-text#10.31219/osf.io/s3k2n. (accessed on 1 January 2022).
63. Potapenko, I.O.; Haakensen, V.D.; Lüders, T.; Helland, Å.; Bukholm, I.; Sørlie, T.; Kristensen, V.N.; Lingjærde, O.C.; Børresen-Dale, A.L. Glycan gene expression signatures in normal and malignant breast tissue; possible role in diagnosis and progression. *Mol. Oncol.* **2010**, *4*, 98–118. [CrossRef] [PubMed]
64. L'Espérance, S.; Popa, I.; Bachvarova, M.; Plante, M.; Patten, N.; Wu, L.; Têtu, B.; Bachvarov, D. Gene expression profiling of paired ovarian tumors obtained prior to and following adjuvant chemotherapy: Molecular signatures of chemoresistant tumors. *Int. J. Oncol.* **2006**, *29*, 5–24. [CrossRef] [PubMed]
65. Thompson, V.C.; Day, T.K.; Bianco-Miotto, T.; Selth, L.A.; Han, G.; Thomas, M.; Buchanan, G.; Scher, H.I.; Nelson, C.C.; Greenberg, N.M.; et al. A gene signature identified using a mouse model of androgen receptor-dependent prostate cancer predicts biochemical relapse in human disease. *Int. J. Cancer* **2012**, *131*, 662–672. [CrossRef] [PubMed]
66. Kim, J.; Yang, P.; Suraokar, M.; Sabichi, A.L.; Llansa, N.D.; Mendoza, G.; Subbarayan, V.; Logothetis, C.J.; Newman, R.A.; Lippman, S.M.; et al. Suppression of prostate tumor cell growth by stromal cell prostaglandin D synthase-derived products. *Cancer Res.* **2005**, *65*, 6189–6198. [CrossRef]
67. Ogretmen, B.; Hannun, Y.A. Biologically active sphingolipids in cancer pathogenesis and treatment. *Nat. Rev. Cancer* **2004**, *4*, 604–616. [CrossRef]
68. Seelan, R.S.; Qian, C.; Yokomizo, A.; Bostwick, D.G.; Smith, D.I.; Liu, W. Human acid ceramidase is overexpressed but not mutated in prostate cancer. *Genes Chromosom. Cancer* **2000**, *29*, 137–146. [CrossRef]
69. Camacho, L.; Meca-Cortés, Ó.; Abad, J.L.; García, S.; Rubio, N.; Díaz, A.; Celiá-Terrassa, T.; Cingolani, F.; Bermudo, R.; Fernández, P.L.; et al. Acid ceramidase as a therapeutic target in metastatic prostate cancer. *J. Lipid Res.* **2013**, *54*, 1207–1220. [CrossRef]
70. Saad, A.F.; Meacham, W.D.; Bai, A.; Anelli, V.; Elojeimy, S.; Mahdy, A.E.M.; Turner, L.S.; Cheng, J.; Bielawska, A.; Bielawski, J.; et al. The functional effects of acid ceramidase overexpression in prostate cancer progression and resistance to chemotherapy. *Cancer Biol. Ther.* **2007**, *6*, 1455–1460. [CrossRef]
71. McCord, J.M.; Edeas, M.A. SOD, oxidative stress and human pathologies: A brief history and a future vision. *Biomed. Pharmacother.* **2005**, *59*, 139–142. [CrossRef]
72. Zheng, S.; Lin, X.; Gan, X.; Wang, X. The impact of SOD3 on prostatic diseases: Elevated SOD3 is a novel biomarker for the diagnosis of chronic nonbacterial prostatiti. *Res. Sq.* **2021**. [CrossRef]
73. Kim, J.; Mizokami, A.; Shin, M.; Izumi, K.; Konaka, H.; Kadono, Y.; Kitagawa, Y.; Keller, E.T.; Zhang, J.; Namiki, M. SOD3 acts as a tumor suppressor in PC-3 prostate cancer cells via hydrogen peroxide accumulation. *Anticancer Res.* **2014**, *34*, 2821–2832.
74. Allocati, N.; Masulli, M.; Di Ilio, C.; Federici, L. Glutathione transferases: Substrates, inihibitors and pro-drugs in cancer and neurodegenerative diseases. *Oncogenesis* **2018**, *7*, 8. [CrossRef]
75. Lin, X.; Tascilar, M.; Lee, W.H.; Vles, W.J.; Lee, B.H.; Veeraswamy, R.; Asgari, K.; Freije, D.; Van Rees, B.; Gage, W.R.; et al. GSTP1 CpG island hypermethylation is responsible for the absence of GSTP1 expression in human prostate cancer cells. *Am. J. Pathol.* **2001**, *159*, 1815–1826. [CrossRef]

76. Nakayama, M.; Bennett, C.J.; Hicks, J.L.; Epstein, J.I.; Platz, E.A.; Nelson, W.G.; De Marzo, A.M. Hypermethylation of the human glutathione S-transferase-π gene (GSTP1) CpG island is present in a subset of proliferative inflammatory atrophy lesions but not in normal or hyperplastic epithelium of the prostate: A detailed study using laser-capture microd. *Am. J. Pathol.* **2003**, *163*, 923–933. [CrossRef]
77. Brooks, J.D.; Weinstein, M.; Lin, X.; Sun, Y.; Pin, S.S.; Bova, G.S.; Epstein, J.I.; Isaacs, W.B.; Nelson, W.G. CG island methylation changes near the GSTP1 gene in prostatic intraepithelial neoplasia. *Cancer Epidemiol. Biomark. Prev.* **1998**, *7*, 531–536.
78. Badowska-Kozakiewicz, A.M.; Budzik, M.P. The multidirectional role of osteopontin in cancer. *Nowotwory* **2018**, *68*, 176–183. [CrossRef]
79. Khodavirdi, A.C.; Song, Z.; Yang, S.; Zhong, C.; Wang, S.; Wu, H.; Pritchard, C.; Nelson, P.S.; Roy-Burman, P. Increased expression of osteopontin contributes to the progression of prostate cancer. *Cancer Res.* **2006**, *66*, 883–888. [CrossRef]
80. Yu, A.; Guo, K.; Qin, Q.; Xing, C.; Zu, X. Clinicopathological and prognostic significance of osteopontin expression in patients with prostate cancer: A systematic review and meta-analysis. *Biosci. Rep.* **2021**, *41*, BSR20203531. [CrossRef]
81. Wiśniewski, T.; Zyromska, A.; Makarewicz, R.; Zekanowska, E. Osteopontin and angiogenic factors as new biomarkers of prostate cancer. *Urol. J.* **2019**, *16*, 134–140. [CrossRef]
82. Prager, A.J.; Peng, C.R.; Lita, E.; Mcnally, D.; Kaushal, A.; Sproull, M.; Compton, K.; Dahut, W.L.; Figg, W.D.; Citrin, D.; et al. Urinary aHGF, IGFBP3 and OPN as diagnostic and prognostic biomarkers for prostate cancer. *Biomark. Med.* **2013**, *7*, 831–841. [CrossRef]
83. Graddis, T.J.; McMahan, C.J.; Tamman, J.; Page, K.J.; Trager, J.B. Prostatic acid phosphatase expression in human tissues. *Int. J. Clin. Exp. Pathol.* **2011**, *4*, 295–306. [CrossRef]
84. Gutman, B.Y.A.B.; Gutman, E.B. An "acid" phosphatase occurring in the serum of patients with metastasizing carcinoma of the prostate gland. *J. Clin. Investig.* **1938**, *17*, 473–478. [CrossRef]
85. Bing, C.; Bao, Y.; Jenkins, J.; Sanders, P.; Manieri, M.; Cinti, S.; Tisdale, M.J.; Trayhurn, P. Zinc-α2-glycoprotein, a lipid mobilizing factor, is expressed in adipocytes and is up-regulated in mice with cancer cachexia. *Proc. Natl. Acad. Sci. USA* **2004**, *101*, 2500–2505. [CrossRef]
86. Bondar, O.P.; Barnidge, D.R.; Klee, E.W.; Davis, B.J.; Klee, G.G. LC-MS/MS quantification of Zn-α2 glycoprotein: A potential serum biomarker for prostate cancer. *Clin. Chem.* **2007**, *53*, 673–678. [CrossRef]
87. Hale, L.P.; Price, D.T.; Sanchez, L.M.; Demark-Wahnefried, W.; Madden, J.F. Zinc α-2-glycoprotein is expressed by malignant prostatic epithelium and may serve as a potential serum marker for prostate cancer. *Clin. Cancer Res.* **2001**, *7*, 846–853.
88. Chintapalli, V.R.; Kato, A.; Henderson, L.; Hirata, T.; Woods, D.J.; Overend, G.; Davies, S.A.; Romero, M.F.; Dow, J.A.T. Transport proteins NHA1 and NHA2 are essential for survival, but have distinct transport modalities. *Proc. Natl. Acad. Sci. USA* **2015**, *112*, 11720–11725. [CrossRef]
89. Shi, W.; Dong, F.; Jiang, Y.; Lu, L.; Wang, C.; Tan, J.; Yang, W.; Guo, H.; Ming, J.; Huang, T. Construction of prognostic microRNA signature for human invasive breast cancer by integrated analysis. *Onco. Targets. Ther.* **2019**, *12*, 1979–2010. [CrossRef]
90. Cui, F.L.; Mahmud, A.N.; Xu, Z.P.; Wang, Z.Y.; Hu, J.P. VASN promotes proliferation of prostate cancer through the YAP/TAZ axis. *Eur. Rev. Med. Pharmacol. Sci.* **2020**, *24*, 6589–6596. [CrossRef]
91. Dho, S.H.; Lim, J.C.; Kim, L.K. Beyond the role of CD55 as a complement component. *Immune Netw.* **2018**, *18*, e11. [CrossRef]
92. Loberg, R.D.; Day, L.S.L.; Dunn, R.; Kalikin, L.M.; Pienta, K.J. Inhibition of decay-accelerating factor (CD55) attenuates prostate cancer growth and survival in vivo. *Neoplasia* **2006**, *8*, 69–78. [CrossRef]
93. Kuefer, R.; Hofer, M.D.; Gschwend, J.E.; Pienta, K.J.; Sanda, M.G.; Chinnaiyan, A.M.; Rubin, M.A.; Day, M.L. The role of an 80 kDa fragment of E-cadherin in the metastatic progression of prostate cancer. *Clin. Cancer Res.* **2003**, *9*, 6447–6452.
94. Iacopino, F.; Pinto, F.; Bertaccini, A.; Calarco, A.; Proietti, G.; Totaro, A.; Martorana, G.; Bassi, P.; Sica, G. Soluble E-cadherin and IL-6 serum levels in patients affected by prostate cancer before and after prostatectomy. *Oncol. Rep.* **2012**, *28*, 370–374. [CrossRef]
95. Banks, R.E.; Porter, W.H.; Whelan, P.; Smith, P.H.; Selby, P.J. Soluble forms of the adhesion molecule E-cadherin in urine. *J. Clin. Pathol.* **1995**, *48*, 179–180. [CrossRef]
96. Katayama, M.; Hirai, S.; Yasumoto, M.; Nishikawa, K.; Nagata, S.; Otsuka, M.; Kato, I.; Kamihagi, K. Soluble fragments of E-cadherin cell adhesion molecule increase in urinary excretion of cancer patients, potentially indicating its shedding from epithelial tumor cells. *Int. J. Oncol.* **1994**, *5*, 1049–1057. [CrossRef]
97. Tsaur, I.; Thurn, K.; Juengel, E.; Gust, K.M.; Borgmann, H.; Mager, R.; Bartsch, G.; Oppermann, E.; Ackermann, H.; Nelson, K.; et al. sE-cadherin serves as a diagnostic and predictive parameter in prostate cancer patients. *J. Exp. Clin. Cancer Res.* **2015**, *34*, 43. [CrossRef]
98. Kuefer, R.; Hofer, M.D.; Zorn, C.S.M.; Engel, O.; Volkmer, B.G.; Juarez-Brito, M.A.; Eggel, M.; Gschwend, J.E.; Rubin, M.A.; Day, M.L. Assessment of a fragment of e-cadherin as a serum biomarker with predictive value for prostate cancer. *Br. J. Cancer* **2005**, *92*, 2018–2023. [CrossRef]
99. Duijvesz, D.; Versluis, C.Y.L.; Van Der Fels, C.A.M.; Vredenbregt-Van Den Berg, M.S.; Leivo, J.; Peltola, M.T.; Bangma, C.H.; Pettersson, K.S.I.; Jenster, G. Immuno-based detection of extracellular vesicles in urine as diagnostic marker for prostate cancer. *Int. J. Cancer* **2015**, *137*, 2869–2878. [CrossRef]
100. Xu, H.; Wang, F.; Li, H.; Ji, J.; Cao, Z.; Lyu, J.; Shi, X.; Zhu, Y.; Zhang, C.; Guo, F. Prostatic acid phosphatase (PAP) predicts prostate cancer progress in a population-based study: The renewal of PAP? *Dis. Markers.* **2019**, *2019*, 7090545. [CrossRef]

101. Fang, L.C.; Dattoli, M.; Taira, A.; True, L.; Sorace, R.; Wallner, K. Prostatic Acid Phosphatase Adversely Affects Cause-Specific Survival in Patients with Intermediate to High-Risk Prostate Cancer Treated with Brachytherapy. *Urology* **2008**, *71*, 146–150. [CrossRef]
102. Alpert, E.; Akhavan, A.; Gruzman, A.; Hansen, W.J.; Lehrer-Graiwer, J.; Hall, S.C.; Johansen, E.; McAllister, S.; Gulati, M.; Lin, M.-F.; et al. Multifunctionality of prostatic acid phosphatase in prostate cancer pathogenesis. *Biosci. Rep.* **2021**, *41*, BSR20211646. [CrossRef]
103. Kote-Jarai, Z.; Amin Al Olama, A.; Leongamornlert, D.; Tymrakiewicz, M.; Saunders, E.; Guy, M.; Giles, G.G.; Severi, G.; Southey, M.; Hopper, J.L.; et al. Identification of a novel prostate cancer susceptibility variant in the KLK3 gene transcript. *Hum. Genet.* **2011**, *129*, 687–694. [CrossRef]
104. Parikh, H.; Wang, Z.; Pettigrew, K.A.; Jia, J.; Daugherty, S.; Yeager, M.; Jacobs, K.B.; Hutchinson, A.; Burdett, L.; Cullen, M.; et al. Fine mapping the KLK3 locus on chromosome 19q13.33 associated with prostate cancer susceptibility and PSA levels. *Hum. Genet.* **2011**, *129*, 675–685. [CrossRef]
105. Gudmundsson, J.; Besenbacher, S.; Sulem, P.; Gudbjartsson, D.F.; Olafsson, I.; Arinbjarnarson, S.; Agnarsson, B.A.; Benediktsdottir, K.R.; Isaksson, H.J.; Kostic, J.P.; et al. Genetic correction of PSA values using sequence variants associated with PSA levels. *Sci. Transl. Med.* **2010**, *2*, 62ra92. [CrossRef]
106. Cotignola, J.; Leonardi, D.B.; Shahabi, A.; Acuña, A.D.; Stern, M.C.; Navone, N.; Scorticati, C.; De Siervi, A.; Mazza, O.; Vazquez, E. Glutathione-S-transferase (GST) polymorphisms are associated with relapse after radical prostatectomy. *Prostate Cancer Prostatic Dis.* **2013**, *16*, 28–34. [CrossRef]
107. Oskina, N.A.; Ermolenko, N.A.; Boyarskih, U.A.; Lazarev, A.F.; Petrova, V.D.; Ganov, D.I.; Tonacheva, O.G.; Lifschitz, G.I.; Filipenko, M.L. Associations between SNPs within antioxidant genes and the risk of prostate cancer in the Siberian region of Russia. *Pathol. Oncol. Res.* **2014**, *20*, 635–640. [CrossRef]
108. Gulfidan, G.; Turanli, B.; Beklen, H.; Sinha, R.; Arga, K.Y. Pan-cancer mapping of differential protein-protein interactions. *Sci. Rep.* **2020**, *10*, 3272. [CrossRef]
109. Engin, B.H.; Guney, E.; Keskin, O.; Oliva, B.; Gursoy, A. Integrating structure to protein-protein interaction networks that drive metastasis to brain and lung in breast cancer. *PLoS ONE* **2013**, *8*, e81035. [CrossRef]
110. Matos, B.; Howl, J.; Jerónimo, C.; Fardilha, M. The disruption of protein-protein interactions as a therapeutic strategy for prostate cancer. *Pharmacol. Res.* **2020**, *161*, 105145. [CrossRef]
111. Foulstone, E.; Prince, S.; Zaccheo, O.; Burns, J.L.; Harper, J.; Jacobs, C.; Church, D.; Hassan, A.B. Insulin-like growth factor ligands, receptors, and binding proteins in cancer. *J. Pathol.* **2005**, *205*, 145–153. [CrossRef]
112. Chatterjee, S.; Sung Park, E.; Soloff, M.S. Proliferation of DU145 prostate cancer cells is inhibited by suppressing insulin-like growth factor binding protein-2. *Int. J. Urol.* **2004**, *11*, 876–884. [CrossRef]
113. Hellawell, G.O.; Turner, G.D.H.; Davies, D.R.; Poulsom, R.; Brewster, S.F.; Macaulay, V.M. Expression of the type 1 insulin-like growth factor receptor is up-regulated in primary prostate cancer and commonly persists in metastatic disease. *Cancer Res.* **2002**, *62*, 2942–2950.
114. Wolk, A.; Mantzoros, C.S.; Andersson, S.O.; Bergström, R.; Signorello, L.B.; Lagiou, P.; Adami, H.O.; Trichopoulos, D. Insulin-like growth factor 1 and prostate cancer risk: A population-based, case-control study. *J. Natl. Cancer Inst.* **1998**, *90*, 911–915. [CrossRef]
115. Heidegger, I.; Kern, J.; Ofer, P.; Klocker, H.; Massoner, P. Oncogenic functions of IGF1R and INSR in prostate cancer include enhanced tumor growth, cell migration and angiogenesis. *Oncotarget* **2014**, *5*, 2723–2735. [CrossRef]
116. Datta, M.W.; Hernandez, A.M.; Schlicht, M.J.; Kahler, A.J.; DeGueme, A.M.; Dhir, R.; Shah, R.B.; Farach-Carson, C.; Barrett, A.; Datta, S. Perlecan, a candidate gene for the CAPB locus, regulates prostate cancer cell growth via the Sonic Hedgehog pathway. *Mol. Cancer* **2006**, *5*, 9. [CrossRef]
117. Mongiat, M.; Sweeney, S.M.; San Antonio, J.D.; Fu, J.; Iozzo, R.V. Endorepellin, a novel inhibitor of angiogenesis derived from the C terminus of perlecan. *J. Biol. Chem.* **2003**, *278*, 4238–4249. [CrossRef]
118. Gonzalez, E.M.; Reed, C.C.; Bix, G.; Fu, J.; Zhang, Y.; Gopalakrishnan, B.; Greenspan, D.S.; Iozzo, R.V. BMP-1/Tolloid-like metalloproteases process endorepellin, the angiostatic C-terminal fragment of perlecan. *J. Biol. Chem.* **2005**, *280*, 7080–7087. [CrossRef]
119. Bix, G.; Castello, R.; Burrows, M.; Zoeller, J.J.; Weech, M.; Iozzo, R.A.; Cardi, C.; Thakur, M.L.; Barker, C.A.; Camphausen, K.; et al. Endorepellin in vivo: Targeting the tumor vasculature and retarding cancer growth and metabolism. *J. Natl. Cancer Inst.* **2006**, *98*, 1634–1646. [CrossRef]
120. Chang, J.W.; Kang, U.B.; Kim, D.H.; Yi, J.K.; Lee, J.W.; Noh, D.Y.; Lee, C.; Yu, M.H. Identification of circulating endorepellin LG3 fragment: Potential use as a serological biomarker for breast cancer. *Proteom.-Clin. Appl.* **2008**, *2*, 23–32. [CrossRef]
121. Parker, T.J.; Sampson, D.L.; Broszczak, D.; Chng, Y.L.; Carter, S.L.; Leavesley, D.I.; Parker, A.W.; Upton, Z. A fragment of the LG3 peptide of endorepellin is present in the urine of physically active mining workers: A potential marker of physical activity. *PLoS ONE* **2012**, *7*, e33714. [CrossRef]
122. Oda, O.; Shinzato, T.; Ohbayashi, K.; Takai, I.; Kunimatsu, M.; Maeda, K.; Yamanaka, N. Purification and characterization of perlecan fragment in urine of end-stage renal failure patients. *Clin. Chim. Acta* **1996**, *255*, 119–132. [CrossRef]
123. Venning, F.A.; Wullkopf, L.; Erler, J.T. Targeting ECM disrupts cancer progression. *Front. Oncol.* **2015**, *5*, 224. [CrossRef]
124. Kobayashi, H.; Shinohara, H.; Fujie, M.; Gotoh, J.; Itoh, M.; Takeuchi, K.; Terao, T. Inhibition of metastasis of lewis lung carcinoma by urinary trypsin inhibitor in experimental and spontaneous metastasis models. *Int. J. Cancer* **1995**, *63*, 455–462. [CrossRef]

125. Suzuki, M.; Kobayashi, H.; Tanaka, Y.; Hirashima, Y.; Kanayama, N.; Takei, Y.; Saga, Y.; Suzuki, M.; Itoh, H.; Terao, T. Suppression of invasion and peritoneal carcinomatosis of ovarian cancer cell line by overexpression of bikunin. *Int. J. Cancer* **2003**, *104*, 289–302. [CrossRef]
126. Geller, A.; Yan, J. The role of membrane bound complement regulatory proteins in tumor development and cancer immunotherapy. *Front. Immunol.* **2019**, *10*, 1074. [CrossRef]
127. Ikeda, Y.; Imai, Y.; Kumagai, H.; Nosaka, T.; Morikawa, Y.; Hisaoka, T.; Manabe, I.; Maemura, K.; Nakaoka, T.; Imamura, T.; et al. Vasorin, a transforming growth factor β-binding protein expressed in vascular smooth muscle cells, modulates the arterial response to injury in vivo. *Proc. Natl. Acad. Sci. USA* **2004**, *101*, 10732–10737. [CrossRef]
128. Zhang, M.; Zhang, Y.Y.; Chen, Y.; Wang, J.; Wang, Q.; Lu, H. TGF-β Signaling and Resistance to Cancer Therapy. *Front. Cell Dev. Biol.* **2021**, *9*, 786728. [CrossRef]
129. Malapeira, J.; Esselens, C.; Bech-Serra, J.J.; Canals, F.; Arribas, J. ADAM17 (TACE) regulates TGFB signaling through the cleavage of vasorin. *Oncogene* **2011**, *30*, 1912–1922. [CrossRef]

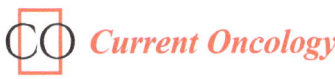

Article

Outcomes of Patients with Metastatic Castration-Resistant Prostate Cancer According to Somatic Damage DNA Repair Gene Alterations

Zoé Neviere [1,*], Elodie Coquan [1], Pierre-Emmanuel Brachet [1], Emeline Meriaux [1], Isabelle Bonnet [1], Sophie Krieger [2], Laurent Castéra [2], Dominique Vaur [2], Flavie Boulouard [2], Alexandra Leconte [3], Justine Lequesne [3], Anais Lelaidier [4], Agathe Ricou [2] and Florence Joly [1,3,5,6]

[1] Oncology Department, Centre François Baclesse, 14000 Caen, France; coque@baclesse.unicancer.fr (E.C.); brape@baclesse.unicancer.fr (P.-E.B.); e.meriaux@baclesse.unicancer.fr (E.M.); i.bonnet@baclesse.unicancer.fr (I.B.); f.joly@baclesse.unicancer.fr (F.J.)

[2] Inserm U1245, Department of Cancer Biology and Genetics, Normandy Centre for Genomic and Personalized Medicine, François Baclesse Center, 14000 Caen, France; s.krieger@baclesse.unicancer.fr (S.K.); l.castera@baclesse.unicancer.fr (L.C.); d.vaur@baclesse.unicancer.fr (D.V.); f.boulouard@baclesse.unicancer.fr (F.B.); a.ricou@baclesse.unicancer.fr (A.R.)

[3] Clinical Reseach Department, Centre François Baclesse, 14000 Caen, France; a.leconte@baclesse.unicancer.fr (A.L.); j.lequesne@baclesse.unicancer.fr (J.L.)

[4] Data Processing Center, the North-West Canceropole, Centre François Baclesse, 14000 Caen, France; a.lelaidier@baclesse.unicancer.fr

[5] Department of Oncology, University Hospital of Caen, 14000 Caen, France

[6] UMR-S1077, Normandy University, Unicaen, Inserm U1086, Anticipe, 14000 Caen, France

* Correspondence: z.neviere@baclesse.unicancer.fr

Abstract: (1) Background: In literature, approximately 20% of mCRPC present somatic DNA damage repair (DDR) gene mutations, and their relationship with response to standard therapies in mCRPC is not well understood. The objective was to evaluate outcomes of mCRPC patients treated with standard therapies according to somatic DDR status. (2) Methods: Eighty-three patients were recruited at Caen Cancer Center (France). Progression-free survival (PFS) after first-line treatment was analyzed according to somatic DDR mutation as primary endpoint. PFS according to first exposure to taxane chemotherapy and PFS2 (time to second event of disease progression) depending on therapeutic sequences were also analyzed. (3) Results: Median first-line PFS was 9.7 months in 33 mutated patients and 8.4 months in 50 non-mutated patients ($p = 0.9$). PFS of first exposure to taxanes was 8.1 months in mutated patients and 5.7 months in non-mutated patients ($p = 0.32$) and significantly longer among patients with ATM/BRCA1/BRCA2 mutations compared to the others (10.6 months vs. 5.5 months, $p = 0.04$). PFS2 was 16.5 months in mutated patients, whatever the sequence, and 11.7 months in non-mutated patients ($p = 0.07$). The mutated patients treated with chemotherapy followed by NHT had a long median PFS (49.8 months). (4) Conclusions: mCRPC patients with BRCA1/2 and ATM benefit from standard therapies, with a long response to taxanes.

Keywords: prostate cancer; molecular profile; homologous repair

1. Introduction

In the area of personalized medicine, the molecular characterization of tumors is becoming an integral feature of new therapeutic strategies, and some genetic alterations may be therapeutic targets [1,2]. Beyond germline mutations, somatic pathogenic variations acquired during the process of tumorigenesis can be found only within the tumor [3].

In prostate cancer, the DNA damage repair (DDR) pathway is one of the major genetic alterations with a potential therapeutic impact. The incidence of somatic alterations in DDR pathways in prostate tumors is higher than that of germline alterations and varies from 19 to 31% in advanced prostate cancer and from 7.4 to 16.2% in germline mutations [1,4–8]. The major alterations concerned are *BRCA1/2* and *ATM* [4,9–12].

In patients with prostate cancer, germline pathogenic *BRCA1/2* variants are usually correlated with poor prognostic characteristics (aggressiveness, castration resistance, lymph node invasion and metastasis at diagnosis, and decreased overall survival) [13–17]. While the predictive impact of somatic *BRCA1/2* and other DDR mutations remains somewhat elusive [13–16], metastatic castration-resistant prostate cancer (mCRPC) patients with DDR mutations are known to have a response to PARP (poly(ADP-Ribose) polymerase) inhibitors [7,17–21].

The predictive impact of DDR gene germline mutations on the response to standard therapies (taxanes and/or new-generation hormone therapy [NHT]) was recently investigated in a first-line setting among mCRPC patients. However, results of the different studies remain conflicting about links between DDR mutations and survival outcomes after NHT and/or taxane treatments [9,11,14,16,22]. Annala et al. evaluated the predictive impact of somatic DDR alterations on circulating tumor DNA (ctDNA) in 115 mCRPC patients treated with first-line NHT [23]. They showed that defects in *BRCA2* and *ATM* were strongly associated with poor time to progression independently of clinical prognostic factors and circulating tumor DNA abundance ($p < 0.001$). Another retrospective study found worse PSA response rates (25%) in 53 mCRPC patients with somatic *BRCA2* mutations treated with docetaxel vs. 71.1% in wild-type mCRPC patients ($p = 0.019$) [24].

Therefore, the predictive value of somatic alterations of DDR pathway genes in mCRPC patients treated with taxanes is still unclear, and sound data on progression-free survival are lacking. The objective of this study was to describe outcomes of mCRPC patients treated with taxanes and/or NHT according to their somatic DDR profile, determined with a large 65-gene panel.

2. Materials and Methods

This was an observational retrospective study conducted at the François Baclesse Center in Caen, France. Patients were screened between 1 January 2017 and 31 December 2018 during multidisciplinary meetings (Figure 1). Criteria of eligibility were all patients with mCRPC adenocarcinoma with evaluable lesions according to the PCWG3 and/or RECIST 1.1 criteria receiving a first-line treatment for mCRPC for at least 3 months, with tumor material available for somatic analysis. Patients may have received more than one line of mCRPC treatment after castration resistance. Patients with tumor types other than adenocarcinoma, with World Health Organization (WHO) performance status <2, or in whom the tumor material was insufficient or unavailable for somatic analysis were excluded.

Data were collected between 1 September 2018 and 15 March 2019 from patients' medical files at the François Baclesse Center. Their characteristics at the initial diagnosis (age at diagnosis, initial PSA, initial TNM, body mass index (BMI), Gleason score, diagnostic modes, different therapeutic lines, best response to castration resistance lines, progression dates after different lines and date of death or last follow-up) were collected. Monitoring ended on 15 March 2019.

Somatic analyses were performed on DNA extracted from the initial biopsy or surgical excision in the Laboratory of Biology and Genetics at the François Baclesse Center. The procedure and the panel are described in Table S1. Only likely pathogenic and pathogenic variations have been considered.

The primary endpoint was progression-free survival (mCRPC-PFS) after first-line castration-resistant treatment, defined as the date of the beginning of castration-resistant first-line treatment and the date of confirmed progression (biochemical as defined by the French Association of Urology and/or radiologic progression according to PCWG3 and/or RECIST 1.1 criteria). The secondary endpoints were PFS of the first mCRPC treatment to taxanes or to first-line hormonal therapy [NHT] during the first two lines of castration-resistant treatment, PFS2 (i.e., the time between the date of initiation of the first line of treatment for mCRPC and the date of progression with the second line of treatment), and overall survival (OS) (calculated from the beginning of the first line of treatment for mCRPC to the date of death or last follow-up). PFS2 was also evaluated according to the therapeutic sequence (NHT treatment for first-line castration resistance followed by taxane chemotherapy (HCS) or first-line chemotherapy followed by second-line NHT (CHS)).

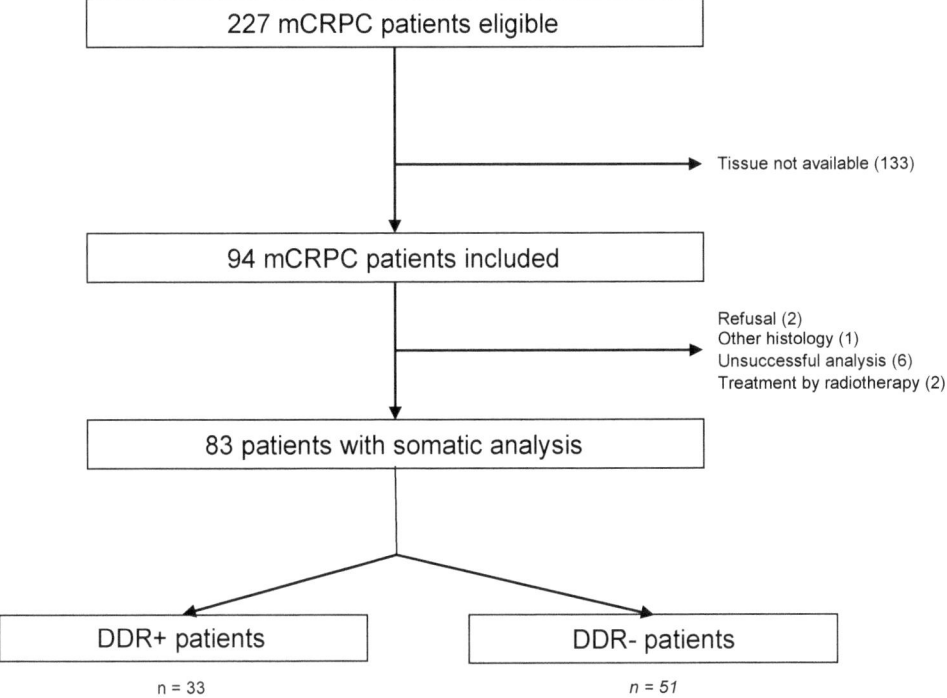

Figure 1. Flow chart of selection of patients. DDR+: mutated patients; DDR−: non-mutated patients; mCRPC: metastatic castration-resistant prostate cancer; n: number of patients.

Comparisons were made between patients with the DDR mutation (DDR+) and those without (DDR−). Analysis also concerned the group of patients with *BRCA1*, *BRCA2*, and/or *ATM* gene alterations (corresponding to the most frequent and already evaluated mutations).

Survival rates were estimated by the Kaplan Meier method. The log-rank test was used to determine factors associated with survival data. The link between the different factors and the molecular data obtained by sequencing the prostate tumors was measured by the Chi2 test in the event of qualitative variables (or Fisher test if necessary) and by the Student test in the event of quantitative variables (or the non-parametric Kruskal Wallis test if the data were not Gaussian). The significance threshold was set at 5% for each statistical analysis and confidence interval.

The Northwest Data Center (CTD-CNO) is acknowledged for managing the data. It is supported by grants from the French National League Against Cancer (LNC) and the French National Cancer Institute (INCa).

The study was approved by the institutional review board. It was conducted in compliance with the French Research Standard MR-004 "Research not involving human participants" (compliance commitment to MR-004 for the Centre François Baclesse n°2214228 v.0, dated from 7 March 2019). All data have been processed anonymously.

3. Results

3.1. Patient Selection

Two hundred and twenty-seven patients with mCRPC were eligible; 94 were included, and 83 patients were finally analyzed. Data regarding treatment group and prostate somatic DDR gene alteration are shown in Figure 1.

3.2. Clinical Characteristics

Table 1 summarizes the clinical characteristics of mCRPC patients according to DDR mutations. Median age was 69.5 years. Thirty-three patients (39.8%) presented the somatic DDR mutation (they represent the DDR+ group). There was no statistical difference between the two groups concerning clinical characteristics. Median follow-up since the date of castration resistance of the 83 patients with somatic analysis was 15.3 months [0.48–83.2].

Table 1. Clinical outcomes of analyzed patients according to somatic DDR+ vs. DDR− alterations BMI: body mass index; DDR+: mutated patients; DDR−: non-mutated patients; n: number of patients; PSA: prostate specific antigen; NHT: new-generation hormonotherapy; PSA: prostate specific antigen.

	Total		DDR+		DDR−		p
Age(years)	69.5	(23–82)	70	(65–76)	69.5	(55–82)	0.43
ECOG							0.21
0	34	(44%)	15	(48%)	19	(41%)	
1	38	(49%)	12	(39%)	26	(55%)	NA
2	6	(8%)	4	(13%)	2	(4%)	NA
BMI	27.5	(23–38)	27.5	(25–31)	27.5	(23–36)	0.71
Previous Treatments							
Surgery	22	(27%)	10	(30%)	12	(24%)	0.74
Chemotherapy	14	(17%)	6	(18%)	8	(16%)	1
Radiotherapy	45	(54%)	19	(58%)	26	(52%)	0.8
First-line Treatment							0.61
NHT	64	(77%)	14	(73%)	40	(80%)	
Taxanes	19	(23%)	9	(27%)	10	(20%)	NA
Gleason							0.47
5 to 7	35	(43%)	12	(36%)	23	(47%)	
8 to 10	47	(57%)	21	(67%)	26	(53%)	NA
TNM							0.85
T1/2	42	(51%)	7	(21%)	14	(28%)	
T3/4	41	(49%)	22	(67%)	30	(60%)	NA
Tx	10	(12%)	4	(12%)	6	(12%)	
N1+	25	(30%)	8	(24%)	17	(34%)	0.55
N0	16	(19%)	6	(18%)	10	(20%)	NA
Nx	42	(51%)	19	(58%)	23	(46%)	NA
M1	43	(52%)	15	(46%)	28	(56%)	0.47
M0/Mx	40	(48%)	18	(54%)	22	(44%)	NA
Initial Pas	28.8	(1–5500)	28.8	(9.7–60)	27.6	(10–232)	0.32
Diagnostic Modes							0.73
Symptoms	49	(62%)	18	(58%)	31	(65%)	
Individual screening	30	(38%)	13	(42%)	17	(35%)	NA
Durtion of Hormonosensitivity (years)	2.07	(0.4–18.1)	2.14	(0.5–18.1)	1.92	(0.4–13.9)	0.5
Time Before Metastasis (years)	0.04	(0–13.8)	0.92	(0–13.8)	0.02	(0–12.1)	0.07

In first-line treatment, 64 mCRPC patients were treated with NHT and 19 with taxanes. Fifty-three patients (64%) received a second-line treatment: 31 patients received taxanes, and 22 patients received NHT second-line mCRPC. Forty-seven (57%) patients received at least one line of taxanes in the first two lines of treatment, and 74 patients received at least one line of NHT (89%). Ten mCRPC patients received chemotherapy followed by NHT, and 28 patients received NHT followed by taxanes. Fourteen patients had received chemotherapy before resistance to castration, and one of them had received taxanes as first-line mCRPC treatment.

Clinical characteristics of the 83 mCRPC patients analyzed and the 136 mCRPC patients excluded are shown in Supplementary Materials (Table S2). Patients included had more aggressive parameters, with more node invasion at diagnosis (30% vs. 17%, $p = 0.001$), higher Gleason score (57% of Gleason 8–10 vs. 39%, $p = 0.013$), and shorter time to metastasis (25 months vs. 0.5 months, $p = 0.05$). They also received more previous loco-regional radiotherapy ($p \leq 0.004$) and first-line taxanes for hormonosensitive disease ($p = 0.028$) and had a shorter median duration of first-line hormonosensitivity ($p = 0.0005$). Prognostic factors were similar between patients treated with taxanes and those with NHT as first line (Table S3).

3.3. Molecular Characteristics of Tumors

Thirty-three (39.7%) patients had at least one DDR alteration. Alterations concerned different genes: 10 patients presented alterations of the ATM gene (12%), 5 BRCA2 (6%), 4 CHEK2 (4.8%), 3 CDK12 and FANCG (3.6% for each gene), 2 MRE11A and PALB2 (2.4% for each gene), 1 BLM, 1 BRCA1, 1 CHEK1, 1 FANCF, 1 FANCI, 1 FANCM, and 1 MDC1 (1.2% for each gene). The subgroup of ATM/BRCA1/BRCA2 patients represented 19.2% of patients and 48.5% of mutated patients. Five samples (6%) had at least two somatic alterations, and one patient had a tumor with four somatic alterations including three pathogenic variants and one likely pathogenic variant. Another alteration was reported that was a likely pathogenic variant and localized on the ATM gene. The mutations are shown in Table 2 (File S1: complementary results).

Table 2. Pathogenic or likely pathogenic variants identified on prostatic tumor somatic analysis among mCRPC cohort.

Patient	Gene	Alteration	Protein	Function	Types
1	ATM	5188C > T	ARG1730*	stop	Pathogenic
2	CDK12	2068DEL	ALA690GLNFS*63	frameshift	Pathogenic
2	CDK12	3046C > T	GLN1016*	stop	Pathogenic
8	ATM	4403T > A	VAL1468ASP	missense	Pathogenic
9	firefox	1100DEL	THR307METFS*15	frameshift	Pathogenic
14	BRCA1	3741DEL	ALA1248LEUFS*16	frameshift	Pathogenic
15	MRE11A	571C > T	ARG191*	stop	Pathogenic
16	ATM	5712DUP	SER1905ILEFS*25	frameshift	Pathogenic
17	BRCA2	-	-	-	Pathogenic
18	CDK12	3566_3575DEL	LEU1189GLNFS*23	frameshift	Pathogenic
19	PALB2	658_659DEL	SER220CYSFS*14	frameshift	Pathogenic
25	BRCA2	5909C > A	SER1970*	stop	Pathogenic
27	CHEK2	1100DEL	THR367METFS*15	frameshift	Pathogenic
28	MDC1	907DEL	VAL303TRPFS*45	frameshift	Pathogenic
30	ATM	9022C > T	ARG3008CYS	missense	Pathogenic
30	ATM	8096C > T	PRO2699LEU	missense	Pathogenic
34	ATM	5293_5302DEL	GLN1765GLUFS*8	frameshift	Pathogenic
38	ATM	8759_8772DEL	ILE2920ARGFS18*	frameshift	Pathogenic
39	BLM	1701G > A	TRP567*	stop	Pathogenic
40	CHEK2	-	TYR370CYS	missense	Pathogenic
51	CHEK1	783DEL	ASP262ILEFS*42	frameshift	Pathogenic
53	FANCM	1827T > G	TYR609*	stop	Pathogenic
53	CDK12	467_470DEL	GLU156GLYFS*10	frameshift	Pathogenic

Table 2. Cont.

Patient	Gene	Alteration	Protein	Function	Types
54	FANCG	1183_1192DEL	GLU375TRPFS*	frameshift	Pathogenic
56	FANCF	1087C > T	GLN363*	stop	Pathogenic
59	ATM	5818G > T	GLU1940*	stop	Pathogenic
60	BRCA2	1597DEL	THR533LEUFS*25	frameshift	Pathogenic
62	MRE11A	1331_1332DEL	VAL444ALAFS*2	frameshift	Pathogenic
63	BRCA2	C.1813DEL	ILE605TYRFS*9	frameshift	Pathogenic
68	FANCG	572T > G	LEU191*	stop	Pathogenic
75	ATM	7306A > G	ARG2436GLY	missense	Pathogenic
76	BRCA2	5073DUP	TRP1692METFS*3	frameshift	Pathogenic
76	FANCI	3184C > T	GLN1082*	stop	Pathogenic
76	FANCG	1143G > C	ARG381SER	missense	Likely pathogenic
76	BRCA2	7307DEL	ASN2436THRFS*33	frameshift	Pathogenic
78	ATM	901G > A	GLY301SER	faux sens	Pathogenic
81	ATM	7031G > A	TRP2344*	stop	Likely pathogenic
81	SMARCA2	4369C > T	ARG1457CYS	missense	Pathogenic
82	PALB2	2850DEL	SER951LEUFS*11	frameshift	Pathogenic
83	CHEK2	1116_1117DEINSTG	LYS373GLU	missense	Pathogenic

3.4. PFS

3.4.1. First-Line PFS

The first-line median PFS of mCRPC patients was 9.7 months. No difference was observed between DDR+ and DDR− patients (9.8 months vs. 8.4 months; $p = 0.91$; Figure 2A). The PFS of the 16 patients with an *ATM/BRCA1/BRCA2* mutation was 14.4 months vs. 8.3 months for the other patients ($p = 0.24$; Figure 2B).

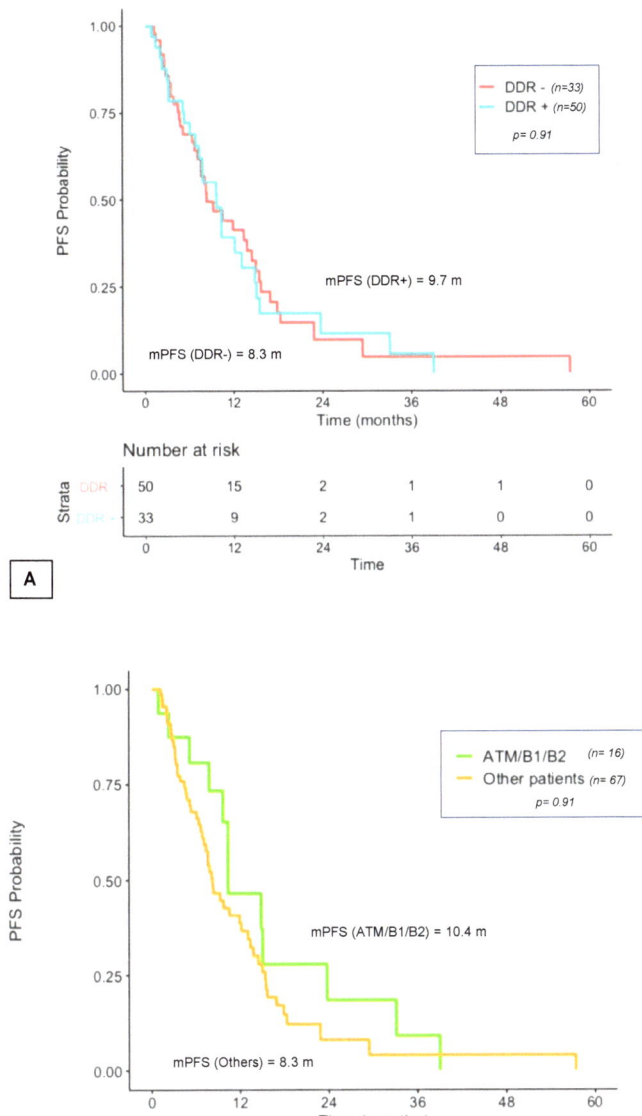

Figure 2. *Cont.*

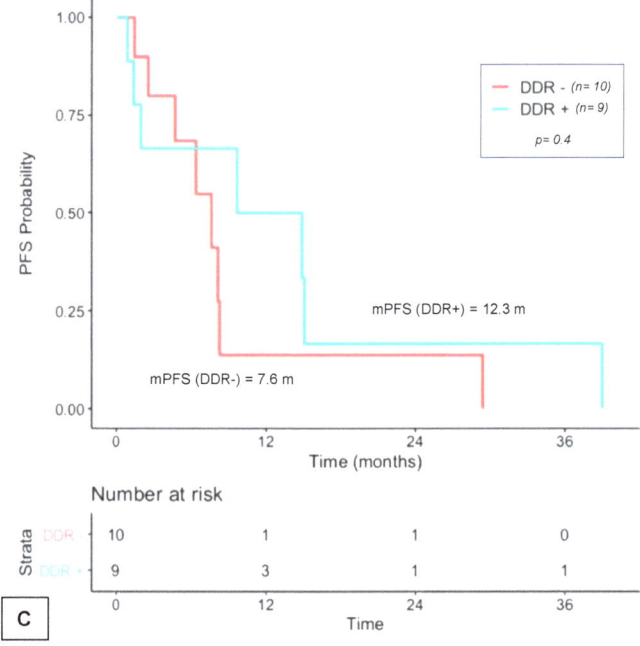

Figure 2. First-line treatment mCRPC PFS according to somatic DDR+ vs. DDR− alterations (**A**), according to ATM/B1/B2-mutated patient vs. other patients (**B**). DDR+: mutated patients; DDR−: non-mutated patients; m: months; mCRPC: metastatic castration-resistant prostate cancer; PFS: progression-free survival; n: number of patients. (**C**) First-line treatment mCRPC PFS according to somatic DDR+ vs. DDR− alterations among patients who received taxanes. DDR+: mutated patients, DDR−: non-mutated patients; m: months; mCRPC: metastatic castration-resistant prostate cancer; mPFS: median progression-free survival; n: number of patients.

For patients treated by taxanes in first line, median PFS of the 9 DDR+ mCRPC patients was 12.3 months, compared to 7.6 months in the 10 DDR− patients ($p = 0.4$; Figure 2C). The PFS of the 6 *ATM/BRCA1/BRCA2* patients treated in first line with taxanes was 14.9 months, compared to 6.4 months for the 13 other patients treated with taxanes with another or no mutation ($p = 0.11$).

For patients treated by NHT in first line, median PFS was 9.8 months for the 24 DDR+ and 12 months for 40 DDR− patients ($p = 0.68$; Figure S1). In patients treated by NHT, median PFS of the 10 *ATM/BRCA1/BRCA2* was 10.4 months vs. 8.3 months for the other patients ($p = 0.43$). No statistical difference between mCRPC first-line PFS of the 6 patients with the somatic *BRCA1/BRCA2* mutation and the 10 patients with *ATM* mutations was observed (respectively 10.3 months and 10.3 months; $p = 0.69$).

3.4.2. PFS with First Exposure to Taxanes and NHT

Among the 47 patients who received at least one line of taxanes in the first two lines of treatment, the PFS with first exposure to taxanes was 8.1 months in DDR+ patients and 5.7 months in DDR− patients ($p = 0.31$; Figure 3A). It was 10.6 months for the 9 *ATM/BRCA1/BRCA2*-mutated patients vs. 5.5 months for the other patients ($p = 0.04$; Figure 3B). Median PFS in the 6 patients with the somatic *ATM* mutation was 9.7 months vs. 15.1 months mPFS in the 3 patients with somatic *BRCA1/2* mutations ($p = 0.14$).

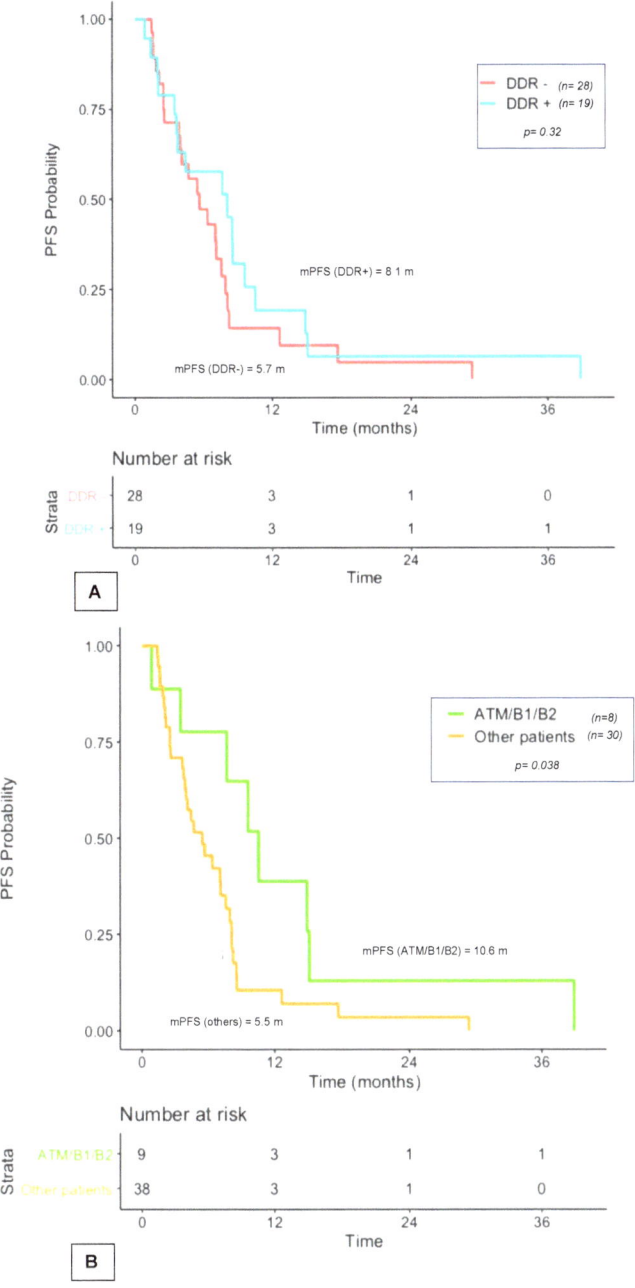

Figure 3. (**A**) First exposure to taxanes among mCRPC patients in first two lines according to somatic DDR+ vs. DDR− alterations (**A**) according to ATM/B1/B2-mutated patients vs. other patients. (**B**) DDR+: mutated patients, DDR−: non-mutated patients; m: months; mCRPC: metastatic castration-resistant prostate cancer; mPFS: median progression-free survival; n: number of patients.

For the 74 patients who received at least one line of NHT, first exposure PFS was similar in the two groups (9.7 months for DDR+ vs. 8.3 months for DDR−; $p = 0.73$; Figure S2A). In this group, PFS was 10.4 months in *ATM/BRCA1/BRCA2*-mutated patients vs. 7.8 months for the other patients ($p = 0.22$; Figure S2B). Median PFS in the 7 patients with the somatic *ATM* mutation was 23.7 months vs. 9 months mPFS in the 6 patients with somatic *BRCA1/2* mutations ($p = 0.056$).

3.5. PFS2

Among all patients who received at least two lines of mCRPC treatment, PFS2 of DDR+ patients was 16.7 months vs. 12.6 months for DDR− patients ($p = 0.88$; Figure S3A). PFS2 of *ATM/BRCA1/BRCA2*-mutated patients was 18.2 months vs. 12.6 months for the others ($p = 0.11$; Figure S3B).

Among the 38 patients who received NHT and chemotherapy during the first two lines for mCRPC, median PFS2 of the 10 patients who received chemotherapy followed by NHT was 11.7 months, and median PFS2 of the 28 mCRPC patients who received NHT followed by taxanes was 13.2 months ($p = 0.56$; Figure 4A). PFS2 of the 3 *ATM/BRCA1/BRCA2*-mutated patients treated with the taxane-NHT sequence was 49.8 months. PFS2 of DDR+ patients was 16.5 months, whatever the sequence, vs. 11.7 months for DDR− patients ($p = 0.07$; Figure 4B). In this chemotherapy and NHT group, the 6 *ATM/BRCA1/BRCA2*-mutated patients had a much longer PFS2 compared to patients with another or no mutation (median PFS2 of 35.7 months vs. 11.7 months; $p = 0.004$). In *ATM/BRCA1/BRCA2*-mutated patients treated by taxane and then the NHT sequence, PFS2 was particularly long (median PFS = 49.8 months) vs. 27.4 months for the reverse sequence ($p = 0.19$). No statistical difference was observed between PFS2 of the 4 patients with the somatic *BRCA1/BRCA2* mutation and the 6 patients with the *ATM* mutation (respectively, 16.5 months and 22.8 months; $p = 0.7$).

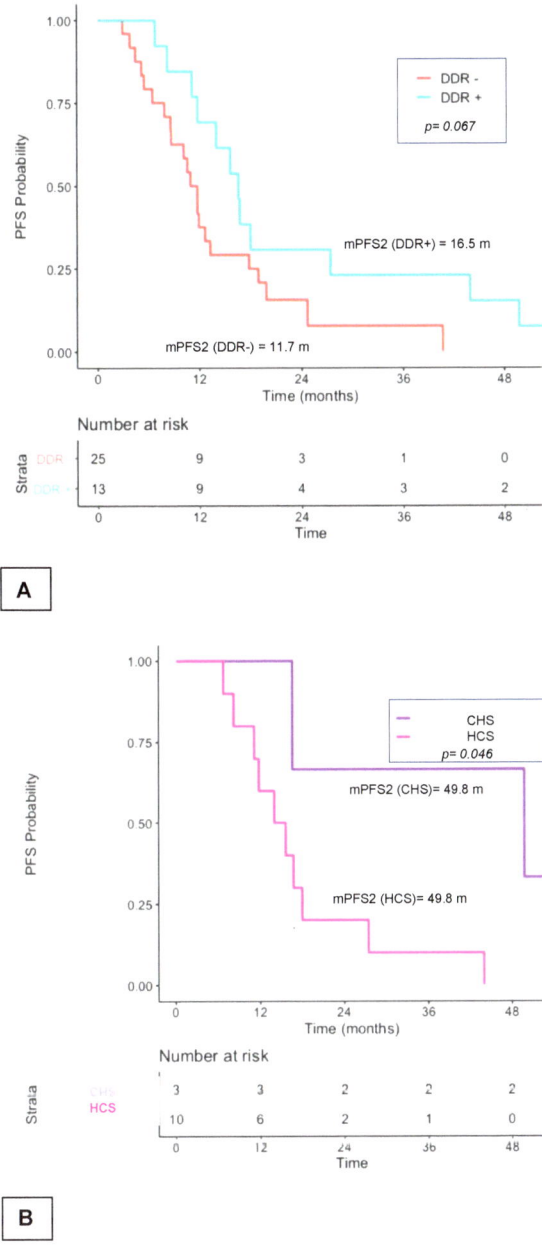

Figure 4. PFS2 according to somatic DDR+ vs. DDR− alterations and among patients who received only CHS or HCS (**A**) and PFS2 among mutated patients who received CHS or HCS according to sequence. (**B**) CHS: chemotherapy followed by NHT sequence; DDR+: mutated patients; DDR−: non-mutated patients; HCS: NHT followed by chemotherapy sequence; m: months; mCRPC: metastatic castration-resistant prostate cancer; median PFS: median progression-free survival; n: number of patients.

3.6. Overall Survival

Of the 83 patients, 35 patients died. Median OS was 2.2 years in DDR− group and was not reached in the DDR+ group ($p = 0.39$) or in the *ATM/BRCA1/BRCA2* group ($p = 0.7$) (Figure S4).

4. Discussion

In our study, patients with somatic mutations of *ATM/BRCA1/BRCA2* genes achieved longer PFS with standard mCRPC treatments than other patients. They seem to receive greater benefit from taxanes. Moreover, alterations of the different DDR genes do not have the same predictive value.

In this series, 40% of mCRPC patients presented a somatic DDR gene alteration. This rate is higher than those previously described in the literature among mCRPC patients, which range from 21% to 32% [1,7,18,25]. While most of those studies focused on a narrow gene panel including only two to 22 genes, we used a much larger panel of 69 genes. On the other hand, *ATM/BRCA1/BRCA2*-mutated patients represent 19% of our cohort, which is consistent with other studies.

Our molecular analysis could not determine whether alterations were mono- or bi-allelic, so the involvement of these alterations in carcinogenesis remains unknown. Some of these alterations might only be passenger mutations with little predictive significance. Moreover, we included patients with aggressive disease; they probably had several somatic mutations. In France, tumor samples are not required to be kept for more than 10 years, so patients with an initial diagnosis dating back over 10 years were usually excluded from our study because of the lack of availability of tumor samples. The patients who were included, therefore, had more aggressive tumors with a short duration of hormonosensitivity (Table S2). This is consistent with the fact that patients with germline *BRCA1/BRCA2* mutations generally develop more aggressive tumors [13,14].

Considering the whole population, outcomes of the DDR+ group and DDR− group were not different, whatever the first-line setting and the sequencing of treatments. This is the first report evaluating first-line mCRPC PFS according to somatic DDR mutations, whatever the treatment, even though the few studies reporting PFS according to heterogenous germline mutations reported the same results [11,22]. Most of the prostatic somatic DDR mutations concerned the *BRCA1/2* and *ATM* genes [1,5]. *BRCA1/BRCA2/ATM* mutations were the first reported molecular alterations conferring sensitivity to PARP inhibitors in prostate cancer and are the most widely studied germline and somatic mutations in this setting [11,26].

To be able to compare our results with previous studies, we also focused on the subgroup of patients with *ATM/BRCA1/BRCA2* mutations. Our study is the first to report data on PFS after mCRPC taxane treatment according to the presence of somatic DDR and *ATM/BRCA1/BRCA2* alterations. Outcomes were better for patients with *ATM/BRCA1/BRCA2* mutations treated with taxanes. These patients with first-taxane exposure had a two-fold longer PFS than those with another or no somatic mutation. Median PFS2 for these mutated patients was also particularly high (around 4 years) with the taxane-NHT sequence. Other studies reported different PFS of mCRPC patients treated with taxanes, but the populations were screened on the basis of germline alterations. Annala et al. did not find any significant difference in PSA-PFS among eight DDR− mutated and 18 non-mutated patients treated by taxanes. Likewise, Mateo et al. did not find any difference in PFS between 44 DDR− mutated patients vs. 238 non-DDR− mutated ones treated with taxanes, and there was no difference according to *BRCA2* mutations. In the study by Castro et al., PFS with first exposure to taxanes and PFS2 with taxanes followed by NHT in the subgroup of 14 *BRCA2*-mutated patients were shorter than those of patients with no germline *BRCA2* mutation [4]. However, it is difficult to draw any conclusions, due to the heterogeneity of those studies. Indeed, our series is a small retrospective singe-center cohort with a brief follow-up time. The other studies also included a limited number of patients selected according to germline mutations and heterogenous panels of genes. In our study, PFS2 was longer when somatic *ATM/BRCA1/BRCA2*-mutated patients were treated by taxanes followed by NHT rather than vice versa. Finally, a small study explored this question of sequence and reported different results: PFS2 of the seven mCRPC patients with the germline *BRCA2* mutation who received taxanes followed by NHT was shorter than that of seven *BRCA2*-mutated patients who received NHT followed by taxanes [4]. However, the subgroup of patients was screened differently, i.e., germline BRCA2-mutated patients vs. somatic *ATM/BRCA1/BRCA2* alterations in our study.

In our series, we did not find any difference between groups treated by NHT. Regarding PFS related to NHT, two other studies confirmed our finding, since they found no strong relationship between mutation and first exposure to NHT [4,11]. Two other studies found different results from ours but with conflicting conclusions. One found better PFS in patients with germline *BRCA2/ATM* mutations treated by NHT than in those without the *BRCA2/ATM* mutation (15.2 vs. 10.8; $p = 0.044$) [22]. On the other hand, Annala et al. found shorter PFS in mutated patients treated with NHT in first line, first in a retrospective study and then in a prospective cohort exploring the predictive impact of *BRCA2* and *ATM* mutations identified in circulating tumor DNA [9,23]. Again, this difference in PFS is likely due to heterogenous gene panels, with either somatic, germline, or circulating tumoral DNA, small series, and follow-up that was too short.

It is difficult to compare these studies because of their heterogeneous populations and screening criteria. Moreover, the panels used were different, and so the predictive impact of the different DDR gene alterations was probably lessened.

In our study, the PFS of *ATM/BRCA1/BRCA2*-mutated patients and of those with other DDR mutations treated with taxanes or NHT was not similar. Patients with an *ATM/BRCA1/BRCA2* mutation had significantly longer PFS2 than those with other mutations when receiving standard treatments. PFS of first exposure to NHT was not statistically different between patients with *ATM* or *BRCA1/BRCA2* mutations, while patients with the *ATM* mutation seemed to have a longer PFS than those with *BRCA1/2* mutations. Contrary results were observed regarding first exposure to taxanes, where PFS was longer in patients with BRCA mutations than in those with ATM mutations. Alterations of the different DDR genes probably do not have the same predictive impact.

This issue has also received attention in patients treated with PARP inhibitors. Marshall et al. observed that PFS in mCRPC patients treated with olaparib with an *ATM* mutation was shorter than that in patients with the *BRCA1/BRCA2* mutation [18]. Gene mutations were germline and/or somatic. The PROFOUND trial compared olaparib to NHT in patients with *ATM/BRCA1/BRCA2* mutations and in those with other DDR mutations screened by a 15-gene panel. Patients with *ATM/BRCA1/BRCA2* mutations had a better PFS with olaparib than with NHT [17]. Exploratory results of PFS by type of mutation showed that *BRCA2*- and *RAD51B*-mutated patients tended to have better PFS than *ATM*- or *BRCA1*-mutated patients. In the TRITON2 trial, which evaluated response to rucaparib in DDR+ mCRPC patients, a limited number of radiographic and PSA responses was observed in patients with *ATM*, *CDK12*, or *CHEK2* gene alterations, whereas responses were observed in patients with alterations in other DDR genes, such as *PALB2*, *BRIP1*, *FANCA*, and *RAD51B*. These studies showed that responses differ according to the somatic DDR alteration [27]. Alteration of the different DDR genes seems to have an independent predictive value for PARP inhibitors and for standard therapies.

Although outcomes were not different between our DDR+ and DDR− patients, whatever the first mCRPC line of treatment setting and the sequencing of treatments, mCRPC patients with the *ATM/BRCA1/BRCA2* mutation benefited from standard therapies, with long responses to taxanes in the BRCA1/2 mutation group and to NHT in patients with the ATM mutation. This reinforces the idea that the predictive impact of the alterations of the different DDR genes varies according to the type of treatment and gene concerned. In the setting of mCRPC, the optimal therapeutic sequence remains elusive. If predictive biomarkers could be established for choosing one particular treatment over another and for knowing the outcomes of standard treatment for the different DDR+ gene, this could help in selecting the best treatment sequence [28,29].

Because this study presents several limitations, such as monocentric and retrospective characteristics, small sample size, and heterogeneous population (prior treatment, metastasis at diagnosis . . .), new prospective studies with more homogenous patients would be needed to confirm these results.

5. Conclusions

Metastatic CRPC patients with the ATM/BRCA1/BRCA2 mutation benefit from standard therapies, with long responses to taxanes. The predictive impact of DDR genes is probably dependent on the gene and the systemic treatment. Future studies are needed to confirm these findings.

In the area of PARP inhibitors, taxane before or after PARP inhibitors should be discussed.

Supplementary Materials: The following supporting information can be downloaded at: https://www.mdpi.com/article/10.3390/curroncol29040226/s1, Table S1—Lists of genes in the panel and methodology. Table S2—Outcomes of analyzed versus excluded patients. Table S3—Clinical outcomes of analyzed patients according to treatments (NHT versus Taxanes). File S1—Annex of molecular results. Figure S1—First-line treatment mCRPC PFS according to somatic DDR+ versus DDR− alterations among patients who received NHT. Figure S2—First exposure to NHT among mCRPC patients in first two lines according to somatic DDR+ versus DDR− alterations and (A) according to ATM/B1/B2-mutated patients versus other patients (B). Figure S3—PFS2 according to somatic DDR+ versus DDR− alterations (A) according to ATM/B1/B2-mutated patients versus other patients (B), according to somatic DDR+ versus DDR−. Figure S4—OS according to somatic DDR+ versus DDR− alterations (A) and according to ATM/B1/B2-mutated patient versus the other patients (B).

Author Contributions: The landscape of personalized medicine is in a large and rapid mutation with molecular profiling. In this article, we propose to explore outcomes of patients with metastatic castration-resistant prostate cancer (mCRPC) according to somatic DNA damage repair genes alterations and standard mCRPC therapies. This is the first paper that proposes outcomes among a mCRPC cohort selected with a large genetic panel screening somatic alterations and standard therapies. Z.N. and F.J. wrote the manuscript and devised the study concept and design. P.-E.B., E.C., E.M. and I.B. edited the paper. J.L. was responsible for overseeing the statistical section. A.L. (Anais Lelaidier) contributed to data collection. A.L. (Alexandra Leconte) took care declarations. A.R., D.V., F.B., L.C. and S.K. carried out somatic analysis. All authors reviewed the paper. All authors have read and agreed to the published version of the manuscript.

Funding: This research received no external funding.

Institutional Review Board Statement: The PROSOTAX retrospective observatory is conducted in accordance with the amended law of 6 January 1978 relating to information technology, files, and freedoms, the EU regulation n 2016/679 relating to data protection ("RGPD"), and the law n 2018-493 of 20 June 2018 relating to personal data protection. The protocol was approved by the Centre François Baclesse, the study promoter. All patients are given global information on potential use of their data registered during their management in the institution; in addition, all patients are specifically informed about this study. Patients are free to express their opposition to the use of their data at any time. This procedure is in line with the French Research Standard MR-004 "Research not involving human participants". The study was approved by the local (internal) IRB from our institution "Centre François Baclesse". This procedure is in line with the French Research Standard MR-004 "Research not involving human participants".

Informed Consent Statement: All patients are given global information on potential use of their data registered during their management in the institution; in addition, all patients are specifically informed about this study. Patients are free to express their opposition to the use of their data at any time.

Data Availability Statement: The datasets used and/or analyzed during the current study are available from the corresponding author on reasonable request.

Acknowledgments: We are grateful to all of the patients and their caregivers. We acknowledge the Data Processing Centre (DPC) of the Northwest Canceropole (Centre de Traitement des Données du Cancéropôle Nord-Ouest) in charge of data management. The investigators are also thanked.

Conflicts of Interest: The authors declare no conflict of interest.

References

1. Robinson, D.; Van Allen, E.M.; Wu, Y.-M.; Schultz, N.; Lonigro, R.J.; Mosquera, J.-M.; Montgomery, B.; Taplin, M.-E.; Pritchard, C.C.; Attard, G.; et al. Integrative Clinical Genomics of Advanced Prostate Cancer. *Cell* **2015**, *161*, 1215–1228. [CrossRef] [PubMed]
2. TCGA Identifies Subtypes of Prostate Cancer. The Cancer Genome Atlas—National Cancer Institute. Available online: https://cancergenome.nih.gov/newsevents/newsannouncements/PRAD_2015 (accessed on 6 March 2017).
3. Jonsson, P.; Bandlamudi, C.; Cheng, M.L.; Srinivasan, P.; Chavan, S.S.; Friedman, N.D.; Rosen, E.Y.; Richards, A.L.; Bouvier, N.; Selcuklu, S.D.; et al. Tumour lineage shapes BRCA-mediated phenotypes. *Nature* **2019**, *571*, 576–579. [CrossRef] [PubMed]
4. Castro, E.; Romero-Laorden, N.; Del Pozo, A.; Lozano, R.; Medina, A.; Puente, J.; Piulats, J.M.; Lorente, D.; Saez, M.I.; Morales-Barrera, R.; et al. PROREPAIR-B: A Prospective Cohort Study of the Impact of Germline DNA Repair Mutations on the Outcomes of Patients with Metastatic Castration-Resistant Prostate Cancer. *J. Clin. Oncol.* **2019**, *37*, 490–503. [CrossRef] [PubMed]
5. Pritchard, C.C.; Mateo, J.; Walsh, M.F.; De Sarkar, N.; Abida, W.; Beltran, H.; Garofalo, A.; Gulati, R.; Carreira, S.; Eeles, R.; et al. Inherited DNA-Repair Gene Mutations in Men with Metastatic Prostate Cancer. *N. Engl. J. Med.* **2016**, *375*, 443–453. [CrossRef]
6. Cancer Genome Atlas Research Network. The Molecular Taxonomy of Primary Prostate Cancer. *Cell* **2015**, *163*, 1011–1025. [CrossRef]
7. Mateo, J.; Carreira, S.; Sandhu, S.; Miranda, S.; Mossop, H.; Perez-Lopez, R.; Nava Rodrigues, D.; Robinson, D.; Omlin, A.; Tunariu, N.; et al. DNA-Repair Defects and Olaparib in Metastatic Prostate Cancer. *N. Engl. J. Med.* **2015**, *373*, 1697–1708. [CrossRef]
8. Armenia, J.; Wankowicz, S.A.M.; Liu, D.; Gao, J.; Kundra, R.; Reznik, E.; Chatila, W.K.; Chakravarty, D.; Han, G.C.; Coleman, I.; et al. The long tail of oncogenic drivers in prostate cancer. *Nat. Genet.* **2018**, *50*, 645–651. [CrossRef]
9. Annala, M.; Struss, W.J.; Warner, E.W.; Beja, K.; Vandekerkhove, G.; Wong, A.; Khalaf, D.; Seppälä, I.-L.; So, A.; Lo, G.; et al. Treatment Outcomes and Tumor Loss of Heterozygosity in Germline DNA Repair-deficient Prostate Cancer. *Eur. Urol.* **2017**, *72*, 34–42. [CrossRef]
10. Grasso, C.S.; Wu, Y.-M.; Robinson, D.R.; Cao, X.; Dhanasekaran, S.M.; Khan, A.P.; Quist, M.J.; Jing, X.; Lonigro, R.J.; Brenner, J.C.; et al. The mutational landscape of lethal castration-resistant prostate cancer. *Nature* **2012**, *487*, 239–243. [CrossRef]
11. Mateo, J.; Cheng, H.H.; Beltran, H.; Dolling, D.; Xu, W.; Pritchard, C.C.; Mossop, H.; Rescigno, P.; Perez-Lopez, R.; Sailer, V.; et al. Clinical Outcome of Prostate Cancer Patients with Germline DNA Repair Mutations: Retrospective Analysis from an International Study. *Eur. Urol.* **2018**, *73*, 687–693. [CrossRef]
12. Wei, Y.; Wu, J.; Gu, W.; Qin, X.; Dai, B.; Lin, G.; Gan, H.; Freedland, S.J.; Zhu, Y.; Ye, D. Germline DNA Repair Gene Mutation Landscape in Chinese Prostate Cancer Patients. *Eur. Urol.* **2019**, *76*, 280–283. [CrossRef] [PubMed]
13. Castro, E.; Goh, C.; Olmos, D.; Saunders, E.; Leongamornlert, D.; Tymrakiewicz, M.; Mahmud, N.; Dadaev, T.; Govindasami, K.; Guy, M.; et al. Germline BRCA Mutations Are Associated with Higher Risk of Nodal Involvement, Distant Metastasis, and Poor Survival Outcomes in Prostate Cancer. *J. Clin. Oncol.* **2013**, *31*, 1748–1757. [CrossRef] [PubMed]
14. Castro, E.; Goh, C.; Leongamornlert, D.; Saunders, E.; Tymrakiewicz, M.; Dadaev, T.; Govindasami, K.; Guy, M.; Ellis, S.; Frost, D.; et al. Effect of BRCA Mutations on Metastatic Relapse and Cause-specific Survival After Radical Treatment for Localised Prostate Cancer. *Eur. Urol.* **2015**, *68*, 186–193. [CrossRef] [PubMed]
15. Gallagher, D.J.; Gaudet, M.M.; Pal, P.; Kirchhoff, T.; Balistreri, L.; Vora, K.; Bhatia, J.; Stadler, Z.; Fine, S.W.; Reuter, V.; et al. Germline BRCA mutations denote a clinicopathologic subset of prostate cancer. *Clin. Cancer Res. Off. J. Am. Assoc. Cancer Res.* **2010**, *16*, 2115–2121. [CrossRef] [PubMed]
16. Gallagher, D.J.; Cronin, A.M.; Milowsky, M.I.; Morris, M.J.; Bhatia, J.; Scardino, P.T.; Eastham, J.A.; Offit, K.; Robson, M.E. Germline BRCA mutation does not prevent response to taxane-based therapy for the treatment of castration-resistant prostate cancer. *Br. J. Urol.* **2011**, *109*, 713–719. [CrossRef]
17. Hussain, M.; Mateo, J.; Fizazi, K.; Saad, F.; Shore, N.D.; Sandhu, S.; Chi, K.N.; Sartor, O.; Agarwal, N.; Olmos, D.; et al. Phase III PROfound Study Evaluates Olaparib in Setting of mCRPC—The ASCO Post. 2019. Available online: https://oncologypro.esmo.org/meeting-resources/esmo-2019-congress/PROfound-Phase-3-study-of-olaparib-versus-enzalutamide-or-abiraterone-for-metastatic-castration-resistant-prostate-cancer-mCRPC-with-homologous-recombination-repair-HRR-gene-alterations (accessed on 11 March 2020).
18. Marshall, C.H.; Sokolova, A.O.; McNatty, A.L.; Cheng, H.H.; Eisenberger, M.A.; Bryce, A.H.; Schweizer, M.T.; Antonarakis, E.S. Differential Response to Olaparib Treatment Among Men with Metastatic Castration-resistant Prostate Cancer Harboring BRCA1 or BRCA2 Versus ATM Mutations. *Eur. Urol.* **2019**, *76*, 452–458. [CrossRef]
19. TRITON2: An International, Multicenter, Open-Label, Phase II Study of the Parp Inhibitor Rucaparib in Patients with Metastatic Castration-Resistant Prostate Cancer (mCRPC) Associated with Homologous Recombination Deficiency (HRD). *J. Clin. Oncol.* **2018**, *36*.

20. Clarke, N.; Wiechno, P.; Alekseev, B.; Sala, N.; Jones, R.; Kocak, I.; Chiuri, V.E.; Jassem, J.; Flechon, A.; Redferm, C.; et al. Olaparib combined with abiraterone in patients with metastatic castration-resistant prostate cancer: A randomised, double-blind, placebo-controlled, phase 2 trial. *Lancet Oncol.* **2018**, *19*, 975–986. [CrossRef]
21. Mateo, J.; Porta, N.; Bianchini, D.; McGovern, U.; Elliott, T.; Jones, R.; Syndikus, I.; Ralph, C.; Jain, S.; Varughese, M.; et al. Olaparib in patients with metastatic castration-resistant prostate cancer with DNA repair gene aberrations (TOPARP-B): A multicentre, open-label, randomised, phase 2 trial. *Lancet Oncol.* **2020**, *21*, 162–174. [CrossRef]
22. Antonarakis, E.S.; Lu, C.; Luber, B.; Liang, C.; Wang, H.; Chen, Y.; Silberstein, J.L.; Piana, D.; Lai, Z.; Chen, Y.; et al. Germline DNA-repair Gene Mutations and Outcomes in Men with Metastatic Castration-resistant Prostate Cancer Receiving First-line Abiraterone and Enzalutamide. *Eur. Urol.* **2018**, *74*, 218–225. [CrossRef]
23. Annala, M.; Vandekerkhove, G.; Khalaf, D.; Taavitsainen, S.; Beja, K.; Warner, E.W.; Sunderland, K.; Kollmannsberger, C.; Eigl, B.J.; Finch, D.; et al. Circulating Tumor DNA Genomics Correlate with Resistance to Abiraterone and Enzalutamide in Prostate Cancer. *Cancer Discov.* **2018**, *8*, 444–457. [CrossRef] [PubMed]
24. Nientiedt, C.; Heller, M.; Endris, V.; Volckmar, A.-L.; Zschäbitz, S.; Tapia-Laliena, M.A.; Duensing, A.; Jäger, D.; Schirmacher, P.; Sültmann, H.; et al. Mutations in BRCA2 and taxane resistance in prostate cancer. *Sci. Rep.* **2017**, *7*, 4574. [CrossRef] [PubMed]
25. Hussain, M.; Daignault-Newton, S.; Twardowski, P.W.; Albany, C.; Stein, M.N.; Kunju, L.P.; Siddiqui, J.; Wu, Y.-M.; Robinson, D.; Lonigro, R.J.; et al. Targeting Androgen Receptor and DNA Repair in Metastatic Castration-Resistant Prostate Cancer: Results From NCI 9012. *J. Clin. Oncol.* **2018**, *36*, 991–999. [CrossRef] [PubMed]
26. Pennington, K.P.; Walsh, T.; Harrell, M.I.; Lee, M.K.; Pennil, C.C.; Rendi, M.H.; Thornton, A.; Norquist, B.M.; Casadei, S.; Nord, A.S.; et al. Germline and Somatic Mutations in Homologous Recombination Genes Predict Platinum Response and Survival in Ovarian, Fallopian Tube, and Peritoneal Carcinomas. *Clin. Cancer Res.* **2014**, *20*, 764–775. [CrossRef]
27. Abida, W.; Campbell, D.; Patnaik, A.; Shapiro, J.D.; Sautois, B.; Vogelzang, N.J.; Voog, E.G.; Bryce, A.H.; McDermott, R.; Ricci, F.; et al. Non-BRCA DNA Damage Repair Gene Alterations and Response to the PARP Inhibitor Rucaparib in Metastatic Castration-Resistant Prostate Cancer: Analysis From the Phase II TRITON2 Study. *Clin. Cancer Res. Off. J. Am. Assoc. Cancer Res.* **2020**, *26*, 2487–2496. [CrossRef]
28. Horwich, A.; Hugosson, J.; de Reijke, T.; Wiegel, T.; Fizazi, K.; Kataja, V.; Parker, C.; Bellmunt, J.; Berthold, D.; Bill-Axelson, A.; et al. Prostate cancer: ESMO Consensus Conference Guidelines 2012. *Ann. Oncol.* **2013**, *24*, 1141–1162. [CrossRef]
29. Rozet, F.; Hennequin, C.; Beauval, J.-B.; Beuzeboc, P.; Cormier, L.; Fromont-Hankard, G.; Mongiat-Artus, P.; Ploussard, G.; Mathieu, R.; Brureau, L.; et al. French ccAFU guidelines—Update 2018-2020: Prostate cancer. *Progres. En. Urol. J. Assoc. Fr. Urol. Soc. Fr. Urol.* **2018**, *28* (Suppl. S1), R81–R132.

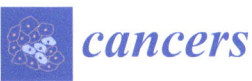

Article

Template-Independent Poly(A)-Tail Decay and RNASEL as Potential Cellular Biomarkers for Prostate Cancer Development

Gordana Kocić [1,*], Jovan Hadzi-Djokić [2], Andrej Veljković [1], Stefanos Roumeliotis [3], Ljubinka Janković-Veličković [4] and Andrija Šmelcerović [5]

1. Department of Biochemistry, Faculty of Medicine, University of Niš, 18000 Niš, Serbia; andrej.veljkovic@medfak.ni.ac.rs
2. Serbian Academy of Sciences and Arts, 11000 Belgrade, Serbia; jovanhdj@sanu.ac.rs
3. Division of Nephrology and Hypertension, 1st Department of Internal Medicine, AHEPA Hospital, School of Medicine, Aristotle University of Thessaloniki, 541 24 Thessaloniki, Greece; roumeliotis@auth.gr
4. Department of Pathology, University Clinical Center Niš, 18000 Niš, Serbia; ljubinka.jankovic.velickovic@medfak.ni.ac.rs
5. Department of Chemistry, Faculty of Medicine, University of Niš, 18000 Niš, Serbia; andrija.smelcerovic@medfak.ni.ac.rs
* Correspondence: gordana.kocic@medfak.ni.ac.rs; Tel.: +381-63-812-2522

Simple Summary: The ultimate need in cancer tissue is to adapt translation machinery to accelerated protein synthesis in a rapidly proliferating environment. Our study was designed with the aim of integrating fundamental and clinical research to find new biomarkers for prostate cancer (PC) with clinical usefulness for the stratification prediction of healthy tissue transition into malignant phenotype. This study revealed: (i) an entirely novel mechanism of the regulatory influence of Poly(A) deadenylase in mRNAs translational activity and the 3′ mRNA untranslated region (3′UTR) length in cancer tissue and its regulation by the poly(A) decay; (ii) the RNASEL interrelationship with the inflammatory pattern of PC and corresponding tumor-adjacent and healthy tissue; and (iii) the sensitivity, specificity, and predictive value of these enzymes. The proposed manuscript is based on the use of specific biochemical and immunoassay methods with the principal research adapted for the use of tissue specimens.

Abstract: The post-transcriptional messenger RNA (mRNA) decay and turnover rate of the template-independent poly(A) tail, localized at the 3′-untranslated region (3′UTR) of mRNA, have been documented among subtle mechanisms of uncontrolled cancer tissue growth. The activity of Poly(A) deadenylase and the expression pattern of RNASEL have been examined. A total of 138 prostate tissue specimens from 46 PC patients (cancer specimens, corresponding adjacent surgically healthy tissues, and in their normal counterparts, at least 2 cm from carcinoma) were used. For the stratification prediction of healthy tissue transition into malignant phenotype, the enzyme activity of tumor-adjacent tissue was considered in relation to the presence of microfocal carcinoma. More than a four-times increase in specific enzyme activity (U/L g.prot) was registered in PC on account of both the dissociation of its inhibitor and genome reprogramming. The obtained ROC curve and Youden index showed that Poly(A) deadenylase identified PC with a sensitivity of 93.5% and a specificity of 94.6%. The RNASEL expression profile was raised significantly in PC, but the sensitivity was 40.5% and specificity was 86.9%. A significantly negative correlation between PC and control tissue counterparts with a higher expression pattern in lymphocyte-infiltrated samples were reported. In conclusion, significantly upregulated Poly(A) deadenylase activity may be a checkpoint for the transition of precancerous lesion to malignancy, while RNASEL may predict chronic inflammation.

Keywords: prostate cancer; poly(A) deadenylase; RNASEL

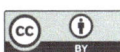

1. Introduction

Prostate cancer (PC) represents a leading cause of cancer-related deaths in men. Known contributing risk factors include old age (50+), race (African American), family history, diet (meat and dairy products), and chronic prostate infections. Different pathogen-associated molecular patterns (PAMP) and damage-associated molecular patterns (DAMP) may induce inflammation, such as bacterial infections, viruses, nutrients, hormones, urine reflux, or autoimmune reactions [1,2]. Along with the study of the subtle molecular mechanisms of carcinoma development, there have been efforts to develop early and reliable diagnostic markers [2,3].

Besides the excessive DNA replication, cancer growth is a consequence of transcriptional deregulation. It has been almost 30 years since Cox and Goding posed a promising hypothesis: "transcription-related research should soon yield major dividends for cancer patients" [4]. Afterwards, the mechanisms of RNA transcription, maturation, and turnover were documented and became mainstream, starting a new trend in cancer research.

The cell-cycle progression, mitotic division, meiotic maturation, embryogenesis, differentiation, and cell response to exposomic factors occur by the modulation of mRNA stability and protein translation machinery. The post-transcriptional messenger RNA (mRNA) maturation, decay, and turnover rate are regulated by the half-life of the template-independent poly(A) tail, localized at the 3′-end of the 3′-untranslated region (3′UTR) of mRNA. In normal cells, remaining in a non-proliferative state, it represents a highly conserved mechanism, a highway of mRNA degradation; afterwards, the mRNA can undergo decapping [5,6]. It is catalyzed by poly(A) deadenylases [7,8]. Minor pathways of decay may be the deadenylation-independent decapping and endoribonucleotidase-catalyzed degradation of mRNA. Besides this, mRNAs can be degraded by a nonsense-mediated decay, a type of accelerated degradation aimed to reduce potential errors in gene expression [9,10].

The most recent approaches that have changed previous paradigms about the decay of 3′UTR poly(A) tail include the following: shorter poly(A) nucleotide tracks and longer mRNA stability, specifically observed in malignant tissues; protein synthesis translated from the shorter mRNA is several times higher than that from the longer mRNA; shorter poly(A) tail mRNA isoforms are capable of producing several times more proteins than the longer ones; mutations resulting in longer poly(A) tracks reduced the protein synthesis rate and mRNA stability; 3′UTR shortening in the mRNAs of proto-oncogenes, which led to their transformation into oncogenic proteins, translated without repressive control of miRNAs [11–13]. In this way, the diminishing of the "polyadenylation code", known as the "survival of the fittest", represents a functional adaptation of malignant cells to escape translational control, by the malignant cell demand. A potential mechanism of their oncogene action has been explained through the loss of microRNA (miRNA) complementary binding sites on mRNAs, which are usually located in the 3′UTR region [14].

Concerning the compartmentation of PC inside of the gland, the peripheral zone (PZ) represents the typical localization for cancer and inflammation. That is why it is not surprising that chronic infection and inflammation very often coexist with cancer. Inflammation may induce tumor growth by causing DNA damage, usually associated with inadequate DNA repair. On the other hand, inflammation may induce the activation of immune defense cells, which may protect tissue from unwanted cells bearing damaged DNA [15,16]. Among diagnostic values, a systemic immune-inflammation index (SII) and neutrophil–lymphocyte ratio (NLR) have been documented [17]. Recent findings suggest that chemokines and cytokine-mediated signaling pathways are intensively involved in PC growth, angiogenesis, endothelial mesenchymal transition, leukocyte infiltration, and hormone resistance in advanced types of PC [18]. Recently, Ribonuclease-L (RNASEL, 2′,5′-oligoisoadenylate synthetase-dependent) has been the subject of intensive research, as the key RNase in a viral RNA decay and inflammation. It triggers the synthesis and secretion of inflammatory cytokines, particularly type I interferon (IFN) [19,20]. The role of RNASEL in hereditary prostate cancer 1 (HPC1) has an intriguing significance. Hereditary mutations in RNASEL may predispose an increased incidence of PC and may determine the aggressiveness of the disease [21–25]. Catalytic action of RNASEL may also produce small non-coding double-stranded RNAs (dsRNAs), important regulators of cell survival via autophagy, versus apoptosis [26]. The role of pleiotropy in PC makes it attractive and currently still mysterious.

The primary focus of our research is the poly(A) decay as a potential checkpoint in PC development and progression. In order to employ the Poly (A) deadenylase as a possible marker of healthy tissue transition into malignant phenotype, it has been detected in carcinoma tissue, adjacent surgically healthy tissue, and in their normal counterparts, at least 2cm from carcinoma. In the present study, we also compared the expression level of RNASEL, in the same tissue specimens. Standard markers of the PC stage and progression (PSA, Gleason Score, and histopathological specimens) were also evaluated. Considering these enzymes as proteins with targeted non-coding RNA regions or non-coding RNAs as substrates, they may represent novel RNA–protein by-pass cellular biomarkers.

2. Patients and Methods

The Research Ethics Committee at the Faculty of Medicine Nis approved this prospective study protocol and waved informed consent (N°12-8818-2/18 on 23 September 2020).

Patient selection: Our pilot study was conducted at University Clinical Center Nis, with 46 consecutive patients with prostate cancer (PC) who underwent radical prostatectomy. The diagnosis was verified by clinical symptoms, abnormal findings on digital rectal examination (DRE), and an increased age-specific reference range of PSA value.

Tissue preparation: After prostatectomy, the parts of the cancer tissue, adjacent surgically healthy tissue, and normal tissue counterpart, at least 2cm from carcinoma, were dissected. The samples obtained were homogenized on ice; 10% of the homogenates were prepared and frozen on $-80\ °C$ until the biochemical examinations were performed.

Enzyme assays: The protocol used for the determination of the activity of Poly(A) deadenylase was optimized in our laboratory, previously published for tissue and cell culture samples and for plasma specimens [27–29]. The method was based on spectrophotometric measurement of released acid-soluble nucleotides at 260 nm, from homopolynucleotide poly(A) as the substrate (purchased from Sigma-Aldrich, Darmstadt, Germany). Enzyme activity was expressed as the total (U/L homogenate) and specific enzyme activity (U/g protein of fresh tumor tissue). For the stratification method for the evaluation of poly(A) deadenylase as a predictive marker of healthy tissue transition into malignant phenotype, the enzyme activity of tumor-adjacent tissue was considered in relation to whether there was a microfocal carcinoma or not.

To evaluate the possible predictive ability of Poly(A) deadenylase-specific activity for identifying PC, we performed receiver operation curves (ROC) and then calculated the Youden index, to determine the optimal cutoff value of Poly (A) deadenylase-specific activity. We then calculated the sensitivity and specificity to predict prostate cancer.

Having in mind the importance of RNase inhibitors for limited cell RNase activity, the activity of latent, i.e., inhibitor-bound RNase, was estimated [30]. The dissociation of Poly(A)deadenylase/inhibitor complex was achieved by using sulfhydryl reagent (0.1mL of 10mM p-chloromercuribenzoate) prior to the determination of enzyme activity [31]. In this way, the enzyme activity was calculated as (i) total (free + inhibitor bound); (ii) free; and (iii) latent, i.e., inhibitor-bound.

The protocol for RNASEL (2′,5′-Oligoisoadenylate Synthetase-Dependent) was based on enzyme-linked immunosorbent assay (kits were purchased from Cloud-Clone Corp., Katy, TX, USA) with a detection range between15.625 and 1000 pg/mL. The specific enzyme expression was calculated according to the tissue protein content (ng/g proteins).

To evaluate the possible predictive ability of the RNASEL-specific expression pattern for identifying PC, we performed receiver operation curves (ROC) and then calculated the Youden index to determine the optimal cutoff value of RNASEL-specific expression. Then, we calculated the sensitivity and specificity to predict the presence of PC.

In order to distinguish enzyme activity in relation to inflammatory conditions, the enzyme activity was considered in relation to whether there was predominantly lymphocyte, macrophage–neutrophil inflammation, or only tissue hypertrophy.

The tissue protein content in homogenates was measured according to the Lowry procedure [32].

Statistical analyses: the results obtained are expressed as the mean ± standard deviation for continuous variables. Data analysis was performed using SPSS (one-way ANOVA) test. To determine the strength of a possible interaction and to quantify a possible association between two variables, a bivariate Pearson correlation coefficient was determined.

3. Results

Clinical characteristics of patients: The clinical characteristics of patients and the level of standard biomarkers are shown in Table 1. A prostate-specific antigen (PSA) test was used to diagnose PC, in which values above 4 ng/mL were suspicious for cancer.

Table 1. The age and level of PSA, Gleason score, and tumor stage in investigated patients with PC.

Investigated Parameters	n%
Age	
<70	28 (60.87%)
>70	18 (39.13%)
Tumor stage	
II	34 (73.91%)
III	12 (26.09%)
pN—lymph node metastasis	
N0	20 (43.48%)
NX	26 (56.52%)
pM-distant metastasis	
M0	22 (47.83%)
MX	24 (52.17%)
Gleason score	
3 + 3	15 (32.6%)
3 + 4	18 (39.13%)
4 + 3	9 (19.56%)
3 + 5	2 (4.35%)
4 + 4	2 (4.35%)
PSA (ng/mL)	
<10	28 (60.87%)
>10	18 (39.13%)

Enzyme assays: Poly(A) deadenylase and RNASEL were measured in PC tissue, adjacent surgically healthy tissue, and in corresponding healthy counterparts, at least 2 cm from carcinoma. The corresponding samples were considered further in relation to a possible influence of tissue transition into malignant phenotype and inflammation; the samples were further subdivided in the corresponding groups.

Poly(A) deadenylase: More than a four-times increase in specific enzyme activity (U/L g.prot) was registered for Poly(A) deadenylase, followed by a more-than twofold increase in its activity in adjacent carcinoma tissue, compared to the control healthy tissue counterparts (Figure 1).

Our preliminary results showed no overlapping value between the PC and control samples, which maybe a prerequisite for considering sensitivity and specificity as well as the cutoff value in a larger series of samples. The enzyme activities for the corresponding prostate tissue specimens for each patient were evaluated with regard to their biomarker potential to distinguish cancer tissue, as a prognostic biomarker of cancer aggressiveness, and as potential predictive biomarkers for the stratification of transition of benign hyperplasia to the malignant process. Following the stratification of benign hyperplasia (BPH) and the appearance of microfocal cancer, apart from the main carcinoma tissue, the appearance of microfocal cancer was registered in 45.65 tumor-adjacent specimens. The enzyme activity was significantly higher in the adjacent tissue with microfocal carcinoma compared to tumor-adjacent tissue bearing only BPH and control specimens but was still significantly lower than that of PC specimens. Poly(A) deadenylase may be considered as an early marker for the transition of benign hyperplasia to a malignant one, when histopathological diagnosis is still insufficient. The evaluation of areas under the curves (AUCs) showed that Poly(A) deadenylase-specific activity (AUC = 0.97, 95% CI = 0.95–1.00, $p < 0.0001$) (Figure 2) predicted PC, and specific activity exhibited a significantly high performance. After determining the optimal cutoff values by Youden's index, we calculated the sensitivity and specificity and found that Poly(A) deadenylase identified prostate cancer with a sensitivity of 93.5% and a specificity of 94.6%.

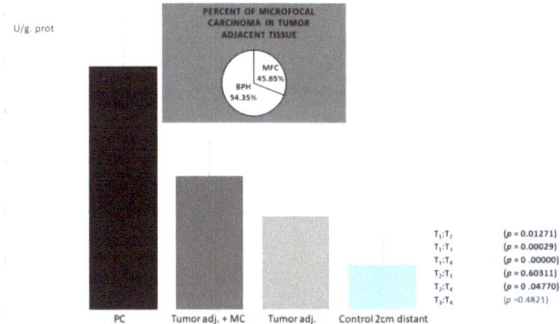

Figure 1. Poly(A) deadenylase specific enzyme activity (U/L g.prot) in PC, tumor adjacent with MC, tumor-adjacent and control healthy counterparts.

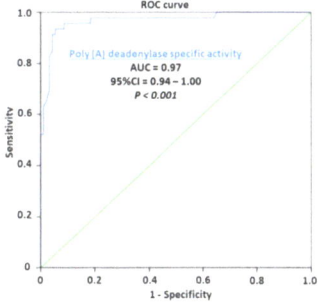

Figure 2. Receiver operating characteristic curve showing the performance of Poly(A) deadenylase specific activity in predicting prostate cancer.

In monitoring the potential specificity of enzyme activity with regard to inflammatory conditions, the histopathological findings of prostatitis caused by infiltration of the prostate tissue by immune cells (lymphocytes, macrophages, or neutrophils) did not have any influence on enzyme activity. It may exclude any inflammatory process as a confounding condition for the increased Poly(A) deadenylase activity.

The dissociation of Poly(A) deadenylase-inhibitor complex by p-chloromercuribenzoate indicated that the main part (59.16%) of Poly(A) deadenylase in control healthy tissue seems to be latent: the inhibitor-bound. No quantity of latent form was detected in PC. The free enzyme in PC specimens was still more than 50% (51.6) higher than the total activity in the control tissue, which may indicate that about 50% of enzyme activity was raised because of genome reprogramming and the consequent increased expression in malignant tissue. Unlike malignant tissue (PC specimens), in tumor-adjacent tissue, only a gradual dissociation of enzymes from its inhibitor complex was documented since the latent form was retained in 35.23% in tumor-adjacent tissue and only in 5.11% in tumor-adjacent tissue with microfocal cancer. Based on the results obtained, it can be assumed that the increased expression of the enzyme may be a checkpoint for the transition to a malignant phenotype (Figure 3).

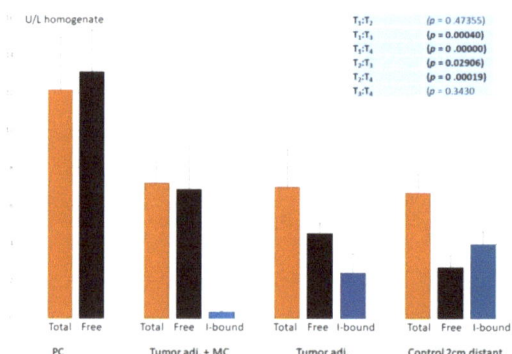

Figure 3. Total, free, and inhibitor-bound (latent) Poly(A) deadenylase activity (U/L) in PC, tumor adjacent with MC, tumor-adjacent, and control healthy counterparts.

RNASEL: A significant difference in RNASEL in investigated groups of samples, concerning the total and specific expression pattern, was observed (Figure 4). The statistical significance was reported in PC specimens only for the total enzyme activity. Since there was no difference in RNASEL concerning the presence of microfocal lesions, tumor-adjacent tissue was not stratified. Based on these results and the difference obtained between the RNASEL expression profile in PC in relation to the control tissue, it would not be considered as an early tumor marker.

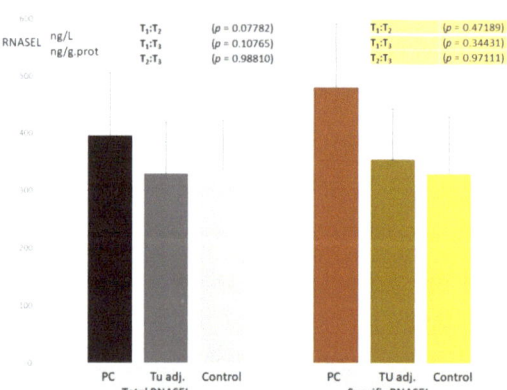

Figure 4. RNASEL total (ng/L) and specific (ng/g.prot) expression level in PC, tumor-adjacent, and control healthy counterparts.

Evaluation of areas under the curves (AUCs) showed that RNASEL specific expression (AUC = 0.64, 95% CI = 0.53–0.74, p = 0.013), (Figure 5) predicted PC. However, the predictive ability of RNASEL was only modest. After determining the optimal cutoff values by Youden's index, we calculated the sensitivity and specificity, which were 40.5% and 86.9%, respectively.

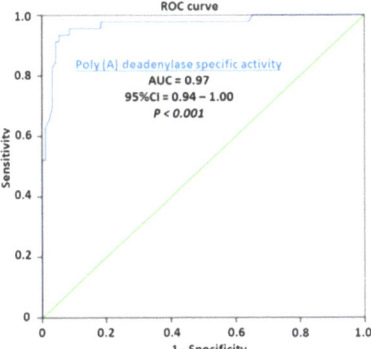

Figure 5. Receiver operating characteristic curve showing the performance of RNASEL-specific expression in predicting prostate cancer.

The on–off switch negative correlation was reported between RNASEL in carcinoma specimens and healthy tissue, since high activity in healthy tissue was followed by a fall in carcinoma tissue, and vice versa (Figure 6), where the correlation coefficient was −0.5.

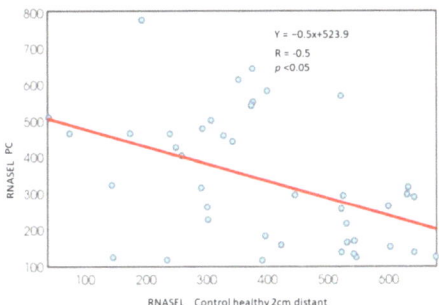

Figure 6. RNASEL correlation between values in PC and corresponding control specimens of healthy tissue.

In monitoring the type of inflammation as the confounding condition for the RNASEL expression profile, the RNASEL was stratified according to the type of inflammation (predominantly chronic lymphocyte infiltration, macrophage/neutrophil infiltration, or the absence of inflammatory cells). Although lymphocytic infiltration tended to be associated with higher RNASEL, it was statistically significant only in control specimens, compared to macrophage/neutrophil infiltration or the absence of inflammatory cells (Figure 7).

The pie charts in Figure 5 explore the percentage influence of lymphocyte infiltration, macrophage/neutrophil infiltration, or the absence of inflammatory cells in different tissue specimens. By analyzing the tissue slices, it seems important to note that only 37% of control samples showed marked inflammation, which decreased in tumor-adjacent tissue to 30% but moderately increased in PC specimens to 54%.

Examples of tissue histopathological findings in the above-mentioned specimens are documented in Figure 8.

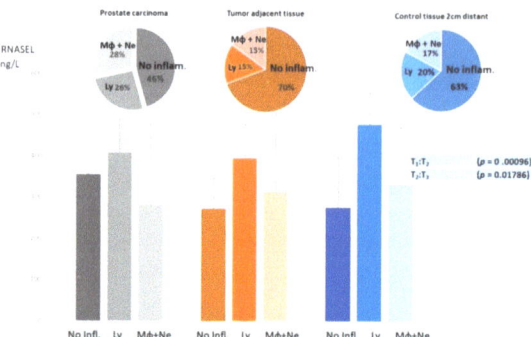

Figure 7. RNASEL in PC, tumor-adjacent and corresponding healthy tissues in relation to the presence and the type of inflammation.

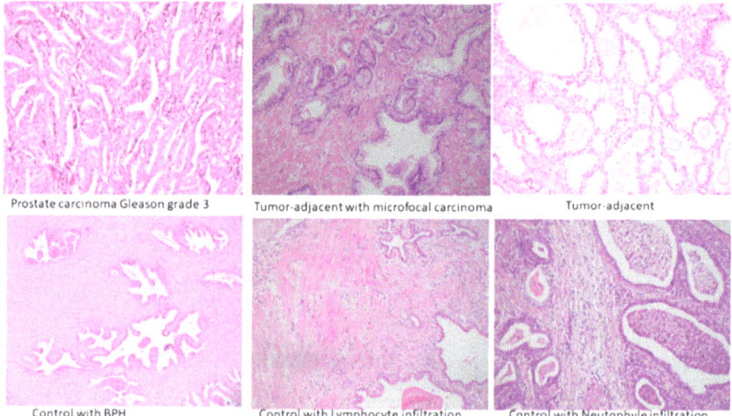

Figure 8. Histological findings of PC, tumor-adjacent tissue with microfocal carcinoma, tumor-adjacent, and control healthy tissue specimens.

4. Discussion

In our study, the Poly(A) deadenylase and RNASEL were determined in PC tissue, adjacent surgically healthy tissue, and in corresponding healthy counterparts, at least 2 cm from carcinoma. The increase in poly(A) deadenylase-specific activity ranged from two to ten times, followed by a more-than twofold increase in its activity in adjacent carcinoma tissue, compared to the control healthy tissue counterparts (Figure 1). The preliminary results obtained may consider Poly(A) deadenylase as a potential surrogate marker for transition of hypertrophic tissue into malignant one, so it is worth paying attention to sensitivity and specificity as well as to cutoff value in a larger series of samples.

From the first understanding of PC development and progression, there has been a tendency to define and establish an ideal or at least an early tumor marker, which would have a key or profound impact on pathogenesis of prostate cancer, early diagnosis, and possible management [1,2]. To define a reliable prostate tumor marker, the National Institute of Standards and Technology (NIST), the American Cancer Society National Prostate Cancer Detection Project, and other relevant associations tried to define criteria for clinical and laboratory prostate tumor marker assessment. According to the biological structure, cancer biomarkers are currently classified as DNA-based, RNA-based, and protein-based. Apart from biochemical structure and cell function, to consider any biomarker for practical clinical use, it should have high diagnostic specificity for detection and for monitoring the stage and prognosis; to be reliable in clinical intervention, recurrence, and survival;

to be easily measurable in biological fluids (plasma, urine);and to be inexpensive. So far, more than fifty biologically active molecules have been identified with more or less proper significance in cancer development, staging, and reaction to therapy and overall survival. To promote one biomolecule as a potential biomarker, the first step is laboratory validation of the method and correlation of clinical significance with standard biomarkers. As routine diagnostic tests for PC development and progression, a prostate-specific antigen (PSA) test and digital rectal examination (DRE) [33,34] are proposed. In the current literature, we did not find any report about Poly(A) deadenylase activity in PC cells at the time this article was prepared. The results obtained about a manifold increase in cancer tissue and in tumor-adjacent tissue may propose Poly(A) deadenylase as a new and potential tumor marker for PC and a possible diagnostic marker for the transition from normal prostate tissue to cancer growth (Figure 1). To evaluate the possible predictive ability of Poly(A) deadenylase-specific activity for identifying PC, the receiver operation curves (ROC) and the Youden index determined the optimal cutoff value. We found that Poly(A) deadenylase identified PC with a sensitivity of 93.5% and a specificity of 94.6% with no overlapping values (Figure 2). Gene reprogramming in cancer occurs through differential expression of cancer-related genes, which leads to differential quantity of specific proteins in cancer tissue. The difference obtained between inhibitory bound and free enzyme activity in PC specimens and control samples may highlight a significant protein reprogramming pattern in prostate carcinoma owing to Poly(A) deadenylase, responsible for at least 50% of its expression (Figure 3).

The active mRNA transcript synthesis occurs through the final structuring of the proper poly(A) tail length. The proper poly(A) tail allows nuclear processing of mRNA and translation initiation after binding to poly(A)-binding protein (PABP). From the other side, the shorter 3′UTR poly(A) tail may diminish the posttranscriptional gene regulation, because they are targets for translational inhibition and mRNA destabilization, assembling into RNA-induced silencing complex (RISC). The rapid deadenylation process may represent a defense system against an aberrant or "unfavorable" mRNAs persistence, which have been found in cancerous tissue [12,13]. Experimental knockout of poly(A) deadenylase gene in a culture of gastric cancer cells resulted in the cell-cycle arrest of G0/G1 phase, followed by the accumulation of p21 tumor suppressor protein [35]. A high expression pattern of Poly(A) deadenylase has been documented in acute leukemias [36]. With regard to specific families, two main families of poly(A) deadenylases were isolated: the DEED types and the exonuclease–endonuclease–phosphatases (EEP) types. The Poly(A)-specific ribonuclease (PARN), POP2 endonuclease, CAF1Z and PAN2 members belong to the DEED family, while CCR4, Nocturinin, ANGEL and 2′ phosphodiesterase (2′PDE) belong to the EEP family [37–40]. Recently, only PARN has been proposed as a potential target of experimental cancer treatment [41]. Transcriptomic analysis of Poly(A) deadenylase expression in squamous cell lung carcinoma referred only PARN and Nocturnin(NOC) type of Poly(A) deadenylase family, significantly over-expressed, with a significant prognostic value in specific subtypes [42]. In this way, Poly(A) deadenylase may represent an integrative part of the cell cycle and survival control checkpoint in tumorigenesis. Aberrant synthesis of many functional "checkpoint" proteins necessary for cell proliferation, together with the synthesis of mutant forms of tumor suppressor proteins, has been documented in cancer pathogenesis [43]. In highlighting the specific role of Poly (A)-specific ribonucleases in reproductive tissues, a specific function in male spermatogenesis, female oogenesis, and fertility was documented [44,45]. Mice with the loss of PARN-regulatory protein (Cnot7-knockout mice), besides compromised deadenylation, suffer from sterility because of oligo-astheno-teratozoospermia and defective maturation of spermatids [46]. These data may point to the crucial importance of the poly(A) tail deadenylation regulation in the reproductive system and prostatic gland function.

In our study, the dissociation of Poly(A)deadenylase-inhibitor complex indicated that the main part (59.16%) of Poly(A) deadenylase in control healthy tissue seemed to be latent: the inhibitor-bound. Since the total activity of enzyme in PC specimens was

51.6% higher than the total activity in the control tissue, it may be calculated that about 50% of enzyme activity was raised because of genome reprogramming and increased expression in malignant tissue. At the same time, it is important to note that the tumor-adjacent tissue may behave like tissue at the crossroads between healthy and malignant phenotype. The appearance of microfocal carcinoma is followed by gradual liberation of the enzyme from its inhibitor complex (from 35.2 to 5.11% of inhibitor-bound enzyme) but still appears to have no effect on tissue reprogramming (Figure 3). The mechanism of enzyme–inhibitor binding has been documented in detail. RNases may make the noncovalent complexes with its natural protein inhibitor in the cell. The proposed roles of RNase inhibitor are the protection, control, and termination of cellular RNA degradation, hence the name "RNAguard". RNase inhibitor proteins are ubiquitous, meaning that they usually follow RNase localization. Regarding the primary structure of inhibitor, it contains highly repetitive leucine-rich amino acid sequences and about 30 reduced cysteine residues of the 32 available. Regarding the tertiary structure, it is made of α-helix and β-strand. Its tertiary horseshoe-like structure, rich in leucine residues, may allow for the tight equimolar interaction with the enzyme [47,48]. The importance of inhibitors in the germinal organs of men is evidenced in the fact that, besides the brain and liver, the testicular germ cells are very rich in RNase inhibitor [49–52]. Due to a large quantity of reduced cysteine, the RNase inhibitor can be inactivated by SH group-modifying reagents, such as PCMB (p-chloromercuriobenzoate), which induces the dissociation of free enzyme and inactive inhibitor [50]. In our earlier results, we documented the influence of steroid hormones on RNase-inhibitor dissociation [53]. Decreased binding of RNase inhibitor was documented in leukemia [54]. In order to explain the potential mechanism of latent enzyme release from the inhibitory complex in PC, we have considered our recent results in relation to the increased generation of free radicals in prostate carcinogenesis, presumably owing to the increased xanthine oxidase/dehydrogenase ratio [55]. Liberated free radicals may oxidize cysteine SH groups in the protein inhibitor, which play a structural and functional role in inhibitor function. Their oxidation can induce conformational changes of inhibitor and can induce the dissociation of enzyme-inhibitor complex [47]; the oxidation of SH groups is a mechanism of in vitro dissociation of latent (inhibitor-bound) enzyme in order to measure latent enzyme.

The mean values of RNASEL in tumor samples were significantly raised, as shown in Figure 4. Evaluation of areas under the curves (AUCs) showed that RNASEL-specific expression may predict PC, but with a low sensitivity of 40.5% and a specificity of 86.9% (Figure 5). A highly negative correlation in cancer vs. corresponding healthy tissue is documented (Figure 6). The possible reason why RNASEL expression was highly negatively correlated in carcinoma tissue to its normal counterpart may be found in the immune-suppressive properties of RNASEL. Besides viral RNAs, RNASEL may initiate the cleavage of other cellular RNAs, which may promote cell apoptosis [20,24,26,56]. Because of apoptotic properties, RNASEL has been proposed as a tumor-suppressor molecule [57,58]. Immunosuppressive properties as the result of increased RNASEL in cancer tissue may be explained as a possible immune-escaping mechanism of cancer tissue, which stands in opposition to more pronounced inflammation. Inflammation as an epigenetic factor may have an influence on DNA damage or the aberrant expression of cell-cycle control proteins [15–18]. It was documented that the type of infiltrates made of inflammatory, innate immune cells and CD4+ T-lymphocyte, may predict cancer progression. The cells of innate immunity, such as macrophages and immune suppressor cells, may predict prostate cancer progression, while surrounding with adaptive immunity cells may act as tumor suppressive cells [56–58]. RNASEL represents a specific type of "housekeeper enzyme", the key switching anti-infective mechanism activated immediately after viral attack, or interferon-receptor binding, through the short 5'-phosphorylated, 2',5'-linked oligoadenylate, known as the 2-5 oligoadenylate system (2-5A). Once activated by 2-5A, the inactive monomeric RNASEL makes a complex 2-5A/RNASEL system, which is responsible for the cleavage of single-stranded regions of RNA, located near the UpUp or UpAp dinucleotides, or double-stranded RNAs, which are typical viral PAMP molecules (pathogen-associated molecular pattern) [59]. The hypothesis has been corroborated by the specific location of the *RNASEL* gene at the chromosome region 1q25, specifically susceptible to rearrangement in some cancer types. Missense point mutations of *RNASEL* gene resulting in aberrant RNASEL structure (arginine to glutamine substitution at position 462) followed by defective function were documented in some families with hereditary prostate cancer [23–26]. The specific Q variant of RNASEL with an almost threefold lower catalytic activity has been registered in about 13% of patients with carcinoma of the prostate, which may be accounted for by the increased risk of prostate cancer in about 50% in the case of heterozygous mutation, while its appearance in a homozygous form may increase the prostate cancer risk two times. Besides a genetic variant, the epigenetic alteration of RNASEL catalytic activity influenced by different inflammatory or infective agents would not be excluded in prostate cancer [19,21–25]. In our study, the statistical significance was reported in PC specimens only for total RNASEL. In monitoring the type of inflammation as the confounding condition for RNASEL expression profile, the RNASEL was stratified according to the type of inflammation (predominantly chronic lymphocyte infiltration, macrophage/neutrophil infiltration or the absence of inflammatory cells). Although lymphocytic infiltration tended to be associated with higher RNASEL, it was statistically significant only in control specimens, compared to macrophage/neutrophil infiltration or the absence of inflammatory cells (Figure 7). The percentage contribution and profile of immune cells infiltration is also shown in Figure 7 in the pie charts. Only 37% of control samples showed marked inflammation, which decreased in tumor-adjacent tissue by 30% but moderately increased in PC specimens by 54%. By comparing the type of immune cells (macrophage, lymphocyte, neutrophil ratio), RNASEL was significantly expressed only in control healthy specimens associated with lymphocyte infiltration.

The study performed has some limitations, the main being a limited number of samples. However, even on the presented number of samples, the consistent conclusions, with regard to sensitivity, specificity, positive predictive value (PPV), negative predictive value (NPV), false-negative rate, and cutoff values, for Poly(A) deadenylase will be drawn. The analysis of enzyme activity in plasma and urine and in liquid biopsies will answer whether there would be any interest for possible noninvasive diagnostic utility and screening.

5. Conclusions

In conclusion, significantly upregulated Poly(A) deadenylase activity in PC tissue and tumor-adjacent tissue associated with microfocal carcinoma highlighted it as a promising RNA–protein bypass biomarker of prostate cancer development. RNASEL may predict lymphocyte infiltration and chronic inflammation of the prostate.

Author Contributions: G.K.: conceptualization, original article preparation; J.H.-D.: supervision of PC cancer patients and biobank validation; A.V.: biochemical methods validation; L.J.-V.: pathohistological diagnostics of PC; S.R.: article proofreading and editing and preparation of statistical analyses; A.Š.: checking analytical methods, final supervision and final text editing. All authors have read and agreed to the published version of the manuscript.

Funding: This work is financed by Science Fund of the Republic of Serbia (IDEAS), project number: 7750154 (NPATPETTMPCB).

Institutional Review Board Statement: The study was conducted in accordance with the Declaration of Helsinki and approved by Ethics Committee of Medical Faculty University of Nis (N12-8818-2/18) approved by Ethical Committee on 29 September 2020 for studies involving humans.

Informed Consent Statement: Informed consent was obtained from all subjects involved in the study.

Data Availability Statement: All data are available in the personal files of BIOBANK patients and results, completed according to the project "IDEAS" needs.

Acknowledgments: The authors are grateful to Basic D for offering PC tissue specimens. The authors are also grateful to Serbian Academy of Science (Branch Nis) for promotion and advancement of our research by current internal projects: O-06-17 (Coordinator M. Colic) and O-28-22 (Coordinator J. Hadzi-Djokic).

Conflicts of Interest: The authors declare no conflict of interest.

References

1. Siegel, R.L.; Miller, K.D.; Jemal, A. Cancer statistics. *CA Cancer J. Clin.* **2016**, *66*, 7–30. [CrossRef] [PubMed]
2. Serrano, N.A.; Anscher, M.S. Favorable vs. Unfavorable Intermediate-Risk Prostate Cancer: A Review of the New Classification System and Its Impact on Treatment Recommendations. *Oncology* **2016**, *30*, 229–236. [PubMed]
3. Kretschmer, A.; Tilki, D. Biomarkers in prostate cancer—Current clinical utility and future perspectives. *Crit. Rev. Oncol. Hematol.* **2017**, *120*, 180–193. [CrossRef] [PubMed]
4. Cox, P.M.; Goding, C.R. Transcription and cancer. *Br. J. Cancer* **1991**, *63*, 651–662. [CrossRef]
5. Garneau, N.L.; Wilusz, J.; Wilusz, C.J. The highways and byways of mRNA decay. *Nat. Rev. Mol. Cell Biol.* **2007**, *8*, 113–126. [CrossRef]
6. Parker, R.; Song, H. The enzymes and control of eukaryotic mRNA turnover. *Nat. Struct. Mol. Biol.* **2004**, *11*, 121–127. [CrossRef]
7. Chen, C.Y.; Shyu, A.B. Mechanisms of deadenylation-dependent decay. *Wiley Interdiscip. Rev. RNA* **2011**, *2*, 167–183. [CrossRef]
8. Goldstrohm, A.C.; Wickens, M. Multifunctional deadenylase complexes diversify mRNA control. *Nat. Rev. Mol. Cell Biol.* **2008**, *9*, 337–344. [CrossRef]
9. Arafat, M.; Sperling, R.A. Quality Control Mechanism of Splice Site Selection Abrogated under Stress and in Cancer. *Cancers* **2022**, *14*, 1750. [CrossRef]
10. Lejeune, F. Nonsense-mediated mRNA decay at the crossroads of many cellular pathways. *BMB Rep.* **2017**, *50*, 175–185. [CrossRef]
11. Sandberg, R.; Neilson, J.R.; Sarma, A.; Sharp, P.A.; Burge, C.B. Proliferating cells express mRNAs with shortened 3′ untranslated regions and fewer microRNA target sites. *Science* **2008**, *320*, 1643–1647. [CrossRef] [PubMed]
12. Morris, A.R.; Bos, A.; Diosdado, B.; Rooijers, K.; Elkon, R.; Bolijn, A.S.; Carvalho, B.; Meijer, G.A.; Agami, R. Alternative cleavage and polyadenylation during colorectal cancer development. *Clin. Cancer Res.* **2012**, *18*, 5256–5266. [CrossRef] [PubMed]
13. Mayr, C.; Bartel, D.P. Widespread shortening of 3′ UTRs by alternative cleavage and polyadenylation activates oncogenes in cancer cells. *Cell* **2009**, *138*, 673–684. [CrossRef] [PubMed]
14. Davis, R.; Shi, Y. The polyadenylation code: A unified model for the regulation of mRNA alternative polyadenylation. *J. Zhejiang Univ. Sci. B* **2014**, *15*, 429–437. [CrossRef] [PubMed]
15. Sciarra, A.; Gentilucci, A.; Salciccia, S.; Pierella, F.; Del Bianco, F.; Gentile, V.; Silvestri, I.; Cattarino, S. Prognostic value of inflammation in prostate cancer progression and response to therapeutic: A critical review. *J. Inflamm.* **2016**, *13*, 35. [CrossRef]
16. Gandaglia, G.; Briganti, A.; Gontero, P.; Mondaini, N.; Novara, G.; Salonia, A.; Sciarra, A.; Montorsi, F. The role of chronic prostatic inflammation in the pathogenesis and progression of benign prostatic hyperplasia. *BJU Int.* **2013**, *112*, 432–441. [CrossRef]
17. Wang, S.; Ji, Y.; Chen, Y.; Du, P.; Cao, Y.; Yang, X.; Ma, J.; Yu, Z.; Yang, Y. The Values of Systemic Immune-Inflammation Index and Neutrophil-Lymphocyte Ratio in the Localized Prostate Cancer and Benign Prostate Hyperplasia: A Retrospective Clinical Study. *Front. Oncol.* **2022**, *11*, 812319. [CrossRef]
18. Mughees, M.; Kaushal, J.B.; Sharma, G.; Wajid, S.; Batra, S.K.; Siddiqui, J.A. Chemokines and Cytokines: Axis and Allies in Prostate Cancer Pathogenesis. *Semin. Cancer Biol.* **2022**. [CrossRef]
19. Silverman, R.H. Implications for RNase L in prostate cancer biology. *Biochemistry* **2003**, *42*, 1805–1812. [CrossRef]
20. Silverman, R.H. A scientific journey through the 2-5A/RNase L system. *Cytokine Growth Factor Rev.* **2007**, *18*, 381–388. [CrossRef]
21. Casey, G.; Neville, P.J.; Plummer, S.J.; Xiang, Y.; Krumroy, L.M.; Klein, E.A.; Catalona, W.J.; Nupponen, N.; Carpten, J.D.; Trent, J.M.; et al. RNASEL Arg462Gln variant is implicated in up to 13% of prostate cancer cases. *Nat. Genet.* **2002**, *32*, 581–583. [CrossRef] [PubMed]
22. Rokman, A.; Ikonen, T.; Seppala, E.H.; Nupponen, N.; Autio, V.; Mononen, N.; Bailey-Wilson, J.; Trent, J.; Carpten, J.; Matikainen, M.P.; et al. Germline alterations of the RNASEL gene, a candidate HPC1 gene at 1q25, in patients and families with prostate cancer. *Am. J. Hum. Genet.* **2002**, *70*, 1299–1304. [CrossRef] [PubMed]
23. Wiklund, F.; Jonsson, B.A.; Brookes, A.J.; Stromqvist, L.; Adolfsson, J.; Emanuelsson, M.; Adami, H.O.; Augustsson-Balter, K.; Gronberg, H. Genetic analysis of the RNASEL gene in hereditary, familial, and sporadic prostate cancer. *Clin. Cancer Res.* **2004**, *10*, 7150–7156. [CrossRef]
24. Maier, C.; Haeusler, J.; Herkommer, K.; Vesovic, Z.; Hoegel, J.; Vogel, W.; Paiss, T. Mutation screening and association study of RNASEL as a prostate cancer susceptibility gene. *Br. J. Cancer* **2005**, *92*, 1159–1164. [CrossRef]
25. Xia, J.; Sun, R. Evidence from 40 Studies that 2 Common Single-Nucleotide Polymorphisms (SNPs) of RNASEL Gene Affect Prostate Cancer Susceptibility: A Preferred Reporting Items for Systematic Reviews and Meta-Analyses (PRISMA)-Compliant Meta-Analysis. *Med. Sci. Monit.* **2019**, *25*, 8315–8325. [CrossRef] [PubMed]
26. Xiang, Y.; Wang, Z.; Murakami, J.; Plummer, S.; Klein, E.A.; Carpten, J.D.; Trent, J.M.; Isaacs, W.B.; Casey, G.; Silverman, R.H. Effects of RNase L mutations associated with prostate cancer on apoptosis induced by 2′,5′-oligoadenylates. *Cancer Res.* **2003**, *63*, 6795–6801. [PubMed]

27. Kocic, G.; Bjelakovic, G.; Pavlovic, D.; Jevtovic, T.; Pavlovic, V.; Sokolovic, D.; Basic, J.; Cekic, S.; Cvetkovic, T.; Kocic, R.; et al. Protective effect of interferon-alpha on the DNA- and RNA-degrading pathway in anti-Fas-antibody induced apoptosis. *Hepatol. Res.* **2007**, *37*, 637–646. [CrossRef]
28. Kocic, G.; Veljkovic, A.; Kocic, H.; Colic, M.; Mihajlovic, D.; Tomovic, K.; Stojanovic, S.; Smelcerovic, A. Depurinized milk downregulates rat thymus MyD88/Akt/p38 function, NF-κB-mediated inflammation, caspase-1 activity but not the endonuclease pathway:in vitro/in vivo study. *Sci. Rep.* **2017**, *7*, 41971. [CrossRef]
29. Kocic, G.; Pavlovic, R.; Nikolic, G.; Veljkovic, A.; Panseri, S.; Chiesa, L.M.; Andjelkovic, T.; Jevtovic-Stoimenov, T.; Sokolovic, D.; Cvetkovic, T.; et al. Effect of commercial or depurinized milk on rat liver growth-regulatory kinases, nuclear factor-kappa B, and endonuclease in experimental hyperuricemia: Comparison with allopurinol therapy. *J. Dairy Sci.* **2014**, *97*, 4029–4042. [CrossRef]
30. Dickson, K.A.; Haigis, M.C.; Raines, R.T. Ribonuclease inhibitor: Structure and function. *Prog. Nucleic Acid Res. Mol. Biol.* **2005**, *80*, 349–374.
31. Cho, S.W.; Joshi, J.G. Ribonuclease inhibitor from pig brain: Purification, characterization, and direct spectrophotometric assay. *Anal. Biochem.* **1989**, *176*, 175–179. [CrossRef]
32. Lowry, O.H.; Rosenbrough, N.J.; Farr, A.J.; Randall, R.J. Protein measurement with the pholin phenol reagent. *J. Biol. Chem.* **1951**, *193*, 265–275. [CrossRef]
33. Hartwell, L.; Mankoff, D.; Paulovich, A.; Ramsey, S.; Swisher, E.M. Cancer biomarkers: A systems approach. *Nat. Biotechnol.* **2006**, *24*, 905–908. [CrossRef] [PubMed]
34. Madu, C.O.; Lu, Y. Novel diagnostic biomarkers for prostate cancer. *J. Cancer* **2010**, *1*, 150–177. [CrossRef] [PubMed]
35. Zhang, L.N.; Yan, Y.B. Depletion of poly(A)-specific ribonuclease (PARN) inhibits proliferation of human gastric cancer cells by blocking cell cycle progression. *Biochim. Biophys. Acta* **2015**, *1853*, 522–534. [CrossRef] [PubMed]
36. Maragozidis, P.; Karangeli, M.; Labrou, M.; Dimoulou, G.; Papaspyrou, K.; Salataj, E.; Pournaras, S.; Matsouka, P.; Gourgoulianis, K.I.; Balatsos, N. Alterations of deadenylase expression in acute leukemias: Evidence for poly(a)-specific ribonuclease as a potential biomarker. *Acta Haematol.* **2012**, *128*, 39–46. [CrossRef]
37. Pavlopoulou, A.; Vlachakis, D.; Balatsos, N.A.; Kossida, S. A comprehensive phylogenetic analysis of deadenylases. *Evol. Bioinform. Online* **2013**, *9*, 491–497. [CrossRef]
38. Virtanen, A.; Henriksson, N.; Nilsson, P.; Nissbeck, M. Poly(A)-specific ribonuclease (PARN): An allosterically regulated, processive and mRNA cap-interacting deadenylase. *Crit. Rev. Biochem. Mol. Biol.* **2013**, *48*, 192–209. [CrossRef]
39. Godwin, A.R.; Kojima, S.; Green, C.B.; Wilusz, J. Kiss your tail goodbye: The role of PARN, Nocturnin, and Angel deadenylases in mRNA biology. *Biochim. Biophys. Acta* **2013**, *1829*, 571–579. [CrossRef]
40. Balatsos, N.A.; Maragozidis, P.; Anastasakis, D.; Stathopoulos, C. Modulation of poly(A)-specific ribonuclease (PARN): Current knowledge and perspectives. *Curr. Med. Chem.* **2012**, *19*, 4838–4849. [CrossRef]
41. Balatsos, N.A.; Nilsson, P.; Mazza, C.; Cusack, S.; Virtanen, A. Inhibition of mRNA deadenylation by the nuclear cap binding complex (CBC). *J. Biol. Chem.* **2006**, *281*, 4517–4522. [CrossRef] [PubMed]
42. Maragozidis, P.; Papanastasi, E.; Scutelnic, D.; Totomi, A.; Kokkori, I.; Zarogiannis, S.G.; Kerenidi, T.; Gourgoulianis, K.I.; Balatsos, N.A.A. Poly(A)-specific ribonuclease and Nocturnin in squamous cell lung cancer: Prognostic value and impact on gene expression. *Mol. Cancer* **2015**, *14*, 187. [CrossRef] [PubMed]
43. Pandolfi, P.P. Aberrant mRNA translation in cancer pathogenesis: An old concept revisited comes finally of age. *Oncogene* **2004**, *23*, 3134–3137. [CrossRef] [PubMed]
44. Morris, J.Z.; Hong, A.; Lilly, M.A.; Lehmann, R. Twin, a CCR4 homolog, regulates cyclin poly(A) tail length to permit Drosophila oogenesis. *Development* **2005**, *132*, 1165–1174. [CrossRef]
45. Berthet, C.; Morera, A.-M.; Asensio, M.-J.; Chauvin, M.-A.; Morel, A.-P.; Dijoud, F.; Magaud, J.-P.; Durand, P.; Rouault, J.-P. CCR4-associated factor CAF1 is an essential factor for spermatogenesis. *Mol. Cell. Biol.* **2004**, *24*, 5808–5820. [CrossRef]
46. Nakamura, T.; Yao, R.; Ogawa, T.; Suzuki, T.; Ito, C.; Tsunekawa, N.; Inoue, K.; Ajima, R.; Miyasaka, T.; Yoshida, Y.; et al. Oligo-astheno-teratozoospermia in mice lacking CNOT7, a regulator of retinoid X receptor β. *Nat. Genet.* **2004**, *36*, 528–533. [CrossRef]
47. Fominaya, J.M.; Hofsteenge, J. Inactivation of ribonuclease inhibitor by thiol–disulfide exchange. *J. Biol. Chem.* **1992**, *267*, 24655–24660. [CrossRef]
48. Hofsteenge, J.; Kieffer, B.; Matthies, R.; Hemmings, B.A.; Stone, S.R. Amino acid sequence of the ribonuclease inhibitor from porcine liver reveals the presence of leucine-rich repeats. *Biochemistry* **1988**, *27*, 8537–8544. [CrossRef]
49. Nadano, D.; Yasuda, T.; Takeshita, H.; Uchide, K.; Kishi, K. Purification and characterization of human brain ribonuclease inhibitor. *Arch. Biochem. Biophys.* **1994**, *312*, 421–428. [CrossRef]
50. Futami, J.; Tsushima, Y.; Murato, Y.; Tada, H.; Sasaki, J.; Seno, M.; Yamada, H. Tissue-specific expression of pancreatic-type RNases and RNase inhibitor in humans. *DNA Cell Biol.* **1997**, *16*, 413–419. [CrossRef]
51. Burton, L.E.; Fucci, N.P. Ribonuclease inhibitors from the liver of five mammalian species. *Int. J. Pept. Protein Res.* **1982**, *19*, 372–379. [CrossRef] [PubMed]
52. Ferreras, M.; Gavilanes, J.G.; Lopez-Otin, C.; Garcia-Segura, J.M. Thiol–disulfide exchange of ribonuclease inhibitor bound to ribonuclease A. Evidence of active inhibitor-bound ribonuclease. *J. Biol. Chem.* **1995**, *270*, 28570–28578. [CrossRef] [PubMed]
53. Bjelakovic, G.; Pavlovic, D.; Nikolic, J.; Kocic, G.; Stankovic, B.; Bjelakovic, B. Effect of pyridoxine on the alkaline ribonuclease activity in the liver of dexamethasone treated rats. *Facta Univ. Ser. Med. Biol.* **1997**, *4*, 17–20.

54. Kraft, N.; Shortman, K. The phylogeny of the ribonuclease-ribonuclease inhibitor system: Its distribution in tissues and its response during leukaemogenesis and aging. *Aust. J. Biol. Sci.* **1970**, *23*, 175–184. [CrossRef] [PubMed]
55. Veljković, A.; Hadži-Dokić, J.; Sokolović, D.; Bašić, D.; Veličković-Janković, L.; Stojanović, M.; Popović, D.; Kocić, G. Xanthine Oxidase/Dehydrogenase Activity as a Source of Oxidative Stress in Prostate Cancer Tissue. *Diagnostics* **2020**, *10*, 668. [CrossRef] [PubMed]
56. Karan, D.; Dubey, S. From Inflammation to Prostate Cancer: The Role of inflammasomes. *Adv. Urol.* **2016**, *2016*, 3140372. [CrossRef] [PubMed]
57. Ammirante, M.; Luo, J.L.; Grivennikov, S.; Nedospasov, S.; Karin, M. B-cell-derived lymphotoxin promotes castration-resistant prostate cancer. *Nature* **2010**, *464*, 302–305. [CrossRef] [PubMed]
58. Gurel, B.; Lucia, M.S.; Thompson, I.M.; Goodman, P.J., Jr.; Tangen, C.M.; Kristal, A.R.; Parnes, H.L.; Hoque, A.; Lippman, S.M.; Sutcliffe, S.; et al. Chronic inflammation in benign prostate tissue is associated with high-grade prostate cancer in the placebo arm of the prostate cancer prevention trial. *Cancer Epidemiol. Biomark. Prev.* **2014**, *23*, 847–856. [CrossRef]
59. Carpten, J.; Nupponen, N.; Isaacs, S.; Sood, R.; Robbins, C.; Xu, J.; Faruque, M.; Moses, T.; Ewing, C.; Gillanders, E.; et al. Germline mutations in the ribonuclease L gene in families showing linkage with HPC1. *Nat. Genet.* **2002**, *30*, 181–184. [CrossRef]

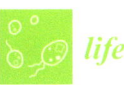 life

Article

SBRT for Localized Prostate Cancer: CyberKnife vs. VMAT-FFF, a Dosimetric Study

Marcello Serra [1,*], Fortuna De Martino [2], Federica Savino [3], Valentina d'Alesio [1], Cecilia Arrichiello [1], Maria Quarto [2], Filomena Loffredo [2], Rossella Di Franco [1], Valentina Borzillo [1], Matteo Muto [4], Gianluca Ametrano [1] and Paolo Muto [1]

[1] Istituto Nazionale Tumori—IRCCS—Fondazione G. Pascale, 80131 Napoli, Italy; valentina.dalesio@istitutotumori.na.it (V.d.); c.arrichiello@istitutotumori.na.it (C.A.); r.difranco@istitutotumori.na.it (R.D.F.); v.borzillo@istitutotumori.na.it (V.B.); gianluca.ametrano@istitutotumori.na.it (G.A.); p.muto@istitutotumori.na.it (P.M.)
[2] Dipartimento di Scienze Biomediche Avanzate, Università degli Studi di Napoli Federico II, 80131 Napoli, Italy; fo.demartino@studenti.unina.it (F.D.M.); maria.quarto@unina.it (M.Q.); filomena.loffredo@unina.it (F.L.)
[3] LB Business Services SRL, 00168 Rome, Italy; savino.federica@gmail.com
[4] Division of Radiotherapy, "S. G. Moscati" Hospital, 83100 Avellino, Italy; matteo.muto@aornmoscati.it
* Correspondence: marcello.serra@istitutotumori.na.it

Abstract: In recent years, stereotactic body radiation therapy (SBRT) has gained popularity among clinical methods for the treatment of medium and low risk prostate cancer (PCa), mainly as an alternative to surgery. The hypo-fractionated regimen allows the administration of high doses of radiation in a small number of fractions; such a fractionation is possible by exploiting the different intrinsic prostate radiosensitivity compared with the surrounding healthy tissues. In addition, SBRT treatment guaranteed a better quality of life compared with surgery, avoiding risks, aftermaths, and possible complications. At present, most stereotactic prostate treatments are performed with the CyberKnife (CK) system, which is an accelerator exclusively dedicated for stereotaxis and it is not widely spread in every radiotherapy centre like a classic linear accelerator (LINAC). To be fair, a stereotactic treatment is achievable also by using a LINAC through Volumetric Modulated Arc Therapy (VMAT), but some precautions must be taken. The aim of this work is to carry out a dosimetric comparison between these two methodologies. In order to pursue such a goal, two groups of patients were selected at Instituto Nazionale Tumori—IRCCS Fondazione G. Pascale: the first group consisting of ten patients previously treated with a SBRT performed with CK; the second one was composed of ten patients who received a hypo-fractionated VMAT treatment and replanned in VMAT-SBRT flattening filter free mode (FFF). The two SBRT techniques were rescaled at the same target coverage and compared by normal tissue sparing, dose distribution parameters and delivery time. All organs at risk (OAR) constraints were achieved by both platforms. CK exhibits higher performances in terms of dose delivery; nevertheless, the general satisfying dosimetric results and the significantly shorter delivery time make VMAT-FFF an attractive and reasonable alternative SBRT technique for the treatment of localized prostate cancer.

Keywords: SBRT; hypofractionation; CyberKnife; VMAT; flattening filter free; prostate cancer

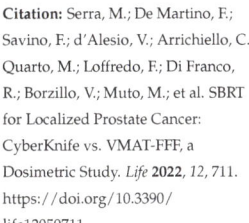

Citation: Serra, M.; De Martino, F.; Savino, F.; d'Alesio, V.; Arrichiello, C.; Quarto, M.; Loffredo, F.; Di Franco, R.; Borzillo, V.; Muto, M.; et al. SBRT for Localized Prostate Cancer: CyberKnife vs. VMAT-FFF, a Dosimetric Study. *Life* 2022, 12, 711. https://doi.org/10.3390/life12050711

Academic Editor: Ana Faustino, Paula A. Oliveira and Lúcio Lara Santos

Received: 31 March 2022
Accepted: 5 May 2022
Published: 10 May 2022

Publisher's Note: MDPI stays neutral with regard to jurisdictional claims in published maps and institutional affiliations.

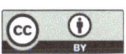

Copyright: © 2022 by the authors. Licensee MDPI, Basel, Switzerland. This article is an open access article distributed under the terms and conditions of the Creative Commons Attribution (CC BY) license (https://creativecommons.org/licenses/by/4.0/).

1. Introduction

Prostate cancer (PCa) is a broad disease affecting male population; it is the second most frequent cancer diagnosed in men after the lung cancer, and it is the fifth cause of death in the world. To understand the extent of the problem, worldwide in 2018, about 1,300,000 new cases of PCa were reported (in Italy, about 36,000 new cases in 2020 [1]), and it caused about 7700 deaths [1,2]. Moreover, the risk to be diagnosed with PCa is strictly linked with aging, and the incidence rate varies across the world but it can be resumed as follows: in men under 39 years old, the probability is about 0.005%; between 40 and 59 years old, the probability rises to 2.2%; between 60 and 79 years old, the probability is 14%; and over 80 years old, the incidence is very high, at about 50% [3]. Given the high incidence of the illness and the lengthening of life expectancy, the population affected by this pathology is estimated to increase; indeed, about 2,300,000 new cases are expected up to 2040 [4]. Today, patients with localized disease and detected at early stage at low to intermediate risk of recurrence have a favorable prognosis: 99% overall survival for 10 years. As matter of fact, the localized PCa shows a high patient's life expectancy, a slow progression rate, and limited metastatic potential; therefore, in this class of patient, comorbidities are considered very significant, since the increase of comorbidities with a poor health status, due to the aging, increase the risk of dying from other causes than PCa [5].

When it comes to the fight against cancer, everyone thinks about surgery [6]; however, for PCa, surgery is not the only way to go. Today, we have different therapeutic approaches, and the best choice is based on the tumor risk class, the patient performance status and, no less important, it depends on the patient's preferences and assessment of side effects. Radiotherapy (RT) is especially effective for the PCa treatment due to the considerable difference of the α/β ratio between the tumor and the surrounding Organ at risk (OAR) [7–9] (bladder, rectum, penile bulb and bowel). Such a difference makes it possible to perform hypofractionated treatment. In 2018, international societies such as ASTRO, ASCO and AUA, after deep studies, reported that there are solid grounds to support the use of the hypofractionated regime for treatment of the PCa for the routine clinical practice [10], and they also recommend the Stereotactic body radiation therapy (SBRT) approach for clinical trials in patients with high risk localized PCa [11,12]. A systematic review of studies where a comparison among SBRT, hypofractionated and normofractionated regimes concluded that SBRT achieves the same results of the other treatment modalities in terms of five years disease free survival, but a reduced gastrointestinal and genitourinary toxicity, <15% and 21% respectively [11].

It is very interesting to investigate if rotational approaches, such as VMAT Volumetric modulated arc therapy (VMAT), can potentially deliver a SBRT treatment as good as that of CyberKnife (CK). The aim of this study is to investigate, retrospectively, the use VMAT with 6-FFF MV for the PCa treatments, and to analyse the differences with the CK system, already adopted in our department. The comparison of these two SBRT will be carried out in terms of tumor coverage and OARs spearing, through relative dosimetric parameters, by analysing and comparing plans and the respective Dose volume histogram (DVH) curves, for the purpose of expanding the use of the SBRT as much as possible, even in radiotherapy centres where a CK system is not available.

2. Materials and Methods

2.1. The CyberKnife System

In RT, the platform specifically designed for the SBRT is the CyberKnife (CK, Accuray Inc., Sunnyvale, CA, USA), and indeed due to its peculiarities, promising outcomes have been achieved. These results are confirmed by 8- to 10- year studies, which support the clinical evidence of the successful employment of SBRT for localized PCa [13–15]. The CK is a linear accelerator of 6 MeV energy installed on a robotic arm with six degrees of freedom; therefore, it is characterized by a non-isocentric dose delivery mode. Moreover, it also ships static circular collimators from 5 to 60 mm, or a dynamic IRIS collimator. In particular, the accelerator can be positioned in 100 nodes and, in each of them, it can take up to a maximum of twelve directions: in that way, 1200 different entry beam directions can be reached. By exploiting its considerable mobility and adaptability of the radiation field, high dose conformation level is achieved; furthermore, CK can deliver the 125% of the prescribed dose in the tumor volume, but at the same time achieving significant OARs sparing.

CK must deliver the dose with surgical precision, otherwise undesired volumes and organs can be reached by high doses and the lesion can be severely underdosed; therefore, CK is equipped with an image-guided system, useful both for the correct positioning of the patient and to monitor the movements of the target during the treatment. The image system is composed by two X-ray tubes stuck to the ceiling by 90° to each other and tilted with respect the patient's axis by 45°; X-ray tubes are correlated to a pair of silicon detectors (flat panel) placed in the floor, next to the treatment bed. The nominal tube voltage is 40 keV–15 MeV. The patient is imaged every 45 s, or at most 60 s, and the live images are digitized and compared to images synthesized from the patient's CT data (digitally reconstructed radiograph (DRR)). This technique allows for determination of intra-fraction target shifts and automatic compensation by the treatment manipulator during treatment delivery. These automatic corrections are achievable for a maximum excursion range: X, Y and Z direction ± 10 mm, pitch, roll and yaw ±5°, ±1°, ±3°, respectively. For shifts greater than these intervals, the treatment is interrupted, and an operator repositions the patient [16].

In order to locate the tumor, in our case the prostate, and to check if its position changes during the treatment, some golden fiducials (usually four) are implanted in the prostate wall; the reconstruction of the prostate position by means of such markers allows adjustments of the accelerator real-time with respect to the target [17–19]. For the sake of completeness, in RT, when an accelerator is supported by an image system, the technology is called image guided radiotherapy (IGRT), and the use of accurate image guidance is crucial to minimize setup errors and facilitate the margins reduction between the gross tumor volume (GTV) and the Planning target volume (PTV), especially for SBRT.

2.2. SBRT-VMAT and FFF Delivery Mode

A SBRT treatment is also achievable by using a state-of-the-art LINAC guided by a software conceived for the VMAT. VMAT combines the intensity modulation of the radiant field with its shape adaptability through a multi-lamellar collimator (MLC). The dose is delivered continuously during the gantry rotation along one or more arcs without interruptions and, over the treatment, the dose rate varies as well. These features allow a dose distribution to be reached that is extremely compliant to the target volume with a greater sparing of normal tissue than static 3D-CRT.

Due to the advent of systems for positioning verification and the movement monitoring of organs and anatomical volumes of interest, it is possible to achieve better safety in the administration of ultra-hypo-fractionated regimens, and therefore it is possible to develop real stereotaxic treatments also with the VMAT technique.

The LINAC used in this work is the Elekta Versa HD; it has photon energy of 6, 10, and 15 MeV, but for the VMAT treatment, just 6 MeV energy is enabled. The maximum field size for a treatment is (40×40) cm^2, defined by a pair of fixed collimators, that can rotate independently of the gantry, mounted orthogonally to the MLC. The MLC consists of 80 pairs of tungsten blades of a projected width of 5 mm at the isocentre, and a small interleaf space less than 0.1 mm. As noted above, in order to perform a SBRT treatment, an IGRT system is required; indeed, in our case, the accelerator is equipped with an ultrasound guidance system released for VMAT treatment: the Clarity System [20] (Elekta, Stockholm, Sweden). It consists of a transperineal ultrasound (not ionizing radiation) probe, which allows real-time prostate visualization during the treatment, and which can stop if the prostate makes too large excursions with respect to the planning Computed tomography (CT). The Clarity System reconstructs a 3D image starting from 2D ultrasound acquisitions. To obtain images, the probe needs to be moved, but during the treatment the radiotherapist is not in the treatment room; therefore, the probe performs automatic scans with a motorized control of the sweeping motion. The probe can scan a complete 75° sweep in 0.5 s. Patients do not feel any discomfort other than a slight vibration, as all motion is internal to the probe housing. Moreover, the probe has an integrated sensor which triggers when it passes through the center. Every sweep is checked for geometrical accuracy [21].

Therefore, such a probe allows a more efficient verification of the position of the tumor and critical structures; indeed, the employment of this technique shows a significant reduction in matching errors compared to standard treatments [20,21]. We want to highlight that this continuous monitoring does not imply a higher dose administration to the patient, since we are dealing with ultrasound images and no additional device needs to be implanted in the patient's prostate [22].

In order to compute and deliver a therapeutic plan which reaches inside the tumor volume, a dose higher than the prescribed dose with a very steep dose gradient, the accelerator must operate in FFF mode; that is, in the absence of the homogenizer filter. The beam emerging from the primary collimator is extremely spiked, due to the greater probability of production of bremsstrahlung photons for small angles with respect to the direction of motion of the incident electron. The result is a non-homogeneous beam, with a maximum of intensity in the centre and a decreasing intensity at the sides. The use of the filter reshapes the beam profile, attenuating it in its central region and widening it by diffusion, thus giving it an almost flat structure. The beam is also hardened since the filter removes most of the low-energy photons by attenuation. On the contrary, when operating in FFF mode, the radiation beam appears narrower and more intense in the central part, which is useful to better conform the dose distribution to the target. Furthermore, the presence of the soft component of the beam leads to an increase in the dose-rate and the consequent reduction in treatment delivery times. This situation helps to minimize the effects of movement of the target and is particularly advantageous in stereotaxic therapies where extremely high doses are delivered and accuracy in the delivery of treatment is of crucial importance.

In general, the beam-on time tends to be longer in SBRT, since higher doses per fraction are prescribed; as a result, the prostate position can change during the treatment, due to rectal activity, bladder filling, muscle clenching and general pelvic motion. As matter of fact, while setting and performing RT, it is important to be able to predict the occurrence and the extent of the prostate movement to establish appropriate planning target volume (PTV) margins, avoiding a missing target. Nevertheless, FFF beams, which have higher dose rates, decrease the treatment time per fraction; therefore, the faster delivery makes the treatment patient-friendly and improves treatment accuracy by preserving the treatment plan quality [23,24], by reducing the intra-fractional motion.

One of the most important aspects of the SBRT is the conical dose distribution with a maximum value that can reach the 125% of the prescribed dose, located near the geometric centre of the target, and a sudden decrease outside the target. Traditional radiotherapy treatments, on the other hand, require a uniform dose on the target, that cannot exceed the 110% of the prescribed dose; small hot spots can sometimes be accepted. From these conceptual differences, it can be derived that the typical dose–volume histogram (DVH) structure of a traditional VMAT treatment is very different to a stereotaxic one. Indeed, in the first case, DVH looks like a step function extending from 0 Gy to the prescription dose value. In a stereotaxic plane, the decreasing part of the graph has a gentler slope, and the maximum dose can reach 125% of the prescribed dose. Such high dose values at the target have precise clinical implications, as they could offer a special advantage in the eradication of radio-resistant hypoxic cells.

To obtain the typical SBRT dose distribution with the VMAT treatment modality, some tricks had to be adopted in the planning process. For each patient, an auxiliary fictitious structure was delineated at the centre of PTV, and the parameters of suited cost functions were given appropriate values. In the inverse planning, these dodges have forced the optimization algorithm to reshape the dose distribution in order to resemble the typical DVH appearance of a stereotaxis treatment (Figure 1).

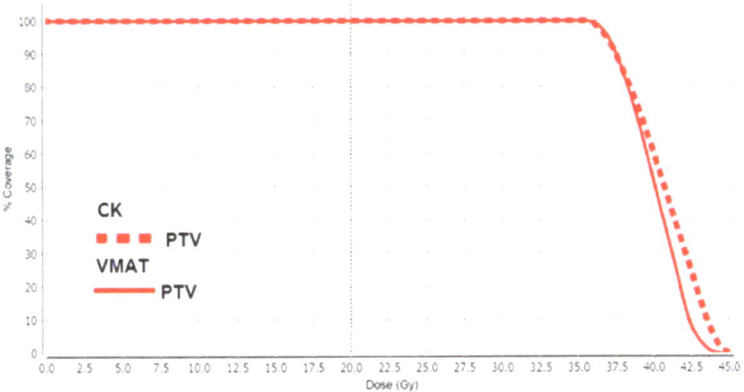

Figure 1. The Planning target volume (PTV) Dose volume histogram (DVH) for the CyberKnife (CK) (dotted line) and Volumetric modulated arc therapy (VMAT)-Flattening Filter Free (FFF) (solid line) techniques. With the specific measures adopted in the planning phase, the VMAT curve looks very similar to the CK one.

2.3. The Dosimetric Study: Patient Selection, Contouring and Planning

Since the two platforms involved in the study have an inherently different way of delivering the dose, and a different IGRT system which can affect the anatomical configuration of the organs, to have a truly representative dosimetric study, we compared patients who were imaged and have received CK treatment with patients who were imaged and received treatment with the VMAT by using the Clarity system. Of course, for the VMAT patients, the therapeutic plans were re-computed in accordance with the ultra hypofractionated prescription: 36.25 Gy in five fractions. At this point, it could be argued that the best or worst results achieved with CK or with SBRT-VMAT would not be directly comparable since they could depend on specific patient anatomical characteristics. Therefore, in order to reduce and smooth such patient's differences, groups of patients were selected, and dosimetric results are expressed as average values.

For sake of completeness, in our institute as actual clinical practice, the patients selected for SBRT with CK satisfy the following settings: age > 18 years; PCa diagnosed with transperineal core biopsy; low risk class (T2a or lower, Prostate Specific Antigen (PSA) $\leq$ 10 ng/mL and Gleason Grade (GG) = 1); intermediate risk class (T2b-2c, PSA $\leq$ 20 ng/mL and GG = 2); prostate volume < 80 cc; uninvolved prostate capsule (documented by prostate multiparametric Magnetic Resonance Imaging (MRI)); performance status: 0–1; TC total body with contrast enhancement bone scintigraphy negative for metastasis (Table 1).

Two groups of patients with a localized PCa, each of them composed of 10 patients treated in Instituto Nazionale Tumori—IRCCS Fondazione G. Pascale in the period between 2016 and 2019, were selected. The first group (Table 1), that from here on it will be named the "CK Group", consisting of ten patients of, on average, 69 years old and having an average prostatic volume of 66 cc, were treated with SBRT realized by the CK system with a dose prescription of 36.25 Gy to the PTV in five fractions. The second one, named the "Clarity Group" (Table 1), comprising of, on average, 76-year-old patients with an average prostatic volume of 44 cc. They were treated with a hypo fractionated VMAT delivered by an Elekta Versa HD matched with the Clarity ultrasound probe, with a dose prescription of 35 Gy to the PTV in five fractions. By taking advantage of the CT scans with the Clarity probe in position, they have been replanned with an optimized template developed for prostate VMAT-SBRT in FFF mode with the same dose prescription and fractionation scheduled for the CK Group.

Table 1. Summarized clinical and demographic characteristics of the population involved in this study.

Patient	Age	Total PSA	Target Volume (cc)	Gleason Score (GS)	Clinical Stage
1 (CK)	72	5.63	51.06	1	1c
2 (CK)	72	10.84	85.82	1	1c
3 (CK)	65	16.6	62.26	1	2b
4 (CK)	70	6.3	44.08	2	2a
5 (CK)	65	7.32	36.48	1	1b
6 (CK)	76	8.63	86.90	1	2a
7 (CK)	63	4	47.08	2	2a
8 (CK)	62	4.5	80.12	2	2b
9 (CK)	72	5.5	66.36	1	2a
10 (CK)	73	7.6	72.35	2	2a
1 (VMAT-FFF)	78	7.29	37.75	2	1c
2 (VMAT-FFF)	78	4.37	31.10	2	2b
3 (VMAT-FFF)	77	10.69	30.78	2	2b
4 (VMAT-FFF)	81	8.71	33	2	
5 (VMAT-FFF)	76	9.6	68.17	1	2b
6 (VMAT-FFF)	78	7.22	36.28	1	2b
7 (VMAT-FFF)	72	12	53.91	1	1c
8 (VMAT-FFF)	72	6.21	44.55	1	2b
9 (VMAT-FFF)	78	11	23.74	2	2b
10 (VMAT-FFF)	70	6.76	79.75	1	2a

Regarding volumes contouring, in both groups, the GTV was defined as prostate without margin, the CTV was set equal to GTV, and the PTV was CTV with 3 mm expansion posteriorly and 5 mm in other directions. The rectum, rectal wall, bladder, bladder wall, bowel, penis bulb and femoral heads were delineated and classified as OARs. The rectal and bladder walls were contoured through a Boolean subtraction between the organ itself and its own contractions, respectively, of 3 mm and 5 mm.

For the IGRT system of the CK Group, four gold fiducials markers have been implanted on prostate surface 7/10 days before CT images acquisition. For Clarity Group patients, the ultrasound probe Clarity was used as a volume monitoring device, and CT images were acquired with the probe in position, compressing perineal region.

The CK treatment planning was performed using the precision inverse treatment planning system (Accuray Inc., Sunnyvale, CA, USA), and the prescription dose was 36.25 Gy at 80% isodose line delivered in five fractions, with a beam energy of 6 MeV, with the dynamic IRIS collimator. The OARs constraints used for planning were $V_{37.5\,Gy} < 5$ cm^3 for the bladder and $V_{36.25\,Gy} < 5\%$ for the rectum, and three concentric shells were used for dose conformation to PTV. VMAT-SBRT treatment plans were computed with Elekta Monaco TPS and the treatments geometrical setup was: 2 arcs of 360° (clockwise and counterclockwise) with a 10° collimator tilt angle and final gantry spacing 3°; in both arches, there was a 0° couch kick. VMAT plans were computed for an Elekta VERSA HD accelerator (Elekta, Crowley, UK) equipped with 6 MeV photon beam in FFF mode and MLC with 5 mm leaf.

In both cases, the dose distribution was renormalized as a 95% prescription dose, covering 95% of the PTV.

3. Statistical Analysis

The VMAT-FFF therapeutic plans were computed by experienced medical physicists, and after, DVHs curves were extracted and analysed with Microsoft Excel. In Table 2, the dose received by a specified volume percentage and the volume that received a certain amount of dose of the respective ROI are presented. Table 3 reports the mean duration of treatment and the parameters characterizing the dose distribution: the homogeneity indexes (HI), the conformality index (CI), and the gradient index (GI).

Table 2. The table summarizes the most significant values of the DVH curves achieved by the two techniques.

	Parameter	CK	VMAT	p-Value
Bladder	D_{MAX} (Gy)	39 ± 2	41 ± 2	0.1
	$D_{1\,CC}$ (Gy)	37 ± 2	38 ± 1	0.05
	$V_{37.5\,Gy} < 5\,cm^3$	1 ± 2	3 ± 2	0.1
	$V_{37\,Gy} < 10\,cm^3$	2 ± 2	4 ± 2	0.2
	$V_{36.25\,Gy} < 10\%$	2 ± 2	3 ± 1	0.2
	$V_{18.125\,Gy} < 40\%$	37 ± 12	35 ± 10	0.7
	$V_{5\,Gy}$ (%)	92 ± 11	68 ± 22	0.02
	$V_{10\,Gy}$ (%)	76 ± 18	57 ± 21	0.06
	$V_{20\,Gy}$ (%)	32 ± 11	30 ± 9	0.7
Bladder wall	D_{MAX} (Gy)	40 ± 2	41 ± 1	0.3
	$D_{10\,cm^3}$ (Gy)	32 ± 3	33 ± 2	0.5
Rectum	D_{MAX} Gy	37 ± 2	37 ± 1	0.3
	$V_{36.25\,Gy} < 5\,cm^3$	0.2 ± 0.3	0.5 ± 0.7	0.1
	$V_{36\,Gy} < 1\,cm^3$	0.1 ± 0.2	0.5 ± 0.6	0.07
	$V_{32.625\,Gy} < 10\%$	4 ± 2	4 ± 3	0.5
	$V_{29\,Gy} < 20\%$	10 ± 4	9 ± 4	0.7
	$V_{18.125\,Gy} < 50\%$	35 ± 8	37 ± 9	0.7
	$V_{5\,Gy}$ (%)	88 ± 12	87 ± 10	0.9
	$V_{10\,Gy}$ (%)	67 ± 15	79 ± 10	0.09
	$V_{20\,Gy}$ (%)	29 ± 7	28 ± 8	0.8
Rectal wall	D_{MAX} (Gy)	37 ± 2	37 ± 2	0.9
Bowel	$V_{30\,Gy} < 1\,cm^3$	1 ± 2	0.02 ± 0.05	0.1
	D_{MAX} (Gy)	24 ± 10	13 ± 11	0.09
	$V_{10\,Gy}$ (%)	4 ± 4	0.2 ± 0.2	0.03
	$V_{20\,Gy}$ (%)	0.3 ± 0.5	0.02 ± 0.05	0.1
LFH	$V_{14.5\,Gy} < 5\%$	1 ± 2	1 ± 2	0.8
	D_{MAX} (Gy)	15 ± 3	14 ± 2	0.5
RFH	$V_{14.5\,Gy} < 5\%$	1 ± 3	0.2 ± 0.5	0.3
	D_{MAX} (Gy)	15 ± 3	13 ± 2	0.3
Penis bulb	$V_{29.5\,Gy} < 50\%$	1 ± 3	13 ± 18	0.08
	$V_{10\,Gy}$ (%)	28 ± 30	62 ± 30	0.04
	$V_{20\,Gy} < 90\%$	8 ± 10	34 ± 30	0.03

Table 3. The conformity index, the homogeneity index, the gradient index and the beam on time for the two SBRT methods are reported.

Parameter	CK	VMAT	p-Value
CI	1.09 ± 0.04	1.01 ± 0.02	0.0006
HI	1.24 ± 0.03	1.2 ± 0.02	0.01
GI_{25}	24 ± 8	22 ± 3	0.01
GI_{50}	5 ± 1	5 ± 1	0.6
GI_{75}	2.7 ± 0.5	2.5 ± 0.2	0.2
Treatment Time (min)	47 ± 9	3 ± 1	≪0.05

Usually, HI deals with the degree of uniformity of dose distribution within target; nevertheless, stereotaxic treatments, by definition, produce an inhomogeneous dose distribution in the target, so in the statistical analysis we referred to a homogeneity index definition that could quantify the dose peak height within the PTV.

For the evaluation of this parameter, we referred to the following equation:

$$HI = \frac{D_{MAX}}{R_{XDose}} \quad (1)$$

D_{MAX} is the maximum dose value at the PTV, and R_{XDose} is the prescription dose value. Theoretically speaking, this value could be 1 in the case of perfect homogeneity, but in our case, we are aware that in an SBRT treatment it is expected to be higher than 1.

CI deals with the degree of compliance of the dose distribution with the target volume; it is defined as the ratio of total volume of tissue treated with a prescription dose over the volume of the tumor treated with the prescription dose:

$$CI = \frac{PIV}{TIV} \quad (2)$$

PIV is the prescription isodose volume (total 3D volume of the isodose line), and TIV is the tumor isodose volume (tumor volume covered by the prescription isodose volume). From a mathematical point of view, CI should be 1 if the prescription dose volume covers the tumor volume perfectly; therefore, a CI closer to 1 is desirable. GI allows to quantify the steepness of the dose fall-off in a stereotaxic treatment. It is defined as the ratio between the volume of a reference isodose and the volume of the prescription isodose:

$$HI = \frac{D_{MAX}}{R_{XDose}} \quad (3)$$

The lower the GI value, the more the considered isodose will adhere to that relating to 100% of the prescribed dose, and the steeper the dose falls outside the target.

4. Results

To give an overview about the treatments, the most relevant constraints used in ultra hypo-fractionated radiotherapy for PCa, and also the values reached by using the two aforementioned technologies, are shown. For OARs, the maximum dose and the most significant values extracted from the DVH curves, the CI, HI and GI indices, and the beam-on time have been reported. They are listed in Tables 2 and 3. In general, from the data analysis emerges a substantial equivalence between the techniques; both of them comply with dose constraints and lead to comparable doses delivered to OARs.

The values in the table indicate that for the bladder: D_{1cc} is the dose absorbed by 1 cc of volume, $V_{37.5}$ and V_{37} are the volumes receiving a dose of 37.5 Gy and 37 Gy, $V_{36.25}$ and $V_{18.125}$ are the volumes receiving the 100% or the 50% of prescription dose, whereas V_5, V_{10} and V_{20} are the volumes receiving 5 Gy, 10 Gy and 20 Gy, respectively. For the rectum, the bladder wall, bowel, penis bulb, left femoral head (LFH) and right femoral head (RFH), listed in the Table 2 as well, different values of dose and volumes are reported, but the indices have the same significance exposed before for the bladder case.

Regarding the bladder, we can assert that both the maximum dose and the reference constraints values are comparable and consistent according to the two-tailed test. The same holds true for the volume of the isodose curves relative to the 20 Gy and 10 Gy dose values. The only significant difference is highlighted at low doses: the VMAT technique shows a greater bladder sparing, which can be displayed by the volume surrounded 5 Gy isoline. The bladder wall takes a comparable dose in the two techniques; instead, the discrepancy between dose values is not significant.

Regarding the rectum and the rectal wall, all values relating to dose and volume constraints are comparable and consistent according to the t-test. Additionally, for the bowel, VMAT shows better organ sparing at low doses, as evidenced by the $V_{10\,Gy}$ isosurface.

Regarding the penis bulb, in the VMAT technique, a larger dose is absorbed, and such a difference becomes more and more appreciable at low doses.

No substantial difference was highlighted for the femoral heads, which for both techniques are well below the dose constraints.

Finally, by looking at Table 3, regarding dose distribution descriptive parameters, a better dose conformation to PTV is evidenced for VMAT as demonstrated by CI values. As expected, the typical conical dose distribution of stereotaxis is more pronounced in the CK case, as can be deduced from HI values. About GI values, they are all comparable, and the discrepancies are not statistically significant (p-value > 0.05). From this, it can be deduced that the trend of the dose gradient outside the PTV is very similar in the two techniques. Regarding the duration of the treatment, the VMAT-FFF allows a much higher dose rate than the CK, enabling a shorter beam-on time.

5. Discussion

As evidenced by the epidemiologic data, PCa is a common disease related to aging with an increasing number of cases projected into the future. RT is carving out more and more space in the fight against the PCa due to its lower invasiveness with respect to surgery. In low risk PCa, exclusive radiotherapy and radical prostatectomy are equivalent and show similar clinical outcomes (overall survival and quality of life) [25]. In the RT field, the gold standard is 2 Gy per fraction, whereas hypofractionation enables higher doses to be reached in fewer sessions. In other words, the α/β for prostate is very low (about 1.5 Gy) if compared to the OARs; therefore, it allows the maximization of the therapeutic effect, and at the same time reduces side effects on OARs as much as possible [26–29], increasing the therapeutic window, i.e., the distance between the tumor control probability (TCP) curve and normal tissue complication probability (NTCP) curve [27]. The evolution of radiotherapy knowledge, and the fast technology improvement, that led to high precision treatments guided by real-time imaging, have allowed the consideration that the SBRT is a promising treatment for this disease. The SBRT is an extremization of the hypofractionated regime, with very few sessions and very high doses; indeed, nowadays, SBRT using a five-fraction schedule appears to be an effective treatment for low- and intermediate- risk PCa in terms of efficacy, safety, patient's quality of life and side effects, as established by the literature [30–33]. As pointed out by other works, the SBRT in an ultra hypofractionated regime is very effective in terms of overall survival and quality of life; indeed, the recent HYPO-RT-PC study provided evidence that 42.7 Gy delivered in seven sessions every other day (6.1 Gy per fraction) has comparable outcomes to standard conventional fractionation of 78 Gy in 2 Gy per fraction [11]. That is, the same result is achieved in fewer sessions, resulting in less stress for the patient and reduced costs for the hospital. Other studies with long term follow up and a large cohort of patients recommend prescription doses between 35 Gy and 36.25 Gy in five fractions [34]. Some authors indicate that patients with low- and intermediate risk disease treated with 31.7 Gy in five fractions and 36.1 Gy in five fractions achieved tumor control probabilities of 90% and 95%, respectively, at five years follow up [35]. Nevertheless, a schedule of 40 Gy in five fractions has shown higher toxicity with respect to the previous radiotherapy programs [36]. In addition, if some works look at a short time window after the treatment time, such results corroborate the idea that the dose escalation could increase the effectiveness of the RT for the PCa, as long as an EQD2 < 100 Gy1.5 is delivered. Furthermore, studies are still in progress to validate the use of even higher doses for high-risk PCa.

SBRT treatment is typically delivered by using a CK, and in the current context its usage is increasing, but technological improvements allowed they delivery of SBRT treatments with isocentric technique, such as VMAT and helical tomotherapy (HT). There is a wide range of literature about comparisons among rotational techniques and CK bringing extremely encouraging outcomes and resulting in a general agreement among different data [37–42]. The SBRT delivered by VMAT is a viable option, and the main differences found in such works are due to the PTV coverage and the margins expansion from the CTV to the PTV. These two points are essential because rotational techniques are routinely used to reach a PTV homogeneous coverage (the perfect PTV-DVH curve could be a step function); however, in a CK-like SBRT, 125% of the prescription dose is deposited in the inner parts of the tumor. If in VMAT and HT no tumor tracking system is used, a wider PTV contouring should be drawn. Hence, even if the two techniques show comparable OARs, sparing the dose in tumor could be significantly lower in VMAT/HT cases with respect to CK ones, and such differences could have important radiobiological consequences; on the other hand, to reach the highest CK doses, if no unsuitable contouring is drawn, dangerous dose spilling is expected. Among rotational techniques for the SBRT, one of the latest developments is the MRI-Linac; it is a Linac equipped with a MRI scanner. Due to the peculiarity of the MRI images to contrast better soft tissues, such technology can deliver high doses with high accuracy. Results reported in the literature show that SBRT treatments supported by MRI images can achieve significant OARs sparing [43,44]. As for some works summarized before, a comparison with our results is not directly practicable, as in MRI-Linac based studies it is accepted that, at most, 107% of the prescription dose reaches the PTV; whereas, in our analysis, we are reaching doses higher than 120% in order to simulate a CyberKnife-like treatment. Nevertheless, even if in this work and MRI-Linac studies the selected constraints for the bladder and rectum are different (but similar), comparable results are reached between the exhibited techniques.

Therefore, to have a significant comparison among the VMAT and CK treatments, we computed VMAT plans in FFF mode in order to obtain the conical dose escalation contemplated by CK, and such plans were worked out on TC with the IGRT system in position so that the same geometrical rules for the PTV delineation could be applied in both cases.

From the results listed in Table 2, the most important discrepancies can be outlined for the bladder and bowel, at low doses; probably such differences could be due to the dose delivery modalities of the two techniques: the freedom of movement of the non-isocentric CK approach implies beam directions coming from a solid angle intercepting larger OARs volume before reaching the prostate with respect to a well delimited strip dose typical of rotational techniques. Such different dose structures may involve the production of low dose spikes that fall extensively within the bowel and bladder volume. It is worth noting that also in previous works there were similar dose structures, with the more interesting differences reached at the lowest or intermediate doses; this should further confirm the idea that the delivering dose modality could also play an important role in the acute and late toxicity.

The other clear disagreement can be found in the penis bulb dose distribution. It can be easily ascribed to the use of the Clarity probe for VMAT IGRT. During the treatment, the ultrasound probe is positioned close to the perineal region, compressing the penis bulb; this arrangement involves an anatomical deformation which brings the penis bulb closer to the prostate, and hence the probe determines a greater absorbed dose to the bulb.

At last, but not the least, the most important difference in the beam is time: VMAT treatments are much faster. This is very important because the time reduction results in greater patient comfort, the natural and uncontrollable organ movements are reduced during the treatment time, and as consequence, a clinical centre could dramatically shorten its waiting list.

We want to highlight that these results are based on small groups of patients (ten for each technique); therefore, to have a more robust statistical significance, the number of patients involved in the dosimetric study should be enlarged. Moreover, in this study, the prostate is not the exclusive target, but in some cases, the PTV is composed of prostate and seminal vesicles. For the sake of completeness, this mix of targets is present in both groups of patients (CK Group and Clarity Group). A further analysis, having at disposal a larger dataset, could be carried out by dividing the low risk PCa patients into two subgroups, in order to analyze if such subdivision can have repercussions on the performance of the two techniques. Finally, none of the patients involved in the study had comorbidities detectable in the TC images, such as diverticula, hernias, etc., which could have influenced the planning process.

6. Conclusions

The authors, with this publication, state that SBRT VMAT-FFF is a noteworthy technique which might substitute, in some cases, the CK. Our data show that VMAT-FFF with the Clarity system could be used for the hypofractionated treatment of PCa with good clinical results and while respecting the recommended constrains. Therefore, the ultra hypofractionated regime, and more generally the SBRT, with its important clinical and managerial implications, might be spread also in smaller radiotherapy centers where a CK is not available.

Author Contributions: Conceptualization, M.S., G.A., F.D.M., R.D.F., V.B., M.M. and P.M.; methodology, M.S., G.A., F.D.M. and C.A.; software, F.D.M., F.S. and V.d.; validation, M.S., G.A., F.D.M., V.d., R.D.F., V.B., M.M. and P.M.; formal analysis, M.S., G.A., F.D.M. and F.S.; investigation, M.S., G.A., F.D.M., V.B. and R.D.F.; resources, V.B., R.D.F., M.M. and P.M.; data curation, M.S., G.A., F.D.M., C.A. and F.L.; writing—original draft preparation, M.S. and F.D.M.; writing—review and editing, M.S., G.A., F.D.M., F.S., C.A., V.d., M.Q., F.L., R.D.F., V.B., M.M. and P.M.; supervision, M.Q. and P.M.; project administration, M.Q. and P.M. All authors have read and agreed to the published version of the manuscript.

Funding: This research received no external funding.

Institutional Review Board Statement: This study is part of the Cypro Trial, approved by the Ethics committee of the National Cancer Institute—G. Pascale Foundation—Naples, Protocol Version 1.0; 27 January 2020. Decision n 105.

Informed Consent Statement: Informed consent for the treatment was obtained from all subjects involved in the study.

Data Availability Statement: In this study we do not use raw data that can be used by other researchers. We elaborated treatment plans by using different approaches.

Conflicts of Interest: The authors declare no conflict of interest.

References

1. AIOM. *I Numeri del Cancro in Italia, 2021*; AIOM Associazione Italiana di Oncologia Medica: Milano, Italy, 2021.
2. Leslie, S.W.; Soon-Sutton, T.L.; Sajjad, H.; Siref, L.E. *Prostate Cancer*; Stat Pearls Publishing: Treasure Island, FL, USA, 2022.
3. Stangelberger, A.; Waldert, M.; Djavan, B. Prostate Cancer in Elderly Men. *Rev. Urol.* **2008**, *10*, 111–119. [PubMed]
4. Rawla, P. Epidemiology of Prostate Cancer. *World J. Oncol.* **2019**, *10*, 63–89. [CrossRef] [PubMed]
5. Rebello, R.J.; Oing, C.; Knudsen, K.E.; Loeb, S.; Johnson, D.C.; Reiter, R.E.; Gillessen, S.; Van der Kwast, T.; Bristow, R.G. Prostate cancer. *Nat. Rev. Dis. Prim.* **2021**, *7*, 9. [CrossRef] [PubMed]
6. Lam, T.B.; MacLennan, S.; Willemse, P.-P.M.; Mason, M.D.; Plass, K.; Shepherd, R.; Baanders, R.; Bangma, C.H.; Bjartell, A.; Bossi, A.; et al. Prostate Cancer Guideline Panel Consensus Statements for Deferred Treatment with Curative Intent for Localised Prostate Cancer from an International Collaborative Study (DETECTIVE Study). *Eur. Urol.* **2019**, *76*, 790–813. [CrossRef]
7. Proust-Lima, C.; Taylor, J.M.; Sécher, S.; Sandler, H.; Kestin, L.; Pickles, T.; Williams, S. Confirmation of a low a/b ratio for prostate cancer treated by external beam radiation therapy alone using a post-treatment repeated measures model for PSA dynamics. *Int. J. Radiat. Oncol. Biol. Phys.* **2010**, *79*, 195e201. [CrossRef]
8. Williams, S.G.; Taylor, J.M.; Liu, N.; Tra, Y.; Duchesne, G.M.; Kestin, L.L.; Sandler, H. Use of individual fraction size data from 3756 patients to directly determine the a/b ratio of prostate cancer. *Int. J. Radiat. Oncol. Biol. Phys.* **2007**, *68*, 24e33. [CrossRef]
9. Cho, L.C.; Timmerman, R.; Kavanagh, B. Hypofractionated External-Beam Radiotherapy for Prostate Cancer. *Prostate Cancer* **2013**, *2013*, 103547. [CrossRef]
10. Morgan, S.C.; Hoffman, K.; Loblaw, D.A.; Buyyounouski, M.K.; Patton, C.; Barocas, D.; Sandler, H. Hypofractionated Radiation Therapy for Localized Prostate Cancer: Executive Summary of an ASTRO, ASCO, and AUA Evidence-Based Guideline. *Pract. Radiat. Oncol.* **2018**, *8*, 354–360. [CrossRef]
11. Fransson, P.; Nilsson, P.; Gunnlaugsson, A.; Beckman, L.; Tavelin, B.; Norman, D.; Thellenberg-Karlsson, C.; Hoyer, M.; Lagerlund, M.; Kindblom, J.; et al. Ultra-hypofractionated versus conventionally fractionated radiotherapy for prostate cancer (HYPO-RT-PC): Patient-reported quality-of-life outcomes of a randomised, controlled, non-inferiority, phase 3 trial. *Lancet Oncol.* **2021**, *22*, 235–245. [CrossRef]
12. Brand, D.H.; Tree, A.C.; Ostler, P.; Van Der Voet, H.; Loblaw, A.; Chu, W.; Ford, D.; Tolan, S.; Jain, S.; Martin, A.; et al. Intensity-modulated fractionated radiotherapy versus stereotactic body radiotherapy for prostate cancer (PACE-B): Acute toxicity findings from an international, randomised, open-label, phase 3, non-inferiority trial. *Lancet Oncol.* **2019**, *20*, 1531–1543. [CrossRef]
13. Wolf, F.; Sedlmayer, F.; Aebersold, D.; Albrecht, C.; Böhmer, D.; Flentje, M.; Ganswindt, U.; Ghadjar, P.; Höcht, S.; Hölscher, T.; et al. Ultrahypofractionation of localized prostate cancer: Statement from the DEGRO working group prostate cancer. *Strahlentherapie Onkologie* **2020**, *197*, 89–96. [CrossRef] [PubMed]
14. Lehrer, E.J.; Kishan, A.U.; Yu, J.B.; Trifiletti, D.M.; Showalter, T.N.; Ellis, R.; Zaorsky, N.G. Ultrahypofractionated versus hypofractionated and conventionally fractionated radiation therapy for localized prostate cancer: A systematic review and meta-analysis of phase III randomized trials. *Radiother. Oncol.* **2020**, *148*, 235–242. [CrossRef] [PubMed]

15. Bijina, T.K.; Ganesh, K.M.; Pichandi, A.; Muthuselvi, C.A. Cyberknife, Helical Tomotherapy and Rapid Arc SIB-SBRT Treatment Plan Comparison for Carcinoma Prostate. *Asian Pac. J. Cancer Prev.* **2020**, *21*, 1149–1154. [CrossRef]
16. Brochure Equipment Specifications—CyberKnife. Available online: http://www.cyberknifelatin.com/pdf/brochure-tecnico.pdf (accessed on 30 March 2022).
17. Di Franco, R.; Borzillo, V.; Alberti, D.; Ametrano, G.; Petito, A.; Coppolaro, A.; Tarantino, I.; Rossetti, S.; Pignata, S.; Iovane, G.; et al. Acute Toxicity in Hypofractionated/Stereotactic Prostate Radiotherapy of Elderly Patients: Use of the Image-guided Radio Therapy (IGRT) Clarity System. *In Vivo* **2021**, *35*, 1849–1856. [CrossRef]
18. Dang, A.; Kupelian, P.A.; Cao, M.; Agazaryan, N.; Kishan, A.U. Image-guided radiotherapy for prostate cancer. *Transl. Androl. Urol.* **2018**, *7*, 308–320. [CrossRef]
19. O'Neill, A.G.M.; Jain, S.; Hounsell, A.R.; O'Sullivan, J.M. Fiducial marker guided prostate radiotherapy: A review. *Br. J. Radiol.* **2016**, *89*, 20160296. [CrossRef]
20. Lachaine, M.; Falco, T. Intrafractional prostate motion management with the clarity autoscan system. *Med. Phys. Int. J.* **2013**, *1*, 72.
21. Grimwood, A.; Rivaz, H.; Zhou, H.; McNair, H.A.; Jakubowski, K.; Bamber, J.C.; Tree, A.C.; Harris, E.J. Improving 3D ultrasound prostate localisation in radiotherapy through increased automation of interfraction matching. *Radiother. Oncol.* **2020**, *149*, 134–141. [CrossRef]
22. Buono, M.; Capussela, T.; Loffredo, F.; Di Pasquale, M.A.; Serra, M.; Quarto, M. Dose-Tracking Software: A Retrospective Analysis of Dosimetric Data in CT Procedures. *Health Phys.* **2022**, *122*, 548–555. [CrossRef]
23. Benedek, H.; Lerner, M.; Nilsson, P.; Knöös, T.; Gunnlaugsson, A.; Ceberg, C. The effect of prostate motion during hypofractionated radiotherapy can be reduced by using flattening filter free beams. *Phys. Imaging Radiat. Oncol.* **2018**, *6*, 66–70. [CrossRef]
24. Scorsetti, M.; Alongi, F.; Clerici, E.; Comito, T.; Fogliata, A.; Iftode, C.; Mancosu, P.; Navarria, P.; Reggiori, G.; Tomatis, S.; et al. Stereotactic body radiotherapy with flattening filter-free beams for prostate cancer: Assessment of patient-reported quality of life. *J. Cancer Res. Clin. Oncol.* **2014**, *140*, 1795–1800. [CrossRef] [PubMed]
25. Buyyounouski, M.K.; Price, R.A.; Harris, E.E.; Miller, R.; Tomé, W.; Schefter, T.; Wallner, P.E. Stereotactic body radiotherapy for primary management of early-stage, low- to intermediate-risk prostate cancer: Report of the American Society for Therapeutic Radiology and Oncology emerging technology committee. *Int. J. Radiat. Oncol. Biol. Phys.* **2010**, *76*, 1297–1304. [CrossRef] [PubMed]
26. Miralbell, R.; Roberts, S.; Zubizarreta, E.; Hendry, J.H. Dose-Fractionation Sensitivity of Prostate Cancer Deduced From Radiotherapy Outcomes of 5,969 Patients in Seven International Institutional Datasets: α/β = 1.4 (0.9–2.2) Gy. *Int. J. Radiat. Oncol. Biol. Phys.* **2012**, *82*, e17–e24. [CrossRef] [PubMed]
27. Nahum, A.E. The radiobiology of hypofractionation. *Clin. Oncol. R. Coll. Radiol.* **2015**, *27*, 260–269. [CrossRef] [PubMed]
28. Fowler, J.F. The radiobiology of prostate cancer including new aspects of fractionated radiotherapy. *Acta Oncol.* **2005**, *44*, 265–276. [CrossRef]
29. Liao, Y.; Joiner, M.; Huang, Y.; Burmeister, J. Hypofractionation: What Does It Mean for Prostate Cancer Treatment? *Int. J. Radiat. Oncol. Biol. Phys.* **2010**, *76*, 260–268. [CrossRef]
30. Hickey, B.E.; James, M.L.; Daly, T.; Soh, F.-Y.; Jeffery, M. Hypofractionation for clinically localized prostate cancer. *Cochrane Database Syst. Rev.* **2019**, *2019*, CD011462. [CrossRef]
31. Kishan, A.U.; Dang, A.; Katz, A.J.; Mantz, C.A.; Collins, S.P.; Aghdam, N.; Chu, F.-I.; Kaplan, I.D.; Appelbaum, L.; Fuller, D.B.; et al. Long-term outcomes of stereotactic body radiotherapy for low-risk and intermediate-risk prostate cancer. *JAMA Netw. Open* **2019**, *2*, e188006. [CrossRef]
32. Tsang, Y.M.; Tharmalingam, H.; Belessiotis-Richards, K.; Armstrong, S.; Ostler, P.; Hughes, R.; Alonzi, R.; Hoskin, P.J. Ultra-hypofractionated radiotherapy for low- and intermediate risk prostate cancer: High-dose-rate brachytherapy vs stereotactic ablative radiotherapy. *Radiother. Oncol.* **2021**, *158*, 184–190. [CrossRef]
33. Kishan, A.U.; King, C.R. Stereotactic Body Radiotherapy for Low- and Intermediate-Risk Prostate Cancer. *Semin. Radiat. Oncol.* **2017**, *27*, 268–278. [CrossRef]
34. Katz, A. Stereotactic Body Radiotherapy for Low-Risk Prostate Cancer: A Ten-Year Analysis. *Cureus* **2019**, *9*, e1668. [CrossRef] [PubMed]
35. Royce, T.J.; Mavroidis, P.; Wang, K.; Falchook, A.D.; Sheets, N.C.; Fuller, D.B.; Collins, S.P.; El Naqa, I.; Song, D.Y.; Ding, G.X.; et al. Tumor control probability modeling and systematic review of the literature of stereotactic body radiation therapy for prostate cancer. *Int. J. Radiat. Oncol. Biol. Phys.* **2020**, *110*, 227–236. [CrossRef] [PubMed]
36. Musunuru, H.B.; Quon, H.; Davidson, M.; Cheung, P.; Zhang, L.; D'Alimonte, L.; DeAbreu, A.; Mamedov, A.; Loblaw, A. Dose-escalation of five-fraction SABR in prostate cancer: Toxicity comparison of two prospective trials. *Radiother. Oncol.* **2016**, *118*, 112–117. [CrossRef] [PubMed]
37. Scobioala, S.; Kittel, C.; Elsayad, K.; Kroeger, K.; Oertel, M.; Samhouri, L.; Haverkamp, U.; Eich, H.T. A treatment planning study comparing IMRT techniques and cyber knife for stereotactic body radiotherapy of low-risk prostate carcinoma. *Radiat. Oncol.* **2019**, *14*, 143. [CrossRef]
38. Serra, M.; Ametrano, G.; Borzillo, V.; Quarto, M.; Muto, M.; Di Franco, R.; Federica, S.; Loffredo, F.; Paolo, M. Dosimetric comparison among cyberknife, helical tomotherapy and VMAT for hypofractionated treatment in localized prostate cancer. *Medicine* **2020**, *99*, e23574. [CrossRef]

39. Chen, C.-Y.; Lee, L.-M.; Yu, H.-W.; Lee, S.P.; Lee, H.-L.; Lin, Y.-W.; Wen, Y.-C.; Chen, Y.-J.; Chen, C.-P.; Tsai, J.-T. Dosimetric and radiobiological comparison of Cyberknife and Tomotherapy in stereotactic body radiotherapy for localized prostate cancer. *J. X-ray Sci. Technol.* **2017**, *25*, 465–477. [CrossRef]
40. Seppälä, J.; Suilamo, S.; Tenhunen, M.; Sailas, L.; Virsunen, H.; Kaleva, E.; Keyriläinen, J. Dosimetric Comparison and Evaluation of 4 Stereotactic Body Radiotherapy Techniques for the Treatment of Prostate Cancer. *Technol. Cancer Res. Treat.* **2017**, *16*, 238–245. [CrossRef]
41. Ślosarek, K.; Osewski, W.; Grządziel, A.; Radwan, M.; Dolla, Ł.; Szlag, M.; Stąpór-Fudzińska, M. Integral dose: Comparison between four techniques for prostate radiotherapy. *Rep. Pr. Oncol. Radiother.* **2014**, *20*, 99–103. [CrossRef]
42. Lin, Y.-W.; Lin, K.-H.; Ho, H.-W.; Lin, H.-M.; Lin, L.-C.; Lee, S.P.; Chui, C.-S. Treatment plan comparison between stereotactic body radiation therapy techniques for prostate cancer: Non-isocentric CyberKnife versus isocentric RapidArc. *Phys. Med.* **2014**, *30*, 654–661. [CrossRef]
43. Alongi, F.; Rigo, M.; Figlia, V.; Cuccia, F.; Giaj-Levra, N.; Nicosia, L.; Ricchetti, F.; Sicignano, G.; De Simone, A.; Naccarato, S.; et al. 1.5 T MR-guided and daily adapted SBRT for prostate cancer: Feasibility, preliminary clinical tolerability, quality of life and patient-reported outcomes during treatment. *Radiat. Oncol.* **2020**, *15*, 69. [CrossRef]
44. Mazzola, R.; Figlia, V.; Rigo, M.; Cuccia, F.; Ricchetti, F.; Giaj-Levra, N.; Nicosia, L.; Vitale, C.; Sicignano, G.; De Simone, A.; et al. Feasibility and safety of 1.5 T MR-guided and daily adapted abdominal-pelvic SBRT for elderly cancer patients: Geriatric assessment tools and preliminary patient-reported outcomes. *J. Cancer Res. Clin. Oncol.* **2020**, *146*, 2379–2397. [CrossRef] [PubMed]

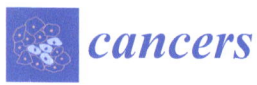 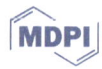

Article

Type 2 Diabetes-Related Variants Influence the Risk of Developing Prostate Cancer: A Population-Based Case-Control Study and Meta-Analysis

José Manuel Sánchez-Maldonado [1,2,3,†], Ricardo Collado [4,†], Antonio José Cabrera-Serrano [1,2,3,†], Rob Ter Horst [5], Fernando Gálvez-Montosa [6], Inmaculada Robles-Fernández [1], Verónica Arenas-Rodríguez [1,7], Blanca Cano-Gutiérrez [7], Olivier Bakker [8], María Inmaculada Bravo-Fernández [4], Francisco José García-Verdejo [6], José Antonio López López [6], Jesús Olivares-Ruiz [4], Miguel Ángel López-Nevot [9], Laura Fernández-Puerta [2], José Manuel Cózar-Olmo [10], Yang Li [5,11], Mihai G. Netea [5,12], Manuel Jurado [1,2,3,13], Jose Antonio Lorente [1,14], Pedro Sánchez-Rovira [6], María Jesús Álvarez-Cubero [1,7] and Juan Sainz [1,2,3,15,*]

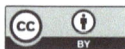

Citation: Sánchez-Maldonado, J.M.; Collado, R.; Cabrera-Serrano, A.J.; Ter Horst, R.; Gálvez-Montosa, F.; Robles-Fernández, I.; Arenas-Rodríguez, V.; Cano-Gutiérrez, B.; Bakker, O.; Bravo-Fernández, M.I.; et al. Type 2 Diabetes-Related Variants Influence the Risk of Developing Prostate Cancer: A Population-Based Case-Control Study and Meta-Analysis. *Cancers* 2022, 14, 2376. https://doi.org/10.3390/cancers14102376

Academic Editors: Paula A. Oliveira, Ana Faustino and Lúcio Lara Santos

Received: 29 March 2022
Accepted: 29 April 2022
Published: 12 May 2022

Publisher's Note: MDPI stays neutral with regard to jurisdictional claims in published maps and institutional affiliations.

Copyright: © 2022 by the authors. Licensee MDPI, Basel, Switzerland. This article is an open access article distributed under the terms and conditions of the Creative Commons Attribution (CC BY) license (https://creativecommons.org/licenses/by/4.0/).

1. Genomic Oncology Area, GENYO, Centre for Genomics and Oncological Research, Pfizer/University of Granada/Andalusian Regional Government, PTS Granada, 18016 Granada, Spain; josemanuel.sanchez@genyo.es (J.M.S.-M.); antonio.cabrera@genyo.es (A.J.C.-S.); inmaculadarobles@gmail.com (I.R.-F.); veronica.arenas@genyo.es (V.A.-R.); manuel.jurado.sspa@juntadeandalucia.es (M.J.); jose.lorente@genyo.es (J.A.L.); mjesusac@ugr.es (M.J.Á.-C.)
2. Hematology Department, Virgen de las Nieves University Hospital, 18012 Granada, Spain; laurafdezpuerta@gmail.com
3. Instituto de Investigación Biosanataria IBs. Granada, 18012 Granada, Spain
4. Medical Oncology Department, Hospital de San Pedro Alcántara, 10003 Cáceres, Spain; ricardo.collado@salud-juntaex.es (R.C.); inmaculada.bravo@salud-juntaex.es (M.I.B.-F.); jesus.olivares@salud-juntaex.es (J.O.-R.)
5. Department of Internal Medicine and Radboud Centre for Infectious Diseases, Radboud University Nijmegen Medical Center, 6525 GA Nijmegen, The Netherlands; rterhorst@cemm.oeaw.ac.at (R.T.H.); yang.li@helmholtz-hzi.de (Y.L.); mihai.netea@radboudumc.nl (M.G.N.)
6. Department of Medical Oncology, Complejo Hospitalario de Jaén, 23007 Jaén, Spain; fernando.galvez.sspa@juntadeandalucia.es (F.G.-M.); francisco.garcia.verdejo.sspa@juntadeandalucia.es (F.J.G.-V.); josea.lopez.l.sspa@juntadeandalucia.es (J.A.L.L.); pedro.sanchez.rovira.sspa@juntadeandalucia.es (P.S.-R.)
7. Department of Biochemistry and Molecular Biology III, Faculty of Medicine, University of Granada, 18016 Granada, Spain; blanca.cano.sspa@juntadeandalucia.es
8. Department of Genetics, University Medical Center Groningen, University of Groningen, 9713 GZ Groningen, The Netherlands; o.b.bakker@umcg.nl
9. Immunology Department, Virgen de las Nieves University Hospital, 18012 Granada, Spain; manevot@ugr.es
10. Urology Department, Virgen de las Nieves University Hospital, 18012 Granada, Spain; josem.cozar.sspa@juntadeandalucia.es
11. Centre for Individualised Infection Medicine (CiiM) & TWINCORE, Joint Ventures between the Helmholtz-Centre for Infection Research (HZI) and the Hannover Medical School (MHH), 30625 Hannover, Germany
12. Department for Immunology & Metabolism, Life and Medical Sciences Institute (LIMES), University of Bonn, 53115 Bonn, Germany
13. Department of Medicine, Faculty of Medicine, University of Granada, 18016 Granada, Spain
14. Department of Legal Medicine, Faculty of Medicine, University of Granada, 18016 Granada, Spain
15. Department of Biochemistry and Molecular Biology I, Faculty of Sciences, University of Granada, 18071 Granada, Spain
* Correspondence: juan.sainz@genyo.es; Tel.: +34-95871-5500 (ext. 126); Fax: +34-9-5863-7071
† These authors contributed equally to this work.

Simple Summary: We investigated the influence of GWAS-identified variants for T2D in modulating prostate cancer (PCa) risk through a meta-analysis of our data with those from the UKBiobank and FinnGEn cohorts and four large European cohorts. We found that genetic variants within the *FTO*, *HNF1B*, and *JAZF1* loci were associated with PCa risk. Our results also suggested, for the first time, a potentially interesting association of SNPs within *NOTCH2* and *RBMS1* genes that need to be further explored and validated. This study also shed some light onto the functional mechanisms behind the observed associations, and demonstrated that the *HNF1B*$_{rs7501939}$ polymorphism correlated with lower levels of SULT1A1, an enzyme responsible for the sulfate conjugation of multiple endogenous and exogenous compounds. Furthermore, we found that SNPs within the *HFN1B*, *NOTCH2*, and *RBMS1* genes impacted PCa risk through the modulation of mRNA gene expression levels of their respective genes. However, given the healthy nature of the subjects included in the cohort used for functional experiments, the link between the *HNF1B* locus and SULT1A1 should be considered still speculative and, therefore, requires further validation.

Abstract: In this study, we have evaluated whether 57 genome-wide association studies (GWAS)-identified common variants for type 2 diabetes (T2D) influence the risk of developing prostate cancer (PCa) in a population of 304 Caucasian PCa patients and 686 controls. The association of selected single nucleotide polymorphisms (SNPs) with the risk of PCa was validated through meta-analysis of our data with those from the UKBiobank and FinnGen cohorts, but also previously published genetic studies. We also evaluated whether T2D SNPs associated with PCa risk could influence host immune responses by analysing their correlation with absolute numbers of 91 blood-derived cell populations and circulating levels of 103 immunological proteins and 7 steroid hormones. We also investigated the correlation of the most interesting SNPs with cytokine levels after in vitro stimulation of whole blood, peripheral mononuclear cells (PBMCs), and monocyte-derived macrophages with LPS, PHA, Pam3Cys, and *Staphylococcus Aureus*. The meta-analysis of our data with those from six large cohorts confirmed that each copy of the $FTO_{rs9939609A}$, $HNF1B_{rs7501939T}$, $HNF1B_{rs757210T}$, $HNF1B_{rs4430796G}$, and $JAZF1_{rs10486567A}$ alleles significantly decreased risk of developing PCa ($p = 3.70 \times 10^{-5}$, $p = 9.39 \times 10^{-54}$, $p = 5.04 \times 10^{-54}$, $p = 1.19 \times 10^{-71}$, and $p = 1.66 \times 10^{-18}$, respectively). Although it was not statistically significant after correction for multiple testing, we also found that the $NOTCH2_{rs10923931T}$ and $RBMS1_{rs7593730}$ SNPs associated with the risk of developing PCa ($p = 8.49 \times 10^{-4}$ and 0.004). Interestingly, we found that the protective effect attributed to the *HFN1B* locus could be mediated by the SULT1A1 protein ($p = 0.00030$), an arylsulfotransferase that catalyzes the sulfate conjugation of many hormones, neurotransmitters, drugs, and xenobiotic compounds. In addition to these results, eQTL analysis revealed that the $HNF1B_{rs7501939}$, $HNF1B_{rs757210}$, $HNF1B_{rs4430796}$, $NOTCH2_{rs10923931}$, and $RBMS1_{rs7593730}$ SNPs influence the risk of PCa through the modulation of mRNA levels of their respective genes in whole blood and/or liver. These results confirm that functional TD2-related variants influence the risk of developing PCa, but also highlight the need of additional experiments to validate our functional results in a tumoral tissue context.

Keywords: prostate cancer; genetic susceptibility; type 2 diabetes-related variants

1. Introduction

Prostate cancer (PCa) is the second most common cancer worldwide and one of the first leading causes of cancer-related deaths in men in developed countries [1]. It accounts for 7.3% of all cancers, with an incidence of 37.5 per 100,000 individuals [2]. Despite the refinements in prevention strategies, a total of 1.4 million new cases were diagnosed in 2020 [2], and the incidence of the disease is increasing over the world, likely due to the interaction of both inherited and modifiable factors [3,4].

Although PCa has a high prevalence among males, only age, family history, and ethnicity have been established as major risk factors for the disease, with an attributable effect ranging from 5 to 9% of the cases [5]. In addition, rare highly penetrant mutations in specific genes, high levels of endogenous androgens, smoking, alcohol consumption, exposure to chemical compounds, sexually transmitted infections, diet, obesity, insulin-like growth factors, and type 2-diabetes (T2D) have been suggested as important modulators of the prostatic tumorigenesis [6]. Among the modifiable risk factors, T2D has attracted significant attention, since it has been consistently identified as a protective factor for PCa development [7–9], but it seems to induce disease progression. Several studies have suggested that the use of anti-diabetic drugs such as metformin might account for this protective effect of T2D on PCa risk [10,11], but other studies were not able to confirm these results in larger cohorts [12], which suggested that the protective effect attributed to T2D on PCa depend on common molecular pathways between these traits rather than the use of anti-diabetic drugs.

Although research on the specific pathways interfering in the development of T2D and PCa traits is still under way, a mounting body of evidence suggests that these diseases might share a genetic component [13–16]. Recent studies have reported that common genetic polymorphisms within T2D-related genes have an important role in modulating the risk of many cancers [17–19], but, so far, only a few studies have investigated the impact of diabetogenic variants on PCa risk, showing controversial results [20–23]. Considering this background, we decided to conduct a population-based case-control study including 994 subjects (304 PCa patients and 686 controls) to evaluate whether 57 diabetogenic variants identified through genome-wide association studies (GWAS) are associated with the risk of developing Pca. In order to validate the association of T2D-related markers with Pca risk, when possible, we performed a meta-analysis with data from previous genetic studies. Finally, we analyzed whether the most interesting markers correlated with absolute numbers of 91 blood-derived cell populations, 106 immunological serum proteins, 7 steroid hormones, and 9 cytokines (IFNγ, IL1β, IL1Ra, IL6, IL8, IL10, IL17, IL22, and TNFα) after stimulation of whole blood, peripheral blood mononuclear cells (PBMCs), and monocyte-derived macrophages with LPS, PHA, Pam3Cys, and *Staphylococcus aureus*.

2. Materials and Methods

2.1. Study Population

The study cohort consisted of 304 Caucasian PCa patients and 686 male healthy controls recruited in the Virgen de las Nieves University hospital (Granada, Spain) and the Complejo Hospitalario de Cáceres (Cáceres, Spain). Only patients without any prior history of malignancy, and who were not treated before blood withdrawal, were enrolled in this study. Patient characteristics are included in Table 1. The diagnosis of PCa was assigned by physicians, and fulfilled the international criteria [24]. Male controls with a mean age of 58.92 were blood donors from the Centro Regional de Transfusiones Sanguíneas de Granada (CRTS) and were selected from the same geographical region of the cases. In accordance with the Declaration of Helsinki, all participants gave their written informed consent to participate in the study and the ethical committees of the participant institutions approved the study.

Table 1. Demographic and clinical characteristics of PCa patients.

Demographic Characteristics		Study Population (n = 990)
Age (years)		62.35 ± 11.51
Clinical assessment		
PSA	PSA (4–10)	137 (46.13)
	PSA (10–20)	68 (22.90)
	PSA (>20)	92 (30.97)
Gleason	Gleason (≤7)	220 (73.58)
	Gleason (8–10)	79 (26.42)
TNM Staging system	T1–T2	209 (76.28)
	T3–T4	65 (23.72)
Risk	High	63 (26.58)
	Intermediate	79 (33.33)
	Low	95 (40.09)

2.2. SNP Selection and Genotyping

An extensive literature search concerning the mechanism of action of T2D-related genes was performed to select candidate genes that might affect the risk of developing PCa. SNPs were assessed on the basis of NCBI data, and were selected according to their known or putative functional consequences, i.e., their modifying influence on the structure of proteins, transcription level, or alternative splicing mechanisms. In total, 57 SNPs in 49 genes were selected for this study (Table 2).

Table 2. Selected type 2 diabetes-related SNPs.

Gene Name	dbSNP rs#	Nucleotide Substitution	GWAS-Identified Risk Allele for T2D	Location/Aa Substitution	References
ADAM30	rs2641348 η	T/C	C	L359P	[25,26]
ADAMTS9	rs4607103	T/C	C	Near gene	[26–28]
ADCY5	rs11708067	T/C	T	Intronic	[29,30]
ADRA2A	rs10885122	G/T	G	Near ADRA2A	[29]
ARAPI, CENTD2	rs1552224	C/A	A	Near gene	[31,32]
CDC123	rs12779790	A/G	G	Near gene	[26–28]
CDKAL1	rs7754840	C/G	C	Intronic	[33–35]
CDKN2A-2B	rs10811661	T/C	T	Near gene	[26–28,33,35–37]
COL5A1	rs4240702	C/T	n/s	Intronic	[38]
CRY2	rs11605924	A/C	A	Intronic	[29]
DCD	rs1153188	A/T	A	Near gene	[26]
EXT2	rs1113132	C/G	C	Intronic	[34,39]
FADS1	rs174550	C/T	T	Intronic	[29]
FAM148B	rs11071657	A/G	A	Near gene	[29,40]
FLJ39370	rs17044137	A/T	A	Near gene	[33]
FTO	rs9939609	A/C	A	Intronic	[27,41,42]
G6PC2	rs560887	G/A	G	Intronic	[29,38,43–45]
GCK	rs1799884	G/A	A	Near gene	[29,38,43–45]
GCKR	rs1260326	A/G	A	Leu446Pro	[46–49]
HHEX	rs1111875	G/A	C	Near gene	[27,33–35,39,41,42]
HMGA2	rs1531343	C/G	C	Near gene	[31,32]
HNF1A, TCF1	rs7957197	A/T	T	Intronic	[31,32]
HNF1B, TCF2	rs7501939 ц	C/T	T	Intronic	[14,50]
HNF1B, TCF2	rs757210	C/T	T	Intronic	[14,31]
HNF1B, TCF2	rs4430796	G/A	G	Intronic	[14]
IGF1	rs35767	C/T	C	Near gene	[29,51]
IGF2BP2	rs4402960	G/T	T	Intronic	[27,33–35,42,52]
IL13	rs20541	C/T	T	R144Q	[33]
IRS1	rs2943641	C/T	C	Near gene	[31,52,53]
JAZF1	rs864745	T/C	T	Intronic	[26,28]
JAZF1	rs10486567	A/G	A	Intronic	[26,28]
KCNJ11	rs5215	T/C	C	V337I	[27,33,35,41,42,54,55]
KCNJ11	rs5219 ε	C/T	T	K23E	
KCNQ1	rs2237897 ȼ	C/T	C	Intronic	
KCNQ1	rs2074196	G/T	G	Intronic	
KCNQ1	rs2237892	C/T	C	Intronic	[36,56–58]
KCNQ1	rs2237895	A/C	C	Intronic	
KCNQ1OT1	rs231362	C/T	G	Intronic	[31,32,57]
LTA	rs10041981	A/C	A	T60N	[59]
MADD	rs7944584	A/T	A	Intronic	[29]
MCR4	rs12970134	A/G	A	Near gene	[40]
MTNR1B	rs1387153	C/T	T	Near gene	[31,38,45]
NOTCH2	rs10923931	G/T	T	Intronic	[26,27]
PKN2	rs6698181	C/T	T	Intergenic	[33]
PPARG	rs1801282	C/G	C	P12A	[26,27,33,35,41,42,54,60]
PRC1	rs8042680	A/C	A	Intronic	[31,32]
PROX1	rs340874	A/G	G	Promoter	[29]
RBMS1	rs7593730	T/C	T	Intronic	[61,62]
SLC2A2	rs11920090	A/T	T	Intronic	[29]
SLC30A8	rs13266634	C/T	C	R325W	[27–29,33–35,39,41,42,63]
TCF7L2	rs7903146 ӄ	C/T	T	Intronic	[27,29,30,33–35,39,41,42,63–65]

Table 2. *Cont.*

Gene Name	dbSNP rs#	Nucleotide Substitution	GWAS-Identified Risk Allele for T2D	Location/Aa Substitution	References
TCF7L2	rs12255372	G/T	T	Intronic	[66]
THADA	rs7578597	T/C	C	Thr1187Ala	[26,67]
TP53INP1	rs896854	T/C	A	Intronic	[31,47,67,68]
TSPAN8, LGR5	rs7961581	C/T	C	Near gene	[69]
VEGFA	rs9472138	C/T	T	Near gene	[26]
WFS1	rs10010131	A/G	G	Intronic	[50]

n/s, not specified; Aa, amino acid; GWAS, genome-wide association studies. η That SNP rs2641348 is in complete linkage disequilibrium with the rs10923931, r^2 = 1.00. ҡ That SNP rs7903146 is in strong linkage disequilibrium with the rs12255372, r^2 = 0.72. ɕ That SNP rs2237897 is in strong linkage disequilibrium with the rs2237892, r^2 = 0.79. ɒ That SNP rs5219 is in complete linkage disequilibrium with the rs5215, r^2 = 1.00. ʯ That SNP rs7501939 is in strong linkage disequilibrium with the rs4430796, r^2 = 0.77.

Selected variants for T2D were genotyped using KASPar® assays (LGC Genomics, London, UK) according to the manufacturer's instructions. For internal quality control, 5% of samples were randomly included as duplicates. Concordance between the original and the duplicate samples for the 57 SNPs was ≥99.0%. Call rates for all SNPs were ≥90.0%.

2.3. Statistical Analysis

The Hardy–Weinberg Equilibrium (HWE) tests were performed in the control group by a standard observed–expected chi-squared (χ^2) test. Logistic regression analyses were used to assess the effects of the genetic polymorphisms on PCa risk using dominant, recessive, and log-additive models of inheritance. Overall analyses were adjusted for age, and conducted using Stata (v12.1). Statistical power was calculated using the Quanto software (vs. 12.4; log-additive model).

In order to account for multiple testing, we calculated an adjusted significance level using data from the SNPclip Tool (https://ldlink.nci.nih.gov/?tab=snpclip, accessed on 8 May 2020), which consider the number of independent marker loci (n = 52). Given the high correlation between the log-additive and dominant models of inheritance, we corrected by log-additive and recessive models, resulting in a significant threshold for the main effect analysis of 0.00048 (0.05/52 SNPs/2 inheritance models). Since a study-wide significance threshold considering all these factors is generally perceived as a too conservative test, we also assessed the magnitude of observed associations between selected SNPs and risk of PCa through a quantile–quantile (QQ) plot generated from the results of the study population. The observed association p-values were ranked in order from smallest to largest on the y-axis and plotted against the expected results from a theoretical $\sim\chi^2$-distribution under the null hypothesis of no association on the x-axis.

2.4. Meta-Analysis

With the aim of assessing the consistency of the association between T2D-related SNPs and the risk of developing PCa, we performed a meta-analysis of our data with those from publicly available GWAS. We downloaded association estimates from the PheWeb site (https://pheweb.sph.umich.edu/, accessed on 11 May 2020) for 6311 PCa cases; 74,685 controls from the FinnGen research project; and 5993 PCa cases and 168,999 controls from the UK Biobank project (UKBiobank TOPMed-imputed). Details on genome-wide associations have been previously reported [70]. Briefly, analyses on binary outcomes were conducted using the SAIGE generalized mixed logistic regression model, adjusting for genetic relatedness, sex, birth year, and the first four principal components. For White British participants of the UK Biobank, endpoint definitions were generated from electronic health-records-derived ICD billing codes, and endpoint definitions for the FinnGen data can be found at risteys.finngen.fi (Risteys = intersection in Finnish). We also validated the association of genetic markers using data from previously published studies that were selected according to the following criteria: (1) GWAS or candidate-gene association studies found in PUBMED (https://www.ncbi.nlm.nih.gov/pubmed, accessed on 13 May 2020) using the following key words: prostate cancer, case-control association study, type 2 diabetes, genetic polymorphisms; (2) Studies using Caucasian populations; (3) Availability of association estimates according to a log-additive model of inheritance; (4) Hardy–Weinberg equilibrium in the control group; and (5) Written in English (Figure 1). We pooled the Odds Ratios (ORs) using a fixed-effect model. Coefficients with a p-value ≤ 0.05 were considered significant. I^2 statistic was used to assess heterogeneity between studies. All statistics were calculated using STATA (v. 12).

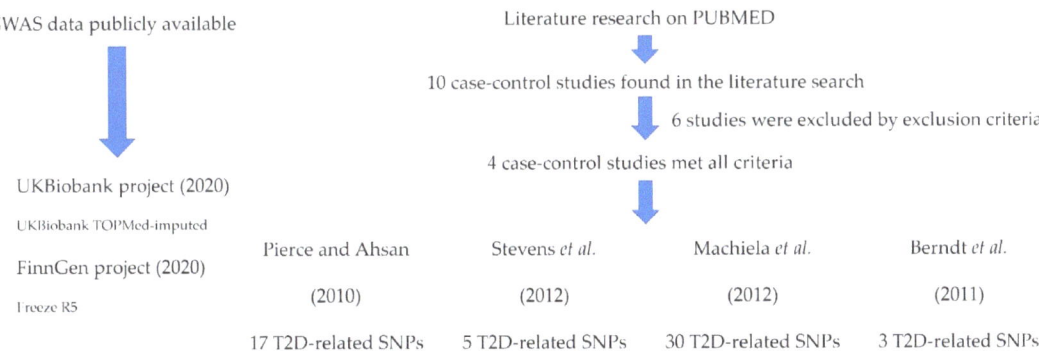

Figure 1. Flow diagram of the study [20–22,71].

2.5. cQTL Analysis of the T2D-Related Variants

Cytokine stimulation experiments were conducted in the 500 Functional Genomics (500FG) cohort from the Human Functional Genomics Project (HFGP; http://www.humanfunctionalgenomics.org/, accessed on 7 July 2020). The HFGP study was approved by the Arnhem-Nijmegen Ethical Committee (no. 42561.091.12), and biological specimens were collected after informed consent was obtained. We investigated whether any of the 57 T2D-related SNPs correlated with cytokine levels (IFNγ, IL1β, IL1Ra, IL6, IL8, IL10, IL17, IL22, and TNFα) after the stimulation of peripheral blood mononuclear cells (PBMCs), macrophages, or whole blood from 172 healthy men with LPS (1 or 100 ng/mL), PHA (10 μg/mL), Pam3Cys (10 μg/mL), and *Staphylococcus aureus*. After log transformation, linear regression analyses adjusted for age were used to determine the correlation of selected SNPs with cytokine expression quantitative trait loci (cQTLs). All analyses were performed using R software (http://www.r-project.org/, accessed on 8 May 2020). In order to account for multiple comparisons, we used a significant threshold of 0.000106 (0.05/52 independent SNPs × 9 cytokines).

Details on PBMCs isolation, macrophage differentiation, and stimulation assays have been reported elsewhere [72–74]. Briefly, PBMCs were washed twice in saline, and suspended in medium (RPMI 1640) supplemented with gentamicin (10 mg/mL), L-glutamine (10 mM), and pyruvate (10 mM). PBMC stimulations were performed with 5×10^5 cells/well in round-bottom 96-well plates (Greiner) for 24 h in the presence of 10% human pool serum at 37 °C and 5% CO_2. Supernatants were collected and stored in −20 °C until used for ELISA. LPS (100 ng/mL), PHA (10 μg/mL), and Pam3Cys (10 μg/mL) were used as stimulators for 24 or 48 h. Whole blood stimulation experiments were conducted using 100 μL of heparin blood that was added to a 48-well plate and subsequently stimulated with 400 μL of LPS and PHA (final volume 500 μL) for 48 h at 37 °C and 5% CO_2. Supernatants were collected and stored in −20 °C until used for ELISA. Concentrations of human cytokines were determined using specific commercial ELISA kits (PeliKine Compact, Amsterdam, The Netherlands or R&D Systems, Minneapolis, MN, USA), following the manufacturer's instructions.

2.6. Correlation between T2D-Related Polymorphisms and Cell Counts of 91 Blood-Derived Immune Cell Populations and 103 Serum/Plasmatic Immunological Proteins

We also investigated whether selected polymorphisms had an impact on blood cell counts by analyzing a set of 91 manually annotated immune cell populations and genotype data from the 500 FG cohort that consisted of 172 healthy men (Supplementary Table S1). Cell populations were measured by 10-color flow cytometry (Navios flow cytometer, Beckman Coulter) after blood sampling (2–3 h), and cell count analysis was performed using the Kaluza software (Beckman Coulter, v. 1.3). In order to reduce inter-experimental noise and increase statistical power, cell count analysis was performed by calculating parental and grandparental percentages, which were defined as the percentage of a certain cell type within the cell populations one or two levels higher in the hierarchical definitions of cell sub-populations [75]. Detailed laboratory protocols for cell isolation, reagents, gating, and flow cytometry analysis have been reported elsewhere [76], and the accession number for the raw flow cytometry data and analyzed data files are available upon request to the authors (http://hfgp.bbmri.nl, accessed on 8 May 2020). A proteomic analysis was also performed in serum and plasma samples from the 500 FG cohort. Circulating proteins were measured using the commercially available Olink® Inflammation panel (Olink, Sweden), which resulted in the measurement of 103 different biomarkers (Supplementary Materials Table S2). Proteins levels were expressed on a log2-scale as normalized protein expression values, and normalized using bridging samples to correct for batch variation. Considering the number of proteins ($n = 103$) and cell populations ($n = 91$) tested, p-values of 9.33×10^{-6} and 1.05×10^{-5} were set as significant thresholds for the proteomic and cell-level variation analysis, respectively.

2.7. Correlation between Steroid Hormone Levels and T2D-Related SNPs

We also measured serum levels of seven steroid hormones (androstenedione, cortisol, 11-deoxy-cortisol, 17-hydroxy progesterone, progesterone, testosterone, and 25 hydroxy vitamin D3) in the 500 FG cohort. Complete protocol details of steroid hormone measurements have been reported elsewhere [74]. Hormone levels and genotyping data were available for a total of 167 subjects. After log-transform, correlation between steroid hormone levels and T2D-related SNPs was evaluated by linear regression analysis adjusted for age. In order to avoid a possible bias, we excluded from the analysis those subjects that were using oral contraceptives, or those subjects in which this information was not available. The significance threshold was set to 0.000137 considering the number of independent SNPs tested ($n = 52$) and the number of hormones determined ($n = 7$).

2.8. In Silico Functional Analysis

Once we assessed the correlation of T2D-related SNPs with cytokine and steroid hormone levels, we used the HaploReg SNP annotation tool to further investigate the functional consequences of each specific variant (http://www.broadinstitute.org/mammals/haploreg/haploreg.php, accessed on 8 July 2020). We also assessed whether any of the potentially interesting markers correlated with mRNA expression levels of their respective genes using data from public eQTL browsers (GTex portal; www.gtexportal.org/home/, accessed on 8 July 2020; https://genenetwork.nl/bloodeqtlbrowser/, accessed on 8 July 2020) [77].

3. Results

3.1. Overall Associations of Selected SNPs with PCa Risk

All SNPs were in HWE in the control group ($p > 0.001$). Logistic regression analysis adjusted for age showed that carriers of the $IGF2BP2_{rs4402960T/T}$, $TCF7L2_{rs12255372T/T}$, and $TSPAN8|LGR5_{rs7961581C/C}$ genotypes had an increased risk of PCa ($p = 0.037$; 0.005 and 0.024), whereas those carrying the $CDKAL1_{rs7754840C}$, $FLJ39370_{rs17044137A}$, $FTO_{rs9939609A}$, $HNF1B_{rs7501939T}$, $HNF1B_{rs757210T}$, $JAZF1_{rs10486567A}$, $KCNQ1_{rs2237897C}$, and $KCNQ1_{rs2237892C}$ alleles showed a decreased risk of developing the disease ($p = 0.022, 0.021, 0.046, 0.030, 0.024,$

0.011, 0.041, and 0.0002; Table 3). Although none of the reported associations remained statistically significant after a stringent correction for multiple testing (p = 0.00048), the QQ plot showed a pronounced and early deviation of identity line, which confirmed that the effect attributed to SNPs in T2D-related loci was more than expected under the null hypothesis and, therefore, might represent true associations (Figure 2).

Table 3. Association of T2D-related variants and risk of developing PCa in the discovery population.

Variant_dbSNP	Gene	Nucleotide Substitution	Risk Allele	OR (95% CI) [†]	p
rs2641348	ADAM30	T/C	C	0.93 (0.66–1.29)	0.66
rs4607103	ADAMTS9	T/C	C	1.06 (0.83–1.37)	0.63
rs11708067	ADCY5	A/G	G	1.08 (0.80–1.48)	0.60
rs10885122	ADRA2A	G/T	T	1.12 (0.81–1.55)	0.49
rs1552224	ARAP1, CENTD2	C/A	A	1.04 (0.76–1.41)	0.82
rs12779790	CDC123, CAMK1D	A/G	G	1.05 (0.80–1.38)	0.73
rs7754840	CDKAL1	C/G	C	0.69 (0.51–0.95) [¥]	0.022
rs10811661	CDKN2A-2B	T/C	T	0.84 (0.64–1.10)	0.22
rs4240702	COL5A1	C/T	T	0.82 (0.66–1.02)	0.082
rs11605924	CRY2	A/C	A	1.03 (0.83–1.28)	0.79
rs1153188	DCD	A/T	T	0.93 (0.73–1.18)	0.55
rs1113132	EXT2	C/G	C	1.02 (0.80–1.30)	0.13
rs174550	FADS1	C/T	C	0.96 (0.76–1.22)	0.75
rs11071657	FAM148B	A/G	G	1.16 (0.94–1.44)	0.16
rs17044137	FLJ39370	A/T	A	0.68 (0.49–0.94) [¥]	0.021
rs9939609	FTO	A/C	A	0.80 (0.63–0.99)	0.046
rs560887	G6PC2	G/A	G	1.15 (0.90–1.46)	0.28
rs1799884	GCK	G/A	A	1.07 (0.80–1.44)	0.65
rs1260326	GCKR	C/T	T	0.93 (0.73–1.20)	0.60
rs1111875	HHEX	C/T	C	0.90 (0.72–1.13)	0.36
rs1531343	HMGA2	C/G	C	0.74 (0.53–1.02)	0.068
rs7957197	HNF1A (TCF1)	A/T	T	0.82 (0.63–1.07)	0.16
rs7501939	HNF1B (TCF2)	C/T	T	0.70 (0.50–0.96) [¥]	0.030
rs757210	HNF1B (TCF2)	C/T	T	0.67 (0.48–0.95) [¥]	0.024
rs4430796	HNF1B (TCF2)	G/A	G	0.73 (0.50–1.06) [¥]	0.10
rs35767	IGF1	C/T	C	0.87 (0.66–1.14)	0.30
rs4402960	IGF2BP2	G/T	T	1.66 (1.03–2.68) [§]	0.037
rs20541	IL13	C/T	T	0.82 (0.60–1.11)	0.20
rs2943641	IRS1	C/T	C	0.97 (0.77–1.21)	0.80
rs864745	JAZF1	T/C	T	1.05 (0.84–1.30)	0.67
rs10486567	JAZF1	A/G	A	0.69 (0.52–0.91)	0.011
rs5215	KCNJ11	T/C	C	0.87 (0.70–1.08)	0.21
rs5219	KCNJ11	C/T	T	0.89 (0.71–1.11)	0.29
rs2237897	KCNQ1	C/T	C	0.66 (0.44–0.98)	0.041
rs2074196	KCNQ1	G/T	T	0.99 (0.53–1.84)	0.97
rs2237892	KCNQ1	C/T	C	0.41 (0.26–0.66)	0.0002
rs2237895	KCNQ1	A/C	C	0.92 (0.73–1.17)	0.50
rs231362	KCNQ1OT1	C/T	C	0.94 (0.75–1.18)	0.61
rs1041981	LTA	A/C	A	0.87 (0.68–1.12)	0.29
rs7944584	MADD	A/T	T	1.16 (0.93–1.46)	0.18
rs12970134	MCR4	A/G	A	0.85 (0.66–1.11)	0.25
rs1387153	MTNR1B	C/T	T	0.81 (0.63–1.04)	0.10
rs10923931	NOTCH2	G/T	T	0.92 (0.66–1.28)	0.63
rs6698181	PKN2	C/T	T	0.90 (0.72–1.13)	0.39
rs1801282	PPARG	C/G	C	0.99 (0.70–1.42)	0.98
rs8042680	PRC1	A/C	A	1.10 (0.87–1.37)	0.40
rs340874	PROX1	A/G	G	0.89 (0.72–1.10)	0.29
rs7593730	RBMS1	C/T	T	0.77 (0.59–1.02)	0.070
rs11920090	SLC2A2	A/T	T	0.81 (0.59–1.12)	0.20
rs13266634	SLC30A8	C/T	C	0.83 (0.65–1.05)	0.11

Table 3. Cont.

Variant_dbSNP	Gene	Nucleotide Substitution	Risk Allele	OR (95% CI) [†]	p
rs7903146	TCF7L2	C/T	T	1.01 (0.80–1.29)	0.91
rs12255372	TCF7L2	G/T	T	1.85 (1.20–2.86) [§]	**0.005**
rs7578597	THADA	T/C	C	0.93 (0.58–1.49)	0.76
rs896854	TP53INP1	G/A	A	0.73 (0.52–1.03) [¥]	0.070
rs7961581	TSPAN8, LGR5	C/T	C	1.72 (1.07–2.76) [§]	**0.024**
rs9472138	VEGFA	C/T	T	1.04 (0.81–1.32)	0.78
rs10010131	WFS1	A/G	G	0.90 (0.72–1.13)	0.39

Abbreviations: OR, odds ratio; CI, confidence interval. Estimates were adjusted for age. $p < 0.05$ in bold. [†] Estimates calculated according to a log-additive model of inheritance and adjusted for age. [¥] Estimates calculated according to a dominant model of inheritance and adjusted for age. [§] Estimates calculated according to a recessive model of inheritance and adjusted for age.

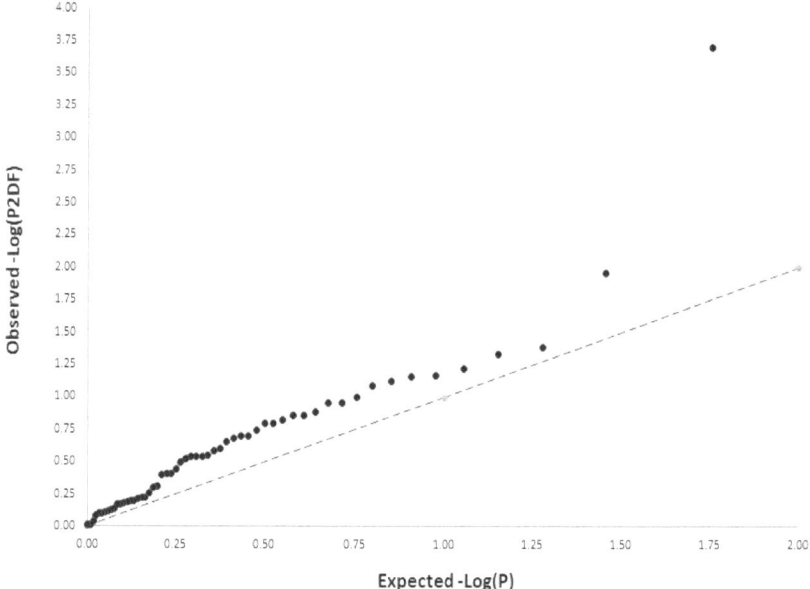

Figure 2. QQ plot showing early deviation of the identity line.

The identity line represents the null hypothesis (no significant association between T2D-related SNPs and PCa risk). Early deviation of the identity line might represent true associations.

3.2. Meta-Analysis

In order to confirm these potentially interesting associations, we conducted a meta-analysis with GWAS data from two large cohorts (UKBiobank and FinnGen) and previously published genetic association studies. After filtering all studies found in the literature according to selected key words, we found that four case-control studies met the eligibility criteria [20–22,71]. The meta-analysis of our data with those from all these studies confirmed that carriers of the $FTO_{rs9939609A}$, $HNF1B_{rs7501939T}$, $HNF1B_{rs757210T}$, $HNF1B_{rs4430796G}$, and $JAZF1_{rs10486567A}$ alleles had a decreased risk of developing PCa ($p = 3.70 \times 10^{-5}$, 9.39×10^{-54}, 5.04×10^{-54}, 1.19×10^{-71}, and 1.66×10^{-18}; Table 4). Although the effect of the FTO and HNF1B loci on PCA risk has been consistently validated in previous studies, this is the first validation study confirming the association of the JAZF1 variant with the risk of developing the disease. In addition, although the association did not remain significant after correction for multiple testing, the meta-analysis suggested modest associations with the risk of developing the disease for SNPs within the *NOTCH2* and *RBMS1* loci ($p = 8.49 \times 10^{-4}$ and 0.004; Table 4). These associations are potentially interesting and need to be further investigated.

3.3. Functional Characterization of T2D-Related Variants in the HFGP Cohort

In order to test the possible functional relevance of the most interesting SNPs, we analyzed data from the HFGP cohort. The proteomic analysis of the immunological serum proteins showed that carriers of the $HNF1B_{rs7501939T}$ allele had decreased circulating levels of ST1A1 protein ($p = 0.00030$; Figure 3). Although this correlation did not survive multiple testing correction, this result supported the implication of the *HNF1B* locus in modulating PCa risk, likely by the regulation of the sulfatation of multiple compounds in the liver. In addition, given the healthy nature of the subjects included in the HFGP cohort, this result is still speculative and needs to be further confirmed in tumor samples of PCa patients. No significant correlation was found between *HFN1B*, *FTO*, *JAZF1*, and *NOTCH2* SNPs and blood-derived cells populations, steroid hormones, or cQTL data, which suggested that these SNPs might affect PCa risk likely through the regulation of mRNA levels of their respective genes.

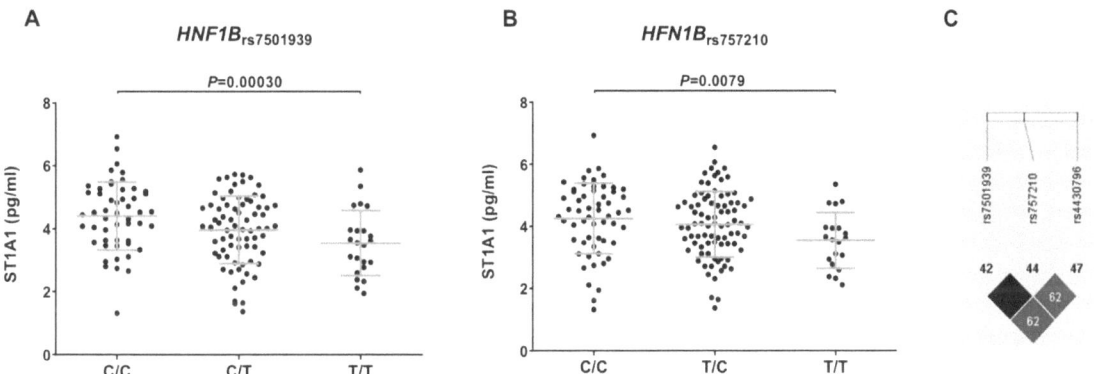

Figure 3. Correlation of the $HFN1B_{rs7501939}$ (**A**) and $HFN1B_{rs757210}$ (**B**) polymorphisms with reduced levels of ST1A1 protein and linkage disequilibrium values among the *HFN1B* SNPs included in the study (**C**). C/C, cytosine/cytosine; C/T, cytosine/thymine; T/T, thymine/thymine; T/C, thymine/cytosine.

Next, we assessed functional information from the HaploReg SNP annotation tool, and we also assessed whether any of the potentially interesting markers correlated with mRNA expression levels of their respective genes using data from public eQTL browsers. We found that, according to Haploreg data, the $HNF1B_{rs7501939}$, $HNF1B_{rs757210}$, and $HNF1B_{rs4430796}$ SNPs were modestly associated with mRNA *HNF1B* expression levels in peripheral whole blood ($p = 9.23 \times 10^{-4}$, 1.00×10^{-3}, and 2.00×10^{-3}) [77], and that they mapped among histone marks (H3K4me1, H3K4me3) in several tissues and changed motifs for CEBPB, DMRT5, p300, HES1, and Maf (Supplementary Table S3). Similarly, we found that the $NOTCH2_{rs10923931}$ and $RBMS1_{rs7593730}$ SNPs also correlated with *NOTCH2* and *RBMS1* mRNA expression levels in peripheral whole blood ($p = 7.3 \times 10^{-6}$ and 3.31×10^{-7}, respectively) [77]. On the other hand, we found that the $FTO_{rs9939609}$ and $JAZF1_{rs10486567}$ SNPs mapped among histone marks in multiple tissues and several immune cells, and changed regulatory motifs for multiple regulatory transcription factors (Supplementary Table S3). In addition, GTEx portal data suggested that the $NOTCH2_{rs10923931}$ SNP is an eQTL in the pancreas and liver.

Table 4. Meta-analysis of association estimates with previous candidate gene association studies according to a log-additive model of inheritance.

SNP	Gene_SNP	Risk Allele	Study Population (304 PCa Cases and 686 Controls) OR (95% CI) [a]	UKBiobank (2020) (5993 PCa Cases and 168,999 Controls) OR (95% CI) [a]	FinnGen (2020) (6311 PCa Cases and 74,685 Controls) OR (95% CI) [a]	Machiela et al. (2012) (2782 PCa Cases and 4458 Controls) OR (95% CI) [a]	Pierce and Ahsan (2010) (1230 PCa Cases and 1160 Controls) OR (95% CI) [a]	Stevens et al. (2010) (2935 PCa Cases and 2932 Controls) OR (95% CI) [a]	Berndt et al. (2011) (10,272 PCa Cases and 9123 Controls) OR (95% CI) [a]	Meta-Analysis (29,827 PCa Cases and 262,042 Controls) OR (95% CI) [a]	p Value	p_{Het}
rs2641348	ADAM30	C	0.93 (0.66–1.29)	0.95 (0.89–1.01)	0.96 (0.90–1.02)	-	0.87 (0.71–1.05)	-	-	**0.95 (0.91–0.99)**	**0.020**	0.826
rs4607103	ADAMTS9	C	1.07 (0.83–1.37)	1.02 (0.97–1.07)	0.97 (0.93–1.02)	0.99 (0.91–1.08)	0.98 (0.85–1.12) η	-	-	0.99 (0.96–1.02)	0.660	0.641
rs11708067	ADCY5	G	1.09 (0.80–1.48)	1.00 (0.96–1.05)	0.99 (0.94–1.05)	**0.91 (0.84–0.99)**	-	-	-	0.98 (0.94–1.02)	0.307	0.217
rs10885122	ADRA2A	T	1.12 (0.81–1.54)	0.99 (0.94–1.05)	1.00 (0.94–1.06)	1.00 (0.91–1.10)	-	-	-	1.00 (0.96–1.04)	0.863	0.750
rs1552224	ARAP1	A	1.04 (0.76–1.41)	1.00 (0.95–1.06)	1.00 (0.95–1.05)	-	-	-	-	1.00 (0.96–1.03)	0.948	0.951
rs12779790	CDC123	G	1.05 (0.80–1.37)	1.04 (0.99–1.09)	0.98 (0.93–1.03)	1.06 (0.97–1.16)	1.03 (0.89–1.19) ξ	-	-	1.02 (0.99–1.05)	0.251	0.441
rs7754840	CDKAL1	C	0.80 (0.63–1.02)	1.00 (0.96–1.05)	1.03 (0.98–1.07)	1.04 (0.97–1.13)	1.00 (0.88–1.14) #	-	-	1.01 (0.98–1.05)	0.316	0.283
rs10811661	CDKN2A-2B	T	0.84 (0.64–1.10)	1.02 (0.97–1.07)	0.95 (0.90–1.01)	**0.91 (0.83–1.00)**	-	-	-	0.98 (0.94–1.01)	0.168	0.063
rs4240702	COL5A1	T	0.83 (0.67–1.03)	1.00 (0.97–1.04)	1.01 (0.97–1.05)	-	-	-	-	1.00 (0.97–1.03)	0.907	0.211
rs11605924	CRY2	A	1.03 (0.82–1.28)	1.01 (0.97–1.04)	1.00 (0.95–1.04)	-	-	-	-	1.01 (0.98–1.03)	0.637	0.924
rs1153188	DCD	T	0.93 (0.73–1.18)	0.97 (0.93–1.02)	0.98 (0.93–1.03)	-	-	-	-	0.97 (0.94–1.01)	0.122	0.892
rs1113132	EXT2	C	0.93 (0.73–1.19)	0.99 (0.95–1.02)	1.01 (0.97–1.06)	-	-	-	-	1.00 (0.97–1.02)	0.890	0.646
rs174550	FADS1	C	0.96 (0.76–1.21)	0.98 (0.94–1.02)	0.98 (0.94–1.03)	-	-	-	-	0.98 (0.95–1.01)	0.182	0.985

Table 4. *Cont.*

SNP	Gene_SNP	Risk Allele	Study Population (304 PCa Cases and 686 Controls) OR (95% CI) [a]	UKBiobank (2020) (5993 PCa Cases and 168,999 Controls) OR (95% CI) [a]	FinnGen (2020) (6311 PCa Cases and 74,685 Controls) OR (95% CI) [a]	Machiela et al. (2012) (2782 PCa Cases and 4458 Controls) OR (95% CI) [a]	Pierce and Ahsan (2010) (1230 PCa Cases and 1160 Controls) OR (95% CI) [a]	Stevens et al. (2010) (2935 PCa Cases and 2932 Controls) OR (95% CI) [a]	Berndt et al. (2011) (10,272 PCa Cases and 9123 Controls) OR (95% CI) [a]	Meta-Analysis (29,827 PCa Cases and 262,042 Controls) OR (95% CI) [a]	p Value	P_{Het}
rs11071657	FAM148B	G	1.16 (0.94–1.44)	1.02 (0.98–1.06)	1.01 (0.96–1.05)	-	-	-	-	1.02 (0.99–1.05)	0.227	0.456
rs17044137	FLJ39370	A	0.79 (0.61–1.03)	1.02 (0.98–1.07)	**0.94 (0.90–0.99)**	-	-	-	-	0.98 (0.95–1.01)	0.199	0.013
rs9939609	FTO	A	**0.30 (0.63–0.99)**	0.96 (0.92–1.00)	0.96 (0.92–1.00)	**0.93 (0.86–1.00)**	**0.87 (0.77–0.98)** δ	0.93 (0.85–1.02) ς	-	**0.95 (0.92–0.97)**	3.70×10^{-5}	0.388
rs560887	G6PC2	G	1.15 (0.90–1.46)	1.02 (0.98–1.07)	0.96 (0.92–1.01)	-	-	-	-	1.00 (0.94–1.06)	0.705	0.088
rs1799884	GCK	A	1.07 (0.80–1.44)	1.03 (0.98–1.08)	0.99 (0.93–1.06)	1.06 (0.96–1.16) ∂	-	-	-	1.02 (0.99–1.06)	0.220	0.643
rs1260326	GCKR	C	1.07 (0.83–1.37)	0.99 (0.96–1.03)	0.98 (0.94–1.02)	0.98 (0.91–1.05) Π	-	-	-	0.99 (0.97–1.00)	0.170	0.889
rs1111875	HHEX	C	0.90 (0.72–1.13)	1.01 (0.97–1.05)	1.01 (0.97–1.05)	1.01 (0.94–1.09)	0.98 (0.87–1.10)	-	-	1.01 (0.98–1.03)	0.586	0.876
rs1531343	HMGA2	C	0.74 (0.53–1.20)	0.98 (0.92–1.04)	1.01 (0.97–1.05)	0.98 (0.88–1.10)	-	-	-	0.99 (0.94–1.03)	0.534	0.512
rs7957197	HNF1A	T	0.82 (0.63–1.07)	1.01 (0.97–1.06)	0.99 (0.94–1.04)	0.96 (0.88–1.05)	-	-	-	0.99 (0.96–1.02)	0.673	0.370
rs7501939	HNF1B	T	0.84 (0.67–1.05)	**0.83 (0.80–0.86)**	**0.83 (0.79–0.87)**	-	-	**0.87 (0.80–0.94)**	**0.84 (0.80–0.87)**	**0.84 (0.82–0.86)**	9.39×10^{-54}	0.873
rs757210	HNF1B	T	0.84 (0.67–1.04)	**0.84 (0.81–0.88)**	**0.82 (0.79–0.86)**	**0.85 (0.79–0.92)**	-	**0.85 (0.79–0.92)**	**0.84 (0.80–0.88)**	**0.84 (0.82–0.86)**	5.04×10^{-54}	0.902
rs4430796	HNF1B	G	0.87 (0.71–1.12)	**0.81 (0.79–0.85)**	**0.82 (0.78–0.85)**	-	**0.87 (0.77–0.97)**	**0.85 (0.79–0.92)**	**0.81 (0.77–0.84)**	**0.82 (0.80–0.84)**	1.19×10^{-71}	0.688
rs35767	IGF1	C	0.87 (0.66–1.13)	0.99 (0.94–1.04)	1.01 (0.96–1.06)	-	-	-	-	1.00 (0.96–1.03)	0.901	0.516

Table 4. Cont.

SNP	Gene_SNP	Risk Allele	Study Population (304 PCa Cases and 686 Controls) OR (95% CI) [a]	UKBiobank (2020) (5993 PCa Cases and 168,999 Controls) OR (95% CI) [a]	FinnGen (2020) (6311 PCa Cases and 74,685 Controls) OR (95% CI) [a]	Machiela et al. (2012) (2782 PCa Cases and 4458 Controls) OR (95% CI) [a]	Pierce and Ahsan (2010) (1230 PCa Cases and 1160 Controls) OR (95% CI) [a]	Stevens et al. (2010) (2935 PCa Cases and 2932 Controls) OR (95% CI) [a]	Berndt et al. (2011) (10,272 PCa Cases and 9123 Controls) OR (95% CI) [a]	Meta-Analysis (29,827 PCa Cases and 262,042 Controls) OR (95% CI) [a]	p Value	p_{Het}
rs4402960	IGF2BP2	T	1.05 (0.83–1.32)	0.99 (0.95–1.03)	1.00 (0.95–1.04)	1.03 (0.95–1.11)	0.91 (0.81–1.04)	-	-	0.99 (0.97–1.02)	0.733	0.552
rs20541	IL13	T	0.82 (0.60–1.11)	0.97 (0.93–1.02)	1.04 (0.99–1.08)	-	-	-	-	1.00 (0.93–1.06)	0.788	0.042
rs2943641	IRS1	C	0.97 (0.77–1.21)	1.01 (0.97–1.05)	1.02 (0.98–1.06)	0.95 (0.88–1.02)	-	-	-	1.01 (0.98–1.03)	0.641	0.403
rs864745	JAZF1	T	1.05 (0.84–1.30)	1.02 (0.98–1.06)	0.99 (0.95–1.03)	1.08 (1.01–1.16)	0.98 (0.87–1.10)	-	-	1.02 (0.99–1.05)	0.269	0.283
rs10486567	JAZF1	A	0.69 (0.52–0.91)	0.87 (0.83–0.91)	0.86 (0.82–0.91)	-	-	0.86 (0.73–0.94)	-	0.86 (0.83–0.89)	1.66×10^{-18}	0.459
rs5215	KCNJ11	C	0.87 (0.70–1.08)	1.02 (0.98–1.06)	0.99 (0.95–1.03)	1.01 (0.94–1.09)	0.89 (0.78–1.00)	-	-	0.99 (0.96–1.03)	0.921	0.182
rs5219	KCNJ11	T	0.89 (0.71–1.11)	1.02 (0.98–1.06)	0.99 (0.95–1.04)	-	-	-	-	1.00 (0.97–1.04)	0.746	0.349
rs2237897	KCNQ1	C	0.66 (0.44–0.98)	0.94 (0.86–1.04)	0.98 (0.91–1.06)	-	-	-	-	0.94 (0.86–1.04)	0.136	0.148
rs2074196	KCNQ1	T	0.99 (0.53–1.84)	1.03 (0.94–1.14)	0.97 (0.88–1.07)	-	-	-	-	1.00 (0.93–1.07)	0.996	0.693
rs2237892	KCNQ1	C	0.41 (0.26–0.66)	0.98 (0.91–1.06)	1.02 (0.93–1.12)	0.85 (0.74–0.98)	0.88 (0.69–1.12)	-	-	0.89 (0.78–1.02)	0.105	0.001
rs2237895	KCNQ1	C	0.92 (0.73–1.16)	0.99 (0.95–1.03)	0.96 (0.92–1.00)	-	-	-	-	0.97 (0.95–1.00)	0.078	0.517
rs231362	KCNQ1OT1	C	0.94 (0.75–1.18)	0.99 (0.96–1.03)	1.03 (0.99–1.08)	0.92 (0.86–0.98)	-	-	-	0.99 (0.94–1.03)	0.515	0.042
rs1041981	LTA	A	0.88 (0.69–1.13)	0.95 (0.91–0.99)	0.99 (0.94–1.04)	-	-	-	-	0.96 (0.93–1.00)	0.028	0.359

Table 4. Cont.

SNP	Gene_SNP	Risk Allele	Study Population (304 PCa Cases and 636 Controls) OR (95% CI) [a]	UKBiobank (2020) (5993 PCa Cases and 168,999 Controls) OR (95% CI) [a]	FinnGen (2020) (6311 PCa Cases and 74,685 Controls) OR (95% CI) [a]	Machiela et al. (2012) (2782 PCa Cases and 4458 Controls) OR (95% CI) [a]	Pierce and Ahsan (2010) (1230 PCa Cases and 1160 Controls) OR (95% CI) [a]	Stevens et al. (2010) (2935 PCa Cases and 2932 Controls) OR (95% CI) [a]	Berndt et al. (2011) (10,272 PCa Cases and 9123 Controls) OR (95% CI) [a]	Meta-Analysis (29,827 PCa Cases and 262,042 Controls) OR (95% CI) [a]	p Value	p_{Het}
rs7944584	MADD	T	1.16 (0.93–1.46)	1.03 (0.99–1.07)	1.04 (0.99–1.10)	-	-	-	-	**1.04 (1.00–1.07)**	**0.026**	0.585
rs12970134	MCR4	A	0.35 (0.65–1.11)	0.99 (0.95–1.04)	0.99 (0.94–1.04)	-	-	-	-	0.99 (0.95–1.02)	0.466	0.541
rs1387153	MTNR1B	T	0.31 (0.63–1.04)	1.02 (0.97–1.06)	0.98 (0.94–1.03)	**1.10 (1.01–1.19)** ᶜ	-	-	-	1.01 (0.96–1.08)	0.517	0.029
rs10923931	NOTCH2	T	0.92 (0.66–1.28)	0.95 (0.90–1.01)	0.95 (0.89–1.01)	**0.86 (0.76–0.96)**	0.87 (0.71–1.05) *	-	-	**0.94 (0.90–0.97)**	**8.49 × 10⁻⁴**	0.552
rs6698181	PKN2	T	0.90 (0.72–1.13)	0.99 (0.96–1.03)	1.01 (0.96–1.06)	-	-	-	-	0.99 (0.97–1.02)	0.732	0.551
rs1801282	PPARG	C	1.00 (0.70–1.42)	1.01 (0.95–1.06)	1.00 (0.94–1.05)	0.96 (0.87–1.07)	0.88 (0.74–1.04)	-	-	0.99 (0.96–1.03)	0.733	0.596
rs8042680	PRC1	A	1.10 (0.87–1.37)	0.99 (0.95–1.03)	**0.96 (0.91–0.99)**	1.04 (0.97–1.12)	-	-	-	0.99 (0.95–1.03)	0.300	0.204
rs340874	PROX1	G	0.89 (0.72–1.10)	1.01 (0.97–1.05)	1.00 (0.96–1.05)	1.01 (0.94–1.08)	-	-	-	1.00 (0.98–1.03)	0.758	0.708
rs7593730	RBMS1	T	0.77 (0.59–1.02)	**1.07 (1.03–1.12)**	1.03 (0.98–1.09)	-	-	-	-	**1.03 (0.96–1.11)**	**0.004**	0.045
rs11920090	SLC2A2	T	0.82 (0.59–1.12)	**0.94 (0.89–0.99)**	0.99 (0.93–1.06)	-	-	-	-	**0.96 (0.92–1.00)**	**0.036**	0.307
rs13266634	SLC30A8	C	0.83 (0.65–1.05)	0.99 (0.95–1.03)	1.00 (0.96–1.05)	1.00 (0.93–1.08)	0.97 (0.86–1.11)	-	-	0.99 (0.96–1.02)	0.551	0.659
rs7903146	TCF7L2	T	1.01 (0.80–1.29)	1.04 (1.00–1.08)	0.99 (0.94–1.04)	**0.90 (0.83–0.97)**	0.97 (0.85–1.10)	-	-	0.98 (0.93–1.03)	0.872	0.047
rs12255372	TCF7L2	T	1.17 (0.94–1.46)	1.02 (0.98–1.06)	0.97 (0.92–1.02)	-	-	-	-	1.00 (0.96–1.06)	0.778	0.123

Table 4. Cont.

SNP	Gene_SNP	Risk Allele	Study Population (304 PCa Cases and 686 Controls) OR (95% CI) [a]	UKBiobank (2020) (5993 PCa Cases and 168,999 Controls) OR (95% CI) [a]	FinnGen (2020) (6311 PCa Cases and 74,685 Controls) OR (95% CI) [a]	Machiela et al. (2012) (2782 PCa Cases and 4458 Controls) OR (95% CI) [a]	Pierce and Ahsan (2010) (1230 PCa Cases and 1160 Controls) OR (95% CI) [a]	Stevens et al. (2010) (2935 PCa Cases and 2932 Controls) OR (95% CI) [a]	Berndt et al. (2011) (10,272 PCa Cases and 9123 Controls) OR (95% CI) [a]	Meta-Analysis (29,827 PCa Cases and 262,042 Controls)		
										OR (95% CI) [a]	p Value	p_{Het}
rs7578597	THADA	T	1.08 (0.67–1.72)	1.05 (0.98–1.11)	1.04 (0.95–1.14)	1.03 (0.91–1.16)	1.10 (0.92–1.32) [†]	-	-	**1.05 (1.00–1.10)**	**0.044**	0.982
rs896854	TP53INP1	T	0.88 (0.71–1.10)	0.99 (0.95–1.02)	0.99 (0.94–1.03)	1.02 (0.95–1.09)	-	-	-	0.99 (0.97–1.02)	0.570	0.615
rs7961581	TSPAN8	C	1.19 (0.94–1.51)	0.98 (0.94–1.02)	1.00 (0.95–1.05)	1.05 (0.97–1.13)	1.04 (0.92–1.19) [τ]	-	-	1.00 (0.97–1.04)	0.924	0.295
rs9472138	VEGFA	T	1.04 (0.82–1.33)	1.01 (0.97–1.05)	0.98 (0.94–1.03)	-	-	-	-	1.00 (0.97–1.03)	0.877	0.586
rs10010131	WFS1	G	0.90 (0.72–1.13)	0.99 (0.95–1.02)	1.01 (0.97–1.05)	1.00 (0.93–1.07)	-	-	-	1.00 (0.97–1.02)	0.859	0.716

Abbreviations: SNP, single nucleotide polymorphism; OR, odds ratio; CI, confidence interval; C, cytosine; T, thymine; A, adenine; G, guanosine; n/s, not specified. a Estimates calculated according to a log-additive model of inheritance and adjusted for age. Meta-analysis was performed assuming a fixed-effect model. $p < 0.05$ in bold. η Authors report the effect found for the rs4411878 (a SNP in complete linkage disequilibrium with the rs4607103, $r^2 = 0.97$). ξ Authors report the effect found for the rs11257655 (a SNP in strong linkage disequilibrium with the rs12779790, $r^2 = 0.82$). # Authors report the effect found for the rs7756992 (a SNP in strong linkage disequilibrium with the rs7754840, $r^2 = 0.75$). δ Authors report the effect found for the rs8050136 (a SNP in complete linkage disequilibrium with the rs9969309, $r^2 = 0.98$). א Authors report the effect found for the rs1635852 (a SNP in complete linkage disequilibrium with the rs864745, $r^2 = 0.98$). * Authors report the effect found for the rs2641348 (a SNP in complete linkage disequilibrium with the rs1092931, $r^2 = 1.00$). ∂ Authors report the effect found for the rs4607517 (a SNP in complete linkage disequilibrium with the rs1799884, $r^2 = 1.00$). Π Authors report the effect found for the rs780094 (a SNP in complete linkage disequilibrium with the rs1260326, $r^2 = 0.92$). † Authors report the effect found for the rs13414140 (a SNP in complete linkage disequilibrium with the rs7578597, $r^2 = 1.00$). ς Authors report the effect found for the rs1353362 (a SNP in strong linkage disequilibrium with the rs7961581, $r^2 = 0.92$). τ Authors report the effect found for the rs10830963 (a SNP in moderate to high linkage disequilibrium with the rs1387153, $r^2 = 0.67$). ς Results from Lewis et al. Plos One 2010; 5: e13485 [78].

4. Discussion

T2D has been consistently identified as protective factor for PCa development and disease progression [7–9]. Several studies have also suggested that both diseases might share a genetic component [13–16], and some others have attempted to demonstrate the impact of diabetogenic variants on PCa risk, showing controversial results [20–23]. With this background, we decided to further investigate the association of diabetogenic variants identified through GWAS with the risk to PCa, and attempted to identify the biological mechanisms underlying the most interesting associations through the analysis of functional data from the HFGP cohort and eQTL browsers.

The meta-analysis of the Spanish cohort with those from the UKBiobank, FinnGen, and previously published studies [20–22] confirmed that carriers of the $FTO_{rs9939609A}$, $HNF1B_{rs7501939T}$, $HNF1B_{rs757210T}$, $HNF1B_{rs4430796G}$, and $JAZF1_{rs10486567A}$ alleles showed a decreased risk of developing the disease. Although the association did not reach the stringent significance threshold, we also found that the $NOTCH2_{rs10923931}$ and $RBMS1_{rs7593730}$ SNPs associated with the risk of developing the disease. The strongest effect on PCa risk was observed for SNPs within the $HNF1B$ locus (rs757210, rs7501939, and rs4430796), which showed a similar direction across all study populations. The $HNF1B$ (TCF2) gene is located at chromosome 17q12, and it encodes for a transcription factor implicated in the control of regulatory networks related to pancreas and kidney development. It has been reported that the $HNF1B$ locus participates not only in the generation of endocrine precursors, but also in the modulation of acinar cell identity and duct morphogenesis. In addition to these functions, it has been consistently reported that the $HNF1B$ locus plays a key role in modulating tumorigenesis in solid [79] and hematological cancers [80], and that its methylation or mRNA expression levels can be used for patient stratification [81] and prediction of disease outcome [82]. The association of the $HNF1B_{rs7501939}$, $HNF1B_{rs757210}$, and $HNF1B_{rs4430796}$ polymorphisms with PCa risk was in agreement with results recently reported in GWAS for PCa [14,83,84], whereas large-scale fine mapping studies have even found additional polymorphisms that might contribute to the development of PCa [71]. These findings, together with our functional results reporting that carriers of the $HNF1B_{rs7501939T}$ and $HNF1B_{rs757210T}$ alleles showed decreased levels of SULT1A1 protein (also known as ST1A1), suggest that the effect of the $HFN1B$ locus on PCa risk might be mediated through the regulation of SULT1A1 expression levels. This protein is an enzyme that catalyzes the sulfate conjugation of many hormones, neurotransmitters, drugs, and xenobiotic compounds, among other compounds. It also has been demonstrated that SULT1A1 regulates the metabolic activation of carcinogenic N-hydroxyarylamines, leading to highly reactive intermediates capable of forming DNA adducts, which could result in mutagenesis [85]. In support of the hypothesis of a tumorigenic effect of the SULT1A1, several studies have shown that an increased expression of the SULT1A1 mRNA expression levels contributes to PCa development [86,87]. Although our functional experiments were conducted in a cohort of healthy donors and, therefore, cannot be directly translated to a disease context, our experimental data are in agreement with previous studies, and suggest that the protective effect attributed to the $HNF1B_{rs7501939}$ and $HNF1B_{rs757210}$ SNPs could be mediated by a reduction in the expression of the SULT1A1 protein. Furthermore, it has been reported that the $HNF1B_{rs7501939}$, $HNF1B_{rs757210}$, and $HNF1B_{rs4430796}$ SNPs are modestly associated with mRNA $HNF1B$ expression levels in peripheral blood, which might help to explain how these genetic variants may influence the risk of developing PCa [77]. However, despite these interesting data, we think that the biological link between the $HNF1B$ locus and SULT1A1 is still speculative and needs to be further explored and validated, since, if confirmed, it might represent a potentially interesting therapeutic target. An option to confirm this hypothesis would be to measure SULT1A1 levels in tumoral tissues.

Besides these results, this study also confirmed the association of the FTO locus with PCa risk. The FTO gene is located on chromosome 16q12.2, and it has been implicated in determining not only obesity, but also other symptoms of the metabolic syndrome. In addition, it has been reported that the FTO gene acts as a tumor suppressor gene by regulating the proliferation, migration, and invasion of PCa cells, and the *FTO* expression level had a relevance with the development of PCa and the prognosis of PCa patients [88]. Although the association of the $FTO_{rs9939609}$ polymorphism with PCa risk was weak in all previous studies, and might depend on different confounding factors, the meta-analysis performed in this study confirmed a strong and consistent association of this intronic variant with a decreased risk of PCa. A recent study also demonstrated that the association of the $FTO_{rs9939609}$ SNP with a decreased risk of PCa was found in non-European populations, and that the presence of this genetic marker tended to be associated with disease severity in patients that were overweighted [89]. These findings, together with the lack of significant results in our functional studies, suggest that the role of the *FTO* locus in determining PCa might be mediated by complex obesogenic and/or diabetogenic mechanisms. In support of this hypothesis, we found that the association of the $FTO_{rs9939609}$ SNP with a decreased risk of PCa showed a similar direction to the one observed in the GWAS for T2D.

Similarly, we also found that the presence of the $JAZF1_{rs10486567}$ SNP was inversely associated with the risk of developing PCa. These results were again in concordance with previous GWAS that have consistently reported that *JAZF1* is a susceptibility locus for PCa [84,90–93]. The JAZF1 gene is located at 7p15, and it encodes for a zinc finger protein that is overexpressed in the human prostate tissue where it induces cell proliferation, migration, and invasion, and tumor development [94]. Even though there is not much evidence about the functional role of the $JAZF1_{rs10486567}$ SNP in PCa, it has been demonstrated that the deletion of the JAZF1 locus is associated with reduced levels of IGF-1 and insulin resistance in mice [95], which suggests that the presence of functional polymorphisms within this locus might act to promote PCa development through diabetogenic mechanisms.

Finally, although the association was not statistically significant after correction for multiple testing, it seems to be reasonable to suggest that genetic variants within the *NOTCH2* and *RBMS1* genes could weakly influence the risk of developing PCa. In this regard, it has been reported that genes of the *NOTCH* family play a relevant role in multiple cancers, including PCa, and that their deregulation may be a key event in tumor onset and disease progression [96–102]. The human *NOTCH2* locus is located in the chromosomal region 1p11.2, and it plays an important role in modulating prostate development and homeostasis, and its deregulation induces proliferation and expansion of both basal and luminal cells in the prostate [97]. In addition, it has been reported that NOTCH activity promotes prostate cancer cell migration [97], invasion [96,97], aggressiveness [98], and metastasis [99], and that its silencing induces apoptosis and increases the chemosensitivity of PCa cells [100]. However, a tumor suppressive role of the NOTCH pathway has also been suggested in the literature [103,104], which points towards the need of additional studies to elucidate the role of these genes in the etiopathogenesis of PCa. On the other hand, the meta-analysis of all study cohorts suggested that carriers of the $RBMS1_{rs7593730T}$ allele had an increased risk of developing PCa. The *RBMS1* gene is located at chromosome 2q24.2, and it encodes for a protein that binds single stranded DNA/RNA and plays an important role in DNA replication, cell cycle progression, gene transcription, and apoptosis. A recent study demonstrated that the *RBMS1* locus acts by regulating the expression of the miR-106b [105], which has been found overexpressed in hepatocellular carcinoma [106], cervical cancer [107], renal carcinoma [108], and gastric cancer [109]. At the same time, Dankert and collaborators have also demostrated that miR-106b can regulate endogenous *RBMS1* expression in PCa cell lines and, thereby, act as a tumor suppressor gene with inhibitory effects on colony formation and cell growth [105]. Despite the lack of evidence linking *RBMS1* SNPs and risk of PCa, it seems to be plausible to suggest that the presence of genetic variants in the *RBMS1* locus might control miR-106b levels and, therefore, favors tumorigenesis. In support of this hypothesis, haploreg data showed that the $RBMS1_{rs7593730}$ SNP is associated with different mRNA *RBMS1* expression levels in several tissues and cells [77], and that it maps among histone marks in multiple tissues and several immune cells, and changed regulatory motifs for multiple regulatory transcription factors. Nonetheless, although interesting, the effect of *NOTCH2* and *RBMS1* SNPs on PCa risk must be considered as preliminary and, therefore, needs to be further confirmed in independent cohorts.

This study has both strengths and weaknesses. The major strength of this study is the large number of genetic markers analyzed that allowed us to perform a well-powered meta-analysis of our data with those from previous studies. The meta-analysis of all study cohorts allowed us to not only confirm previous associations between T2D-related polymorphisms and PCa risk, but also to identify potentially interesting genetic markers for the disease. Although the discovery population was relatively small and the influence of diabetogenic variants on the risk of the disease was expected to be modest, our study was sufficiently powered to detect such small effects. Based on the genotype frequencies observed in our study cohort, we had 80% of power (log-additive model) to detect an odds ratio of 1.59 at alpha = 0.00048 (multiple testing threshold) for a polymorphism with a minor allele frequency of 0.25. Likewise, we comprehensively analyzed the impact of T2D-related SNPs in modulating immune responses, blood cell counts, steroid hormones, and serum and plasma metabolites in a relatively large cohort of healthy subjects. However, we also have important limitations. One of them was the fact that functional characterization of the most interesting SNPs was conducted in a healthy control cohort rather than in PCa patients. In addition, we did not have access to medication history, T2D status, and BMI for a substantial number of PCa cases included in the meta-analyses, which did not allow us to adjust our analyses for these confounding variables and, consequently, to rule out the possibility that some of the reported associations could arise as a result of a different distributions of diabetic and/or obese subjects between PCa cases and controls, or because of the effect of diabetes medication rather than the diabetes condition itself. Nonetheless, previous studies have reported that the effect of T2D-related variants on the risk of PCa was independent of T2D status and BMI.

5. Conclusions

In conclusion, our study indicates that T2D-related variants within the *HNF1B*, *FTO*, and *JAZF1* genes influence the risk of PCa likely through the modulation of diabetogenic pathways, and suggests, for the first time, an association of SNPs within the *NOTCH2* and *RBMS1* loci that need to be validated in independent cohorts. This study also suggests that the effect of the *HFN1B* SNPs on PCa risk might be mediated by not only the ST1A1 protein, but also *HFN1B* mRNA expression levels, whereas the effect of the *FTO*, *JAZF1*, *NOTCH2*, and *RBMS1* SNPs on PCa risk seem to be involved in the regulation of mRNA expression levels of their respective genes.

Supplementary Materials: The following supporting information can be downloaded at: https://www.mdpi.com/article/10.3390/cancers14102376/s1. Table S1: Cell types analyzed either in whole blood or peripheral mononuclear blood cells; Table S2: Serum and plasma metabolites measured in the HFGP cohort; Table S3: Summary of functional and regulatory annotation of the most significant SNPs.

Author Contributions: J.S. and M.J.Á.-C. conceived the study and participated in its design and coordination. R.C., A.J.C.-S., F.J.G.-V., F.G.-M., J.A.L.L., I.R.-F., V.A.-R., B.C.-G., P.S.-R., M.I.B.-F., J.O.-R., M.Á.L.-N., L.F.-P., J.M.C.-O., M.J., J.A.L. and M.J.Á.-C. coordinated patient recruitment and provided the clinical data. J.M.S.-M. performed the genetic experiments and R.T.H., O.B., M.G.N. and Y.L. provided functional data. J.S. and A.J.C.-S. performed all statistical analyses and drafted the manuscript. All authors have read and agreed to the published version of the manuscript.

Funding: This study was supported by grants from the FIBAO foundation (Granada, Spain) and from the Instituto de Salud Carlos III (PI12/02688, PI17/02256 and PI20/01845; Madrid, Spain).

Institutional Review Board Statement: The study was conducted according to the guidelines of the Declaration of Helsinki, and approved by the Institutional Review Boards of all institutions participating in patient recruitment (Virgen de las Nieves University Hospital, 18012, Granada, Spain; Hospital de San Pedro Alcántara, 10003, Cáceres, Spain).

Informed Consent Statement: Informed consent was obtained from all subjects involved in the study.

Data Availability Statement: The genotype data used in the present study are available from the corresponding authors upon reasonable request. Functional data used in this project have been meticulously catalogued and archived in the BBMRI-NL data infrastructure (https://hfgp.bbmri.nl/, accessed on 7 July 2020) using the MOLGENIS open-source platform for scientific data [52]. This allows flexible data querying and download, including sufficiently rich metadata and interfaces for machine processing (R statistics, REST API), and using FAIR principles to optimize findability, accessibility, interoperability, and reusability [53,54].

Acknowledgments: We kindly thank all individuals who agreed to participate in the study, as well as all cooperating physicians and students.

Conflicts of Interest: The authors declare no conflict of interest.

References

1. Siegel, R.L.; Fedewa, S.A.; Miller, K.D.; Goding-Sauer, A.; Pinheiro, P.S.; Martinez-Tyson, D.; Jemal, A. Cancer statistics for Hispanics/Latinos, 2015. *CA Cancer J. Clin.* **2015**, *65*, 457–480. [CrossRef]
2. Sung, H.; Ferlay, J.; Siegel, R.L.; Laversanne, M.; Soerjomataram, I.; Jemal, A.; Bray, F. Global Cancer Statistics 2020: GLOBOCAN Estimates of Incidence and Mortality Worldwide for 36 Cancers in 185 Countries. *CA Cancer. J. Clin.* **2021**, *71*, 209–249. [CrossRef]
3. Weiner, A.B.; Matulewicz, R.S.; Eggener, S.E.; Schaeffer, E.M. Increasing incidence of metastatic prostate cancer in the United States (2004–2013). *Prostate Cancer Prostatic Dis.* **2016**, *19*, 395–397. [CrossRef]
4. Wong, M.C.; Goggins, W.B.; Wang, H.H.; Fung, F.D.; Leung, C.; Wong, S.Y.; Ng, C.F.; Sung, J.J. Global Incidence and Mortality for Prostate Cancer: Analysis of Temporal Patterns and Trends in 36 Countries. *Eur. Urol.* **2016**, *70*, 862–874. [CrossRef]
5. Hodson, R. Prostate cancer: 4 big questions. *Nature* **2015**, *528*, S137. [CrossRef] [PubMed]
6. Eeles, R.; Goh, C.; Castro, E.; Bancroft, E.; Guy, M.; Al Olama, A.A.; Easton, D.; Kote-Jarai, Z. The genetic epidemiology of prostate cancer and its clinical implications. *Nat. Rev. Urol.* **2014**, *11*, 18–31. [CrossRef] [PubMed]
7. Khan, A.E.; Gallo, V.; Linseisen, J.; Kaaks, R.; Rohrmann, S.; Raaschou-Nielsen, O.; Tjonneland, A.; Johnsen, H.E.; Overvad, K.; Bergmann, M.M.; et al. Diabetes and the risk of non-Hodgkin's lymphoma and multiple myeloma in the European Prospective Investigation into Cancer and Nutrition. *Haematologica* **2008**, *93*, 842–850. [CrossRef] [PubMed]
8. Richardson, P.G.; Sonneveld, P.; Schuster, M.W.; Stadtmauer, E.A.; Facon, T.; Harousseau, J.L.; Ben-Yehuda, D.; Lonial, S.; Goldschmidt, H.; Reece, D.; et al. Reversibility of symptomatic peripheral neuropathy with bortezomib in the phase III APEX trial in relapsed multiple myeloma: Impact of a dose-modification guideline. *Br. J. Haematol.* **2009**, *144*, 895–903. [CrossRef]
9. Castillo, J.J.; Mull, N.; Reagan, J.L.; Nemr, S.; Mitri, J. Increased incidence of non-Hodgkin lymphoma, leukemia, and myeloma in patients with diabetes mellitus type 2: A meta-analysis of observational studies. *Blood* **2012**, *119*, 4845–4850. [CrossRef]
10. Haring, A.; Murtola, T.J.; Talala, K.; Taari, K.; Tammela, T.L.; Auvinen, A. Antidiabetic drug use and prostate cancer risk in the Finnish Randomized Study of Screening for Prostate Cancer. *Scand. J. Urol.* **2017**, *51*, 5–12. [CrossRef]
11. Murtola, T.J.; Tammela, T.L.; Lahtela, J.; Auvinen, A. Antidiabetic medication and prostate cancer risk: A population-based case-control study. *Am. J. Epidemiol.* **2008**, *168*, 925–931. [CrossRef]
12. Haggstrom, C.; Van Hemelrijck, M.; Zethelius, B.; Robinson, D.; Grundmark, B.; Holmberg, L.; Gudbjornsdottir, S.; Garmo, H.; Stattin, P. Prospective study of Type 2 diabetes mellitus, anti-diabetic drugs and risk of prostate cancer. *Int. J. Cancer* **2017**, *140*, 611–617. [CrossRef]
13. Frayling, T.M.; Colhoun, H.; Florez, J.C. A genetic link between type 2 diabetes and prostate cancer. *Diabetologia* **2008**, *51*, 1757–1760. [CrossRef]
14. Gudmundsson, J.; Sulem, P.; Steinthorsdottir, V.; Bergthorsson, J.T.; Thorleifsson, G.; Manolescu, A.; Rafnar, T.; Gudbjartsson, D.; Agnarsson, B.A.; Baker, A.; et al. Two variants on chromosome 17 confer prostate cancer risk, and the one in TCF2 protects against type 2 diabetes. *Nat. Genet.* **2007**, *39*, 977–983. [CrossRef]
15. Winckler, W.; Weedon, M.N.; Graham, R.R.; McCarroll, S.A.; Purcell, S.; Almgren, P.; Tuomi, T.; Gaudet, D.; Bostrom, K.B.; Walker, M.; et al. Evaluation of common variants in the six known maturity-onset diabetes of the young (MODY) genes for association with type 2 diabetes. *Diabetes* **2007**, *56*, 685–693. [CrossRef]
16. Horikawa, Y.; Iwasaki, N.; Hara, M.; Furuta, H.; Hinokio, Y.; Cockburn, B.N.; Lindner, T.; Yamagata, K.; Ogata, M.; Tomonaga, O.; et al. Mutation in hepatocyte nuclear factor-1 beta gene (TCF2) associated with MODY. *Nat. Genet.* **1997**, *17*, 384–385. [CrossRef]
17. Rios, R.; Lupianez, C.B.; Campa, D.; Martino, A.; Martinez-Lopez, J.; Martinez-Bueno, M.; Varkonyi, J.; Garcia-Sanz, R.; Jamroziak, K.; Dumontet, C.; et al. Type 2 diabetes-related variants influence the risk of developing multiple myeloma: Results from the IMMEnSE consortium. *Endocr.-Relat. Cancer* **2015**, *22*, 545–559. [CrossRef]
18. Sainz, J.; Rudolph, A.; Hoffmeister, M.; Frank, B.; Brenner, H.; Chang-Claude, J.; Hemminki, K.; Forsti, A. Effect of type 2 diabetes predisposing genetic variants on colorectal cancer risk. *J. Clin. Endocrinol. Metab.* **2012**, *97*, E845–E851. [CrossRef]
19. Zhao, Z.; Wen, W.; Michailidou, K.; Bolla, M.K.; Wang, Q.; Zhang, B.; Long, J.; Shu, X.O.; Schmidt, M.K.; Milne, R.L.; et al. Association of genetic susceptibility variants for type 2 diabetes with breast cancer risk in women of European ancestry. *Cancer Causes Control* **2016**, *27*, 679–693. [CrossRef]
20. Pierce, B.L.; Ahsan, H. Genetic susceptibility to type 2 diabetes is associated with reduced prostate cancer risk. *Hum. Hered.* **2010**, *69*, 193–201. [CrossRef]

21. Stevens, V.L.; Ahn, J.; Sun, J.; Jacobs, E.J.; Moore, S.C.; Patel, A.V.; Berndt, S.I.; Albanes, D.; Hayes, R.B. HNF1B and JAZF1 genes, diabetes, and prostate cancer risk. *Prostate* **2010**, *70*, 601–607. [CrossRef]
22. Machiela, M.J.; Lindstrom, S.; Allen, N.E.; Haiman, C.A.; Albanes, D.; Barricarte, A.; Berndt, S.I.; Bueno-de-Mesquita, H.B.; Chanock, S.; Gaziano, J.M.; et al. Association of type 2 diabetes susceptibility variants with advanced prostate cancer risk in the Breast and Prostate Cancer Cohort Consortium. *Am. J. Epidemiol.* **2012**, *176*, 1121–1129. [CrossRef]
23. Waters, K.M.; Wilkens, L.R.; Monroe, K.R.; Stram, D.O.; Kolonel, L.N.; Henderson, B.E.; Le Marchand, L.; Haiman, C.A. No association of type 2 diabetes risk variants and prostate cancer risk: The multiethnic cohort and PAGE. *Cancer Epidemiol. Biomark. Prev.* **2011**, *20*, 1979–1981. [CrossRef]
24. Mottet, N.; Bellmunt, J.; Bolla, M.; Briers, E.; Cumberbatch, M.G.; De Santis, M.; Fossati, N.; Gross, T.; Henry, A.M.; Joniau, S.; et al. EAU-ESTRO-SIOG Guidelines on Prostate Cancer. Part 1: Screening, Diagnosis, and Local Treatment with Curative Intent. *Eur. Urol.* **2017**, *71*, 618–629. [CrossRef]
25. Lyssenko, V.; Nagorny, C.L.; Erdos, M.R.; Wierup, N.; Jonsson, A.; Spegel, P.; Bugliani, M.; Saxena, R.; Fex, M.; Pulizzi, N.; et al. Common variant in MTNR1B associated with increased risk of type 2 diabetes and impaired early insulin secretion. *Nat. Genet.* **2009**, *41*, 82–88. [CrossRef]
26. Zeggini, E.; Scott, L.J.; Saxena, R.; Voight, B.F.; Marchini, J.L.; Hu, T.; de Bakker, P.I.; Abecasis, G.R.; Almgren, P.; Andersen, G.; et al. Meta-analysis of genome-wide association data and large-scale replication identifies additional susceptibility loci for type 2 diabetes. *Nat. Genet.* **2008**, *40*, 638–645. [CrossRef]
27. Mohlke, K.L.; Boehnke, M.; Abecasis, G.R. Metabolic and cardiovascular traits: An abundance of recently identified common genetic variants. *Hum. Mol. Genet.* **2008**, *17*, R102–R108. [CrossRef]
28. Shu, X.O.; Long, J.; Cai, Q.; Qi, L.; Xiang, Y.B.; Cho, Y.S.; Tai, E.S.; Li, X.; Lin, X.; Chow, W.H.; et al. Identification of new genetic risk variants for type 2 diabetes. *PLoS Genet.* **2010**, *6*, e1001127. [CrossRef] [PubMed]
29. Dupuis, J.; Langenberg, C.; Prokopenko, I.; Saxena, R.; Soranzo, N.; Jackson, A.U.; Wheeler, E.; Glazer, N.L.; Bouatia-Naji, N.; Gloyn, A.L.; et al. New genetic loci implicated in fasting glucose homeostasis and their impact on type 2 diabetes risk. *Nat. Genet.* **2010**, *42*, 105–116. [CrossRef] [PubMed]
30. Saxena, R.; Hivert, M.F.; Langenberg, C.; Tanaka, T.; Pankow, J.S.; Vollenweider, P.; Lyssenko, V.; Bouatia-Naji, N.; Dupuis, J.; Jackson, A.U.; et al. Genetic variation in GIPR influences the glucose and insulin responses to an oral glucose challenge. *Nat. Genet.* **2010**, *42*, 142–148. [CrossRef] [PubMed]
31. Voight, B.F.; Scott, L.J.; Steinthorsdottir, V.; Morris, A.P.; Dina, C.; Welch, R.P.; Zeggini, E.; Huth, C.; Aulchenko, Y.S.; Thorleifsson, G.; et al. Twelve type 2 diabetes susceptibility loci identified through large-scale association analysis. *Nat. Genet.* **2010**, *42*, 579–589. [CrossRef]
32. Nielsen, T.; Sparso, T.; Grarup, N.; Jorgensen, T.; Pisinger, C.; Witte, D.R.; Diabetes Genetics, R.; Meta-analysis, C.; Hansen, T.; Pedersen, O. Type 2 diabetes risk allele near CENTD2 is associated with decreased glucose-stimulated insulin release. *Diabetologia* **2011**, *54*, 1052–1056. [CrossRef]
33. Saxena, R.; Voight, B.F.; Lyssenko, V.; Burtt, N.P.; de Bakker, P.I.; Chen, H.; Roix, J.J.; Kathiresan, S.; Hirschhorn, J.N.; Daly, M.J.; et al. Genome-wide association analysis identifies loci for type 2 diabetes and triglyceride levels. *Science* **2007**, *316*, 1331–1336. [CrossRef]
34. Florez, J.C.; Manning, A.K.; Dupuis, J.; McAteer, J.; Irenze, K.; Gianniny, L.; Mirel, D.B.; Fox, C.S.; Cupples, L.A.; Meigs, J.B. A 100K genome-wide association scan for diabetes and related traits in the Framingham Heart Study: Replication and integration with other genome-wide datasets. *Diabetes* **2007**, *56*, 3063–3074. [CrossRef]
35. Scott, L.J.; Mohlke, K.L.; Bonnycastle, L.L.; Willer, C.J.; Li, Y.; Duren, W.L.; Erdos, M.R.; Stringham, H.M.; Chines, P.S.; Jackson, A.U.; et al. A genome-wide association study of type 2 diabetes in Finns detects multiple susceptibility variants. *Science* **2007**, *316*, 1341–1345. [CrossRef]
36. Yamauchi, T.; Hara, K.; Maeda, S.; Yasuda, K.; Takahashi, A.; Horikoshi, M.; Nakamura, M.; Fujita, H.; Grarup, N.; Cauchi, S.; et al. A genome-wide association study in the Japanese population identifies susceptibility loci for type 2 diabetes at UBE2E2 and C2CD4A-C2CD4B. *Nat. Genet.* **2010**, *42*, 864–868. [CrossRef]
37. Takeuchi, F.; Serizawa, M.; Yamamoto, K.; Fujisawa, T.; Nakashima, E.; Ohnaka, K.; Ikegami, H.; Sugiyama, T.; Katsuya, T.; Miyagishi, M.; et al. Confirmation of multiple risk Loci and genetic impacts by a genome-wide association study of type 2 diabetes in the Japanese population. *Diabetes* **2009**, *58*, 1690–1699. [CrossRef]
38. Bouatia-Naji, N.; Bonnefond, A.; Cavalcanti-Proenca, C.; Sparso, T.; Holmkvist, J.; Marchand, M.; Delplanque, J.; Lobbens, S.; Rocheleau, G.; Durand, E.; et al. A variant near MTNR1B is associated with increased fasting plasma glucose levels and type 2 diabetes risk. *Nat. Genet.* **2009**, *41*, 89–94. [CrossRef]
39. Sladek, R.; Rocheleau, G.; Rung, J.; Dina, C.; Shen, L.; Serre, D.; Boutin, P.; Vincent, D.; Belisle, A.; Hadjadj, S.; et al. A genome-wide association study identifies novel risk loci for type 2 diabetes. *Nature* **2007**, *445*, 881–885. [CrossRef]
40. Chambers, J.C.; Elliott, P.; Zabaneh, D.; Zhang, W.; Li, Y.; Froguel, P.; Balding, D.; Scott, J.; Kooner, J.S. Common genetic variation near MC4R is associated with waist circumference and insulin resistance. *Nat. Genet.* **2008**, *40*, 716–718. [CrossRef]
41. Wellcome Trust Case Control Consortium. Genome-wide association study of 14,000 cases of seven common diseases and 3000 shared controls. *Nature* **2007**, *447*, 661–678. [CrossRef]

42. Zeggini, E.; Weedon, M.N.; Lindgren, C.M.; Frayling, T.M.; Elliott, K.S.; Lango, H.; Timpson, N.J.; Perry, J.R.; Rayner, N.W.; Freathy, R.M.; et al. Replication of genome-wide association signals in UK samples reveals risk loci for type 2 diabetes. *Science* **2007**, *316*, 1336–1341. [CrossRef]
43. Bouatia-Naji, N.; Rocheleau, G.; Van Lommel, L.; Lemaire, K.; Schuit, F.; Cavalcanti-Proenca, C.; Marchand, M.; Hartikainen, A.L.; Sovio, U.; De Graeve, F.; et al. A polymorphism within the G6PC2 gene is associated with fasting plasma glucose levels. *Science* **2008**, *320*, 1085–1088. [CrossRef]
44. Chen, W.M.; Erdos, M.R.; Jackson, A.U.; Saxena, R.; Sanna, S.; Silver, K.D.; Timpson, N.J.; Hansen, T.; Orru, M.; Grazia Piras, M.; et al. Variations in the G6PC2/ABCB11 genomic region are associated with fasting glucose levels. *J. Clin. Investig.* **2008**, *118*, 2620–2628. [CrossRef]
45. Prokopenko, I.; Langenberg, C.; Florez, J.C.; Saxena, R.; Soranzo, N.; Thorleifsson, G.; Loos, R.J.; Manning, A.K.; Jackson, A.U.; Aulchenko, Y.; et al. Variants in MTNR1B influence fasting glucose levels. *Nat. Genet.* **2009**, *41*, 77–81. [CrossRef]
46. Vujkovic, M.; Keaton, J.M.; Lynch, J.A.; Miller, D.R.; Zhou, J.; Tcheandjieu, C.; Huffman, J.E.; Assimes, T.L.; Lorenz, K.; Zhu, X.; et al. Discovery of 318 new risk loci for type 2 diabetes and related vascular outcomes among 1.4 million participants in a multi-ancestry meta-analysis. *Nat. Genet.* **2020**, *52*, 680–691. [CrossRef]
47. Kichaev, G.; Bhatia, G.; Loh, P.R.; Gazal, S.; Burch, K.; Freund, M.K.; Schoech, A.; Pasaniuc, B.; Price, A.L. Leveraging Polygenic Functional Enrichment to Improve GWAS Power. *Am. J. Hum. Genet.* **2019**, *104*, 65–75. [CrossRef] [PubMed]
48. Mahajan, A.; Taliun, D.; Thurner, M.; Robertson, N.R.; Torres, J.M.; Rayner, N.W.; Payne, A.J.; Steinthorsdottir, V.; Scott, R.A.; Grarup, N.; et al. Fine-mapping type 2 diabetes loci to single-variant resolution using high-density imputation and islet-specific epigenome maps. *Nat. Genet.* **2018**, *50*, 1505–1513. [CrossRef]
49. Mahajan, A.; Wessel, J.; Willems, S.M.; Zhao, W.; Robertson, N.R.; Chu, A.Y.; Gan, W.; Kitajima, H.; Taliun, D.; Rayner, N.W.; et al. Refining the accuracy of validated target identification through coding variant fine-mapping in type 2 diabetes. *Nat. Genet.* **2018**, *50*, 559–571. [CrossRef]
50. Sandhu, M.S.; Weedon, M.N.; Fawcett, K.A.; Wasson, J.; Debenham, S.L.; Daly, A.; Lango, H.; Frayling, T.M.; Neumann, R.J.; Sherva, R.; et al. Common variants in WFS1 confer risk of type 2 diabetes. *Nat. Genet.* **2007**, *39*, 951–953. [CrossRef]
51. Pechlivanis, S.; Wagner, K.; Chang-Claude, J.; Hoffmeister, M.; Brenner, H.; Forsti, A. Polymorphisms in the insulin like growth factor 1 and IGF binding protein 3 genes and risk of colorectal cancer. *Cancer Detect. Prev.* **2007**, *31*, 408–416. [CrossRef] [PubMed]
52. Rung, J.; Cauchi, S.; Albrechtsen, A.; Shen, L.; Rocheleau, G.; Cavalcanti-Proenca, C.; Bacot, F.; Balkau, B.; Belisle, A.; Borch-Johnsen, K.; et al. Genetic variant near IRS1 is associated with type 2 diabetes, insulin resistance and hyperinsulinemia. *Nat. Genet.* **2009**, *41*, 1110–1115. [CrossRef] [PubMed]
53. Tang, Y.; Han, X.; Sun, X.; Lv, C.; Zhang, X.; Guo, W.; Ren, Q.; Luo, Y.; Zhang, X.; Zhou, X.; et al. Association study of a common variant near IRS1 with type 2 diabetes mellitus in Chinese Han population. *Endocrine* **2013**, *43*, 84–91. [CrossRef] [PubMed]
54. Willer, C.J.; Bonnycastle, L.L.; Conneely, K.N.; Duren, W.L.; Jackson, A.U.; Scott, L.J.; Narisu, N.; Chines, P.S.; Skol, A.; Stringham, H.M.; et al. Screening of 134 single nucleotide polymorphisms (SNPs) previously associated with type 2 diabetes replicates association with 12 SNPs in nine genes. *Diabetes* **2007**, *56*, 256–264. [CrossRef]
55. Gloyn, A.L.; Weedon, M.N.; Owen, K.R.; Turner, M.J.; Knight, B.A.; Hitman, G.; Walker, M.; Levy, J.C.; Sampson, M.; Halford, S.; et al. Large-scale association studies of variants in genes encoding the pancreatic beta-cell KATP channel subunits Kir6.2 (KCNJ11) and SUR1 (ABCC8) confirm that the KCNJ11 E23K variant is associated with type 2 diabetes. *Diabetes* **2003**, *52*, 568–572. [CrossRef]
56. Unoki, H.; Takahashi, A.; Kawaguchi, T.; Hara, K.; Horikoshi, M.; Andersen, G.; Ng, D.P.; Holmkvist, J.; Borch-Johnsen, K.; Jorgensen, T.; et al. SNPs in KCNQ1 are associated with susceptibility to type 2 diabetes in East Asian and European populations. *Nat. Genet.* **2008**, *40*, 1098–1102. [CrossRef]
57. Tsai, F.J.; Yang, C.F.; Chen, C.C.; Chuang, L.M.; Lu, C.H.; Chang, C.T.; Wang, T.Y.; Chen, R.H.; Shiu, C.F.; Liu, Y.M.; et al. A genome-wide association study identifies susceptibility variants for type 2 diabetes in Han Chinese. *PLoS Genet.* **2010**, *6*, e1000847. [CrossRef]
58. Yasuda, K.; Miyake, K.; Horikawa, Y.; Hara, K.; Osawa, H.; Furuta, H.; Hirota, Y.; Mori, H.; Jonsson, A.; Sato, Y.; et al. Variants in KCNQ1 are associated with susceptibility to type 2 diabetes mellitus. *Nat. Genet.* **2008**, *40*, 1092–1097. [CrossRef]
59. Hamid, Y.H.; Urhammer, S.A.; Glumer, C.; Borch-Johnsen, K.; Jorgensen, T.; Hansen, T.; Pedersen, O. The common T60N polymorphism of the lymphotoxin-alpha gene is associated with type 2 diabetes and other phenotypes of the metabolic syndrome. *Diabetologia* **2005**, *48*, 445–451. [CrossRef]
60. Altshuler, D.; Hirschhorn, J.N.; Klannemark, M.; Lindgren, C.M.; Vohl, M.C.; Nemesh, J.; Lane, C.R.; Schaffner, S.F.; Bolk, S.; Brewer, C.; et al. The common PPARgamma Pro12Ala polymorphism is associated with decreased risk of type 2 diabetes. *Nat. Genet.* **2000**, *26*, 76–80. [CrossRef]
61. Qi, L.; Cornelis, M.C.; Kraft, P.; Stanya, K.J.; Linda Kao, W.H.; Pankow, J.S.; Dupuis, J.; Florez, J.C.; Fox, C.S.; Pare, G.; et al. Genetic variants at 2q24 are associated with susceptibility to type 2 diabetes. *Hum. Mol. Genet.* **2010**, *19*, 2706–2715. [CrossRef]
62. Morris, A.P.; Voight, B.F.; Teslovich, T.M.; Ferreira, T.; Segre, A.V.; Steinthorsdottir, V.; Strawbridge, R.J.; Khan, H.; Grallert, H.; Mahajan, A.; et al. Large-scale association analysis provides insights into the genetic architecture and pathophysiology of type 2 diabetes. *Nat. Genet.* **2012**, *44*, 981–990. [CrossRef]

63. Steinthorsdottir, V.; Thorleifsson, G.; Reynisdottir, I.; Benediktsson, R.; Jonsdottir, T.; Walters, G.B.; Styrkarsdottir, U.; Gretarsdottir, S.; Emilsson, V.; Ghosh, S.; et al. A variant in CDKAL1 influences insulin response and risk of type 2 diabetes. *Nat. Genet.* **2007**, *39*, 770–775. [CrossRef]
64. Grant, S.F.; Thorleifsson, G.; Reynisdottir, I.; Benediktsson, R.; Manolescu, A.; Sainz, J.; Helgason, A.; Stefansson, H.; Emilsson, V.; Helgadottir, A.; et al. Variant of transcription factor 7-like 2 (TCF7L2) gene confers risk of type 2 diabetes. *Nat. Genet.* **2006**, *38*, 320–323. [CrossRef]
65. Scott, L.J.; Bonnycastle, L.L.; Willer, C.J.; Sprau, A.G.; Jackson, A.U.; Narisu, N.; Duren, W.L.; Chines, P.S.; Stringham, H.M.; Erdos, M.R.; et al. Association of transcription factor 7-like 2 (TCF7L2) variants with type 2 diabetes in a Finnish sample. *Diabetes* **2006**, *55*, 2649–2653. [CrossRef]
66. Peng, S.; Zhu, Y.; Lu, B.; Xu, F.; Li, X.; Lai, M. TCF7L2 gene polymorphisms and type 2 diabetes risk: A comprehensive and updated meta-analysis involving 121,174 subjects. *Mutagenesis* **2013**, *28*, 25–37. [CrossRef]
67. Zhao, W.; Rasheed, A.; Tikkanen, E.; Lee, J.J.; Butterworth, A.S.; Howson, J.M.M.; Assimes, T.L.; Chowdhury, R.; Orho-Melander, M.; Damrauer, S.; et al. Identification of new susceptibility loci for type 2 diabetes and shared etiological pathways with coronary heart disease. *Nat. Genet.* **2017**, *49*, 1450–1457. [CrossRef]
68. Chen, J.; Spracklen, C.N.; Marenne, G.; Varshney, A.; Corbin, L.J.; Luan, J.; Willems, S.M.; Wu, Y.; Zhang, X.; Horikoshi, M.; et al. The trans-ancestral genomic architecture of glycemic traits. *Nat. Genet.* **2021**, *53*, 840–860. [CrossRef]
69. Grarup, N.; Andersen, G.; Krarup, N.T.; Albrechtsen, A.; Schmitz, O.; Jorgensen, T.; Borch-Johnsen, K.; Hansen, T.; Pedersen, O. Association testing of novel type 2 diabetes risk alleles in the JAZF1, CDC123/CAMK1D, TSPAN8, THADA, ADAMTS9, and NOTCH2 loci with insulin release, insulin sensitivity, and obesity in a population-based sample of 4516 glucose-tolerant middle-aged Danes. *Diabetes* **2008**, *57*, 2534–2540. [CrossRef]
70. Gagliano Taliun, S.A.; VandeHaar, P.; Boughton, A.P.; Welch, R.P.; Taliun, D.; Schmidt, E.M.; Zhou, W.; Nielsen, J.B.; Willer, C.J.; Lee, S.; et al. Exploring and visualizing large-scale genetic associations by using PheWeb. *Nat. Genet.* **2020**, *52*, 550–552. [CrossRef]
71. Berndt, S.I.; Sampson, J.; Yeager, M.; Jacobs, K.B.; Wang, Z.; Hutchinson, A.; Chung, C.; Orr, N.; Wacholder, S.; Chatterjee, N.; et al. Large-scale fine mapping of the HNF1B locus and prostate cancer risk. *Hum. Mol. Genet.* **2011**, *20*, 3322–3329. [CrossRef]
72. Li, Y.; Oosting, M.; Smeekens, S.P.; Jaeger, M.; Aguirre-Gamboa, R.; Le, K.T.T.; Deelen, P.; Ricano-Ponce, I.; Schoffelen, T.; Jansen, A.F.M.; et al. A Functional Genomics Approach to Understand Variation in Cytokine Production in Humans. *Cell* **2016**, *167*, 1099–1110.e1014. [CrossRef]
73. Schirmer, M.; Smeekens, S.P.; Vlamakis, H.; Jaeger, M.; Oosting, M.; Franzosa, E.A.; Horst, R.T.; Jansen, T.; Jacobs, L.; Bonder, M.J.; et al. Linking the Human Gut Microbiome to Inflammatory Cytokine Production Capacity. *Cell* **2016**, *167*, 1897.e113. [CrossRef]
74. Ter Horst, R.; Jaeger, M.; Smeekens, S.P.; Oosting, M.; Swertz, M.A.; Li, Y.; Kumar, V.; Diavatopoulos, D.A.; Jansen, A.F.M.; Lemmers, H.; et al. Host and Environmental Factors Influencing Individual Human Cytokine Responses. *Cell* **2016**, *167*, 1111–1124. [CrossRef]
75. Orru, V.; Steri, M.; Sole, G.; Sidore, C.; Virdis, F.; Dei, M.; Lai, S.; Zoledziewska, M.; Busonero, F.; Mulas, A.; et al. Genetic variants regulating immune cell levels in health and disease. *Cell* **2013**, *155*, 242–256. [CrossRef]
76. Aguirre-Gamboa, R.; Joosten, I.; Urbano, P.C.M.; van der Molen, R.G.; van Rijssen, E.; van Cranenbroek, B.; Oosting, M.; Smeekens, S.; Jaeger, M.; Zorro, M.; et al. Differential Effects of Environmental and Genetic Factors on T and B Cell Immune Traits. *Cell Rep* **2016**, *17*, 2474–2487. [CrossRef]
77. Westra, H.J.; Peters, M.J.; Esko, T.; Yaghootkar, H.; Schurmann, C.; Kettunen, J.; Christiansen, M.W.; Fairfax, B.P.; Schramm, K.; Powell, J.E.; et al. Systematic identification of trans eQTLs as putative drivers of known disease associations. *Nat. Genet.* **2013**, *45*, 1238–1243. [CrossRef]
78. Lewis, S.J.; Murad, A.; Chen, L.; Davey Smith, G.; Donovan, J.; Palmer, T.; Hamdy, F.; Neal, D.; Lane, J.A.; Davis, M.; et al. Associations between an obesity related genetic variant (FTO rs9939609) and prostate cancer risk. *PLoS ONE* **2010**, *5*, e13485. [CrossRef]
79. Yu, D.D.; Guo, S.W.; Jing, Y.Y.; Dong, Y.L.; Wei, L.X. A review on hepatocyte nuclear factor-1beta and tumor. *Cell Biosci.* **2015**, *5*, 58. [CrossRef]
80. Rios Tamayo, R.; Lupianez, C.B.; Campa, D.; Hielscher, T.; Weinhold, N.; Martinez-Lopez, J.; Jerez, A.; Landi, S.; Jamroziak, K.; Dumontet, C.; et al. A common variant within the HNF1B gene is associated with overall survival of multiple myeloma patients: Results from the IMMEnSE consortium and meta-analysis. *Oncotarget* **2016**, *7*, 59029–59048. [CrossRef] [PubMed]
81. Silva, T.D.; Vidigal, V.M.; Felipe, A.V.; JM, D.E.L.; Neto, R.A.; Saad, S.S.; Forones, N.M. DNA methylation as an epigenetic biomarker in colorectal cancer. *Oncol. Lett.* **2013**, *6*, 1687–1692. [CrossRef] [PubMed]
82. Kim, L.; Liao, J.; Zhang, M.; Talamonti, M.; Bentrem, D.; Rao, S.; Yang, G.Y. Clear cell carcinoma of the pancreas: Histopathologic features and a unique biomarker: Hepatocyte nuclear factor-1beta. *Mod. Pathol.* **2008**, *21*, 1075–1083. [CrossRef] [PubMed]
83. Eeles, R.A.; Kote-Jarai, Z.; Giles, G.G.; Olama, A.A.; Guy, M.; Jugurnauth, S.K.; Mulholland, S.; Leongamornlert, D.A.; Edwards, S.M.; Morrison, J.; et al. Multiple newly identified loci associated with prostate cancer susceptibility. *Nat. Genet.* **2008**, *40*, 316–321. [CrossRef] [PubMed]
84. Thomas, G.; Jacobs, K.B.; Yeager, M.; Kraft, P.; Wacholder, S.; Orr, N.; Yu, K.; Chatterjee, N.; Welch, R.; Hutchinson, A.; et al. Multiple loci identified in a genome-wide association study of prostate cancer. *Nat. Genet.* **2008**, *40*, 310–315. [CrossRef]
85. Chou, H.C.; Lang, N.P.; Kadlubar, F.F. Metabolic activation of N-hydroxy arylamines and N-hydroxy heterocyclic amines by human sulfotransferase(s). *Cancer Res.* **1995**, *55*, 525–529.

86. Nowell, S.; Ratnasinghe, D.L.; Ambrosone, C.B.; Williams, S.; Teague-Ross, T.; Trimble, L.; Runnels, G.; Carrol, A.; Green, B.; Stone, A.; et al. Association of SULT1A1 phenotype and genotype with prostate cancer risk in African-Americans and Caucasians. *Cancer Epidemiol. Biomark. Prev.* **2004**, *13*, 270–276. [CrossRef]
87. Al-Buheissi, S.Z.; Patel, H.R.; Meinl, W.; Hewer, A.; Bryan, R.L.; Glatt, H.; Miller, R.A.; Phillips, D.H. N-Acetyltransferase and sulfotransferase activity in human prostate: Potential for carcinogen activation. *Pharmacogenet. Genom.* **2006**, *16*, 391–399. [CrossRef]
88. Zhu, K.; Li, Y.; Xu, Y. The FTO m(6)A demethylase inhibits the invasion and migration of prostate cancer cells by regulating total m(6)A levels. *Life Sci.* **2021**, *271*, 119180. [CrossRef]
89. Salgado-Montilla, J.L.; Rodriguez-Caban, J.L.; Sanchez-Garcia, J.; Sanchez-Ortiz, R.; Irizarry-Ramirez, M. Impact of FTO SNPs rs9930506 and rs9939609 in Prostate Cancer Severity in a Cohort of Puerto Rican Men. *Arch. Cancer Res.* **2017**, *5*, 148. [CrossRef]
90. Hoffmann, T.J.; Van Den Eeden, S.K.; Sakoda, L.C.; Jorgenson, E.; Habel, L.A.; Graff, R.E.; Passarelli, M.N.; Cario, C.L.; Emami, N.C.; Chao, C.R.; et al. A large multiethnic genome-wide association study of prostate cancer identifies novel risk variants and substantial ethnic differences. *Cancer Discov.* **2015**, *5*, 878–891. [CrossRef]
91. Hoffmann, T.J.; Passarelli, M.N.; Graff, R.E.; Emami, N.C.; Sakoda, L.C.; Jorgenson, E.; Habel, L.A.; Shan, J.; Ranatunga, D.K.; Quesenberry, C.P.; et al. Genome-wide association study of prostate-specific antigen levels identifies novel loci independent of prostate cancer. *Nat. Commun.* **2017**, *8*, 14248. [CrossRef]
92. Conti, D.V.; Darst, B.F.; Moss, L.C.; Saunders, E.J.; Sheng, X.; Chou, A.; Schumacher, F.R.; Olama, A.A.A.; Benlloch, S.; Dadaev, T.; et al. Trans-ancestry genome-wide association meta-analysis of prostate cancer identifies new susceptibility loci and informs genetic risk prediction. *Nat. Genet.* **2021**, *53*, 65–75. [CrossRef]
93. Schumacher, F.R.; Al Olama, A.A.; Berndt, S.I.; Benlloch, S.; Ahmed, M.; Saunders, E.J.; Dadaev, T.; Leongamornlert, D.; Anokian, E.; Cieza-Borrella, C.; et al. Association analyses of more than 140,000 men identify 63 new prostate cancer susceptibility loci. *Nat. Genet.* **2018**, *50*, 928–936. [CrossRef]
94. Sung, Y.; Park, S.; Park, S.J.; Jeong, J.; Choi, M.; Lee, J.; Kwon, W.; Jang, S.; Lee, M.H.; Kim, D.J.; et al. Jazf1 promotes prostate cancer progression by activating JNK/Slug. *Oncotarget* **2018**, *9*, 755–765. [CrossRef]
95. Lee, H.J.D. Early growth retardation and insulin resistance in JAZF1 KO Mice. *Diabetes* **2011**, *60*, A103.
96. Bin Hafeez, B.; Adhami, V.M.; Asim, M.; Siddiqui, I.A.; Bhat, K.M.; Zhong, W.; Saleem, M.; Din, M.; Setaluri, V.; Mukhtar, H. Targeted knockdown of Notch1 inhibits invasion of human prostate cancer cells concomitant with inhibition of matrix metalloproteinase-9 and urokinase plasminogen activator. *Clin. Cancer Res.* **2009**, *15*, 452–459. [CrossRef]
97. Wang, Z.; Li, Y.; Banerjee, S.; Kong, D.; Ahmad, A.; Nogueira, V.; Hay, N.; Sarkar, F.H. Down-regulation of Notch-1 and Jagged-1 inhibits prostate cancer cell growth, migration and invasion, and induces apoptosis via inactivation of Akt, mTOR, and NF-kappaB signaling pathways. *J. Cell Biochem.* **2010**, *109*, 726–736. [CrossRef]
98. Kashat, M.; Azzouz, L.; Sarkar, S.H.; Kong, D.; Li, Y.; Sarkar, F.H. Inactivation of AR and Notch-1 signaling by miR-34a attenuates prostate cancer aggressiveness. *Am. J. Transl. Res.* **2012**, *4*, 432–442.
99. Zhu, H.; Zhou, X.; Redfield, S.; Lewin, J.; Miele, L. Elevated Jagged-1 and Notch-1 expression in high grade and metastatic prostate cancers. *Am. J. Transl. Res.* **2013**, *5*, 368–378.
100. Ye, Q.F.; Zhang, Y.C.; Peng, X.Q.; Long, Z.; Ming, Y.Z.; He, L.Y. Silencing Notch-1 induces apoptosis and increases the chemosensitivity of prostate cancer cells to docetaxel through Bcl-2 and Bax. *Oncol. Lett.* **2012**, *3*, 879–884. [CrossRef]
101. Than, B.L.; Goos, J.A.; Sarver, A.L.; O'Sullivan, M.G.; Rod, A.; Starr, T.K.; Fijneman, R.J.; Meijer, G.A.; Zhao, L.; Zhang, Y.; et al. The role of KCNQ1 in mouse and human gastrointestinal cancers. *Oncogene* **2014**, *33*, 3861–3868. [CrossRef] [PubMed]
102. Jacobs, D.I.; Mao, Y.; Fu, A.; Kelly, W.K.; Zhu, Y. Dysregulated methylation at imprinted genes in prostate tumor tissue detected by methylation microarray. *BMC Urol.* **2013**, *13*, 37. [CrossRef] [PubMed]
103. Shou, J.; Ross, S.; Koeppen, H.; de Sauvage, F.J.; Gao, W.Q. Dynamics of notch expression during murine prostate development and tumorigenesis. *Cancer Res.* **2001**, *61*, 7291–7297. [PubMed]
104. Whelan, J.T.; Kellogg, A.; Shewchuk, B.M.; Hewan-Lowe, K.; Bertrand, F.E. Notch-1 signaling is lost in prostate adenocarcinoma and promotes PTEN gene expression. *J. Cell. Biochem.* **2009**, *107*, 992–1001. [CrossRef]
105. Dankert, J.T.; Wiesehofer, M.; Wach, S.; Czyrnik, E.D.; Wennemuth, G. Loss of RBMS1 as a regulatory target of miR-106b influences cell growth, gap closing and colony forming in prostate carcinoma. *Sci. Rep.* **2020**, *10*, 18022. [CrossRef]
106. Gu, H.; Gu, S.; Zhang, X.; Zhang, S.; Zhang, D.; Lin, J.; Hasengbayi, S.; Han, W. miR-106b-5p promotes aggressive progression of hepatocellular carcinoma via targeting RUNX3. *Cancer Med.* **2019**, *8*, 6756–6767. [CrossRef]
107. Zong, S.; Liu, X.; Zhou, N.; Yue, Y. E2F7, EREG, miR-451a and miR-106b-5p are associated with the cervical cancer development. *Arch. Gynecol. Obstet.* **2019**, *299*, 1089–1098. [CrossRef]
108. Miao, L.J.; Yan, S.; Zhuang, Q.F.; Mao, Q.Y.; Xue, D.; He, X.Z.; Chen, J.P. miR-106b promotes proliferation and invasion by targeting Capicua through MAPK signaling in renal carcinoma cancer. *OncoTargets Ther.* **2019**, *12*, 3595–3607. [CrossRef]
109. Yuan, C.; Zhang, Y.; Tu, W.; Guo, Y. Integrated miRNA profiling and bioinformatics analyses reveal upregulated miRNAs in gastric cancer. *Oncol. Lett.* **2019**, *18*, 1979–1988. [CrossRef]

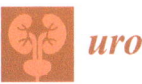 uro

Review

Recent Advances in Prostate Cancer (PCa) Diagnostics

Ahmad Abdelrazek [1,*], Ahmed M. Mahmoud [2,*], Vidhu B. Joshi [3], Mohamed Habeeb [4], Mohamed E. Ahmed [2], Khaled Ghoniem [1], Arleen Delgado [5], Nazih Khater [6], Eugene Kwon [2] and A. Tuba Kendi [1]

1. Department of Radiology, Division of Nuclear Medicine, Mayo Clinic, Rochester, MN 55905, USA; ghoniem.khaled@mayo.edu (K.G.); kendi.ayse@mayo.edu (A.T.K.)
2. Department of Urology, Mayo Clinic, Rochester, MN 55905, USA; mohamed.ahmed@mayo.edu (M.E.A.); kwon.eugene@mayo.edu (E.K.)
3. Department of Biochemistry and Molecular Biology, Mayo Clinic, Rochester, MN 55905, USA; joshi.vidhu@mayo.edu
4. Department of Medical Oncology, King Abdullah Medical City, Mecca 24246, Saudi Arabia; dr.m.habeeb@live.com
5. Department of Pediatrics, Woodhull Medical Center, Brooklyn, NY 11206, USA; arleendelgadomd@gmail.com
6. Department of Urology, Louisiana State University Health Shreveport, Shreveport, LA 71103, USA; nazih.khater@lsuhs.edu
* Correspondence: abdelrazek.ahmad@mayo.edu (A.A.); mahmoud.ahmed@mayo.edu (A.M.M.); Tel.: +1-480-819-1343 (A.A.)

Citation: Abdelrazek, A.; Mahmoud, A.M.; Joshi, V.B.; Habeeb, M.; Ahmed, M.E.; Ghoniem, K.; Delgado, A.; Khater, N.; Kwon, E.; Kendi, A.T. Recent Advances in Prostate Cancer (PCa) Diagnostics. *Uro* **2022**, *2*, 109–121. https://doi.org/10.3390/uro2020014

Academic Editors: Ana Faustino, Paula A. Oliveira, Lúcio Lara Santos and Tommaso Cai

Received: 6 May 2022
Accepted: 30 May 2022
Published: 1 June 2022

Publisher's Note: MDPI stays neutral with regard to jurisdictional claims in published maps and institutional affiliations.

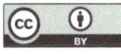

Copyright: © 2022 by the authors. Licensee MDPI, Basel, Switzerland. This article is an open access article distributed under the terms and conditions of the Creative Commons Attribution (CC BY) license (https://creativecommons.org/licenses/by/4.0/).

Abstract: Prostate cancer (PCa), which is among the most prevalent types of cancer in men, is a prominent topic in imaging research. The primary aim of PCa imaging is to acquire more accurate characterizations of the disease. More precise imaging of the local stage progression, early discovery of metastatic cancers, reliable diagnosis of oligometastatic cancer, and optimum treatment response evaluation are areas in which contemporary imaging is quickly improving and developing. Imaging techniques, such as magnetic resonance imaging (MRI) for the whole body and molecular imaging with combined positron emission tomography (PET), computed tomography (CT), and MRI, enable imaging to support and enhance treatment lines in patients with local and advanced PCa. With the availability of multiple imaging modalities for the management of PCa, we aim in this review to offer a multidisciplinary viewpoint on the appropriate function of contemporary imaging in the identification of PCa.

Keywords: prostate cancer; diagnostic tests; imaging techniques

1. Introduction

PCa is a heterogeneous disease with a longer natural history than other solid tumors and a wide range of behavioral and biological activity ranging from inactive to aggressive behavior [1,2]. According to the American Cancer Society, there were 248,530 new cases of PCa and more than 3.1 million survivors in the United States in 2021. Prostate cancer was considered the second leading cause of cancer-related death among men in the United States in 2021, after lung cancer [3]. Additionally, males of African ancestry have a greater risk of PCa than those of European ancestry [4]. Despite the early diagnosis of PCa, the risk/benefit ratio of the treatment remains uncertain and is one of the most challenging and disputed areas of medicine because of the significant morbidity associated with the therapy [5,6].

Historically, imaging had a minimal role in diagnosing locally advanced PCa. Transrectal ultrasound (TRUS) was the only modality that was successfully employed during diagnosis and was primarily used to guide biopsies [6]. The bone scan (BS) and computed tomography (CT) are typically used in patients who are at an increased risk of developing advanced disease. However, PET/CT scanning with tracers, high-field endorectal coil MRI, and contrast-enhanced TRUS improve the detection of locally progressed PCa [7]. Each imaging method has its own set of pros and cons and a subset of indications for best uses within the setting of PCa [8]. In our review, we try to summarize each imaging modality's role and its impact on the management of PCa.

2. Localized PCa Diagnosis

2.1. Digital Rectal Examination (DRE)

DRE is one of the most frequently used methods for the early identification of PCa. The DRE is a low-cost test that evaluates the prostate's size, consistency, mobility, and form abnormalities. However, we cannot rely on size alone as a PCa risk indicator, and there is no correlation between DRE-estimated prostate volume and TRUS-measured volume [9,10]. Furthermore, similar indurations may be caused by calculi or benign prostatic hypertrophy (BPH), whereas carcinomas are felt as hard irregular nodules. This implies that when any induration is felt the provider must request more tests, such as TRUS, and repeat the DRE regularly to identify any changes or advancement [11]. Additionally, the DRE requires technical proficiency. Not all examiners can palpate the prostate's whole posterior surface [12,13].

There is considerable doubt that early detection approaches such as the digital rectal examination (DRE) and serum PSA testing contributed significantly to the decades-long decline in PCa stage progression [14]. Since 1988, the rate of metastatic disease detected through standard physical examinations has decreased considerably [15]. At the time of diagnosis, 70% to 80% of PCa are organ-confined, pathologically. Recent studies show that PSA screening of early-stage prostate cancer patients is more often prostate-confined than those found only through DRE [14,16].

The value of DRE may be questioned due to conflicting findings regarding the effectiveness of PCa screening in reducing morbidity and mortality. Nonetheless, due to the disease's prevalence and the potential to detect it while it is curable, many patients and clinicians opt for screening [13]. A recent meta-analysis showed that the pooled sensitivity and specificity of DRE conducted by primary care practitioners to detect PCa were 0.51 and 0.59, respectively. The aggregated positive predictive value (PPV) was 0.41, and the aggregated negative predictive value (NPV) was 0.64 [10]. As determined by Grades of Recommendation Assessment, Development, and Evaluation (GRADE), the quality of evidence was inferior.

Additionally, when DRE is performed to screen males over the age of 50 for PCa, the cancer detection rate is 3.2%, with a 21% PPV, a sensitivity of 21%, and a specificity of 86% [17]. Thus, DRE should be used in combination with a prostate-specific antigen (PSA) test in PCa screening to increase the overall sensitivity. Whereas DRE detected PCa at a rate of 3.2%, PSA detected it at a rate of 4.6%, and the two procedures together detected it at a rate of 5.8%. Notably, the two tests' detection rates separately are slightly close, and when combined, they identify a higher number of instances with PCa [13,18].

2.2. Transrectal Ultrasound (TRUS)

Holm and Gammelgaard established TRUS-guided biopsies as the gold standard technique for prostate cancer diagnosis [19]. Due to its widespread availability and low cost, TRUS is the most often utilized clinical imaging modality for PCa. TRUS is primarily used to determine the prostate's volume, guide biopsy placement, and implant brachytherapy seeds. However, it is deemed insufficient for detecting or staging prostate cancer. Of note, contrast agents and computer-assisted methods have been examined as ways to enhance TRUS diagnostic performance.

While gray-scale TRUS is ineffective in detecting prostate cancer consistently and therefore cannot be used in place of systematic biopsies, it has established itself as the gold standard for prostate biopsy guidance. Since PCa can present with different intensities such as hypo-, iso-, or hyperechoic [20], the sensitivity (46–91%) and specificity (18–96%) are relatively varied [21]. The increasing number of patients with elevated PSA but normal

DRE highlights the critical need to develop more accurate TRUS-based procedures to improve the diagnostic equipment predictive values, specificity, and sensitivity [22,23].

Due to increased tumor vascularity, contrast-enhanced TRUS utilizing intravenously administered microbubble contrast agents has been demonstrated to improve PCa detection [24]. The bulk of modern ultrasound machines are equipped with ultrasonic technology capable of scanning microbubble contrast agents. In addition, because cancers are often associated with increased blood flow, targeted prostate biopsies may be conducted [25]. A study of 1776 males scheduled for their first or subsequent biopsy showed that collecting five targeted biopsy cores from hypervascular areas in the peripheral zone resulted in a slightly better detection rate (26.8%) than doing ten systematic core biopsies (23.1%) [26]. However, the specificity of this approach is hampered by benign prostatic hyperplasia and prostatitis hypervascularity, which might provide false-positive findings [27].

However, Taverner et al. randomly assigned 300 patients with a negative DRE and a PSA level less than 10 ng/mL to one of three groups: systematic biopsy guided by TRUS, color Doppler ultrasound-guided biopsy, or color Doppler ultrasound-guided biopsy prior to and during contrast agent injection. According to the authors, there was no statistically significant variance in the frequency of PCa detection between the three methods [28].

In another study, Loch et al. created a computer-based TRUS signal analysis (C-TRUS) approach for collecting signal information from serial static TRUS pictures independent of the ocular gray scale, hence improving PCa diagnostic imaging [29]. Further technological advancements resulted in the development of a network-compatible module that enables remote users to input photographs, which are then re-transmitted as tagged images through the internet after analysis [24,30]. C-TRUS offers the benefit of requiring no extra equipment aside from a storage system for digital ultrasound pictures. Sensitivity, specificity, positive predictive value (PPV), and negative predictive value (NPV) were 83%, 64%, 80%, and 68%, respectively, when preoperative C-TRUS pictures were compared to tumor localization in 28 patients having radical prostatectomies [31]. Combining multiparametric MRI with C-TRUS appeared to improve PCa detection in a study of twenty individuals suspected of having the disease. In this analysis, PCa was detected in 58% of instances, which is comparable to the results of large-scale C-TRUS investigations [32].

Furthermore, ultrasonography was combined with real-time elastography, which is a technique that uses physical compression and relaxation to detect changes in tissue compliance. The sensitivity, specificity, PPV, and NPV of this approach were previously reported to be 50%, 72%, 76%, and 44%, respectively [21]. Another study employed elastography and contrast-enhanced ultrasound (CEUS). Elastography indicated a sensitivity of 49% and a specificity of 74% in 86 PCa patients. The percentage of false positives was lowered from 34.9% to 10.3% when elastography was combined with CEUS, while the PPV for cancer diagnosis increased from 65.1% to 89.7% [33]. However, the findings show that elastography is less effective when the gland volume is larger and the lesions are located anteriorly. Additionally, it has been demonstrated that elastography is more sensitive to identifying PCa lesions with a higher Gleason score, a diameter greater than 5 mm, and extracapsular extension [34,35].

2.3. Magnetic Resonance Imaging (MRI)

MRI plays a critical role in detecting PCa [36]. Regarding traditional (T2W) MRI, Hambrock et al. [37] found that 59% of prostate cancer patients with a minimum of two prior negative biopsy sessions could be identified using a 3-Tesla scanner and an average of just four sample cores. However, it is crucial to stress that the majority of these tumors (57%) were detected in the ventral transitional zone and the anterior horns of the peripheral zone (11%), suggesting a carefully selected group of participants. Before the biopsy, conducting an MRI resulted in a 41.2% PPV and an 83.0% sensitivity [38].

Multiparametric MRI has made dramatic inroads into the management of localized PCa over the last five years. International rules are steadily promoting the use of MRI before the biopsy. This presents a widespread shift in the management of localized PCa, which has traditionally been guided by biopsy histology rather than imaging [39].

The current findings indicate that including prebiopsy MRI into the diagnostic tool kit for clinically suspected PCa enhances the detection of clinically relevant illness, lowers biopsy-related complications, and may even eliminate unnecessary biopsies in some patients [40]. New guidelines for PCa analysis and management from the United Kingdom National Institute for Health and Care Excellence (NICE) recommend that all persons with suspected clinically localized PCa undergo multiparametric MRI as a first-line investigation [41]. However, the American Urological Association (AUA) guidance suggests that there is a lack of sufficient evidence to support routine MRI use in each biopsy-naïve subject and confined its utility to males whose clinical examinations for biopsy are undefined (normal PSA with abnormal DRE, minimal PSA elevated, or very young or old subjects) [42].

Multiparametric MRI gives biopsy target data and can serve as guidance for conducting a focused prostate biopsy [43,44]. In this situation, an MRI-guided biopsy of the prostate will detect clinically significant cancer in 34% to 41% of males with a previous negative biopsies. In addition, numerous meta-analyses have reported that targeted biopsies have resulted in increasing identification rates of clinically relevant PCa compared to systemic biopsies in a repeat biopsy context [45–47].

In a recent systematic review, MRI had a pooled sensitivity of 72% and a pooled specificity of 96% compared to a template-guided biopsy. In contrast, the pooled sensitivity for systematic biopsy was 62%, and the specificity was 100% [47]. With time, we anticipate that advancements in MRI will make further contributions to PCa diagnosis.

2.4. Computed Tomography (CT)

CT has a minor role in the identification of PCa and is not advised for reasons such as low prostate soft-tissue resolution and poorly defined gland margins. However, CT is sometimes used for nodal staging of PCa [48]. A recent study showed that CT, in conjunction with deep learning, has the potential to perform comparably to diagnostic pipelines based on MRI [49], suggesting enhancements in the diagnostic capability of CT are potentially forthcoming.

3. Advanced PCa Diagnosis

3.1. Positron Emission Tomography (PET)

PET has displayed significant superiority in the recognition of extra-prostatic disease (Figure 1) [50]. Multiple PET tracers are available for PCa detection. The clinically available tracers include 18F-*sodium fluoride* (18F-NaF), fludeoxyglucose (FDG), 18F-choline, 11C-choline, 68Ga-prostate-specific membrane antigen (PSMA), and 18F-fluciclovine, a tracer newly approved by the U.S. Food and Drug Administration (FDA) [51].

Despite its poor sensitivity of 33% for detecting primary lesions, FDG caught nodal or bone metastatic disease in six out of nine participants [52]. Notably, FDG is more sensitive in detecting metastatic lesions than primary lesions, which might be explained by the increased metabolic activity of metastatic lesions [53].

In a study involving 24 patients who had a biochemical relapse and underwent FDG PET before the dissection of pelvic lymph nodes, the authors found that specificity, sensitivity, PPV, and NPP were 100%, 75.0%, 100%, and 67.7%, respectively, for nodal detection [54]. However, in a prospective study involving 37 patients with a biochemical relapse but negative findings on imaging, the investigators noticed a superior detection rate using NaF PET/CT compared to FDG PET/CT, which has limited efficacy in detecting metastases [55].

Concerning choline PET/CT, two large meta-analyses examining its utility in the staging of nodal disease showed high specificity with variable sensitivity; however, sensitivity increased in higher-risk cases with nodal disease [56,57]. In one meta-analysis of 609 patients, choline PET/CT demonstrated a pooled specificity of 92% and a sensitivity of 62% in assessing pelvic nodal disease at staging [56]. In another study of 1270 cases, C-11-choline PET/CT showed a pooled assessment rate of 62%, specificity of 89%, and sensitivity of 89% in detecting any relapsed disease [58].

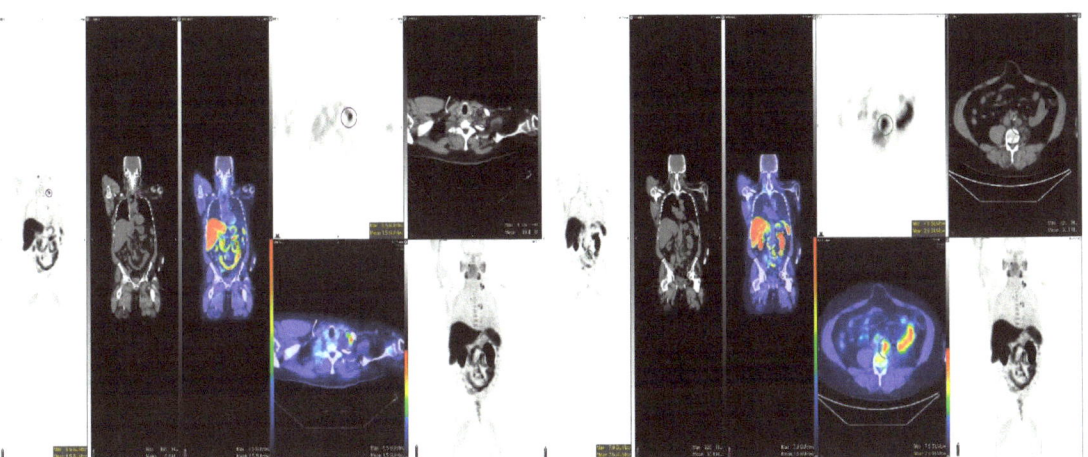

Figure 1. Choline PET/CT shows the extra-prostatic extension of PCa with involvement of left supraclavicular and retroperitoneal lymph nodes.

Although 16 trials using 18F-choline with or without 11C-choline demonstrated a satisfactory pooled sensitivity of 75.4% and a specificity of 82%, additional studies have shown that MRI remains the preferable approach in detecting local recurrence [59].

The PSA levels influence the disease detection with choline PET/CT in biochemical relapse. A study of C11-choline PET/CT in 4426 cases showed that a PSA level greater than 1.16 ng/mL was a positive predictor of the scan. The positive 11C-choline scan rate increased with high PSA levels in 358 cases with biochemical relapse. With PSA levels between 0.2 and 1 ng/mL, the detection rate of the 11C-choline scan was 19%, and for PSA levels between 1 and 3 ng/mL, 46% of scans were positive. Finally, with a PSA level >3 ng/mL, 82% of scans were positive [60].

Another imaging modality is prostate-specific membrane antigen (PSMA) PET/CT scan, which is a surface protein found on prostate cells expressed differently than in other tissues. PSMA overexpression is reported in PCa cells and can be detected using gallium-68-labeled PSMA ligands via PET/CT imaging (PSMA-PET/CT) [61]. The PSMA-PET/CT lymph node (LN) staging sensitivity and specificity were 65.9% and 98.9%, respectively, according to a retrospective study of 130 intermediate- to high-risk PCa patients who also underwent radical prostatectomy (RP) with pelvic LN dissection [62]. According to a meta-analysis, the PSMA-PET/CT sensitivity and specificity were recently reported to be 71% and 95%, respectively, in pelvic LN metastasis detection [63]. PSMA-PET scan is considered a promising mode of imaging for diagnosing positive lymph nodes.

Hybrid PSMA PET/mp-MRI improves the diagnosis of suspicious lesions on MRI and may also assist in better fusion biopsy guidance in patients who have previously had negative biopsies and had intratumoral bleeding, as intratumoral bleeding would impact mp-MRI results. Notably, PSMA has a higher sensitivity than choline or acetate PET in detecting nodal and distant metastasis [64].

The combination of mp-MRI and PSMA PET also has the potential to serve as a single comprehensive staging modality in intermediate- to high-risk PCa. However, PSMA PET has mainly been investigated in the context of detecting disease recurrence [65]. In a study of 248 patients who underwent RP and experienced biochemical recurrence, Eiber et al. observed an 89.5% detection rate using 68Ga-PSMA PET. Faster PSA velocity and levels of more than 2 ng/mL correlated with the highest detection rate [66]. In both post-RP and post-RT patients, 68Ga-PSMA PET had higher detection rates than choline PET in detecting local and distant recurrence [66,67]. This was especially evident during the early stages of PSA rise (0.5–1 ng/mL) when choline PET was only shown to be positive in a few cases [2,65].

18F-DCFPyL is another PSMA-based PET ligand with exceptional staging performance in clinical trials (Figure 2). For example, in a study of over 400 patients with PC of all Gleason grades, 18F-DCFPyL demonstrated a detection rate of over 90% in patients with a PSA of 0.5 ng/mL and approximately 50% for PSA levels <0.5 ng/mL [68]. One of the drawbacks of PSMA is its uptake in a diverse range of nonmalignant conditions such as bone-related conditions, inflammatory and infectious processes, and benign tumors; however, many factors should be considered to decrease the bias in reporting, such as topography, distribution, and PSMA uptake intensity [68,69].

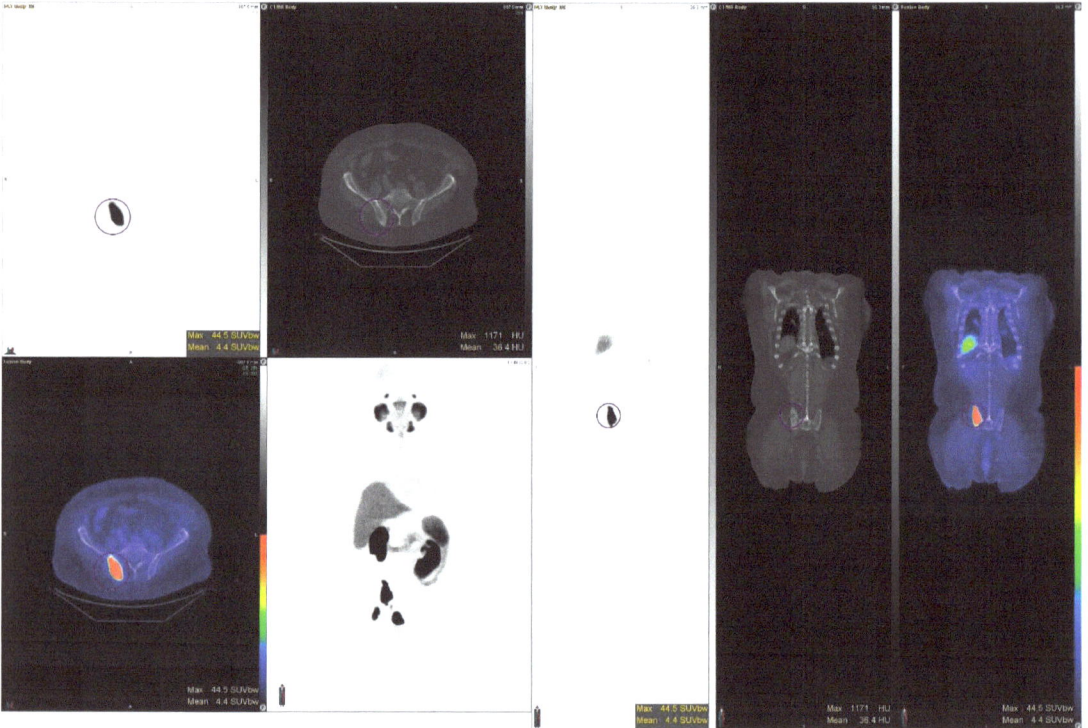

Figure 2. F-18 Pyl PSMA PET/CT demonstrates the distribution of PCa *metastasis* at pelvic bones.

Another PSMA-based PET ligand is 64Cu-PSMA PET/CT. A prospective cohort of 23 individuals with intermediate- to high-risk prostate cancer who had radical prostatectomy with extensive pelvic LN dissection was studied. The researchers discovered that 64Cu-PSMA PET/CT had a sensitivity of 87.5 percent, specificity of 100%, PPV of 100%, and NPV of 93.7% in identifying LN metastasis [70].

3.2. Bone Scan (BS)

A meta-analysis that included 12 articles investigating the BS revealed a pooled sensitivity of 0.79 and a specificity of 0.82 for bone metastases diagnosis [71]. However, the sensitivity and specificity were enhanced when combined with a minimal CT dose or single-photon emission computed tomography (SPECT) with CT. The combination of

SPECT-CT with BS raised the sensitivity from 70% to 87–92% [72]. Of note, metastases are not directly imaged by BS, but instead, this modality detects the osteoblastic response to the presence of tumor cells. However, a bone scan only detects bone metastases in <1% of cases with PSA < 20 ng/mL (Figure 3) [73,74]. Notably, the detection rate of bone scans rises in concordance with increased PSA levels. Specifically, the detection rates for the metastases were 2.3% in cases with a PSA level of ≤10 ng/mL, 5.3% in cases with a PSA level of 10.1–19.9 ng/mL, and 16.2% in cases with a PSA level of 20.0–49.9 ng/mL [75].

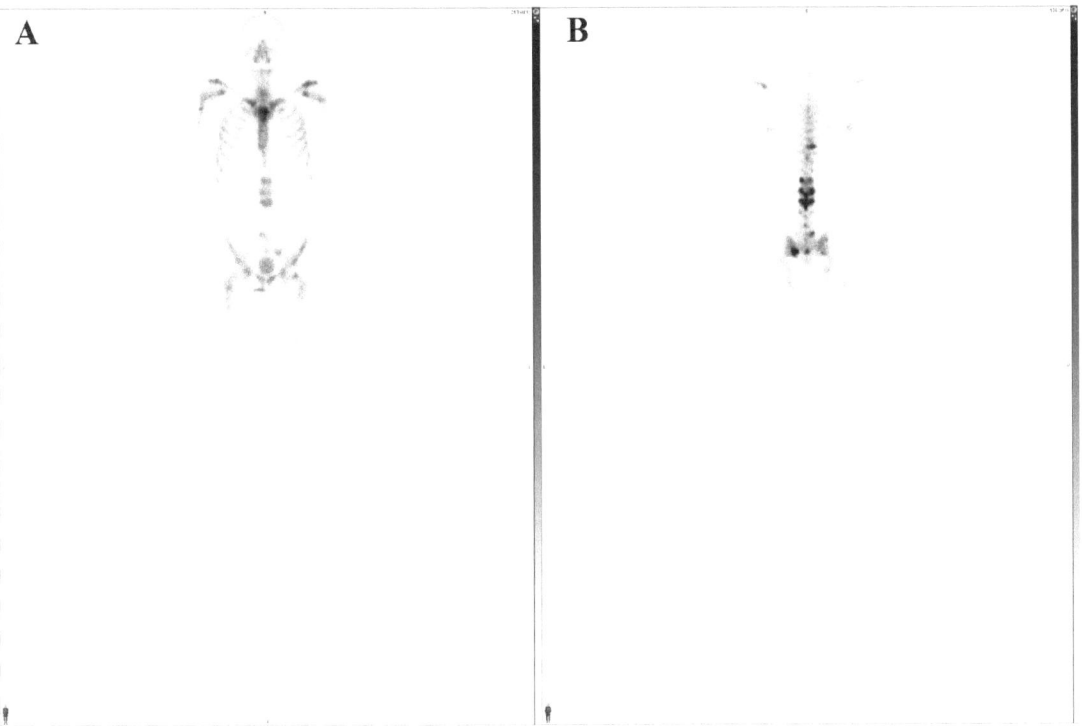

Figure 3. Anterior (**A**) and posterior (**B**) planar views of a whole-body bone scan show multiple radiotracer avid bone metastases at both axial and appendicular skeleton, most located at the spine.

3.3. Conventional CT Imaging

Conventional CT has a poor performance in detecting lymph node involvement due to the similarities in the size of benign reactive versus metastatic nodes [48]. In addition, CT diagnostic sensitivity and standard anatomic T1- or T2-weighted MRI sequences are less than 40% sensitive in identifying nodal metastases (0.5–2 cm on a shorter axis) in patients with PCa due to the common occurrence of micrometastases [76]. As a result, clinical nomography has played a vital role in deciding whether or not to perform lymph node dissection (LND) during primary PCa surgery.

The most frequently used technique for detecting and evaluating bone metastases in patients with prostate cancer is technetium 99 m (99 mTc) diphosphonate BS. Nonetheless, early metastases located in the bone marrow may lack tracer absorption, making disease detection more complex [77]. The SPECT to planar imaging inclusion can increase diagnostic accuracy, particularly when employing hybrid SPECT/CT cameras. On a per-patient basis, a meta-analysis of 1102 PCa patients across 12 studies using 99 mTc planar BS and 3 studies using SPECT found that the sensitivity and specificity of PCa diagnosis using planar BS were 59% and 75% per lesion, respectively, compared to 90% and 85%, respectively, by adding SPECT [71].

3.4. MRI

Multiparametric MRI shows usefulness in differentiating between residual local disease and distant metastases. In addition, MRI is utilized for detecting seminal vesicle invasion and extraprostatic extension in patient candidates for salvage prostatectomy based on high-risk features. MRI studies after radiotherapy to the prostate seem effective in cases with suspected clinical local recurrence based on elevated PSA. However, MRI is not suggested for monitoring therapeutic responses until clinical evidence of disease recurrence exists [78,79].

Diffusion-weighted (DW) MRI detects changes in water mobility between tissues and allows the apparent diffusion coefficient (ADC) to be calculated. However, in malignant lymph nodes, it has been shown that ADC values did not differ significantly from benign nodes [80]. According to a meta-analysis, DW MRI accompanied with ultrasmall superparamagnetic iron oxide (USPIO) demonstrated higher sensitivity in terms of the diagnosis of lymph node metastasis in PCa than utilizing USPIO-MRI alone. The use of DW MRI combined with a USPIO enhanced both the diagnostic sensitivity, with a range of 65–75%, and the specificity, with a range of 93–96%, compared with USPIO-MRI alone (sensitivity ranged from 55–65% and specificity ranged from 71–91%) [81]. Furthermore, in a study of 2993 normal-sized lymph nodes in patients with prostate or bladder cancer, combined USPIO-DW-MRI had sensitivity and specificity ranges of 65–75% and 93–96%, respectively, and was found to be superior to MRI with a USPIO alone (sensitivity ranged from 55–65%, and specificity ranged from 71–91%) [82].

In bone metastasis detection, whole-body MRI was more sensitive than BS and choline PET/CT; however, choline PET/CT exhibited better specificity [71]. The addition of DW MRI to modern whole-body MRI increases bone metastasis diagnosis by including morphologic sequences (e.g., T1- or T2-weighted sequences, short inversion time inversion-recovery sequence). In a study involving 30 patients, the whole-body DW MRI demonstrated a higher sensitivity (100%) and specificity (100%) in detecting bone or node metastases compared with the combination of BS and CT, which demonstrated a sensitivity and specificity of 85% and 88%, respectively [83]. A whole-body MRI approach, which incorporates both conventional and diffusion-weighted imaging, offers a high detection sensitivity in bone and visceral metastases [84,85].

4. Conclusions

While various novel imaging techniques have been developed in recent years, an unmet need exists for improved PCa diagnosis and staging. Concerning diagnosis, advancements in imaging technology have the potential to enable us to abandon spontaneous biopsies in favor of targeted biopsies in the future. Combining several imaging modalities may be one approach to enhance our current standards in diagnosing PCa.

Author Contributions: Conceptualization, M.E.A.; resources, A.T.K.; writing—original draft preparation, A.A.; writing—review and editing, A.M.M., M.H., K.G., V.B.J., A.D. and N.K.; supervision, A.T.K. and E.K. All authors have read and agreed to the published version of the manuscript.

Funding: This research received no external funding.

Informed Consent Statement: Informed consent was obtained from all subjects involved in the review in order to retrieve their scans.

Conflicts of Interest: The authors declare no conflict of interest.

References

1. Rawla, P. Epidemiology of Prostate Cancer. *World J. Oncol.* **2019**, *10*, 63–89. Available online: http://www.ncbi.nlm.nih.gov/pubmed/31068988 (accessed on 11 April 2022). [CrossRef]
2. Jadvar, H.; Alavi, A. Role of Imaging in Prostate Cancer. *PET Clin.* **2009**, *4*, 135–138. Available online: http://www.ncbi.nlm.nih.gov/pubmed/20161047 (accessed on 11 April 2022). [CrossRef]
3. Siegel, R.L.; Miller, K.D.; Fuchs, H.E.; Jemal, A. Cancer Statistics, 2021. *CA Cancer J. Clin.* **2021**, *71*, 7–33. Available online: http://www.ncbi.nlm.nih.gov/pubmed/33433946. (accessed on 11 April 2022). [CrossRef]
4. Giri, V.N.; Morgan, T.M.; Morris, D.S.; Berchuck, J.E.; Hyatt, C.; Taplin, M.-E. Genetic testing in prostate cancer management: Considerations informing primary care. *CA Cancer J. Clin.* **2022**, online ahead of print. Available online: http://www.ncbi.nlm.nih.gov/pubmed/35201622 (accessed on 11 April 2022). [CrossRef]
5. Desai, M.M.; Cacciamani, G.E.; Gill, K.; Zhang, J.; Liu, L.; Abreu, A.; Gill, I.S. Trends in Incidence of Metastatic Prostate Cancer in the US. *JAMA Netw. Open* **2022**, *5*, e222246. Available online: http://www.ncbi.nlm.nih.gov/pubmed/35285916 (accessed on 11 April 2022). [CrossRef]
6. Cuzick, J.; Thorat, M.A.; Andriole, G.; Brawley, O.W.; Brown, P.H.; Culig, Z.; Eeles, R.A.; Ford, L.G.; Hamdy, F.C.; Holmberg, L.; et al. Prevention and early detection of prostate cancer. *Lancet Oncol.* **2014**, *15*, e484-92. Available online: http://www.ncbi.nlm.nih.gov/pubmed/25281467 (accessed on 11 April 2022). [CrossRef]
7. Turkbey, B.; Albert, P.S.; Kurdziel, K.; Choyke, P.L. Imaging localized prostate cancer: Current approaches and new developments. *AJR. Am. J. Roentgenol.* **2009**, *192*, 1471–1480. Available online: http://www.ncbi.nlm.nih.gov/pubmed/19457807 (accessed on 11 April 2022). [CrossRef]
8. Ghafoor, S.; Burger, I.A.; Vargas, A.H. Multimodality Imaging of Prostate Cancer. *J. Nucl. Med.* **2019**, *60*, 1350–1358. Available online: http://www.ncbi.nlm.nih.gov/pubmed/31481573 (accessed on 11 April 2022). [CrossRef]
9. Soares, S.C.M.; de Camargo Cancela, M.; Migowski, A.; de Souza, D.L.B. Digital rectal examination and its associated factors in the early detection of prostate cancer: A cross-sectional population-based study. *BMC Public Health* **2019**, *19*, 1573. Available online: http://www.ncbi.nlm.nih.gov/pubmed/31775710 (accessed on 11 April 2022). [CrossRef]
10. Naji, L.; Randhawa, H.; Sohani, Z.; Dennis, B.; Lautenbach, D.; Kavanagh, O.; Bawor, M.; Banfield, L.; Profetto, J. Digital Rectal Examination for Prostate Cancer Screening in Primary Care: A Systematic Review and Meta-Analysis. *Ann. Fam. Med.* **2018**, *16*, 149–154. Available online: http://www.ncbi.nlm.nih.gov/pubmed/29531107 (accessed on 11 April 2022). [CrossRef]
11. Izawa, J.I.; Klotz, L.; Siemens, D.R.; Kassouf, W.; So, A.; Jordan, J.; Chetner, M.; Iansavichene, A.E. Prostate cancer screening: Canadian guidelines 2011. *Can. Urol. Assoc. J.* **2011**, *5*, 235–240. Available online: http://www.ncbi.nlm.nih.gov/pubmed/21801679 (accessed on 11 April 2022). [CrossRef]
12. Koulikov, D.; Mamber, A.; Fridmans, A.; Abu Arafeh, W.; Shenfeld, O.Z. Why I cannot find the prostate? Behind the subjectivity of rectal exam. *ISRN Urol.* **2012**, *2012*, 456821. Available online: http://www.ncbi.nlm.nih.gov/pubmed/22530153 (accessed on 11 April 2022). [CrossRef]
13. Zhang, A.; Fear, T.; Ahmed, H. Digital rectal examination in prostate cancer screening. *Univ. West. Ont. Med. J.* **2013**, *82*, 10–11. Available online: https://ojs.lib.uwo.ca/index.php/uwomj/article/view/4626 (accessed on 11 April 2022). [CrossRef]
14. Kawachi, M.H.; Bahnson, R.R.; Barry, M.; Busby, J.E.; Carroll, P.R.; Carter, H.B.; Catalona, W.J.; Cookson, M.S.; Epstein, J.I.; Etzioni, R.B.; et al. NCCN clinical practice guidelines in oncology: Prostate cancer early detection. *J. Natl. Compr. Cancer Netw.* **2010**, *8*, 240–262. Available online: http://www.ncbi.nlm.nih.gov/pubmed/20141680 (accessed on 11 April 2022). [CrossRef]
15. Adhyam, M.; Gupta, A.K. A Review on the Clinical Utility of PSA in Cancer Prostate. *Indian J. Surg. Oncol.* **2012**, *3*, 120–129. Available online: http://www.ncbi.nlm.nih.gov/pubmed/23730101 (accessed on 11 April 2022). [CrossRef]
16. Miller, D.C.; Hafez, K.S.; Stewart, A.; Montie, J.E.; Wei, J.T. Prostate carcinoma presentation, diagnosis, and staging: An update form the National Cancer Data Base. *Cancer* **2003**, *98*, 1169–1178. Available online: http://www.ncbi.nlm.nih.gov/pubmed/12973840 (accessed on 11 April 2022). [CrossRef]
17. Richie, J.P.; Catalona, W.J.; Ahmann, F.R.; Hudson, M.A.; Scardino, P.T.; Flanigan, R.C.; DeKernion, J.B.; Ratliff, T.L.; Kavoussi, L.R.; Dalkin, B.L.; et al. Effect of patient age on early detection of prostate cancer with serum prostate specific antigen and digital rectal examination. *Urology* **1993**, *42*, 365–374. Available online: http://www.ncbi.nlm.nih.gov/pubmed/7692657 (accessed on 11 April 2022). [CrossRef]
18. Catalona, W.J.; Richie, J.P.; Ahmann, F.R.; Hudson, M.A.; Scardino, P.T.; Flanigan, R.C.; DeKernion, J.B.; Ratliff, T.L.; Kavoussi, L.R.; Dalkin, B.L.; et al. Comparison of Digital Rectal Examination and Serum Prostate Specific Antigen in the Early Detection of Prostate Cancer: Results of a Multicenter Clinical Trial of 6630 Men. *J. Urol.* **2017**, *197*, S200–S207. Available online: http://www.ncbi.nlm.nih.gov/pubmed/28012755 (accessed on 11 April 2022). [CrossRef]
19. Anastasi, G.; Subba, E.; Pappalardo, R.; Macchione, L.; Ricotta, G.; Muscarà, G.; Lembo, F.; Magno, C. Transrectal ultrasound (TRUS) guided prostate biopsy: Three different types of local anesthesia. *Arch. Ital. Urol. Androl.* **2016**, *88*, 308–310. Available online: http://www.ncbi.nlm.nih.gov/pubmed/28073199 (accessed on 11 April 2022). [CrossRef]
20. Dähnert, W.F.; Hamper, U.M.; Eggleston, J.C.; Walsh, P.C.; Sanders, R.C. Prostatic evaluation by transrectal sonography with histopathologic correlation: The echopenic appearance of early carcinoma. *Radiology* **1986**, *158*, 97–102. Available online: http://www.ncbi.nlm.nih.gov/pubmed/3510032 (accessed on 11 April 2022). [CrossRef]

21. Brock, M.; von Bodman, C.; Sommerer, F.; Löppenberg, B.; Klein, T.; Deix, T.; Palisaar, J.R.; Noldus, J.; Eggert, T. Comparison of real-time elastography with grey-scale ultrasonography for detection of organ-confined prostate cancer and extra capsular extension: A prospective analysis using whole mount sections after radical prostatectomy. *BJU Int.* **2011**, *108 Pt 2*, E217–E222. Available online: http://www.ncbi.nlm.nih.gov/pubmed/21819532 (accessed on 11 April 2022). [CrossRef]
22. Trevethan, R. Sensitivity, Specificity, and Predictive Values: Foundations, Pliabilities, and Pitfalls in Research and Practice. *Front. Public Health* **2017**, *5*, 307. Available online: http://www.ncbi.nlm.nih.gov/pubmed/29209603 (accessed on 11 April 2022). [CrossRef]
23. Pummer, K.; Rieken, M.; Augustin, H.; Gutschi, T.; Shariat, S.F. Innovations in diagnostic imaging of localized prostate cancer. *World J. Urol.* **2014**, *32*, 881–890. Available online: http://www.ncbi.nlm.nih.gov/pubmed/24078105 (accessed on 11 April 2022). [CrossRef]
24. Wildeboer, R.R.; Postema, A.W.; Demi, L.; Kuenen, M.P.J.; Wijkstra, H.; Mischi, M. Multiparametric dynamic contrast-enhanced ultrasound imaging of prostate cancer. *Eur. Radiol.* **2017**, *27*, 3226–3234. Available online: http://www.ncbi.nlm.nih.gov/pubmed/28004162 (accessed on 11 April 2022). [CrossRef]
25. Carpagnano, F.A.; Eusebi, L.; Carriero, S.; Giannubilo, W.; Bartelli, F.; Guglielmi, G. Prostate Cancer Ultrasound: Is Still a Valid Tool? *Curr. Radiol. Rep.* **2021**, *9*, 7. Available online: https://link.springer.com/10.1007/s40134-021-00382-6 (accessed on 11 April 2022). [CrossRef]
26. Mitterberger, M.J.; Aigner, F.; Horninger, W.; Ulmer, H.; Cavuto, S.; Halpern, E.J.; Frauscher, F. Comparative efficiency of contrast-enhanced colour Doppler ultrasound targeted versus systematic biopsy for prostate cancer detection. *Eur. Radiol.* **2010**, *20*, 2791–2796. Available online: http://www.ncbi.nlm.nih.gov/pubmed/20571801 (accessed on 11 April 2022). [CrossRef]
27. Halpern, E.J. Contrast-enhanced ultrasound imaging of prostate cancer. *Rev. Urol.* **2006**, *8* (Suppl. 1), S29–S37. Available online: http://www.ncbi.nlm.nih.gov/pubmed/17021624 (accessed on 11 April 2022).
28. Taverna, G.; Morandi, G.; Seveso, M.; Giusti, G.; Benetti, A.; Colombo, P.; Minuti, F.; Grizzi, F.; Graziotti, P. Colour Doppler and microbubble contrast agent ultrasonography do not improve cancer detection rate in transrectal systematic prostate biopsy sampling. *BJU Int.* **2011**, *108*, 1723–1727. Available online: http://www.ncbi.nlm.nih.gov/pubmed/21756276 (accessed on 11 April 2022). [CrossRef]
29. Loch, T. Computerized transrectal ultrasound (C-TRUS) of the prostate: Detection of cancer in patients with multiple negative systematic random biopsies. *World J. Urol.* **2007**, *25*, 375–380. Available online: http://www.ncbi.nlm.nih.gov/pubmed/17694312 (accessed on 11 April 2022). [CrossRef]
30. van der Aa, A.A.M.A.; Mannaerts, C.K.; Gayet, M.C.W.; van der Linden, J.C.; Schrier, B.P.; Sedelaar, J.P.M.; Mischi, M.; Beerlage, H.P.; Wijkstra, H. Three-dimensional greyscale transrectal ultrasound-guidance and biopsy core preembedding for detection of prostate cancer: Dutch clinical cohort study. *BMC Urol.* **2019**, *19*, 23. Available online: https://bmcurol.biomedcentral.com/articles/10.1186/s12894-019-0455-7 (accessed on 11 April 2022). [CrossRef]
31. Walz, J.; Loch, T.; Salomon, G.; Wijkstra, H. Imaging of the prostate. *Die Urol.* **2013**, *52*, 490–496. Available online: http://www.ncbi.nlm.nih.gov/pubmed/23494334 (accessed on 11 April 2022).
32. Strunk, T.; Decker, G.; Willinek, W.; Mueller, S.C.; Rogenhofer, S. Combination of C-TRUS with multiparametric MRI: Potential for improving detection of prostate cancer. *World J. Urol.* **2014**, *32*, 335–339. Available online: http://www.ncbi.nlm.nih.gov/pubmed/22885659 (accessed on 11 April 2022). [CrossRef]
33. Brock, M.; Eggert, T.; Palisaar, R.J.; Roghmann, F.; Braun, K.; Löppenberg, B.; Sommerer, F.; Noldus, J.; von Bodman, C. Multiparametric ultrasound of the prostate: Adding contrast enhanced ultrasound to real-time elastography to detect histopathologically confirmed cancer. *J. Urol.* **2013**, *189*, 93–98. Available online: http://www.ncbi.nlm.nih.gov/pubmed/23164379 (accessed on 11 April 2022). [CrossRef]
34. Sigrist, R.M.S.; Liau, J.; El Kaffas, A.; Chammas, M.C.; Willmann, J.K. Ultrasound Elastography: Review of Techniques and Clinical Applications. *Theranostics* **2017**, *7*, 1303–1329. Available online: http://www.ncbi.nlm.nih.gov/pubmed/28435467 (accessed on 11 April 2022). [CrossRef] [PubMed]
35. Zhu, Y.; Chen, Y.; Qi, T.; Jiang, J.; Qi, J.; Yu, Y.; Yao, X.; Guan, W. Prostate cancer detection with real-time elastography using a bi-plane transducer: Comparison with step section radical prostatectomy pathology. *World J. Urol.* **2014**, *32*, 329–333. Available online: http://www.ncbi.nlm.nih.gov/pubmed/22885658 (accessed on 11 April 2022). [CrossRef]
36. Yuan, J.; Poon, D.M.C.; Lo, G.; Wong, O.L.; Cheung, K.Y.; Yu, S.K. A narrative review of MRI acquisition for MR-guided-radiotherapy in prostate cancer. *Quant. Imaging Med. Surg.* **2022**, *12*, 1585–1607. Available online: http://www.ncbi.nlm.nih.gov/pubmed/35111651 (accessed on 11 April 2022). [CrossRef]
37. Hambrock, T.; Somford, D.M.; Hoeks, C.; Bouwense, S.A.W.; Huisman, H.; Yakar, D.; van Oort, I.M.; Witjes, J.A.; Fütterer, J.J.; Barentsz, J.O. Magnetic resonance imaging guided prostate biopsy in men with repeat negative biopsies and increased prostate specific antigen. *J. Urol.* **2010**, *183*, 520–527. Available online: http://www.ncbi.nlm.nih.gov/pubmed/20006859 (accessed on 11 April 2022). [CrossRef]
38. Choi, M.S.; Choi, Y.S.; Yoon, B.I.; Kim, S.J.; Cho, H.J.; Hong, S.H.; Lee, J.Y.; Hwang, T.-K.; Kim, S.W. The Clinical Value of Performing an MRI before Prostate Biopsy. *Korean J. Urol.* **2011**, *52*, 572–577. Available online: http://www.ncbi.nlm.nih.gov/pubmed/21927706 (accessed on 11 April 2022). [CrossRef]
39. Laurence Klotz, C.M. Can high resolution micro-ultrasound replace MRI in the diagnosis of prostate cancer? *Eur. Urol. Focus* **2020**, *6*, 419–423. Available online: http://www.ncbi.nlm.nih.gov/pubmed/31771935 (accessed on 11 April 2022). [CrossRef]

40. Schoots, I.G.; Padhani, A.R. Delivering Clinical impacts of the MRI diagnostic pathway in prostate cancer diagnosis. *Abdom. Radiol. (N. Y.)* **2020**, *45*, 4012–4022. Available online: http://www.ncbi.nlm.nih.gov/pubmed/32356003 (accessed on 11 April 2022). [CrossRef]
41. Available online: https://www.ncbi.nlm.nih.gov/books/NBK544759/?report=reader (accessed on 11 April 2022).
42. Bjurlin, M.A.; Carroll, P.R.; Eggener, S.; Fulgham, P.F.; Margolis, D.J.; Pinto, P.A.; Rosenkrantz, A.B.; Rubenstein, J.N.; Rukstalis, D.B.; Taneja, S.S.; et al. Update of the Standard Operating Procedure on the Use of Multiparametric Magnetic Resonance Imaging for the Diagnosis, Staging and Management of Prostate Cancer. *J. Urol.* **2020**, *203*, 706–712. Available online: http://www.ncbi.nlm.nih.gov/pubmed/31642740 (accessed on 11 April 2022). [CrossRef] [PubMed]
43. Siddiqui, M.M.; Rais-Bahrami, S.; Turkbey, B.; George, A.K.; Rothwax, J.; Shakir, N.; Okoro, C.; Raskolnikov, D.; Parnes, H.L.; Linehan, W.M.; et al. Comparison of MR/ultrasound fusion-guided biopsy with ultrasound-guided biopsy for the diagnosis of prostate cancer. *JAMA* **2015**, *313*, 390–397. Available online: http://www.ncbi.nlm.nih.gov/pubmed/25626035 (accessed on 11 April 2022). [CrossRef] [PubMed]
44. Penzkofer, T.; Tuncali, K.; Fedorov, A.; Song, S.-E.; Tokuda, J.; Fennessy, F.M.; Vangel, M.G.; Kibel, A.S.; Mulkern, R.V.; Wells, W.M.; et al. Transperineal in-bore 3-T MR imaging-guided prostate biopsy: A prospective clinical observational study. *Radiology* **2015**, *274*, 170–180. Available online: http://www.ncbi.nlm.nih.gov/pubmed/25222067 (accessed on 11 April 2022). [CrossRef] [PubMed]
45. Moore, C.M.; Robertson, N.L.; Arsanious, N.; Middleton, T.; Villers, A.; Klotz, L.; Taneja, S.S.; Emberton, M. Image-guided prostate biopsy using magnetic resonance imaging-derived targets: A systematic review. *Eur. Urol.* **2013**, *63*, 125–140. Available online: http://www.ncbi.nlm.nih.gov/pubmed/22743165 (accessed on 16 April 2022). [CrossRef] [PubMed]
46. Wegelin, O.; van Melick, H.H.E.; Hooft, L.; Bosch, J.L.H.R.; Reitsma, H.B.; Barentsz, J.O.; Somford, D.M. Comparing Three Different Techniques for Magnetic Resonance Imaging-targeted Prostate Biopsies: A Systematic Review of In-bore versus Magnetic Resonance Imaging-transrectal Ultrasound fusion versus Cognitive Registration. Is There a Preferred Technique? *Eur. Urol.* **2017**, *71*, 517–531. Available online: http://www.ncbi.nlm.nih.gov/pubmed/27568655 (accessed on 16 April 2022). [CrossRef]
47. Drost, F.-J.H.; Osses, D.F.; Nieboer, D.; Steyerberg, E.W.; Bangma, C.H.; Roobol, M.J.; Schoots, I.G. Prostate MRI, with or without MRI-targeted biopsy, and systematic biopsy for detecting prostate cancer. *Cochrane Database Syst. Rev.* **2019**, *4*, CD012663. Available online: http://www.ncbi.nlm.nih.gov/pubmed/31022301 (accessed on 16 April 2022). [CrossRef]
48. Hövels, A.M.; Heesakkers, R.A.M.; Adang, E.M.; Jager, G.J.; Strum, S.; Hoogeveen, Y.L.; Severens, J.L.; Barentsz, J.O. The diagnostic accuracy of CT and MRI in the staging of pelvic lymph nodes in patients with prostate cancer: A meta-analysis. *Clin. Radiol.* **2008**, *63*, 387–395. Available online: http://www.ncbi.nlm.nih.gov/pubmed/18325358 (accessed on 16 April 2022). [CrossRef]
49. Korevaar, S.; Tennakoon, R.; Page, M.; Brotchie, P.; Thangarajah, J.; Florescu, C.; Sutherland, T.; Kam, N.M.; Bab-Hadiashar, A. Incidental detection of prostate cancer with computed tomography scans. *Sci. Rep.* **2021**, *11*, 7956. Available online: http://www.ncbi.nlm.nih.gov/pubmed/33846450 (accessed on 16 April 2022). [CrossRef]
50. Rowe, S.P.; Gorin, M.A.; Allaf, M.E.; Pienta, K.J.; Tran, P.T.; Pomper, M.G.; Ross, A.E.; Cho, S.Y. PET imaging of prostate-specific membrane antigen in prostate cancer: Current state of the art and future challenges. *Prostate Cancer Prostatic Dis.* **2016**, *19*, 223–230. Available online: http://www.ncbi.nlm.nih.gov/pubmed/27136743 (accessed on 16 April 2022). [CrossRef]
51. Wang, R.; Shen, G.; Huang, M.; Tian, R. The Diagnostic Role of 18F-Choline, 18F-Fluciclovine and 18F-PSMA PET/CT in the Detection of Prostate Cancer With Biochemical Recurrence: A Meta-Analysis. *Front. Oncol.* **2021**, *11*, 684629. Available online: http://www.ncbi.nlm.nih.gov/pubmed/34222008 (accessed on 16 April 2022). [CrossRef]
52. Liu, Y. Diagnostic role of fluorodeoxyglucose positron emission tomography-computed tomography in prostate cancer. *Oncol. Lett.* **2014**, *7*, 2013–2018. Available online: http://www.ncbi.nlm.nih.gov/pubmed/24932281 (accessed on 16 April 2022). [CrossRef] [PubMed]
53. Wallitt, K.L.; Khan, S.R.; Dubash, S.; Tam, H.H.; Khan, S.; Barwick, T.D. Clinical PET Imaging in Prostate Cancer. *Radiographics* **2017**, *37*, 1512–1536. Available online: http://www.ncbi.nlm.nih.gov/pubmed/28800286 (accessed on 16 April 2022). [CrossRef]
54. Chang, C.-H.; Wu, H.-C.; Tsai, J.J.P.; Shen, Y.-Y.; Changlai, S.-P.; Kao, A. Detecting metastatic pelvic lymph nodes by 18F-2-deoxyglucose positron emission tomography in patients with prostate-specific antigen relapse after treatment for localized prostate cancer. *Urol. Int.* **2003**, *70*, 311–315. Available online: http://www.ncbi.nlm.nih.gov/pubmed/12740497 (accessed on 16 April 2022). [CrossRef]
55. Jadvar, H.; Desai, B.; Ji, L.; Conti, P.S.; Dorff, T.B.; Groshen, S.G.; Gross, M.E.; Pinski, J.K.; Quinn, D.I. Prospective evaluation of 18F-NaF and 18F-FDG PET/CT in detection of occult metastatic disease in biochemical recurrence of prostate cancer. *Clin. Nucl. Med.* **2012**, *37*, 637–643. Available online: http://www.ncbi.nlm.nih.gov/pubmed/22691503 (accessed on 16 April 2022). [CrossRef] [PubMed]
56. von Eyben, F.E.; Kairemo, K. Meta-analysis of (11)C-choline and (18)F-choline PET/CT for management of patients with prostate cancer. *Nucl. Med. Commun.* **2014**, *35*, 221–230. Available online: http://www.ncbi.nlm.nih.gov/pubmed/24240194 (accessed on 16 April 2022). [CrossRef] [PubMed]
57. Evangelista, L.; Guttilla, A.; Zattoni, F.; Muzzio, P.C.; Zattoni, F. Utility of choline positron emission tomography/computed tomography for lymph node involvement identification in intermediate- to high-risk prostate cancer: A systematic literature review and meta-analysis. *Eur. Urol.* **2013**, *63*, 1040–1048. Available online: http://www.ncbi.nlm.nih.gov/pubmed/23036576 (accessed on 16 April 2022). [CrossRef] [PubMed]

58. Fanti, S.; Minozzi, S.; Castellucci, P.; Balduzzi, S.; Herrmann, K.; Krause, B.J.; Oyen, W.; Chiti, A. PET/CT with (11)C-choline for evaluation of prostate cancer patients with biochemical recurrence: Meta-analysis and critical review of available data. *Eur. J. Nucl. Med. Mol. Imaging* **2016**, *43*, 55–69. Available online: http://www.ncbi.nlm.nih.gov/pubmed/26450693 (accessed on 16 April 2022). [CrossRef]
59. Evangelista, L.; Zattoni, F.; Guttilla, A.; Saladini, G.; Zattoni, F.; Colletti, P.M.; Rubello, D. Choline PET or PET/CT and biochemical relapse of prostate cancer: A systematic review and meta-analysis. *Clin. Nucl. Med.* **2013**, *38*, 305–314. Available online: http://www.ncbi.nlm.nih.gov/pubmed/23486334 (accessed on 16 April 2022). [CrossRef]
60. Graziani, T.; Ceci, F.; Castellucci, P.; Polverari, G.; Lima, G.M.; Lodi, F.; Morganti, A.G.; Ardizzoni, A.; Schiavina, R.; Fanti, S. (11)C-Choline PET/CT for restaging prostate cancer. Results from 4426 scans in a single-centre patient series. *Eur. J. Nucl. Med. Mol. Imaging* **2016**, *43*, 1971–1979. Available online: http://www.ncbi.nlm.nih.gov/pubmed/27277279 (accessed on 16 April 2022). [CrossRef]
61. Jones, W.; Griffiths, K.; Barata, P.C.; Paller, C.J. PSMA Theranostics: Review of the Current Status of PSMA-Targeted Imaging and Radioligand Therapy. *Cancers* **2020**, *12*, 1367. Available online: http://www.ncbi.nlm.nih.gov/pubmed/32466595 (accessed on 16 April 2022). [CrossRef]
62. Ferraro, D.A.; Garcia Schüler, H.I.; Muehlematter, U.J.; Eberli, D.; Müller, J.; Müller, A.; Gablinger, R.; Kranzbühler, H.; Omlin, A.; Kaufmann, P.A.; et al. Impact of 68Ga-PSMA-11 PET staging on clinical decision-making in patients with intermediate or high-risk prostate cancer. *Eur. J. Nucl. Med. Mol. Imaging* **2020**, *47*, 652–664. Available online: http://www.ncbi.nlm.nih.gov/pubmed/31802175 (accessed on 16 April 2022). [CrossRef]
63. Luiting, H.B.; van Leeuwen, P.J.; Busstra, M.B.; Brabander, T.; van der Poel, H.G.; Donswijk, M.L.; Vis, A.N.; Emmett, L.; Stricker, P.D.; Roobol, M.J. Use of gallium-68 prostate-specific membrane antigen positron-emission tomography for detecting lymph node metastases in primary and recurrent prostate cancer and location of recurrence after radical prostatectomy: An overview of the current literature. *BJU Int.* **2020**, *125*, 206–214. Available online: http://www.ncbi.nlm.nih.gov/pubmed/31680398 (accessed on 16 April 2022). [CrossRef]
64. Maurer, T.; Eiber, M.; Schwaiger, M.; Gschwend, J.E. Current use of PSMA-PET in prostate cancer management. *Nat. Rev. Urol.* **2016**, *13*, 226–235. Available online: http://www.ncbi.nlm.nih.gov/pubmed/26902337 (accessed on 16 April 2022). [CrossRef]
65. Razik, A.; Das, C.J.; Sharma, S. PET-CT and PET-MR in urological cancers other than prostate cancer: An update on state of the art. *Indian J. Urol.* **2018**, *34*, 20–27. Available online: http://www.ncbi.nlm.nih.gov/pubmed/29343908 (accessed on 16 April 2022).
66. Eiber, M.; Maurer, T.; Souvatzoglou, M.; Beer, A.J.; Ruffani, A.; Haller, B.; Graner, F.-P.; Kübler, H.; Haberkorn, U.; Eisenhut, M.; et al. Evaluation of Hybrid 68Ga-PSMA Ligand PET/CT in 248 Patients with Biochemical Recurrence After Radical Prostatectomy. *J. Nucl. Med.* **2015**, *56*, 668–674. Available online: http://www.ncbi.nlm.nih.gov/pubmed/25791990 (accessed on 16 April 2022). [CrossRef]
67. Einspieler, I.; Rauscher, I.; Düwel, C.; Krönke, M.; Rischpler, C.; Habl, G.; Dewes, S.; Ott, A.; Wester, H.-J.; Schwaiger, M.; et al. Detection Efficacy of Hybrid 68Ga-PSMA Ligand PET/CT in Prostate Cancer Patients with Biochemical Recurrence After Primary Radiation Therapy Defined by Phoenix Criteria. *J. Nucl. Med.* **2017**, *58*, 1081–1087. Available online: http://www.ncbi.nlm.nih.gov/pubmed/28209912 (accessed on 16 April 2022). [CrossRef]
68. Pan, K.-H.; Wang, J.-F.; Wang, C.-Y.; Nikzad, A.A.; Kong, F.Q.; Jian, L.; Zhang, Y.-Q.; Lu, X.-M.; Xu, B.; Wang, Y.-L.; et al. Evaluation of 18F-DCFPyL PSMA PET/CT for Prostate Cancer: A Meta-Analysis. *Front. Oncol.* **2020**, *10*, 597422. Available online: http://www.ncbi.nlm.nih.gov/pubmed/33680924 (accessed on 16 April 2022). [CrossRef]
69. Hartrampf, P.E.; Petritsch, B.; Buck, A.K.; Serfling, S.E. Pitfalls in PSMA-PET/CT: Intensive bone marrow uptake in a case with polycythemia vera. *Eur. J. Nucl. Med. Mol. Imaging* **2021**, *48*, 1669–1670. Available online: http://www.ncbi.nlm.nih.gov/pubmed/33111182 (accessed on 16 April 2022). [CrossRef]
70. Cantiello, F.; Gangemi, V.; Cascini, G.L.; Calabria, F.; Moschini, M.; Ferro, M.; Musi, G.; Butticè, S.; Salonia, A.; Briganti, A.; et al. Diagnostic Accuracy of 64Copper Prostate-specific Membrane Antigen Positron Emission Tomography/Computed Tomography for Primary Lymph Node Staging of Intermediate- to High-risk Prostate Cancer: Our Preliminary Experience. *Urology* **2017**, *106*, 139–145. Available online: http://www.ncbi.nlm.nih.gov/pubmed/28438628 (accessed on 16 April 2022). [CrossRef]
71. Shen, G.; Deng, H.; Hu, S.; Jia, Z. Comparison of choline-PET/CT, MRI, SPECT, and bone scintigraphy in the diagnosis of bone metastases in patients with prostate cancer: A meta-analysis. *Skelet. Radiol.* **2014**, *43*, 1503–1513. Available online: http://www.ncbi.nlm.nih.gov/pubmed/24841276 (accessed on 16 April 2022). [CrossRef]
72. Beheshti, M.; Langsteger, W.; Fogelman, I. Prostate cancer: Role of SPECT and PET in imaging bone metastases. *Semin. Nucl. Med.* **2009**, *39*, 396–407. Available online: http://www.ncbi.nlm.nih.gov/pubmed/19801219 (accessed on 16 April 2022). [CrossRef] [PubMed]
73. O'Sullivan, J.M.; Norman, A.R.; Cook, G.J.; Fisher, C.; Dearnaley, D.P. Broadening the criteria for avoiding staging bone scans in prostate cancer: A retrospective study of patients at the Royal Marsden Hospital. *BJU Int.* **2003**, *92*, 685–689. Available online: http://www.ncbi.nlm.nih.gov/pubmed/14616446 (accessed on 16 April 2022). [CrossRef] [PubMed]
74. Lin, K.; Szabo, Z.; Chin, B.B.; Civelek, A.C. The value of a baseline bone scan in patients with newly diagnosed prostate cancer. *Clin. Nucl. Med.* **1999**, *24*, 579–582. Available online: http://www.ncbi.nlm.nih.gov/pubmed/10439178 (accessed on 16 April 2022). [CrossRef]

75. Abuzallouf, S.; Dayes, I.; Lukka, H. Baseline staging of newly diagnosed prostate cancer: A summary of the literature. *J. Urol.* **2004**, *171 Pt 1*, 2122–2127. Available online: http://www.ncbi.nlm.nih.gov/pubmed/15126770 (accessed on 16 April 2022). [CrossRef] [PubMed]
76. Harisinghani, M.G.; Barentsz, J.; Hahn, P.F.; Deserno, W.M.; Tabatabaei, S.; van de Kaa, C.H.; de la Rosette, J.; Weissleder, R. Noninvasive detection of clinically occult lymph-node metastases in prostate cancer. *N. Engl. J. Med.* **2003**, *348*, 2491–2499. Available online: http://www.ncbi.nlm.nih.gov/pubmed/12815134 (accessed on 16 April 2022). [CrossRef]
77. Perez-Lopez, R.; Tunariu, N.; Padhani, A.R.; Oyen, W.J.G.; Fanti, S.; Vargas, H.A.; Omlin, A.; Morris, M.J.; de Bono, J.; Koh, D.-M. Imaging Diagnosis and Follow-up of Advanced Prostate Cancer: Clinical Perspectives and State of the Art. *Radiology* **2019**, *292*, 273–286. Available online: http://www.ncbi.nlm.nih.gov/pubmed/31237493 (accessed on 16 April 2022). [CrossRef]
78. Westphalen, A.C.; Reed, G.D.; Vinh, P.P.; Sotto, C.; Vigneron, D.B.; Kurhanewicz, J. Multiparametric 3T endorectal mri after external beam radiation therapy for prostate cancer. *J. Magn. Reson. Imaging* **2012**, *36*, 430–437. Available online: http://www.ncbi.nlm.nih.gov/pubmed/22535708 (accessed on 16 April 2022). [CrossRef]
79. Pucar, D.; Shukla-Dave, A.; Hricak, H.; Moskowitz, C.S.; Kuroiwa, K.; Olgac, S.; Ebora, L.E.; Scardino, P.T.; Koutcher, J.A.; Zakian, K.L. Prostate cancer: Correlation of MR imaging and MR spectroscopy with pathologic findings after radiation therapy-initial experience. *Radiology* **2005**, *236*, 545–553. Available online: http://www.ncbi.nlm.nih.gov/pubmed/15972335 (accessed on 16 April 2022). [CrossRef]
80. Thoeny, H.C.; Froehlich, J.M.; Triantafyllou, M.; Huesler, J.; Bains, L.J.; Vermathen, P.; Fleischmann, A.; Studer, U.E. Metastases in normal-sized pelvic lymph nodes: Detection with diffusion-weighted MR imaging. *Radiology* **2014**, *273*, 125–135. Available online: http://www.ncbi.nlm.nih.gov/pubmed/24893049 (accessed on 16 April 2022). [CrossRef]
81. Woo, S.; Suh, C.H.; Kim, S.Y.; Cho, J.Y.; Kim, S.H. The Diagnostic Performance of MRI for Detection of Lymph Node Metastasis in Bladder and Prostate Cancer: An Updated Systematic Review and Diagnostic Meta-Analysis. *Am. J. Roentgenol.* **2018**, *210*, W95–W109. Available online: http://www.ncbi.nlm.nih.gov/pubmed/29381380 (accessed on 16 April 2022). [CrossRef]
82. Birkhäuser, F.D.; Studer, U.E.; Froehlich, J.M.; Triantafyllou, M.; Bains, L.J.; Petralia, G.; Vermathen, P.; Fleischmann, A.; Thoeny, H.C. Combined ultrasmall superparamagnetic particles of iron oxide-enhanced and diffusion-weighted magnetic resonance imaging facilitates detection of metastases in normal-sized pelvic lymph nodes of patients with bladder and prostate cancer. *Eur. Urol.* **2013**, *64*, 953–960. Available online: http://www.ncbi.nlm.nih.gov/pubmed/23916692 (accessed on 16 April 2022). [CrossRef] [PubMed]
83. Pasoglou, V.; Larbi, A.; Collette, L.; Annet, L.; Jamar, F.; Machiels, J.-P.; Michoux, N.; Vande Berg, B.C.; Tombal, B.; Lecouvet, F.E. One-step TNM staging of high-risk prostate cancer using magnetic resonance imaging (MRI): Toward an upfront simplified "all-in-one" imaging approach? *Prostate* **2014**, *74*, 469–477. Available online: http://www.ncbi.nlm.nih.gov/pubmed/24375774 (accessed on 16 April 2022). [CrossRef] [PubMed]
84. Padhani, A.R.; Lecouvet, F.E.; Tunariu, N.; Koh, D.-M.; De Keyzer, F.; Collins, D.J.; Sala, E.; Schlemmer, H.P.; Petralia, G.; Vargas, H.A.; et al. METastasis Reporting and Data System for Prostate Cancer: Practical Guidelines for Acquisition, Interpretation, and Reporting of Whole-body Magnetic Resonance Imaging-based Evaluations of Multiorgan Involvement in Advanced Prostate Cancer. *Eur. Urol.* **2017**, *71*, 81–92. Available online: http://www.ncbi.nlm.nih.gov/pubmed/27317091 (accessed on 16 April 2022). [CrossRef] [PubMed]
85. Barnes, A.; Alonzi, R.; Blackledge, M.; Charles-Edwards, G.; Collins, D.J.; Cook, G.; Coutts, G.; Goh, V.; Graves, M.; Kelly, C.; et al. UK quantitative WB-DWI technical workgroup: Consensus meeting recommendations on optimisation, quality control, processing and analysis of quantitative whole-body diffusion-weighted imaging for cancer. *Br. J. Radiol.* **2018**, *91*, 20170577. Available online: http://www.ncbi.nlm.nih.gov/pubmed/29076749 (accessed on 16 April 2022). [CrossRef]

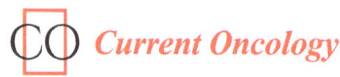 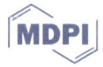

Case Report

Isolated Peritoneal Metastasis of Prostate Cancer Presenting with Massive Ascites: A Case Report

Hee Ryeong Jang [1], Kyoungyul Lee [2] and Kyu-Hyoung Lim [1,*]

[1] Department of Internal Medicine, Kangwon National University Hospital, Kangwon National University School of Medicine, Chuncheon-si 24289, Gangwon-do, Korea; jangheeryeong@kangwon.ac.kr
[2] Department of Pathology, Kangwon National University Hospital, Kangwon National University School of Medicine, Chuncheon-si 24289, Gangwon-do, Korea; pathkyl@kangwon.ac.kr
* Correspondence: kyuhyoung.lim@kangwon.ac.kr

Abstract: The peritoneal carcinomatosis of prostate cancer without bone or other visceral organ involvement is extremely rare. We report a case of an isolated peritoneal metastasis of prostate cancer in a patient without other metastatic sites and a history of prostate surgery. A 63-year-old male with locally advanced prostate cancer without known distant metastasis on androgen deprivation therapy presented with abdominal distension that had persisted for a month. Abdominopelvic computed tomography (CT) showed gastric wall thickening and a moderate amount of ascites. The gastroscopy showed hyperemic mucosal patches on the antrum body. A cytological examination of the ascites fluid was negative for malignant cells. Diagnostic laparoscopy showed multiple nodules in the peritoneum. A biopsy was performed. Histological findings were compatible with metastatic carcinoma of the prostate, which was immunohistochemically positive for pan-cytokeratin, the androgen receptor, and prostate-specific antigen (PSA). The patient was then treated with abiraterone acetate. After 1 month of treatment, both ascites and the PSA value decreased. We describe an extremely rare case of isolated peritoneal carcinomatosis from prostate cancer without any organ metastasis or history of surgery. Clinicians should be aware of these very rare metastases of prostate cancer. Hormonal therapy may be helpful for such cases.

Keywords: prostate cancer; peritoneal carcinomatosis; abiraterone acetate

1. Introduction

Prostate cancer is the second most common cancer and one of the leading causes of cancer-associated death in men. At the time of diagnosis, approximately 80% of prostate cancer is localized and fully contained within the prostate gland, with a minority of patients having locoregional metastasis (15%) or distant metastasis (5%) [1].

The most common sites of prostate cancer metastasis are locoregional lymph nodes (99%) and bones (84%). Distant lymph nodes (10.6%) and visceral organs such as the liver (~10%), lungs (9.1%), and brain (<2%) are uncommon sites of metastases [2].

Peritoneal carcinomatosis from prostate cancer is very rare, especially when there are no other visceral organ or bone metastases. Thirteen cases of isolated peritoneal carcinomatosis from prostate cancer in patients without a history of surgery have been reported to date. Some cases of peritoneal metastasis after prostate surgery have also been reported [3–5].

Herein, we report a case of an isolated peritoneal carcinomatosis from prostate cancer in a patient without visceral organ or skeletal metastases and no history of previous surgery.

2. Case Description

A 61-year-old male patient complained of urinary frequency in September 2019. The patient had an elevated prostate-specific antigen (PSA) value of 60.2 ng/mL. Abdominopelvic computed tomography (CT) showed the multifocal subcapsular extension of the entire prostate and an invasion of the bladder wall and the right distal ureter. He underwent a transrectal biopsy, and the pathology revealed a Gleason score nine (5 + 4) prostate adenocarcinoma. Whole-body bone scans were negative for skeletal involvement. The locally advanced prostate cancer had been treated with androgen deprivation therapy (ADT), leuprolide, and flutamide since September 2019. During the treatment period, his urinary frequency disappeared, and his PSA level decreased to below the normal range. ADT was maintained for 26 months until November 2021.

In December 2021, the patient was referred to our institute, presenting with gradually worsening abdominal distension that had persisted for a month. His PSA at that time was 586 ng/mL. An abdominal CT showed thickening of the gastric antrum wall and a moderate amount of ascites with peritoneal nodules, suggesting possible gastric cancer with peritoneal metastasis (Figure 1a,b). A gastroscopy showed hyperemic mucosal patches on the antrum body. A histological analysis of the endoscopic biopsy revealed chronic gastritis with intestinal metaplasia. A cytological examination of the ascites was negative for malignant cells. A bone scan showed no evidence of skeletal metastasis.

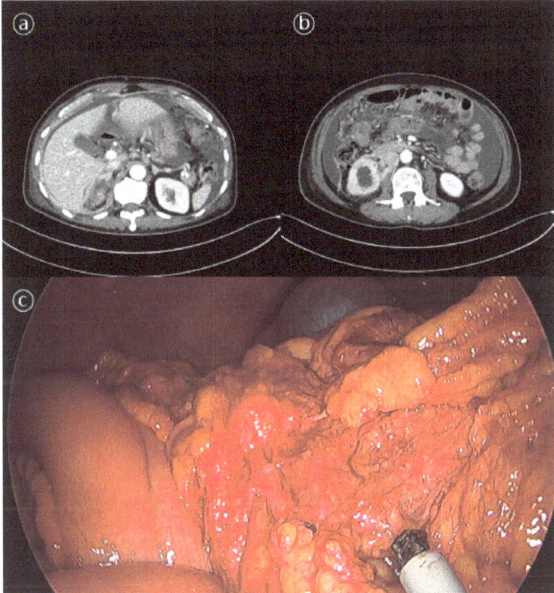

Figure 1. Abdominal computed tomography (**a**,**b**) and diagnostic laparoscopic biopsy (**c**) results. (**a**) Abdominal computed tomography showing metastatic lymph nodes in left gastric, retrocaval, aortocaval, and left paraaortic areas. (**b**) Abdominal computed tomography showing massive ascites and peritoneal seeding. (**c**) Diagnostic laparoscopic biopsy showing multiple nodular lesions in the omentum.

The patient underwent diagnostic laparoscopic exploration to determine the cause of the ascites. Multiple nodular lesions in the omentum were observed and biopsied (Figure 1c). As a pathologic finding, tumor cells with a diffuse sheet-like growth pattern were observed. Most tumor cells had a solid growth pattern, with some having a glandular differentiation. Additional immunohistochemical staining was negative for CK7, CK20, TTF-1, and CDX2, whereas staining results for pan-CK, the androgen receptor (AR), AMACR (alpha-methylacyl-CoA racemase), and PSA were positive (Figure 2). These results were consistent with metastatic carcinoma of the prostate.

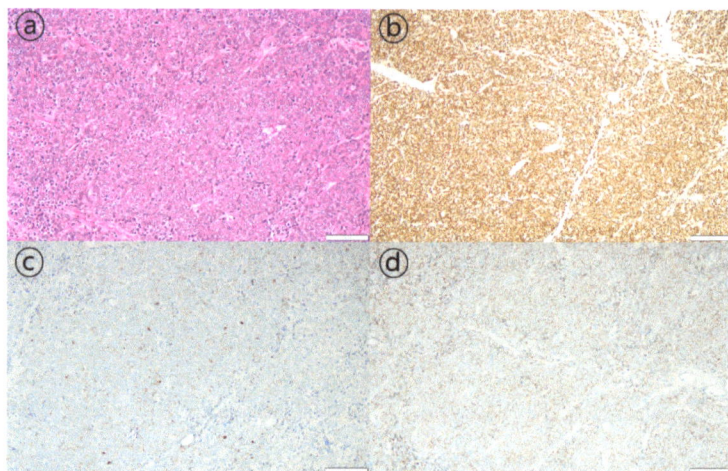

Figure 2. Histopathological findings of peritoneal carcinomatosis of prostate cancer. (**a**) Hematoxylin-eosin staining of the peritoneal nodule at a magnification of 200×. (**b–d**) Results of immunohistochemistry revealing the tumor was androgen-receptor-positive (magnification 100×), prostate-specific-antigen-positive, and alpha-methylacyl-CoA-racemase-positive (magnification 200×).

The patient started second-line treatment with abiraterone acetate alone in January 2022. One month after the start of abiraterone acetate, ascites significantly decreased, and the PSA level dropped to 1.22 ng/mL (the reference level). The patient is still being followed up with in the outpatient clinic. He continues the treatment with abiraterone acetate.

3. Discussion

The peritoneum is a rare metastatic site for prostate cancer. Previously reported studies on peritoneal carcinomatosis of prostate cancer can be categorized into three groups. First, two studies performed a postmortem analysis. Only 5 cases of peritoneal carcinomatosis from prostate cancer were found in 176 postmortem cases [6]. Thirteen isolated peritoneal cases were observed in the autopsy cases of 523 patients with prostate cancer [4]. Second, review studies have shown that peritoneal carcinomatosis of prostate cancer is related to surgical intervention. Approximately 15 reports of iatrogenic peritoneal carcinomatosis associated with prostate cancer surgery were found [4,5]. Third, Delchambre et al. reviewed 13 cases of isolated peritoneal carcinomatosis of prostate cancer without history of surgery [3].

The mechanism of peritoneal prostate cancer metastases is unknown. Based on previously reported studies, iatrogenic peritoneal seeding after surgery can cause rare metastases in patients with prostate cancer. However, cases of isolated peritoneal carcinomatosis without history of previous surgery are presumed to be due to other risk factors of peritoneal metastases. Including our case, 7 of 14 patients had Gleason scores ≥ 9 at the initial cancer histological analysis [3]. Patient age, initial PSA level, and initial staging at diagnosis have not been shown to be factors predicting isolated peritoneal carcinomatosis in patients with prostate cancer. Further studies such as genomics are necessary to identify the aggressive variants associated with progression to peritoneal carcinomatosis.

The early detection of metastasis in prostate cancer is also important to determine the optimal treatment plan. Including the current patient, a biopsy of metastatic lesion is usually performed to confirm the origin of metastasis. Recently, ^{68}Ga-prostate-specific membrane antigen (PSMA) PET, a new imaging modality, has received attention because of it being less invasive with higher sensitivity than the conventional modality in patients with prostate cancer. Especially, ^{68}Ga-PSMA PET has been reported to be more sensitive than a CT scan in detecting the early lymph node metastasis of prostate cancer, including the peritoneal carcinomatosis of prostate cancer [7,8].

The optimal management for the isolated peritoneal dissemination of prostate cancer has not been established yet. The majority of patients received docetaxel-based chemotherapy. Their overall survival time ranged from 3 weeks to 33 months [3]. Only three patients with isolated peritoneal carcinomatosis were treated with abiraterone acetate. Two of them showed a rapid response as in our case. The other one showed a radiological response for more than 4 years [3,9,10].

Visceral metastases occur mainly in the late stages of cancer. They are correlated with poor outcomes [2]. However, whether patients with isolated peritoneal carcinomatosis have a worse prognosis than those with other visceral metastases of prostate cancer is unknown. Therefore, active attempts to diagnose the cause of atypical presentations of prostate cancer and radical treatment strategies should be considered to control the related symptoms and improve the quality of life.

4. Conclusions

We presented a rarely described case of an isolated peritoneal carcinomatosis from prostate cancer in a patient without a previous history of surgery. After treatment with abiraterone acetate, ascites disappeared and the PSA level rapidly decreased within a month. This case highlights the importance of not only a thorough workup process for a very rare presentation of an isolated peritoneal carcinomatosis from prostate cancer, but also a proper therapeutic strategy with abiraterone acetate treatment. Physicians should be aware of this rare case of prostate cancer metastasis. Further studies are needed to identify predictive markers and the optimal treatment for isolated peritoneal carcinomatosis from prostate cancer.

Author Contributions: Writing-original draft preparation, H.R.J. and K.-H.L. Writing-review and editing, H.R.J. and K.-H.L. Performed histopathology exams and Writing-review, K.L. All authors have read and agreed to the published version of the manuscript.

Funding: This research received no external funding.

Institutional Review Board Statement: This study was conducted in accordance with the Declaration of Helsinki. It was approved by the Institutional Review Board of Kangwon National University Hospital (KNUH-2022-05-011).

Informed Consent Statement: Informed consent was obtained from the patient for the publication of this case report and related images.

Data Availability Statement: The data presented in this study are available on request from the corresponding author. The data are not publicly available due to patient confidentiality.

Conflicts of Interest: We have read and understood the current oncology policy on disclosing conflict of interests. We have no conflict of interest relevant to this study to disclose.

References

1. Siegel, R.L. Cancer Statistics, 2021. *CA Cancer J. Clin.* **2021**, *71*, 7–33. [CrossRef]
2. Litwin, M.S.; Tan, H.-J. The Diagnosis and Treatment of Prostate Cancer: A Review. *JAMA* **2017**, *317*, 2532–2542. [CrossRef] [PubMed]
3. Delchambre, E.; Rysselinck, S.; Pairet, G.; Confente, C.; Seront, E. Isolated peritoneal carcinomatosis in prostate cancer: From a successful hormonal management to a review of the literature. *Future Sci. OA* **2021**, *7*, FSO707. [CrossRef]
4. Motterle, G.; Ahmed, M.E.; Andrews, J.R.; Moschini, M.; Kwon, E.D.; Karnes, R.J. Tumor Seeding after Robot-Assisted Radical Prostatectomy: Literature Review and Experience from a Single Institution. *J. Urol.* **2020**, *203*, 1141–1146. [CrossRef] [PubMed]
5. Achard, V.; Achard, G.; Friedlaender, A.; Roth, A.; Tille, J.C.; Miralbell, R.; Zilli, T. Prostate cancer nonascitic peritoneal carcinomatosis after robot-assisted laparoscopic radical prostatectomy: 3 case reports and review of the literature. *Urology* **2020**, *137*, 121–125. [CrossRef] [PubMed]
6. FK, A. Carcinoma of the prostate; a study of the postmortem findings in 176 cases. *J. Urol.* **1948**, *60*, 599–603.

7. Maurer, T.; Gschwend, J.E.; Rauscher, I.; Souvatzoglou, M.; Haller, B.; Weirich, G.; Wester, H.-J.; Heck, M.; Kübler, H.; Eiber, M.; et al. Diagnostic Efficacy of ^{68}Gallium-PSMA Positron Emission Tomography Compared to Conventional Imaging for Lymph Node Staging of 130 Consecutive Patients with Intermediate to High Risk Prostate Cancer. *J. Urol.* **2016**, *195*, 1436–1443. [CrossRef] [PubMed]
8. Roach, P.J.; Francis, R.; Emmett, L.; Hsiao, E.; Kneebone, A.; Hruby, G.; Eade, T.; Nguyen, Q.A.; Thompson, B.D.; Scott, A.M.; et al. The Impact of ^{68}Ga-PSMA PET/CT on Management Intent in Prostate Cancer: Results of an Australian Prospective Multicenter Study. *J. Nucl. Med.* **2018**, *59*, 82–88. [CrossRef] [PubMed]
9. Sheng, J.; Findley, T.W.; Sadeghi-Nejad, H. Isolated non-ascitic peritoneal carcinomatosis from metastatic prostate cancer. *Urol. Case Rep.* **2017**, *10*, 14–15. [CrossRef] [PubMed]
10. İki, R.Y.R.P.S. Two unique cases of peritoneal carcinomatosis following robotic assisted radical prostatectomy. *J. Urol. Surg.* **2019**, *6*, 152–155.

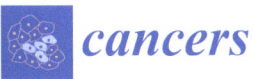

Article

New Insights into the Multivariate Analysis of SER Spectra Collected on Blood Samples for Prostate Cancer Detection: Towards a Better Understanding of the Role Played by Different Biomolecules on Cancer Screening: A Preliminary Study

Vlad Cristian Munteanu [1,2,3,†], Raluca Andrada Munteanu [3,4,†], Diana Gulei [4], Radu Mărginean [4], Vlad Horia Schițcu [1], Anca Onaciu [3,4], Valentin Toma [4], Gabriela Fabiola Știufiuc [5], Ioan Coman [2,6] and Rareș Ionuț Știufiuc [4,7,*]

[1] Department of Urology, The Oncology Institute "Prof Dr. Ion Chiricuta", 400015 Cluj-Napoca, Romania; vladcristian.munteanu@gmail.com (V.C.M.); schitcu@yahoo.com (V.H.S.)
[2] Department of Urology, "Iuliu Hatieganu" University of Medicine and Pharmacy, 400012 Cluj-Napoca, Romania; jcoman@yahoo.com
[3] "Iuliu Hatieganu" University of Medicine and Pharmacy, 400012 Cluj-Napoca, Romania; muresan.raluca.andrada@gmail.com (R.A.M.); anca.onaciu@umfcluj.ro (A.O.)
[4] MedFuture—Research Center for Advanced Medicine, "Iuliu Hatieganu" University of Medicine and Pharmacy, 400337 Cluj-Napoca, Romania; diana.c.gulei@gmail.com (D.G.); margi.radu@outlook.com (R.M.); valentin.toma@umfcluj.ro (V.T.)
[5] Faculty of Physics, "Babes Bolyai" University, 400084 Cluj-Napoca, Romania; gabriela.stiufiuc@ubbcluj.ro
[6] Department of Urology, Clinical Municipal Hospital, 400139 Cluj-Napoca, Romania
[7] Department of Pharmaceutical Physics-Biophysics, "Iuliu Hațieganu" University of Medicine and Pharmacy, 400349 Cluj-Napoca, Romania
* Correspondence: rares.stiufiuc@umfcluj.ro; Tel.: +40-726-340-278
† These authors contributed equally to this work.

Simple Summary: In recent years, research on biofluids using Raman and SERS has expanded dramatically, indicating the enormous promise of this technology as a high-throughput tool for identifying cancer and other disorders. In the investigations thus far, researchers have concentrated on a specific illness or condition, but the techniques employed to acquire experimental spectra prevent direct comparison of the data. This necessitates comparative research of a variety of diseases and an increase in scientific cooperation to standardize experimental conditions. In our study, positive results were reached by applying a combined SERS multivariate analysis (MVA) to the urgent problem of prostate cancer diagnosis that was directly linked to real-world settings in healthcare. Moreover, in comparison to the prostate-specific antigen (PSA) test, which has a high sensitivity but limited specificity, our combined SERS-MVA method has greater specificity, which may assist in preventing the overtreatment of patients.

Abstract: It is possible to obtain diagnostically relevant data on the changes in biochemical elements brought on by cancer via the use of multivariate analysis of vibrational spectra recorded on biological fluids. Prostate cancer and control groups included in this research generated almost similar SERS spectra, which means that the values of peak intensities present in SERS spectra can only give unspecific and limited information for distinguishing between the two groups. Our diagnostic algorithm for prostate cancer (PCa) differentiation was built using principal component analysis and linear discriminant analysis (PCA-LDA) analysis of spectral data, which has been widely used in spectral data management in many studies and has shown promising results so far. In order to fully utilize the entire SERS spectrum and automatically determine the most meaningful spectral features that can be used to differentiate PCa from healthy patients, we perform a multivariate analysis on both the entire and specific spectral intervals. Using the PCA-LDA model, the prostate cancer and control groups are clearly distinguished in our investigation. The separability of the following two data sets is also evaluated using two alternative discrimination techniques: principal

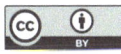

least squares discriminant analysis (PLS-DA) and principal component analysis—support vector machine (PCA-SVM).

Keywords: prostate cancer; Raman; SERS; multivariate analysis

1. Introduction

Prostate cancer is a major public health problem. It represents the second most diagnosed neoplasm and occupies sixth place in terms of mortality. In 2018, there were approximately 1.3 million cases and 359,000 deaths worldwide due to prostate cancer (PCa). In Europe, the estimated incidence of PCa in the same year was 449,800 cases and 107,300 deaths. This trend is stationary in many countries and is in a slow decline in high-income countries [1].

Before the discovery of prostatic specific antigen (PSA) in the 1970s and screening studies in the late 1980s, there was no way of screening for prostate cancers. Most of the patients first presented with metastatic disease, because nonmetastatic tumors are asymptomatic. Once PSA was discovered and used on a global scale, PCa became curable [2]. As such, urologists introduced new PSA-based screening procedures for PCa detection and soon started overdiagnosing and overtreating not only aggressive cases but cases that later proved to be indolent cancers. Unfortunately, PSA is organ-specific and not disease-specific, having high sensitivity but low specificity. PSA-based screening tests identify a lot of indolent cancers and have minimal impact on identifying aggressive tumors. To this day, PSA represents the cornerstone of prostate cancer diagnosis [3], and the ultimate goal remains to identify and treat only aggressive cancers [4,5].

The classical PCa detection scenario, based on PSA and prostate biopsy, has a detection rate of 20–40% accuracy [6], which is quite low compared to the incidence of this disease. In recent years, a lot of new alternative diagnostic modalities aroused such as blood and urine tests, and imaging modalities. Some of them even proved to be superior to PSA in detecting significant PCa cases [7]. Still, the challenge is to find a reliable, affordable, and accurate biomarker [8].

On the other hand, one of the most promising tools in the arsenal of developing new strategies for PCa diagnosis is Raman and its counterpart, surface-enhanced Raman spectroscopy (SERS). Raman spectroscopy has the capacity to provide specific molecular data (molecular fingerprint) that could have a major impact in the medical field, such as assisting new biomarker identification regarding cancer development [9]. These optical techniques are based on the inelastic scattering of the photons after the monochromatic laser beam interacts with specific molecules present in the biological sample. The difference between the energy of the photons before and after interacting with the sample, measured in wavenumbers, represents the Raman shift. These shifts, taken together, form the Raman spectrum, with each peak being assigned to a specific vibrational mode encountered in the sample [10]. Although Raman spectroscopy is able to detect a considerable number of biological molecules and offers support in the medical diagnosis area, its applicability can be limited by analyte concentration, which affects the intensity of the signal. Moreover, depending on the protocol strategy, the distribution of the molecules will not be homogenous, and the spectral bands will be preponderately assigned to proteins and other high molecular weight biomolecules present in the sample [11].

In the case of SERS, the procedure implies the use of metallic plasmonic substrates whose role is to enhance the Raman signal of the molecules present in the very close vicinity (<10 nm) of the plasmonic nanoparticles that compose the substrates. Depending on the adsorption geometry of the sample molecules onto these surfaces, their bands' intensity varies, which slightly complicates spectra interpretation. Several SERS-based cancer studies performed on blood samples derivatives reported an accuracy of over 90% in differentiating between PCa groups and controls [12–14]. Silver and/or gold nanoparticles are widely used as plasmonic substrates for such investigations. By carefully engineering substrates' composition and morphology, it was shown that SERS has the capacity to identify nanoscale molecular interactions responsible for chiral discrimination [15–17]. The use of low concentrations analytes is another major advantage of SERS analysis. However, similar to in most of the cases, these advantages come with a cost, and in the case of SERS performed on biological samples, the most important drawback is the lack of signal reproducibility. Very recently, our research group developed a new type of plasmonic solid substrate based on tangential flow filtered (TFF) silver nanoparticles capable of generating reproducible spectra that have been further analyzed by means of multivariate analysis (MVA) in order to develop an early-stage diagnostic tool for breast cancer [18].

In the last years, our research group has demonstrated that a combined SERS-MVA analysis can be successfully applied for the diagnosis of different types of solid tumors [19], including prostate cancer [11], using serum samples collected from cancer patients. Moreover, such implementations have been extensively involved in various statistical algorithms used to differentiate between normal and cancerous tissue from biopsies [20,21]. It has been shown that a SERS analysis on serum samples was able to discriminate between prostate cancer and benign prostatic hyperplasia (BPH) in an attempt to decrease the number of unnecessary biopsies [12]. In these cases, the SERS substrate was used in a colloidal formulation.

However, many difficulties can be encountered in the case of biofluid analysis due to their complex molecular composition. Very recently, Fornasaro et al., 2021, have shown that ergothioneine, which is a dietary amino acid present in different biological samples, has a great impact on the SERS spectra collected on various biofluids (e.g., erythrocytes lysates, serum, gingival crevicular fluid, seminal plasma, cerebrospinal fluid). This phenomenon may occur due to its high affinity for the plasmonic substrates, highlighting once more the major role played by the nanoscale interactions of the biomolecules with the plasmonic nanostructure in SERS analysis [22].

To overcome this drawback and to try to understand the influence of different molecular species on cancer discrimination using the here-proposed SERS-MVA analysis, in this study, we have employed a twofold strategy. Firstly, we have recorded, using our solid plasmonic substrates, very reproducible SERS spectra on serum and plasma samples collected from healthy (Controls) and prostate cancer donors (Patients) that were further compared and analyzed by means of MVA. Secondly, complete MVA studies have been performed not only on the entire spectra but also on specific spectral regions where the most intense vibrational bands have been assigned to proteins and/or other biomolecules in order to understand if these vibrational bands can be used for proper discrimination between cancer and control samples. In the end, the separability of the two data sets was evaluated using the following two alternative discrimination techniques: principal least squares discriminant analysis (PLS-DA) and principal component analysis—support vector machine (PCA-SVM).

To the best of our knowledge, such a comprehensive SERS-MVA analysis of vibrational spectra collected on plasma and serum for cancer discrimination has not been reported so far in the scientific literature.

2. Materials and Methods

2.1. Sample Collection

Between July 2018 and March 2020 we collected blood and prostate tissue samples from 103 patients treated in the Institute of Oncology "Prof. Dr. Ion Chiricuta" in Cluj-Napoca, Romania, in conformity with the ethical accordance 119/20 March 2020 from the University of Medicine and Pharmacy "Iuliu Hatieganu" Cluj-Napoca. All patients were previously diagnosed with prostate cancer through prostate biopsy. We excluded patients with other known diseases or those who had previous prostate cancer treatment (radiotherapy or androgen deprivation therapy). Regarding the PCa patient's cohort, the average age was 61 (min 52, maximum 68). In the case of the healthy donors' cohort, were selected individuals who were referred by the general practitioner to perform routine urological check-ups with an average age of over 50 years old.

Collected blood samples were immediately processed. For the processing of plasma, blood samples were immediately centrifuged for 10 min at 4000 rpm and the resulting supernatant (plasma) was transferred to a new tube that was stored at $-80\ °C$ until further processing. For serum, the blood collection tubes were left at room temperature for 30 min and then centrifuged for 10 min at 4000 rpm. The supernatant was transferred to a new tube and stored at $-80\ °C$ until further processing. All tubes were anonymously annotated based on patient's codes and additional variables.

2.2. Synthesis of Silver Nanoparticles

The silver nanoparticles were synthesized using the protocol developed by Leopold and Lendl, 2003 [23]. All the solutions were prepared using ultrapure water (18.2 MΩ × cm, ELGA Labwater from PURELAB Chorus, Buckinghamshire, UK). Briefly, 5 mL of 30 mM $NH_2OH \cdot HCl$ solution was mixed with 5 mL of 63.5 mM NaOH and 80 mL ultrapure water under vigorous stirring conditions (400 rpm). Then 10 mL of 10 mM $AgNO_3$ solution was carefully incorporated, under continuous stirring for 10 min until it was observed a brown to yellowish coloration. The resulting silver colloid was subjected to tangential flow filtration (TFF, Pall Corporation, New York, NY, USA) and physical characterization for further plasmonic substrate assembly.

2.3. SERS Substrates Preparation

Solid plasmonic SERS substrate preparation was performed according to a procedure described by Stiufiuc et al., 2020 [18]. This included several cleaning steps of CaF_2 Raman grade glass (Crystran, Poole, UK) using acetone, ethanol, and ultrapure water. After 15 min, the port-probe was heated at 40 °C using a plate heater and 1 µL of concentrated silver colloids was added to this site and let dry for 2 min. The obtained solid substrates were ready to use for SERS analysis after cooling down at room temperature.

2.4. SERS Measurements

For SERS measurements, 1 µL of serum, respectively, 1 µL plasma, were poured on the top of plasmonic substrates and were left to dry for 30 min at room temperature before acquiring the SERS signal. Both spectra types were recorded at maximum 50 µm distance from the sample ring edges. The analysis was performed using the Renishaw™ inVia Reflex Raman (Renishaw plc, Gloucestershire, UK) confocal multilaser spectrometer at a resolution of 2 cm^{-1}. The spectrograph was equipped with a 600 lines/mm grating and a charge-coupled device camera (CCD). An internal silicon reference was used for calibration. The 50× (N.A = 0.75) objective lens was used to record the spectra. A 785 nm diode laser was used for excitation. In the case of SERS, the acquisition time was set at 20 s (exposure time 5 s and 4 accumulations) while the laser power to the surface of the sample was 2 mW. Baseline correction was applied to all SERS spectra in order to eliminate the fluorescence background. The baseline correction was performed by using the Wire 4.2 software provided by Renishaw (Gloucestershire, UK) and final data processing was performed with aid of OriginPro 2019 software platform. The final spectrum represents the average of 20 spectral acquisitions.

2.5. Data Analysis

To inspect whether there is a separation between patient and control sample sets, we use a multivariate approach that is suitable for comparing high-dimensional objects such as spectral data. Thus, we apply principal component analysis—linear discriminant analysis (PCA-LDA) to the spectra, a method that combines dimensionality reduction with multivariate classification.

As a preprocessing step for the multivariate analysis, we align the spectra by sampling at equal 1 cm^{-1} intervals and normalizing them using the standard normal variate method, where each spectrum's intensities are scaled and offset such that they have zero mean and unit standard deviation.

Due to the curse of dimensionality, high-dimensional objects cannot be reliably compared in small samples. For this reason, we show that most of the information contained within our data is contained in a small number of dimensions—the principal components obtained via principal component analysis (PCA). Thus, by using PCA, we project the data onto a low-dimensional space by filtering out the noisy dimensions. This allows us to proceed with linear discriminant analysis (LDA), a method that finds a plane that separates data points belonging to different classes by optimizing for the maximum ratio of between-class and within-class variances.

The resulting LDA plane separates the projected spectra into two classes—patient and control. To assess the quality of this separation, we employ a leave-one-out cross-validation (LOOCV) scheme to efficiently use our relatively small dataset.

For completeness, we also evaluate the separability of the following two spectra sets (in LOOCV fashion) using alternative discrimination techniques: principal least squares discriminant analysis (PLS-DA), and principal component analysis—support vector machine (PCA-SVM).

We also perform a univariate analysis, where we test the separability hypothesis at each sampled wave number using a t-test. To account for multiple testing, we also apply a Benjamini-Hochberg correction with the false discovery rate set at 5% [24].

3. Results

3.1. Subject Data and Pathological Classification

One hundred and three patients were screened for enrolment in the study. After applying the exclusion criteria based on previous treatments and additional pathological status, as well as sample technical eligibility, 29 PCa patients were included. The clinical data for the patients are summarized in Table 1. The control cohort was formed of 14 samples. For all donors, both serum and plasma samples were analyzed.

Table 1. Clinical data of patients group.

Number of Patients: 29		
Age (years old)		
Min.	Max.	Mean
52	68	61
PSA (ng/mL)		
Min.	Max.	Mean
5.8	39.82	13.36
Pre-operative Gleason Score		
6		9 patients
7(3 + 4)		12 patients
7(4 + 3)		5 patients
8		1 patient
9		2 patients
Post-operative Gleason Score		
N+		2 patients
M+		0 patients
L+		2 patients
R+		4 patients

Legend: N+ (node positive); M+ (positive metastases); L+ (lymphatic invasion); R+ (tumoral margins).

3.2. SERS Analysis of Plasma and Serum Samples

Plasma and serum SERS spectra were recorded at a maximum 50 μm distance from the analyte ring edges and normalized to the integrated area under the curve in the 350–2200 cm^{-1} spectral interval. Figure 1 shows the average SERS spectra recorded on blood plasma samples collected from healthy and PCa patients. One can notice that the spectra are dominated by the following vibrational peaks: 390, 498, 596, 642, 728, 815, 893, 1010, 1075, 1136, 1209, 1256, 1336, 1369, 1406, 1447, 1508, 1577, 1617, and 1662 cm^{-1}. From these, 1256, 1336, 1506, 1617, and 1662 cm^{-1} bands are more intense in the case of the healthy group compared to the PCa group. Three prominent peaks that display the strongest SERS signal among both groups are located at 642, 1136, and 1662 cm^{-1}.

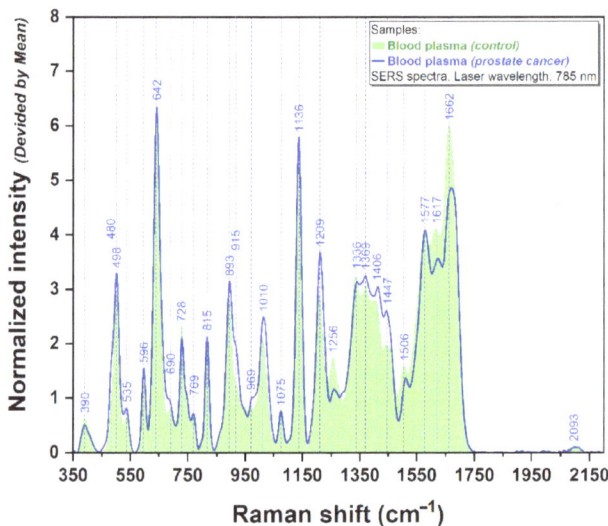

Figure 1. The average SERS plasmatic spectra obtained from PCa patients (n = 27, blue spectrum) and healthy donors (n = 14, green spectrum), using a 785 nm laser.

The SERS spectra of the serum samples, recorded using exactly the same experimental conditions and substrates, are presented in Figure 2. It can be noticed that the same three peaks dominate the spectra, as in the case of plasma samples. A distinct vibrational band located at 1099 cm^{-1} can be remarked only in the case of serum spectra collected from PCa patients. Moreover, slight differences can be observed regarding the intensity of several bands, which are more prominent for the healthy group (728, 1334, 1447, 1506, 1580, and 1662 cm^{-1}) than for the patients' group.

When visually comparing the plasmatic and serum SERS spectra, one can observe that serum samples offer a better separation between control and PCa groups.

3.3. Data Analysis

The PCA-LDA analysis uses two principal components for projecting the spectra. The number of components was chosen for the robustness to noise and amount of information contained within (explained variance). For plasma samples, the two components explain 76% of the variance (99% is explained by 14 components), while for serum samples, the two components explain 78% of the variance (99% is explained by 13 components).

The spectra projected onto the two principal components (PCs) are used as input for the discrimination step of the PCA-LDA analysis. For the plasma set of samples, our dataset consists of 14 controls and 27 patients, while for the serum samples it consists of 14 controls and 29 patients. The results of the PCA-LDA analysis, as evaluated using the LOOCV strategy, are shown in the following table (Table 2).

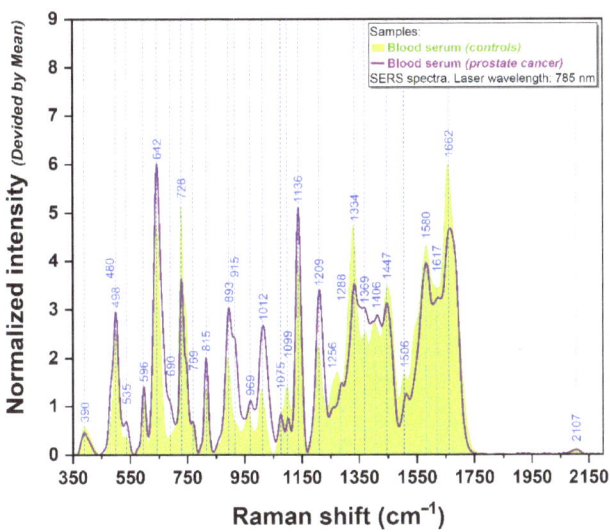

Figure 2. The average serum SERS spectra of PCa patients (n = 29, magenta spectrum) and healthy donors (n = 14, green spectrum), using a 785 nm laser.

Table 2. PCA-LDA results on plasma and serum samples.

Sample	Accuracy	Precision	Sensitivity	Specificity	True Pos.	True Neg.	False Pos.	False Neg.
Plasma	87.8%	86.7%	96.3%	71.4%	26	10	4	1
Serum	97.7%	100.0%	96.6%	100.0%	28	14	0	1

Additionally, we also performed a PCA-LDA analysis under the same set-up on a restricted band of wavenumbers, between 1200 cm^{-1} and 1700 cm^{-1}. Table 3 shows the obtained results.

Table 3. PCA-LDA results on plasma and serum samples for 1200–1700 cm^{-1} spectral region.

Sample	Accuracy	Precision	Sensitivity	Specificity	True Pos.	True Neg.	False Pos.	False Neg.
Plasma	80.5%	85.2%	85.2%	71.4%	23	10	4	4
Serum	93.0%	96.4%	93.1%	92.9%	27	13	1	2

We ran experiments with more principal components as well, and adding more PCs generally improves the obtained results. Nevertheless, given the size of our dataset, we decided to use a small number of PCs to avoid the potential overfitting of complex multivariate models to our data. Specifically, with two PCs, we see negligible differences in the classification performance obtained via LOOCV and the training folds (Figure 3). With larger numbers of PCs, this difference is more pronounced, suggesting that the more complex PCA models do not generalize as well from our limited data set.

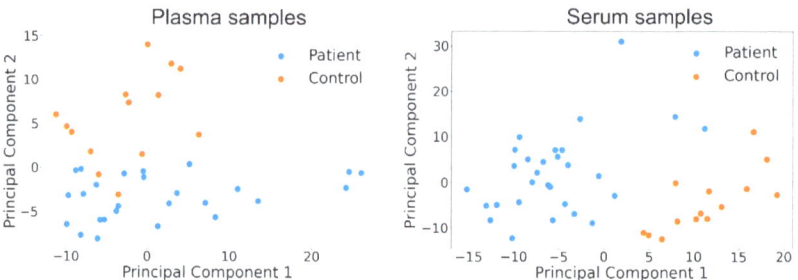

Figure 3. Score-score plots for the first two principal components obtained from plasma and serum samples LOOCV analysis.

Table S2 shows the accuracy obtained with different models (PCA-LDA and PLSDA) for both train and test samples. We used accuracy for ease of measurement and clarity—the same relative train/test differences can be observed across other metrics as well.

Finally, to validate further the observed separations, we also classify the spectra using principal least squares discriminant analysis (PLSDA) with two intermediate dimensions, similar to our PCA-LDA setup. The following table (Table 4) shows the obtained results.

Table 4. PLSDA results on plasma and serum samples.

Sample	Accuracy	Precision	Sensitivity	Specificity	True Pos.	True Neg.	False Pos.	False Neg.
Plasma	90.2%	89.7%	96.3%	78.6%	26	11	3	1
Serum	95.3%	100.0%	93.1%	100.0%	27	14	0	2

The use of the PLSDA method allowed us to compute the importance of wavenumbers in the classification decision by using the variable importance in projection (VIP) score, which measures the relative contribution of each variable (wavenumber) in the classification decision. A VIP score greater than 1.0 is conventionally considered to be the threshold for selecting important variables. In the following figures (Figures 3 and 4), we show the bands of important variables as instructed by the VIP score, as well as the bands of wavenumbers where the univariate difference in mean intensity between the patient and control sets is deemed significant by a Benjamini-Hochberg (BH)-corrected t-test using a false discovery rate (FDR) set at 5%.

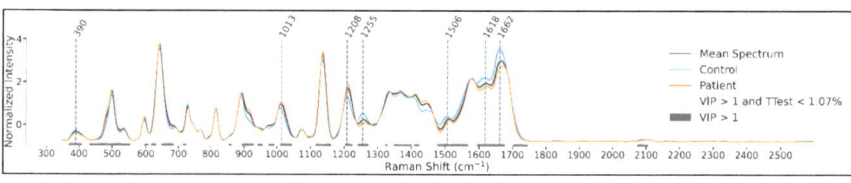

Figure 4. Mean spectra with emphasized t-test significance and VIP > 1 for plasma samples.

We also mark the significant peaks identified in these mean spectra. The identified peaks can differ slightly between the class-wise and grouped charts since the control and patient mean spectra can have peaks that do not perfectly overlap (in the charts only one of the peaks is shown for figure legibility), and these will determine a different peak in the grouped spectrum.

For the plasma samples, we see significant peaks around the 390, 1012, 1210, 1260, 1622, and 1666 cm^{-1} spectral regions (Figure 4).

For the serum samples, we see significant peaks around the 390, 499, 643, 729, 815, 892, 1012, 1100, 1137, 1210, 1331, 1368, 1412, 1511, 1582, and 1660 cm^{-1}, and in the range above 1700 cm^{-1} spectral bands (Figure 5).

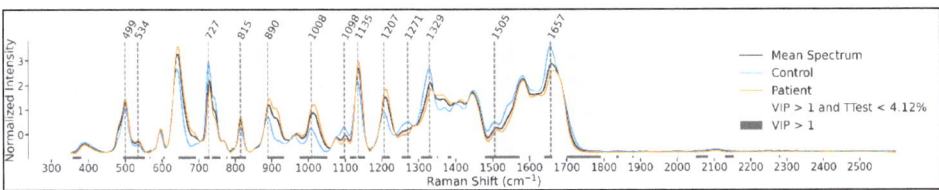

Figure 5. Mean spectra with emphasized t-test significance and VIP > 1 for serum samples.

We observe that for both plasma and serum samples, there is a significant overlap between the wavenumbers considered important in the univariate and multivariate analysis.

The classification results of PCA-SVM using 2 PCs and a linear kernel for the SVM, SVM using a linear kernel and no dimensionality reduction, and LDA with no dimensionality reduction are presented in Table S3. Figures S1 and S2 show the mean spectrum and the first two principal components of the plasma and serum samples.

4. Discussion

Liquid biopsies, including plasma, serum, or urine, offer a valuable platform in determining new biomarkers for prostate cancer diagnosis, leading to time efficiency and enlarging the treatment options, therefore improving the quality of life for such patients.

Cell-free nucleic acids (cfNA), which may be detected in the blood plasma, have been the subject of most liquid biopsy investigations aimed at identifying biomarkers that are predictive, diagnostic, and/or prognostic in cancer [25]. Other elements, such as circulating proteins, analytes, and exosomes, have received less research attention, however. Cancer patients' circulating DNA, tumor cells, and exosomes may all be detected using liquid biopsy methods that have yet to be used in the clinical setting [26–28].

This study's aim was to explore the outstanding properties of univariate and multivariate analysis performed on plasmatic and serum SERS spectra in discriminating between PCa patients and healthy donors. We also wanted to investigate the role of the most important vibrational bands, assigned to different biomolecules present in blood samples, in the discrimination process.

SERS is an ultrasensitive technique that can achieve a diagnostic value by enabling the spectral analysis of biological samples and molecules. Most of the SERS analyses on blood samples are performed on colloidal nanoparticles. The affinity of the molecules toward the plasmonic substrate plays a crucial role in the recording process of SERS spectra. Very recently, it has been shown that there is a strong possibility that much of the SERS spectra collected on blood samples reported so far in the literature are dominated by a dietary amino acid (ergothioneine) that has a great affinity for the plasmonic substrates used in SERS experiments [22]. In order to reduce the possibility of the occurrence of such experimental artifacts, all the spectra included in this study have been recorded on solid plasmonic substrates prepared using a procedure developed in our laboratory that proved their capacity to generate specific and reproducible SERS spectra of blood plasma and serum based on their ability to act as a "spectroscopic filter" [18].

The multivariate analysis of these spectral data offers the advantage of determining more accurately and realistically the factors that influence the variability between the two groups of samples. In addition, the univariate analysis represents a strong descriptive method that can clearly elucidate the differences between the two types of samples investigated in this study. Moreover, such algorithms are still needed to be implemented in the diagnosis steps for a better correlation with molecular modifications associated with cancer development and progression.

Our multivariate analysis, performed on the entire spectral window (350–2200 cm^{-1}), supports the idea that the use of serum samples instead of plasma ones can improve the discrimination process between PCa patients and healthy donors. The results obtained on serum samples offered a better accuracy (97.7% vs. 87.8%), precision (100% vs. 86.7%), sensitivity (96.6% vs. 96.3%), and specificity (100% vs. 71.4%) as compared to those obtained on plasma samples.

We have performed a univariate analysis, where we test the separability hypothesis at each sampled wavenumber using a *t*-test. To account for multiple testing, we also applied a BH correction with the FDR set at 5%. In other words, we have tested the hypothesis that the mean intensity is significantly different between the two groups (control and patients) at each individual wave number. The univariate nature of the analysis is due to the lack of interaction between the different variables (wavenumbers) in the analysis. We have reported our results as charts of the mean spectrum (both class-wise and grouped), where we have emphasized the regions of wave numbers that were identified as being significant with respect to the BH-corrected t-test.

Plasma sample spectral data analysis detected 6 major regions in the SERS spectra corresponding to 350–400, 740–870, 990–1030, 1220–1300, 1390–1410, and 1750–1760 cm^{-1} bands, achieving an AUROC (area under the receiver operating characteristic curve) value of 0.9 or higher. In addition, we also identified three other isolated spectral windows (centered at 970, 1180, and 1710 cm^{-1}) that could play a role in discrimination. On the other hand, our univariate analysis identified the presence of the following 6 major peaks relevant for SERS-based discrimination between PCa and controls: 390, 1012, 1210, 1260, 1622, and 1666 cm^{-1}. They can be assigned as follows: ~390—uric acid [29], ~1012—breathing mode of aromatic amino acids and nucleic acids [18,30–33], ~1210—proteins, aromatic amino acids [34–38], ~1260—proteins, amide III [29,32,36,39], ~1666 cm^{-1}—proteins, amide I α-helix [11,30,35,40,41].

Concerning serum samples, the univariate analysis reveals a broad area (350–1750 cm^{-1}) in the spectra that can be used successfully in differentiating PCa from controls. This region is composed of the following 3 windows: 350–1550, 1600–1700, and 1750 cm^{-1}. The univariate analysis indicates the presence of the following 16 important peaks for PCa and normal sample differentiation, located at: 390, 499, 643, 729, 815, 892, 1012, 1100, 1137, 1210, 1331, 1368, 1412, 1511, 1582, 1660 cm^{-1}. These can be assigned as follows: 390—uric acid [29], 499—proteins, amino acids [29,40,42,43], 643—DNA bases, ring stretching of uric acid and hypoxanthine [18,31,36,37,43], 729—DNA/RNA bases, ring stretching in uric acid and hypoxanthine [30,31,43,44], 815—collagen, uric acid [18,41,45], 892—deoxyribose phosphate backbone, glutathione, uric acid [18,43,46], 1012—aromatic amino acids and nucleic acids [18,30–33], 1100—proteins, phospholipids and carbohydrates [36,38,43,46], 1137—aminoacids, phopsholipids [18,41,42,45], 1210—aromatic amino acids [34–38], 1331—nucleic acid bases, phospholipids, proteins, amide linkages [18,35,36], 1368—pyridine bases, amide III, phospholipids [36,47], 1412—collagen, lipids and phospholipids [31,36], 1511—DNA/RNA bases, amide II, phenylalanine [36], 1582—phenylalanine [18,31,36,43], DNA/RNA bases, 1660 cm^{-1}—amide I α-helix [11,30,35,40,41]. Most of these bands are attributed to nucleic acid bases and proteins, which may indicate that a PCa complex metabolism has a crucial role in disease development. For a more accurate determination, we have prepared a tentative assignment in Table S1 for all the recorded SERS spectra of plasma and serum samples according to the available literature [19,29–67].

498, 642, 815, 893, 1010, 1137, 1210, 1368, and 1412 cm^{-1} vibrational bands show high intensities in PCa serum samples compared to normal samples. On the other hand, we notice that 729, 1100, 1331, 1511, 1582, and 1660 cm^{-1} show higher intensities in normal samples compared to PCa samples.

At first glance, we can observe that the following 4 major peaks are common in both serum and plasma samples: 390, 1010, 1210, and 1662 cm^{-1}. The 1010 and 1210 cm^{-1} followed a similar increased pattern regarding intensities in PCa samples, while the

390 and 1662 cm^{-1} bands' increased intensity is specific for normal samples. Moreover, an overview of both SERS spectra considering the results obtained from the univariate analysis indicates a very uniform tendency respecting the bands' intensities.

In the case of PCa plasma and serum samples, 1010 cm^{-1} symmetric ring breathing mode of phenylalanine and 1210 cm^{-1} protein bands showed an increased signal than those of normal samples. On the other hand, the amide I bands (1600–1700 cm^{-1}) were lower compared to normal plasma and serum samples. A slight difference can be observed in the case of amide III regions regarding the relevant peaks in discriminating between PCa patients and healthy donors. The 1260 cm^{-1} peak was determined to be relevant for normal plasma samples, where it presents a higher intensity than PCa samples. Concerning serum samples, the 1368 cm^{-1} peak showed an increased behavior for PCa compared to normal samples. Analyzing both SERS spectra, these two peaks followed similar intensities in both types of samples investigated.

These similarities between both plasma and serum samples may be due to abnormal metabolism associated with cancer, implying the activation of alternative metabolic systems to create ATP, proteins, nucleosides, and lipids for cellular growth [68]. Cancers of the peripheral prostatic epithelium may have a similar, citrate-oriented metabolism to that of normal prostate tissue. The oxidative phosphorylation in primary prostate tumors seems to be increased, although glycolysis is restricted. Prostate cancer also seems to be connected with the synthesis of fatty acids in the form of lipogenesis [69]. Advanced castrate-resistant prostate cancer is characterized by increased glycolysis. Maintaining the amino acid pool and converting it to glucose, lipids, and precursors of nitrogen-containing metabolites such as purines or pyrimidines for nucleic acid synthesis are all important aspects of amino acid metabolism in prostate cancer growth [70].

PCa has been previously linked to a buildup of cholesterol and has been shown to synthesize fatty acids by means of de novo lipid synthesis [71]. It is well known that freshly generated fatty acids enhance cellular pathways that promote cell growth and survival in cancer patients [72,73]. Lipogenesis has been demonstrated to increase the saturation of membrane lipids, which has implications for membrane dynamics and the absorption and effectiveness of chemotherapy [74].

The bands situated between 900 and 1300 cm^{-1} are mostly generated by carbohydrates and phosphates found in nucleic acids [36]. Carbohydrates are represented by the C-COO$^-$ stretching vibration at the band 915 cm^{-1} [39,53]. Biopsies of prostate cancer tissue and cervical cancer tissue have shown that glycogen concentration is lower in prostate cancer tissue and cervical adenocarcinoma cells [75]. It is known that in malignant cells, the cause of decreased glycogen can be an implication of increased metabolic activity [75–77].

Due to the C=O and C-N stretching vibrations, the amide I band (1600–1700 cm^{-1}) gives information on the secondary structure of proteins [78–80], which has been thoroughly studied in several research studies. There is, however, a correlation between the peak at 1617 cm^{-1} assigned to C=O, C=C, and NH$_2$ stretching vibrations [30,42,59] and the existence of protein aggregates [79,81]. Protein misfolding and subsequent aggregation are caused by conditions that cause cancer cells to be subjected to stress [82]. Cancer cells and tumors may develop protein aggregates of the tumor suppressor gene p53 [83–85], which may play an essential role in the development of cancer [86]. It has been shown that the loss of proteostasis in cancer growth is linked to platinum resistance and the stem cell characteristics of certain ovarian cancers [87]. As an example, PNT1A and PNT2 normal prostate cell lines are characterized by spectral assignments of 1653 and 1636 cm^{-1}, respectively, which are associated with α-helices and parallel sheets [71]. There are fewer β-sheets in proteins that are generally more soluble and less prone to congregating [88], which may be due to the fact that most proteins have a combination of β-sheets and α-helices as secondary structures [80].

5. Conclusions

The discrimination between PCa and healthy donors based on liquid biopsy still remains a challenging analysis since it needs multiple examinations. However, to our knowledge, this is the first study that has evaluated blood plasma and serum provided by PCa patients and healthy donors using a combined SERS, multivariate and univariate analyses in order to establish which analyte can offer a better diagnostic value. Our results show that serum samples have a better diagnostic capacity compared to plasma samples. The best values have been obtained when performing the multivariate analysis of the full spectrum as well as the two spectral intervals of 825–1050 and 1506–1750 cm^{-1}.

The spectrum is dominated by aromatic amino acids (tryptophan, tyrosine, phenylalanine, serine) and protein vibrational bands, which have been shown to achieve a valuable potential as biomarkers [70,89]. There are several studies that engaged the use of chromatography and mass spectrometry techniques to determine the free amino acid profiles from liquid samples such as urine, serum, or plasma [89–95]. These are indicating that the amount of some specific amino acids in such biological samples may gain more insights into PCa diagnosis purposes. Therefore, we believe that a combination between SERS and proteomics and metabolomics methods together with multivariate and univariate analyses tools will elevate the standard diagnostic (PSA level evaluation and prostate tissue biopsy) properties.

There are some drawbacks to this research, the most significant of which being the limited number of patients included in the study. In order to obtain the most accurate results, we only included individuals with prostatic adenocarcinoma confirmed by biopsy. Our study also eliminated individuals with other chronic illnesses, patients with unconfirmed tumors, or patients with confirmed tumors but not eligible for surgery (advanced cancers), since their serology would have remained unchanged. However, since this is a pilot study whose major goal is to estimate average values and variability in order to design larger later investigations, we believe that the sample sizes were sufficient.

Our study shows promising results since SERS analysis can be performed on small amounts of liquid samples with high specificity and reproducibility as a direct consequence of the use of our solid plasmonic substrate [18]. Moreover, the implementation of multivariate and univariate analysis allowed us to determine that serum samples offer more accurate results in discriminating between PCa patients and healthy donors when compared to plasma samples. Another advantage of this design refers to the minimal invasiveness of the technique, which is supported by easy handling and fast results generation. At the same time, there is still a need for such investigations on large cohorts in order to establish the necessity of needle biopsy and histopathological examination.

Supplementary Materials: The following are available online at https://www.mdpi.com/article/10.3390/cancers14133227/s1, Table S1: The SERS peaks tentative assignments of major vibrational bands in plasma and serum samples from PCa patients and healthy donors. Table S2: Different models (PCA-LDA and PLSDA) for both train and test samples. Table S3: The classification results of PCA-SVM, SVM, and LDA analyses. Figure S1: Mean spectrum and first two principal components for plasma spectra. Figure S2: Mean spectrum and first two principal components for serum spectra. Reference [96] is cited in the supplementary materials.

Author Contributions: Conceptualization, V.C.M., I.C. and R.I.Ș.; methodology, V.C.M. and R.I.Ș.; software, V.T. and R.M.; validation, V.C.M., I.C. and R.I.Ș.; formal analysis, V.C.M., R.A.M., D.G., A.O., V.T. and G.F.Ș.; investigation, V.C.M., R.A.M., V.H.S., A.O., V.T., G.F.Ș., and R.I.Ș.; resources, V.C.M., R.A.M., D.G., and R.I.Ș.; data curation, I.C. and R.I.Ș.; writing—original draft preparation, V.C.M., R.A.M., D.G., A.O., V.T., R.M. and R.I.Ș.; writing—review and editing, V.C.M., R.A.M., A.O. and R.I.Ș.; visualization, V.C.M., V.T. and R.M.; supervision, R.I.Ș.; project administration, V.C.M. and R.I.Ș.; funding acquisition, R.A.M., D.G. and R.I.Ș. All authors have read and agreed to the published version of the manuscript.

Funding: This work was supported by the Executive Agency for Higher Education, Research, Development and Innovation Funding (UEFISCDI), Romanian Ministry of Education and Research, grant no. PN-III-P4-ID-PCCF-2016-0112, research grant No. PCE 185/18.02.2021 "Validation of epigenetic reprogramming of lung cancer models and anti-cancer activity through serial administration of repositioned 5-Azacytidine-AZUR", PN-III-P4-ID-PCE-2020-1957, "MicroRNAs in prostate adenocarcinoma. Diagnostic, prognostic and therapeutic role"-PCD1530/43 funded by "Iuliu Hatieganu" University of Medicine and Pharmacy, Cluj-Napoca, Romania and "Role and evaluation of new therapeutic targets in prostatic adenocarcinoma"—PCD 2461/48, funded by "Iuliu Hatieganu" University of Medicine and Pharmacy, Cluj-Napoca, Romania.

Institutional Review Board Statement: The study was conducted according to the guidelines of the Declaration of Helsinki, and approved Ethics Committee of University of Medicine and Pharmacy, Cluj-Napoca, Romania, and The Oncology Institute "Prof Dr. Ion Chiricuta", protocol code 145/19 September 2019.

Informed Consent Statement: Informed consent was obtained from all subjects involved in the study. Written informed consent has been obtained from all the patients to publish this paper.

Data Availability Statement: The data presented in this study are available on request from the corresponding author. The processed data is contained within the article.

Acknowledgments: This work was granted by project PDI-PFE-CDI 2021, entitled Increasing the Performance of Scientific Research, Supporting Excellence in Medical Research and Innovation, PROGRES, no. 40PFE/30 December 2021.

Conflicts of Interest: The authors declare no conflict of interest. The funders had no role in the design of the study; in the collection, analyses, or interpretation of data; in the writing of the manuscript, or in the decision to publish the results.

References

1. Culp, M.B.; Soerjomataram, I.; Efstathiou, J.A.; Bray, F.; Jemal, A. Recent Global Patterns in Prostate Cancer Incidence and Mortality Rates. *Eur. Urol.* **2020**, *77*, 38–52. [CrossRef] [PubMed]
2. Carlsson, S.V.; Vickers, A.J. Screening for Prostate Cancer. *Med. Clin. N. Am.* **2020**, *104*, 1051–1062. [CrossRef] [PubMed]
3. Albertsen, P.C. Prostate cancer screening and treatment: Where have we come from and where are we going? *BJU Int.* **2020**, *126*, 218–224. [CrossRef] [PubMed]
4. Pellegrino, F.; Coghi, A.; Lavorgna, G.; Cazzaniga, W.; Guazzoni, E.; Locatelli, I.; Villa, I.; Bolamperti, S.; Finocchio, N.; Alfano, M.; et al. A mechanistic insight into the anti-metastatic role of the prostate specific antigen. *Transl. Oncol.* **2021**, *14*, 101211. [CrossRef]
5. Gatto, F.; Bratulic, S.; Cavarretta, I.T.R.; Alfano, M.; Maccari, F.; Galeotti, F.; Volpi, N.; Edqvist, P.-H.; Levin, M.; Nyman, J.; et al. Detection of any-stage cancer using plasma and urine glycosaminoglycans. *J. Clin. Oncol.* **2021**, *39*, 3034. [CrossRef]
6. Wu, Q.; Chen, G.; Qiu, S.; Feng, S.; Lin, D. A target-triggered and self-calibration aptasensor based on SERS for precise detection of a prostate cancer biomarker in human blood. *Nanoscale* **2021**, *13*, 7574–7582. [CrossRef]
7. Munteanu, V.C.; Munteanu, R.A.; Gulei, D.; Schitcu, V.H.; Petrut, B.; Berindan Neagoe, I.; Achimas Cadariu, P.; Coman, I. PSA Based Biomarkers, Imagistic Techniques and Combined Tests for a Better Diagnostic of Localized Prostate Cancer. *Diagnostics* **2020**, *10*, 806. [CrossRef]
8. Tan, G.H.; Nason, G.; Ajib, K.; Woon, D.T.S.; Herrera-Caceres, J.; Alhunaidi, O.; Perlis, N. Smarter screening for prostate cancer. *World J. Urol.* **2019**, *37*, 991–999. [CrossRef]
9. Zhou, Y.; Liu, C.; Wu, B.; Zhang, C.; Yu, X.; Cheng, G.; Chen, H.; Li, S.; Liang, Q.; Zhang, M.; et al. Invited Article: Molecular biomarkers characterization for human brain glioma grading using visible resonance Raman spectroscopy. *APL Photonics* **2018**, *3*, 120802. [CrossRef]
10. Crow, P.; Stone, N.; Kendall, C.A.; Uff, J.S.; Farmer, J.A.M.; Barr, H.; Wright, M.P.J. The use of Raman spectroscopy to identify and grade prostatic adenocarcinoma in vitro. *Br. J. Cancer* **2003**, *89*, 106–108. [CrossRef]
11. Stefancu, A.; Moisoiu, V.; Couti, R.; Andras, I.; Rahota, R.; Crisan, D.; Pavel, I.E.; Socaciu, C.; Leopold, N.; Crisan, N. Combining SERS analysis of serum with PSA levels for improving the detection of prostate cancer. *Nanomedicine* **2018**, *13*, 2455–2467. [CrossRef] [PubMed]
12. Chen, N.; Rong, M.; Shao, X.; Zhang, H.; Liu, S.; Dong, B.; Xue, W.; Wang, T.; Li, T.; Pan, J. Surface-enhanced Raman spectroscopy of serum accurately detects prostate cancer in patients with prostate-specific antigen levels of 4–10 ng/mL. *Int. J. Nanomed.* **2017**, *12*, 5399–5407. [CrossRef] [PubMed]
13. Shao, X.; Pan, J.; Wang, Y.; Zhu, Y.; Xu, F.; Shangguan, X.; Dong, B.; Sha, J.; Chen, N.; Chen, Z.; et al. Evaluation of expressed prostatic secretion and serum using surface-enhanced Raman spectroscopy for the noninvasive detection of prostate cancer, a preliminary study. *Nanomed. Nanotechnol. Biol. Med.* **2017**, *13*, 1051–1059. [CrossRef] [PubMed]

14. Li, S.; Zhang, Y.; Xu, J.; Li, L.; Zeng, Q.; Lin, L.; Guo, Z.; Liu, Z.; Xiong, H.; Liu, S. Noninvasive prostate cancer screening based on serum surface-enhanced Raman spectroscopy and support vector machine. *Appl. Phys. Lett.* **2014**, *105*, 091104. [CrossRef]
15. Stiufiuc, R.; Iacovita, C.; Stiufiuc, G.; Bodoki, E.; Chis, V.; Lucaciu, C.M. Surface mediated chiral interactions between cyclodextrins and propranolol enantiomers: A SERS and DFT study. *Phys. Chem. Chem. Phys.* **2015**, *17*, 1281–1289. [CrossRef]
16. Știufiuc, G.F.; Toma, V.; Onaciu, A.; Chiș, V.; Lucaciu, C.M.; Știufiuc, R.I. Proving Nanoscale Chiral Interactions of Cyclodextrins and Propranolol Enantiomers by Means of SERS Measurements Performed on a Solid Plasmonic Substrate. *Pharmaceutics* **2021**, *13*, 1594. [CrossRef]
17. Bodoki, E.; Oltean, M.; Bodoki, A.; Știufiuc, R. Chiral recognition and quantification of propranolol enantiomers by surface enhanced Raman scattering through supramolecular interaction with β-cyclodextrin. *Talanta* **2012**, *101*, 53–58. [CrossRef]
18. Știufiuc, G.F.; Toma, V.; Buse, M.; Mărginean, R.; Morar-Bolba, G.; Culic, B.; Tetean, R.; Leopold, N.; Pavel, I.; Lucaciu, C.M.; et al. Solid Plasmonic Substrates for Breast Cancer Detection by Means of SERS Analysis of Blood Plasma. *Nanomaterials* **2020**, *10*, 1212. [CrossRef]
19. Moisoiu, V.; Stefancu, A.; Gulei, D.; Boitor, R.; Magdo, L.; Raduly, L.; Pasca, S.; Kubelac, P.; Mehterov, N.; Chis, V.; et al. SERS-based differential diagnosis between multiple solid malignancies: Breast, colorectal, lung, ovarian and oral cancer. *Int. J. Nanomed.* **2019**, *14*, 6165–6178. [CrossRef]
20. Wu, B.; Liu, C.-H.; Boydston-White, S.; Beckman, H.; Sriramoju, V.; Sordillo, L.; Zhang, C.; Zhang, L.; Shi, L.; Smith, J.; et al. Statistical analysis and machine learning algorithms for optical biopsy. In Proceedings of the Optical Biopsy XVI: Toward Real-Time Spectroscopic Imaging and Diagnosis, San Francisco, CA, USA, 19 February 2018; Alfano, R.R., Demos, S.G., Eds.; SPIE: Bellingham, WA, USA, 2018; p. 28.
21. Bendau, E.; Smith, J.; Zhang, L.; Ackerstaff, E.; Kruchevsky, N.; Wu, B.; Koutcher, J.A.; Alfano, R.; Shi, L. Distinguishing metastatic triple-negative breast cancer from nonmetastatic breast cancer using second harmonic generation imaging and resonance Raman spectroscopy. *J. Biophotonics* **2020**, *13*, e202000005. [CrossRef]
22. Fornasaro, S.; Sergo, V.; Bonifacio, A. The key role of ergothioneine in label-free surface-enhanced Raman scattering spectra of biofluids: A retrospective re-assessment of the literature. *FEBS Lett.* **2022**, *596*, 1348–1355. [CrossRef] [PubMed]
23. Leopold, N.; Lendl, B. A New Method for Fast Preparation of Highly Surface-Enhanced Raman Scattering (SERS) Active Silver Colloids at Room Temperature by Reduction of Silver Nitrate with Hydroxylamine Hydrochloride. *J. Phys. Chem. B* **2003**, *107*, 5723–5727. [CrossRef]
24. Benjamini, Y.; Hochberg, Y. Controlling the False Discovery Rate: A Practical and Powerful Approach to Multiple Testing. *J. R. Stat. Soc. Ser. B* **1995**, *57*, 289–300. [CrossRef]
25. Rapisuwon, S.; Vietsch, E.E.; Wellstein, A. Circulating biomarkers to monitor cancer progression and treatment. *Comput. Struct. Biotechnol. J.* **2016**, *14*, 211–222. [CrossRef] [PubMed]
26. Diehl, F.; Li, M.; Dressman, D.; He, Y.; Shen, D.; Szabo, S.; Diaz, L.A.; Goodman, S.N.; David, K.A.; Juhl, H.; et al. Detection and quantification of mutations in the plasma of patients with colorectal tumors. *Proc. Natl. Acad. Sci. USA* **2005**, *102*, 16368–16373. [CrossRef] [PubMed]
27. Miyamoto, D.T.; Zheng, Y.; Wittner, B.S.; Lee, R.J.; Zhu, H.; Broderick, K.T.; Desai, R.; Fox, D.B.; Brannigan, B.W.; Trautwein, J.; et al. RNA-Seq of single prostate CTCs implicates noncanonical Wnt signaling in antiandrogen resistance. *Science* **2015**, *349*, 1351–1356. [CrossRef]
28. Balaj, L.; Lessard, R.; Dai, L.; Cho, Y.-J.; Pomeroy, S.L.; Breakefield, X.O.; Skog, J. Tumour microvesicles contain retrotransposon elements and amplified oncogene sequences. *Nat. Commun.* **2011**, *2*, 180. [CrossRef]
29. Tefas, C.; Mărginean, R.; Toma, V.; Petrushev, B.; Fischer, P.; Tanțău, M.; Știufiuc, R. Surface-enhanced Raman scattering for the diagnosis of ulcerative colitis: Will it change the rules of the game? *Anal. Bioanal. Chem.* **2021**, *413*, 827–838. [CrossRef]
30. Premasiri, W.R.; Lee, J.C.; Ziegler, L.D. Surface-Enhanced Raman Scattering of Whole Human Blood, Blood Plasma, and Red Blood Cells: Cellular Processes and Bioanalytical Sensing. *J. Phys. Chem. B* **2012**, *116*, 9376–9386. [CrossRef]
31. Otto, C.; van den Tweel, T.J.J.; de Mul, F.F.M.; Greve, J. Surface-enhanced Raman spectroscopy of DNA bases. *J. Raman Spectrosc.* **1986**, *17*, 289–298. [CrossRef]
32. Bonifacio, A.; Dalla Marta, S.; Spizzo, R.; Cervo, S.; Steffan, A.; Colombatti, A.; Sergo, V. Surface-enhanced Raman spectroscopy of blood plasma and serum using Ag and Au nanoparticles: A systematic study. *Anal. Bioanal. Chem.* **2014**, *406*, 2355–2365. [CrossRef] [PubMed]
33. Aroca, R.; Bujalski, R. Surface enhanced vibrational spectra of thymine. *Vib. Spectrosc.* **1999**, *19*, 11–21. [CrossRef]
34. Bankapur, A.; Zachariah, E.; Chidangil, S.; Valiathan, M.; Mathur, D. Raman Tweezers Spectroscopy of Live, Single Red and White Blood Cells. *PLoS ONE* **2010**, *5*, e10427. [CrossRef] [PubMed]
35. Auner, G.W.; Koya, S.K.; Huang, C.; Broadbent, B.; Trexler, M.; Auner, Z.; Elias, A.; Mehne, K.C.; Brusatori, M.A. Applications of Raman spectroscopy in cancer diagnosis. *Cancer Metastasis Rev.* **2018**, *37*, 691–717. [CrossRef]
36. Medipally, D.K.R.; Cullen, D.; Untereiner, V.; Sockalingum, G.D.; Maguire, A.; Nguyen, T.N.Q.; Bryant, J.; Noone, E.; Bradshaw, S.; Finn, M.; et al. Vibrational spectroscopy of liquid biopsies for prostate cancer diagnosis. *Ther. Adv. Med. Oncol.* **2020**, *12*, 175883592091849. [CrossRef]
37. Dingari, N.C.; Horowitz, G.L.; Kang, J.W.; Dasari, R.R.; Barman, I. Raman Spectroscopy Provides a Powerful Diagnostic Tool for Accurate Determination of Albumin Glycation. *PLoS ONE* **2012**, *7*, e32406. [CrossRef]

38. González-Solís, J. Discrimination of different cancer types clustering Raman spectra by a super paramagnetic stochastic network approach. *PLoS ONE* **2019**, *14*, e0213621. [CrossRef]
39. Gao, N.; Wang, Q.; Tang, J.; Yao, S.; Li, H.; Yue, X.; Fu, J.; Zhong, F.; Wang, T.; Wang, J. Non-invasive SERS serum detection technology combined with multivariate statistical algorithm for simultaneous screening of cervical cancer and breast cancer. *Anal. Bioanal. Chem.* **2021**, *413*, 4775–4784. [CrossRef]
40. Feng, S.; Lin, D.; Lin, J.; Li, B.; Huang, Z.; Chen, G.; Zhang, W.; Wang, L.; Pan, J.; Chen, R.; et al. Blood plasma surface-enhanced Raman spectroscopy for non-invasive optical detection of cervical cancer. *Analyst* **2013**, *138*, 3967. [CrossRef]
41. Lin, D.; Pan, J.; Huang, H.; Chen, G.; Qiu, S.; Shi, H.; Chen, W.; Yu, Y.; Feng, S.; Chen, R. Label-free blood plasma test based on surface-enhanced Raman scattering for tumor stages detection in nasopharyngeal cancer. *Sci. Rep.* **2015**, *4*, 4751. [CrossRef]
42. Ryzhikova, E.; Ralbovsky, N.M.; Halámková, L.; Celmins, D.; Malone, P.; Molho, E.; Quinn, J.; Zimmerman, E.A.; Lednev, I.K. Multivariate Statistical Analysis of Surface Enhanced Raman Spectra of Human Serum for Alzheimer's Disease Diagnosis. *Appl. Sci.* **2019**, *9*, 3256. [CrossRef]
43. Prescott, B.; Steinmetz, W.; Thomas, G.J. Characterization of DNA structures by laser Raman spectroscopy. *Biopolymers* **1984**, *23*, 235–256. [CrossRef] [PubMed]
44. Cao, X.; Wang, Z.; Bi, L.; Zheng, J. Label-Free Detection of Human Serum Using Surface-Enhanced Raman Spectroscopy Based on Highly Branched Gold Nanoparticle Substrates for Discrimination of Non-Small Cell Lung Cancer. *J. Chem.* **2018**, *2018*, 9012645. [CrossRef]
45. Wu, Q.; Qiu, S.; Yu, Y.; Chen, W.; Lin, H.; Lin, D.; Feng, S.; Chen, R. Assessment of the radiotherapy effect for nasopharyngeal cancer using plasma surface-enhanced Raman spectroscopy technology. *Biomed. Opt. Express* **2018**, *9*, 3413. [CrossRef] [PubMed]
46. Schneider, F.W.; Frank, S. Parker: Applications of Infrared, Raman, and Resonance Raman Spectroscopy in Biochemistry. In *Berichte der Bunsengesellschaft für Phys. Chemie*; Plenum Press: New York, NY, USA; London, UK, 1984; Volume 88, pp. 1167–1168. [CrossRef]
47. Xue, L.; Yan, B.; Li, Y.; Tan, Y.; Luo, X.; Wang, M. Surface-enhanced Raman spectroscopy of blood serum based on gold nanoparticles for tumor stages detection and histologic grades classification of oral squamous cell carcinoma. *Int. J. Nanomed.* **2018**, *13*, 4977–4986. [CrossRef]
48. Tan, Y.; Yan, B.; Xue, L.; Li, Y.; Luo, X.; Ji, P. Surface-enhanced Raman spectroscopy of blood serum based on gold nanoparticles for the diagnosis of the oral squamous cell carcinoma. *Lipids Health Dis.* **2017**, *16*, 73. [CrossRef] [PubMed]
49. De Gelder, J.; De Gussem, K.; Vandenabeele, P.; Moens, L. Reference database of Raman spectra of biological molecules. *J. Raman Spectrosc.* **2007**, *38*, 1133–1147. [CrossRef]
50. Westley, C.; Xu, Y.; Thilaganathan, B.; Carnell, A.J.; Turner, N.J.; Goodacre, R. Absolute Quantification of Uric Acid in Human Urine Using Surface Enhanced Raman Scattering with the Standard Addition Method. *Anal. Chem.* **2017**, *89*, 2472–2477. [CrossRef]
51. Garcia-Rico, E.; Alvarez-Puebla, R.A.; Guerrini, L. Direct surface-enhanced Raman scattering (SERS) spectroscopy of nucleic acids: From fundamental studies to real-life applications. *Chem. Soc. Rev.* **2018**, *47*, 4909–4923. [CrossRef]
52. Barhoumi, A.; Zhang, D.; Tam, F.; Halas, N.J. Surface-Enhanced Raman Spectroscopy of DNA. *J. Am. Chem. Soc.* **2008**, *130*, 5523–5529. [CrossRef]
53. Fan, C.; Hu, Z.; Mustapha, A.; Lin, M. Rapid detection of food- and waterborne bacteria using surface-enhanced Raman spectroscopy coupled with silver nanosubstrates. *Appl. Microbiol. Biotechnol.* **2011**, *92*, 1053–1061. [CrossRef] [PubMed]
54. Domenici, F.; Bizzarri, A.R.; Cannistraro, S. Surface-enhanced Raman scattering detection of wild-type and mutant p53 proteins at very low concentration in human serum. *Anal. Biochem.* **2012**, *421*, 9–15. [CrossRef] [PubMed]
55. Xiaoming, D.; Yoshinori, Y.; Hiroshi, Y.; Harumi, U.; Ozaki, Y. Biological Applications of Anti-Stokes Raman Spectroscopy: Quantitative Analysis of Glucose in Plasma and Serum by a Highly Sensitive Multichannel Raman Spectrometer. *Appl. Spectrosc.* **1996**, *50*, 1301–1306.
56. Kamińska, A.; Winkler, K.; Kowalska, A.; Witkowska, E.; Szymborski, T.; Janeczek, A.; Waluk, J. SERS-based Immunoassay in a Microfluidic System for the Multiplexed Recognition of Interleukins from Blood Plasma: Towards Picogram Detection. *Sci. Rep.* **2017**, *7*, 10656. [CrossRef]
57. Grubisha, D.S.; Lipert, R.J.; Park, H.-Y.; Driskell, J.; Porter, M.D. Femtomolar Detection of Prostate-Specific Antigen: An Immunoassay Based on Surface-Enhanced Raman Scattering and Immunogold Labels. *Anal. Chem.* **2003**, *75*, 5936–5943. [CrossRef]
58. Jarvis, R.M.; Brooker, A.; Goodacre, R. Surface-Enhanced Raman Spectroscopy for Bacterial Discrimination Utilizing a Scanning Electron Microscope with a Raman Spectroscopy Interface. *Anal. Chem.* **2004**, *76*, 5198–5202. [CrossRef]
59. Atkins, C.G.; Buckley, K.; Blades, M.W.; Turner, R.F.B. Raman Spectroscopy of Blood and Blood Components. *Appl. Spectrosc.* **2017**, *71*, 767–793. [CrossRef]
60. Xie, Y.; Xu, L.; Wang, Y.; Shao, J.; Wang, L.; Wang, H.; Qian, H.; Yao, W. Label-free detection of the foodborne pathogens of Enterobacteriaceae by surface-enhanced Raman spectroscopy. *Anal. Methods* **2013**, *5*, 946–952. [CrossRef]
61. Wang, G.; Lipert, R.J.; Jain, M.; Kaur, S.; Chakraboty, S.; Torres, M.P.; Batra, S.K.; Brand, R.E.; Porter, M.D. Detection of the potential pancreatic cancer marker MUC4 in serum using surface-enhanced Raman scattering. *Anal. Chem.* **2011**, *83*, 2554–2561. [CrossRef]

62. Maquelin, K.; Choo-Smith, L.-P.; van Vreeswijk, T.; Endtz, H.P.; Smith, B.; Bennett, R.; Bruining, H.A.; Puppels, G.J. Raman Spectroscopic Method for Identification of Clinically Relevant Microorganisms Growing on Solid Culture Medium. *Anal. Chem.* **2000**, *72*, 12–19. [CrossRef]
63. Bulkin, B.J. Raman spectroscopic study of human erythrocyte membranes. *Biochim. Biophys. Acta-Biomembr.* **1972**, *274*, 649–651. [CrossRef]
64. Munro, C.H.; Smith, W.E.; Garner, M.; Clarkson, J.; White, P.C. Characterization of the Surface of a Citrate-Reduced Colloid Optimized for Use as a Substrate for Surface-Enhanced Resonance Raman Scattering. *Langmuir* **1995**, *11*, 3712–3720. [CrossRef]
65. Schuster, K.C.; Urlaub, E.; Gapes, J.R. Single-cell analysis of bacteria by Raman microscopy: Spectral information on the chemical composition of cells and on the heterogeneity in a culture. *J. Microbiol. Methods* **2000**, *42*, 29–38. [CrossRef]
66. Maiti, N.C.; Apetri, M.M.; Zagorski, M.G.; Carey, P.R.; Anderson, V.E. Raman Spectroscopic Characterization of Secondary Structure in Natively Unfolded Proteins: α-Synuclein. *J. Am. Chem. Soc.* **2004**, *126*, 2399–2408. [CrossRef] [PubMed]
67. Huefner, A.; Kuan, W.-L.; Mason, S.L.; Mahajan, S.; Barker, R.A. Serum Raman spectroscopy as a diagnostic tool in patients with Huntington's disease. *Chem. Sci.* **2020**, *11*, 525–533. [CrossRef]
68. Wehbe, K.; Pineau, R.; Eimer, S.; Vital, A.; Loiseau, H.; Déléris, G. Differentiation between normal and tumor vasculature of animal and human glioma by FTIR imaging. *Analyst* **2010**, *135*, 3052. [CrossRef]
69. Flavin, R.; Zadra, G.; Loda, M. Metabolic alterations and targeted therapies in prostate cancer. *J. Pathol.* **2011**, *223*, 284–295. [CrossRef]
70. Strmiska, V.; Michalek, P.; Eckschlager, T.; Stiborova, M.; Adam, V.; Krizkova, S.; Heger, Z. Prostate cancer-specific hallmarks of amino acids metabolism: Towards a paradigm of precision medicine. *Biochim. Biophys. Acta-Rev. Cancer* **2019**, *1871*, 248–258. [CrossRef]
71. Santos, F.; Magalhães, S.; Henriques, M.C.; Silva, B.; Valença, I.; Ribeiro, D.; Fardilha, M.; Nunes, A. Understanding Prostate Cancer Cells Metabolome: A Spectroscopic Approach. *Curr. Metab.* **2019**, *6*, 218–224. [CrossRef]
72. Flier, J.S.; Underhill, L.H.; Griffin, J.E. Androgen Resistance—The Clinical and Molecular Spectrum. *N. Engl. J. Med.* **1992**, *326*, 611–618. [CrossRef]
73. Menendez, J.A.; Lupu, R. Fatty acid synthase and the lipogenic phenotype in cancer pathogenesis. *Nat. Rev. Cancer* **2007**, *7*, 763–777. [CrossRef] [PubMed]
74. Rysman, E.; Brusselmans, K.; Scheys, K.; Timmermans, L.; Derua, R.; Munck, S.; Van Veldhoven, P.P.; Waltregny, D.; Daniëls, V.W.; Machiels, J.; et al. De novo Lipogenesis Protects Cancer Cells from Free Radicals and Chemotherapeutics by Promoting Membrane Lipid Saturation. *Cancer Res.* **2010**, *70*, 8117–8126. [CrossRef] [PubMed]
75. Neviliappan, S.; Fang Kan, L.; Tiang Lee Walter, T.; Arulkumaran, S.; Wong, P.T.T. Infrared Spectral Features of Exfoliated Cervical Cells, Cervical Adenocarcinoma Tissue, and an Adenocarcinoma Cell Line (SiSo). *Gynecol. Oncol.* **2002**, *85*, 170–174. [CrossRef] [PubMed]
76. Gazi, E.; Dwyer, J.; Gardner, P.; Ghanbari-Siahkali, A.; Wade, A.; Miyan, J.; Lockyer, N.; Vickerman, J.; Clarke, N.; Shanks, J.; et al. Applications of Fourier transform infrared microspectroscopy in studies of benign prostate and prostate cancer. A pilot study. *J. Pathol.* **2003**, *201*, 99–108. [CrossRef]
77. Clemens, G.; Hands, J.R.; Dorling, K.M.; Baker, M.J. Vibrational spectroscopic methods for cytology and cellular research. *Analyst* **2014**, *139*, 4411–4444. [CrossRef]
78. Magalhães, S.; Graça, A.; Tavares, J.; Santos, M.A.S.; Delgadillo, I.; Nunes, A. Saccharomyces cerevisiae as a Model to Confirm the Ability of FTIR to Evaluate the Presence of Protein Aggregates. *Spectr. Anal. Rev.* **2018**, *6*, 81120. [CrossRef]
79. Shivu, B.; Seshadri, S.; Li, J.; Oberg, K.A.; Uversky, V.N.; Fink, A.L. Distinct β-Sheet Structure in Protein Aggregates Determined by ATR–FTIR Spectroscopy. *Biochemistry* **2013**, *52*, 5176–5183. [CrossRef]
80. Miller, L.M.; Bourassa, M.W.; Smith, R.J. FTIR spectroscopic imaging of protein aggregation in living cells. *Biochim. Biophys. Acta-Biomembr.* **2013**, *1828*, 2339–2346. [CrossRef]
81. Kumar, S.; Srinivasan, A.; Nikolajeff, F. Role of Infrared Spectroscopy and Imaging in Cancer Diagnosis. *Curr. Med. Chem.* **2018**, *25*, 1055–1072. [CrossRef]
82. Hetz, C.; Chevet, E.; Oakes, S.A. Proteostasis control by the unfolded protein response. *Nat. Cell Biol.* **2015**, *17*, 829–838. [CrossRef]
83. Koo, E.H.; Lansbury, P.T.; Kelly, J.W. Amyloid diseases: Abnormal protein aggregation in neurodegeneration. *Proc. Natl. Acad. Sci. USA* **1999**, *96*, 9989–9990. [CrossRef] [PubMed]
84. Levy, C.B.; Stumbo, A.C.; Ano Bom, A.P.D.; Portari, E.A.; Carneiro, Y.; Silva, J.L.; De Moura-Gallo, C.V. Co-localization of mutant p53 and amyloid-like protein aggregates in breast tumors. *Int. J. Biochem. Cell Biol.* **2011**, *43*, 60–64. [CrossRef] [PubMed]
85. Xu, J.; Reumers, J.; Couceiro, J.R.; De Smet, F.; Gallardo, R.; Rudyak, S.; Cornelis, A.; Rozenski, J.; Zwolinska, A.; Marine, J.-C.; et al. Gain of function of mutant p53 by coaggregation with multiple tumor suppressors. *Nat. Chem. Biol.* **2011**, *7*, 285–295. [CrossRef] [PubMed]
86. Yang-Hartwich, Y.; Bingham, J.; Garofalo, F.; Alvero, A.B.; Mor, G. Detection of p53 Protein Aggregation in Cancer Cell Lines and Tumor Samples. In *Apoptosis and Cancer*; Methods in Molecular Biology; Mor, G., Alvero, A., Eds.; Humana Press: New York, NY, USA, 2015; Volume 1219, pp. 75–86. [CrossRef]
87. Yang-Hartwich, Y.; Soteras, M.G.; Lin, Z.P.; Holmberg, J.; Sumi, N.; Craveiro, V.; Liang, M.; Romanoff, E.; Bingham, J.; Garofalo, F.; et al. p53 protein aggregation promotes platinum resistance in ovarian cancer. *Oncogene* **2015**, *34*, 3605–3616. [CrossRef]

88. Barth, A.; Zscherp, C. What vibrations tell about proteins. *Q. Rev. Biophys.* **2002**, *35*, 369–430. [CrossRef]
89. Dereziński, P.; Klupczynska, A.; Sawicki, W.; Pałka, J.A.; Kokot, Z.J. Amino Acid Profiles of Serum and Urine in Search for Prostate Cancer Biomarkers: A Pilot Study. *Int. J. Med. Sci.* **2017**, *14*, 1–12. [CrossRef]
90. Miyagi, Y.; Higashiyama, M.; Gochi, A.; Akaike, M.; Ishikawa, T.; Miura, T.; Saruki, N.; Bando, E.; Kimura, H.; Imamura, F.; et al. Plasma Free Amino Acid Profiling of Five Types of Cancer Patients and Its Application for Early Detection. *PLoS ONE* **2011**, *6*, e24143. [CrossRef]
91. Shamsipur, M.; Naseri, M.T.; Babri, M. Quantification of candidate prostate cancer metabolite biomarkers in urine using dispersive derivatization liquid–liquid microextraction followed by gas and liquid chromatography–mass spectrometry. *J. Pharm. Biomed. Anal.* **2013**, *81*, 65–75. [CrossRef]
92. Heger, Z.; Cernei, N.; Gumulec, J.; Masarik, M.; Eckschlager, T.; Hrabec, R.; Zitka, O.; Adam, V.; Kizek, R. Determination of common urine substances as an assay for improving prostate carcinoma diagnostics. *Oncol. Rep.* **2014**, *31*, 1846–1854. [CrossRef]
93. Jentzmik, F.; Stephan, C.; Miller, K.; Schrader, M.; Erbersdobler, A.; Kristiansen, G.; Lein, M.; Jung, K. Sarcosine in Urine after Digital Rectal Examination Fails as a Marker in Prostate Cancer Detection and Identification of Aggressive Tumours. *Eur. Urol.* **2010**, *58*, 12–18. [CrossRef]
94. Bartolomeo, M.P.; Maisano, F. Validation of a reversed-phase HPLC method for quantitative amino acid analysis. *J. Biomol. Tech.* **2006**, *17*, 131–137. [PubMed]
95. Shimbo, K.; Oonuki, T.; Yahashi, A.; Hirayama, K.; Miyano, H. Precolumn derivatization reagents for high-speed analysis of amines and amino acids in biological fluid using liquid chromatography/electrospray ionization tandem mass spectrometry. *Rapid Commun. Mass Spectrom.* **2009**, *23*, 1483–1492. [CrossRef] [PubMed]
96. Moisoiu, V.; Stefancu, A.; Iancu, S.D.; Moisoiu, T.; Loga, L.; Dican, L.; Alecsa, C.D.; Boros, I.; Jurj, A.; Dima, D.; et al. SERS assessment of the cancer-specific methylation pattern of genomic DNA: Towards the detection of acute myeloid leukemia in patients undergoing hematopoietic stem cell transplantation. *Anal. Bioanal. Chem.* **2019**, *411*, 7907–7913. [CrossRef] [PubMed]

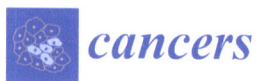

Review

Liquid Biopsy in Prostate Cancer Management—Current Challenges and Future Perspectives

Felice Crocetto [1], Gianluca Russo [2], Erika Di Zazzo [3,*], Pasquale Pisapia [2], Benito Fabio Mirto [1], Alessandro Palmieri [1], Francesco Pepe [2], Claudio Bellevicine [2], Alessandro Russo [4], Evelina La Civita [5], Daniela Terracciano [5], Umberto Malapelle [2], Giancarlo Troncone [2] and Biagio Barone [1]

[1] Department of Neurosciences, Reproductive Sciences and Odontostomatology, University of Naples "Federico II", 80131 Naples, Italy; felice.crocetto@unina.it (F.C.); fmirto22@gmail.com (B.F.M.); alessandro.palmieri@unina.it (A.P.); biagio.barone@unina.it (B.B.)
[2] Department of Public Health, University of Naples Federico II, 80131 Naples, Italy; gianlucar93@libero.it (G.R.); pasquale.pisapia@unina.it (P.P.); francesco.pepe4@unina.it (F.P.); claudio.bellevicine@unina.it (C.B.); umberto.malapelle@unina.it (U.M.); giancarlo.troncone@unina.it (G.T.)
[3] Department of Medicine and Health Sciences "V. Tiberio", University of Molise, 86100 Campobasso, Italy
[4] Medical Oncology Unit, Papardo Hospital, 98121 Messina, Italy; alessandrorusso@aopapardo.it
[5] Department of Translational Medical Sciences, University of Naples "Federico II", 80131 Naples, Italy; eva.lacivita@gmail.com (E.L.C.); daniela.terracciano@unina.it (D.T.)
* Correspondence: erika.dizazzo@unimol.it

Simple Summary: Prostate cancer (PCa) is a widespread malignancy, representing the second leading cause of cancer-related death in men. In the last years, liquid biopsy has emerged as an attractive and promising strategy complementary to invasive tissue biopsy to guide PCa diagnosis, follow-up and treatment response. Liquid biopsy is employed to assess several body fluids biomarkers, including circulating tumor cells (CTCs), extracellular vesicles (EVs), circulating tumor DNA (ctDNA) and RNA (ctRNA). This review dissects recent advancements and future perspectives of liquid biopsy, highlighting its strength and weaknesses in PCa management.

Abstract: Although appreciable attempts in screening and diagnostic approaches have been achieved, prostate cancer (PCa) remains a widespread malignancy, representing the second leading cause of cancer-related death in men. Drugs currently used in PCa therapy initially show a potent anti-tumor effect, but frequently induce resistance and PCa progresses toward metastatic castration-resistant forms (mCRPC), virtually incurable. Liquid biopsy has emerged as an attractive and promising strategy complementary to invasive tissue biopsy to guide PCa diagnosis and treatment. Liquid biopsy shows the ability to represent the tumor microenvironment, allow comprehensive information and follow-up the progression of the tumor, enabling the development of different treatment strategies as well as permitting the monitoring of therapy response. Liquid biopsy, indeed, is endowed with a significant potential to modify PCa management. Several blood biomarkers could be analyzed for diagnostic, prognostic and predictive purposes, including circulating tumor cells (CTCs), extracellular vesicles (EVs), circulating tumor DNA (ctDNA) and RNA (ctRNA). In addition, several other body fluids may be adopted (i.e., urine, sperm, etc.) beyond blood. This review dissects recent advancements and future perspectives of liquid biopsies, highlighting their strength and weaknesses in PCa management.

Keywords: liquid biopsy; prostate cancer; cancer biomarkers; circulating tumor cells; extracellular vesicles; cell-free nucleic acids; circulating nucleic acids; cell-free DNA; cell-free RNA

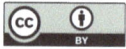

1. Introduction

Prostate cancer (PCa) affects millions of men worldwide, representing the second most common type of malignancy in men, with 1.4 million of newly diagnosed cancers per year, and one of the leading causes of cancer-related death in men, accounting for 350,000 deaths per year globally [1,2].

In developed and industrialized countries, the incidence of PCa increases progressively with the age of the worldwide population. It has been estimated, indeed, that all-age incidence was 31 per 100,000 males, with a lifetime cumulative risk of 3.9% and more than 1 in 4 men over 75 years is affected by PCa [3,4]. PCa shows an extreme geographical variation both in incidence and mortality rates, being widely spread in developed countries (such as Europe, the United States of America, Canada, Australia and Middle-Southern Africa), while it is less common in developing ones. These differences could be mostly related to disparities in diagnostic tests frequency and potency among countries as well as lifestyle factors, as evidenced by migration studies [5]. An emblematic study by Shimizu et al. showed how an increased PCa incidence and mortality rate was observed among men migrating from Asian countries with a low-risk of PCa onset to European and North American countries with a high PCa risk, compared to men remaining in their native countries [6,7].

Nevertheless, despite the widespread prevalence of this disease, about 80% of cancers at diagnosis are limited to the anatomical bounds of the prostate gland with an estimated life expectancy of localized PCa patients up to 99% over 10 years [4,8]. However, on the other side, a minority of patients have local positive lymph nodes (about 15%) or distant metastasis (5%) at the diagnosis, reducing the 5 years survival rate at 30–40% [9].

Although PCa etiology is still not yet fully understood, it is recognized that both environmental (modifiable) and innate factors (unmodifiable) play a pivotal role in PCa onset [10].

Among unmodifiable factors, age is strongly and linearly associated with the PCa risk [11]. Similarly, Afro-Americans show an increased PCa risk, due to high levels of serum testosterone and insulin-like growth factor-1 (IGF-1) [12].

Finally, about 9% of PCa are hereditary forms, i.e., the affected patients have at least two relatives with a PCa diagnosis before the age of 55. Interestingly, genes involved in DNA damage repair mechanisms, are involved in PCa, such as *BRCA 1/2*, *HOXB13* and *RNaseL* (1q24-25) [13–15].

Among modifiable factors, the dysregulation of hormonal pathways, due to several environmental factors, such as metabolic syndrome, obesity, hypercholesterolemia and processed foods intake, leads to increased serum insulin levels, inflammatory cytokines and estradiol, which predisposes to an increased high-grade PCa risk [16–22].

The current clinical approaches in PCa diagnosis include digital rectal examination (DRE), prostate-specific antigen (PSA) measurement, imaging (transrectal ultrasound and multiparametric magnetic resonance imaging of the prostate) and prostate biopsies [23].

Although inexpensive, easy to perform and relatively noninvasive, the effectiveness of DRE, with a predictive positive value between 5% and 30%, is contingent on the experience and skill of the examiner [24]. Conversely, PCa diagnosis has been revolutionized by the introduction of serum PSA testing, being an early, comfortably and relatively inexpensive marker. However, PSA is an organ but not a cancer-specific marker, whose expression level is influenced by age and increases also in non-malignant conditions (e.g., benign prostatic hyperplasia, prostatitis, genito-urinary infections, DRE). Furthermore, the PSA cut-off level is still not standardized, and despite its role as PCa independent predictor, its use alone could be misleading [25–28]. PSA sensitivity ranges between 67.5% and 80%, while specificity is up to 40%. Therefore, about 20–30% of PCa could not be diagnosed if PSA is used as the only diagnostic test. To address this need, several new laboratory tests have been developed, with a clear tendency to combine panels biomarkers. Among these, the most promising laboratory tests are Phi (Beckman Coulter s.r.l., Milano, Italia) 4K score (BioReference Laboratories, Inc. Elmwood Park, NJ, USA) and Stockholm 3 (A3P Biomedical AB, Stockholm, Sweden) as circulating biomarkers, Mi-prostate score (MLabs, Ann Arbor, MI, USA), Exo DX Prostate (Exosome Diagnostics, Martinsried, Germany) and Select MD-X MDxHealth, Irvine, CA, USA as urinary biomarkers and Confirm MDx

(Veracyte Headquarters, South San Francisco, CA, USA) Oncotype Dx (Exact Sciences, London, UK,), Prolaris (Myriad Genetics Corporate Headquarters, Salt Lake City, UT, USA) and Decipher (GenomeDx Biosciences, San Diego, CA, USA) as tissue biomarkers. These tests aimed to minimize overdiagnosis without missing the identification of clinically significant PCa [29].

Regarding the imaging, the use of the standard transrectal ultrasound sonography (TRUS) alone, albeit having improved the diagnostic capabilities in urological clinical practice, prior to the introduction of multiparametric magnetic resonance imaging (mpMRI), is still not reliable in detecting PCa, due to its limitations in recognizing only hypoechoic lesions in the peripheral zone of the prostate [30].

The mpMRI scan represents the game-changer of PCa diagnosis, due to its high sensitivity and specificity, reporting a negative predictive value between 92% and 100% for clinically significant tumors. In addition, mpMRI provides detailed anatomical and functional information on the prostate via the use of several standards weighed sequences, such as T1 (T1w), T2 (T2w) and diffusion (DWI), permitting to evaluate also the potential capsular and seminal vesicles infiltration of PCa. Nevertheless, the main limitations of the mpMRI are the high cost of this equipment and the limited number of radiologists experts in its interpretation [31,32].

Prostate biopsy represents the only procedure which allows a certain diagnosis and it is currently performed, under ultrasound guidance, transperineally or transrectally. A combined approach involving the use of coupled TRUS and mpMRI imaging (Fusion biopsy), has permitted to increase the overall accuracy of PCa diagnosis, especially in biopsy-naïve patients, reaching concordance rates with the definitive histologic report up to 52.3% (for targeted biopsy) and 85.5% (for systematic biopsy) [33].

Nevertheless, this approach shows several risks, such as hematuria, hematochezia and hematospermia up to a month after examination, increased body temperature, abscesses, bacteriemia, sepsis or lesions of the prostatic urethra and urinary retention [34,35].

Consequently, less-invasive methods aimed to reduce biopsy complications without lowering the detection rate of the procedure, are strongly needed.

In the past few years, liquid biopsy has emerged as a new diagnostic and prognostic tool to trace cancer [36,37]. The term "liquid biopsy" refers, indeed, to a non-invasive analysis of biomarkers in biological fluids (such as blood, plasma, urine, liquor and saliva) to allow the detection, and the longitudinal follow-up, of cancers, avoiding the limitations of invasive procedures and, contextually, obtaining enough molecular information than those derived from tissue biopsies (Figure 1) [38].

The biomarkers commonly obtained from a liquid biopsy are circulating cell-free tumor DNA (ctDNA), circulating cell-free tumor RNA (ctRNA), proteins, peptides, metabolites, circulating tumor cells (CTCs) and extracellular vesicles (EVs), which incorporate genomic, epigenomic, transcriptomic and proteomic information of tumors. Furthermore, a single specimen could be used in multiple assays [39,40].

Another advantage of circulating biomarkers' analysis is related to the reduction of intra-tumor heterogeneity, permitting to overcome the variability of molecular information obtained by tissue analysis which could be dependent on tumor localization and accessibility. Moreover, liquid biopsy displays the tumor microenvironment behavior. Finally, liquid biopsy provides a tool for monitoring tumor progression, predicting prognosis, overall survival and treatment efficacy, dictating a tailored therapy [41]. Figure 2 shows the advantages and limitations of tissue versus liquid biopsy (Figure 2).

This current review aims to summarize the potential implications of circulating serum and urine biomarkers analysis in PCa management, delineating current challenges and perspectives of the employment of liquid biopsy in clinical practice.

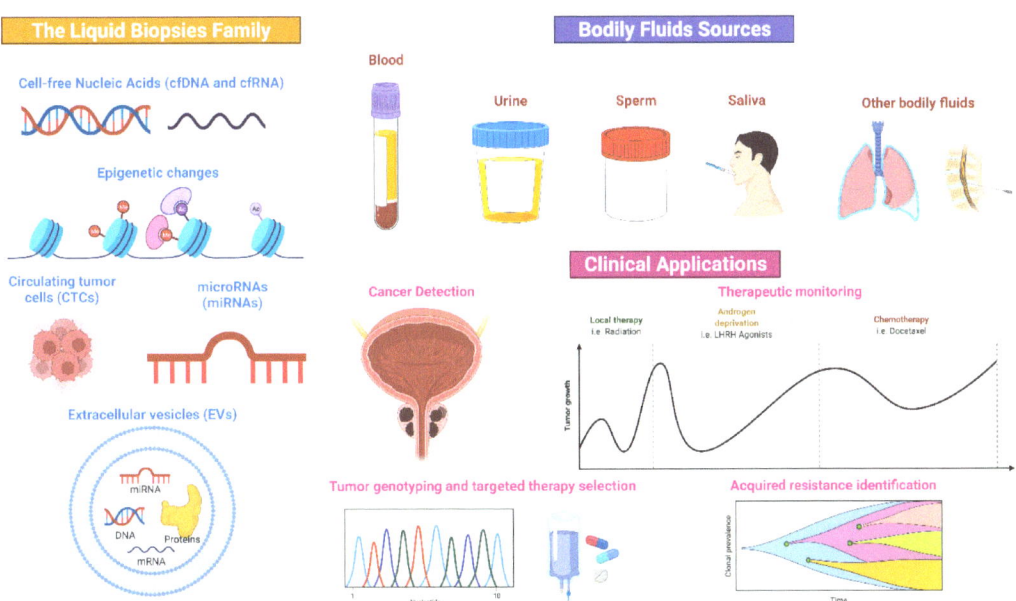

Figure 1. Schematic representation of liquid biopsy composition and application. Credit: Created with BioRender.com (accessed on 3 June 2022).

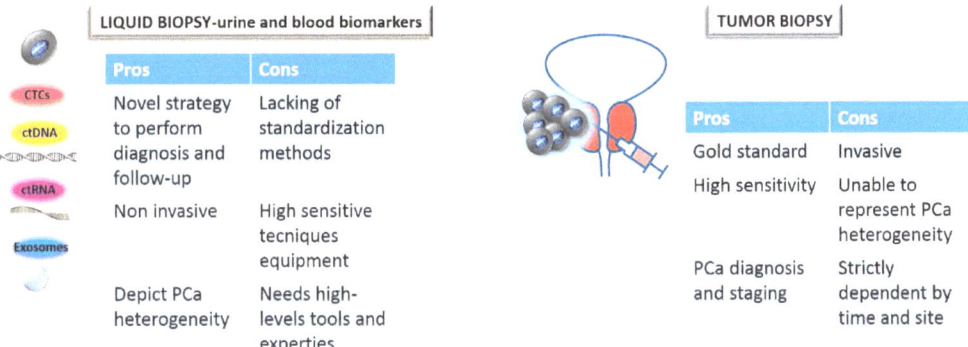

Figure 2. Comparison of the advantages and limitations of tissue versus liquid biopsy.

2. Blood and Serum Biomarkers in the Detection of PCa

The limitation met in the recovery of tissue biopsy highlighted the necessity to implement alternative biological sources [42,43]. The introduction in routine diagnostic practice of highly sensitive techniques encouraged the comprehension of tumor landscape, analyzing circulating tumor nucleic acids (ctNA), circulating tumor cells (CTCs) and tumor-derived extracellular vesicles (EVs) released by cancer cells by using blood samples [43–46]. A comprehensive table summarizes the blood, serum and urinary biomarkers reported in this review (Table 1).

Table 1. Summary of blood, serum and urine biomarkers.

	Variables	Test Name	Manufacturer	Assay Type	Molecular Targets	References
Blood Biomarkers	ctDNA	Qubit 3.0 Fluorometer and dsDNA HS AssayKit	Life Technologies, Carlsbad, CA, USA	dsDNA Quantitation	dsDNA	[47]
	ctDNA	2100 Bioanalyzer with High Sensitivity DNA Chips	Agilent Technologies, Santa Clara, CA, USA	dsDNA Quantitation purity and fragment size	dsDNA	
	ctDNA	Fluorometer and Qubit™ dsDNA HS Assay Kit	Thermo Fisher Scientific, Waltham, MA, USA	dsDNA Quantitation	dsDNA	[48]
	ctDNA	Agilent High Sensitivity D5000 ScreenTape System on Agilent-4200 TapeStation	Agilent Technologies; Santa Clara, CA, USA	dsDNA Qualitative analysis	dsDNA	
	ctDNA	ABI 7900HT system	Applied Biosystems, Foster City, CA, USA	qPCR analysis of repeated genomic ALU sequences to detect and quantify cfDNA	dsDNA	[49]
	ctDNA	Microfluidic electrophoresis using the Agilent 2100 Bioanalyzer and High Sensitivity DNA Chips	Agilent technologies Inc., Palo Alto, CA, USA	DNA fragment length analysis	dsDNA	
	Gene promoters' methylation	ND	ND	Sodium bisulfite-PCR	GSTP1, RARB2	
	ctDNA	iCycler iQ Real-Time PCR	Biorad, Hercules, CA, USA	qPCR analysis of long interspersed nuclear elements (LINE1) for ctDNA quantification	dsDNA	[50]
	ctDNA	Quant-IT Picogreen HS DNA kit and BioTek microplate spectrophotometer at 480ex/520em	Thermo Fisher, Waltham, MA, USA	dsDNA Quantification	dsDNA	[51]
	ctDNA	Illumina MiSeq (V3 600 cycle kit) or HiSeq 2500 (V4 250 cycle kit)	Illumina Inc., Towne Centre Drive, San Diego, CA, USA	ctDNA sequencing	AR, SPOP, TP53, PTEN, RB1, APC, CDKN1B, BRCA2, and PIK3R1	[52]

243

Table 1. Cont.

Variables	Test Name	Manufacturer	Assay Type	Molecular Targets	References
ctRNA	ExiLENT SYBR® Greenassay (Exiqon, Denmark) qPCR was performed on QuantStudio 6 Real-Time PCR System	Applied Biosystems, Foster City, CA, USA	qRT-PCR analysis	miR-141, 375, 21, 30c, 145, 26b, 223, 24, and let-7a	[53]
ctRNA	TaqMan MicroRNA Assay, TaqMan PCR master mix and TaqMan probes. ABI Prism Model 7900 HT instrument was used to perform the qRT-PCR.	Applied Biosystems, Foster City, CA, USA	qRT-PCR analysis	miR-200c, miR-605, miR-135a, miR-433, and miR-106a	[54]
ctRNA	Sso Advanced Universal SYBR Green Supermix (Bio-Rad, USA). The reaction was performed on the 7900HT Fast Real-Time PCR System Thermocycler	Applied Biosystems, Foster City, CA, USA	qRT-PCR analysis	OR51E2, SIM2	[55]
CTC	ISET®-CTC Test and Immuno-Cyto-Chemistry (ICC)	Rarecells Diagnostics, Paris, France	immuno-cyto-chemistry	PSA	[56]
CTC	CELLSEARCH assay	Menarini, Silicon Biosystems Inc., Bologna, Italy	immuno-cyto-chemistry	epithelial cell adhesion molecule (EpCAM), cytokeratins, CD45	[57]
EV	CD63 Exo ELISA Kit (EXOEL-CD63A-1)	System Biosciences, Mountain View, CA, USA	ELISA	CD63	[58]
EV	CD63 Exo ELISA KitEXOEL-CD63A-1); human glutamate carboxypeptidase 2 (FOLH1) ELISA kit (MBS901525)	System Biosciences, Mountain View, CA, USA;MY BioSource, Inc., San Diego, CA, USA	ELISA	prostate-specific membrane antigen (PSMA)	[58]
EV	Mx-3000 or Mx 3005 instrument	Stratagene, Amsterdam, The Netherlands	qRT-PCR analysis for EV quantification		[59]

Table 1. Cont.

	Variables	Test Name	Manufacturer	Assay Type	Molecular Targets	References
	CTC	CellSearch Instrument	Janssen Diagnostics Inc. Huntington Valley, PA, USA	CTC Enumeration	EpCAM+CK+CD45-	[60]
Urine Biomarkers	ctDNA	Qiamp DNA minikit; IQ SYBR green;Rotor Gene 6000 detection system	Qiagen, Milan, Italy; Biorad, Milan, Italy; Corbett Research, St. Neots, UK	qPCR analysis for ctDNA fragmentation index evaluation	c-Myc, BCAS1, HER2, STOX1	[61]
	ctDNA	Qiamp DNA minikit; IQ SYBR green;Rotor Gene 6000 detection system	Qiagen, Milan, Italy; Biorad, Milan, Italy; Corbett Research, St. Neots, UK	qPCR analysis for ctDNA fragmentation index evaluation	c-Myc, AR, HER2, STOX1	[62]
	ucfRNA	RNeasy Micro kit; Omni-Plex Whole Transcriptome Amplification (WTA) kit	Qiagen, Inc., Valencia, CA, USA; Rubicon Genomics, Ann Arbor, MI, USA	qRT-PCR	TMPRSS2:ERG gene fusion	[63]
	EV	ExoDx Prostate IntelliScore urine exosome assay; QIAGEN Rotor-Gene Q MDx System	Exosome Diagnostics, Waltham, MA, USA; Qiagen, Venlo, The Netherlands	qRT-PCR	ERG, PCA3, SPDEF	[64]
	CTC	MIL-38 immunofluorescence assay (IFA)	Minomic International Ltd., Sydney, Australia	immunofluorescence	glycoprotein glypican 1 (GPC-1)	[65]

2.1. ctDNA

Circulating cell-free DNA (cfDNA) analysis has gained relevance also in the setting of PCa. cfDNA represents DNA fragments released in blood by normal and tumor cells [66]. Remarkably, DNA released by tumor cells represents a small fraction of cfDNA, called ctDNA, which shows a smaller size than cfDNA released by normal cells [67,68]. From a prognostic point of view, ctDNA concentration in blood could potentially be complementary to PSA tests or replace it. High ctDNA concentration, indeed, correlates with poor PCa outcome [69]. Corbetta et al. reported a transient ctDNA concentration and fragment lengths increase after prostate biopsy at different time points [48]. Recently, Chen et al. have demonstrated that advanced stage PCa patients have a higher ctDNA concentration compared to those with localized disease or healthy controls. In this study, ctDNA was quantified with a Qubit 3.0 fluorometer and a DNA dsDNA HS Assay Kit (Life Technologies, Carlsbad, CA, USA), and the 2100 Bioanalyzer with High Sensitivity DNA Chips (Agilent Technologies, Santa Clara, CA, USA) was applied to assess purity, concentration and fragment size of sample analyzed [47]. In addition, the authors highlighted that ctDNA amount was remarkably increased (from 3.9- to 164-fold) after the surgical approach. Moreover, it was also estimated that cfDNA was characterized by a larger fraction of di-, tri- and multi-nucleosome associated DNA fragments [47]. Similarly, Kwee et al. observed, by RT-PCR analysis of the methylated promoter of the PCa-related genes *GSTP1* and *RARB2*, a significant ctDNA concentration increase after chemotherapy [49]. In fact, it has been demonstrated that specific hypermethylation of *RARB2* and *GSTP1* CpG sites may be adopted for PCa diagnosis [70]. According to cfDNA level modification as a clinical biomarker in PCa patients, in another experience, Patsch et al. evaluated a rapid decline of ctDNA amount quantified for long interspersed nuclear elements (LINE1) with qPCR approach after chemotherapy [50]. The phase III FIRSTANA and PROSELICA clinical trials revealed that ctDNA concentration may be considered an independent prognostic biomarker in advanced stage PCa. A higher ctDNA baseline concentration has been, indeed, associated with shorter progression-free survival (PFS) and overall survival (OS) after chemotherapy. Conversely, a total ctDNA concentration reduction during the first 9 weeks of treatment correlated with drug response therapy [51]. ctDNA analysis could represent a valid cost-effective alternative to tissue biomarkers analysis in advanced stage PCa. Interestingly, this approach could be useful to identify predictive biomarkers that can be further assessed in future clinical trials [67]. As an example, Wyatt et al., by comparing PCa ctDNA alterations with matched tissue, detected several genetic alterations, including Androgen Receptor (*AR*) amplifications, *SPOP* mutations and *TP53*, *PTEN*, *RB1*, *APC*, *CDKN1B*, *BRCA2* and *PIK3R1* genes inactivation, which may be further studied in these patients from a predictive point of view. In this setting, the remarkable concordance of ctDNA and metastatic tissue biopsies in advanced stage PCa patients suggests that ctDNA assays could be used for molecular stratification of patients for prognostic and predictive purposes [52,71].

2.2. ctRNA

Similarly to DNA fragments, tumor cells shade RNA-derived fragments in blood, known as circulating tumor RNA (ctRNA), ctRNA- messenger RNA (mRNA), microRNA (miRNA) and long non-coding RNA, may similarly represent a fascinating biosource for molecular analysis. In particular, the miRNAs expression profiling analysis is increasing to perform diagnosis, staging, progression, prognosis and treatment response [72,73]. miRNA can be extracted from ribonucleoprotein complexes or EVs [72,74]. Mitchell et al. firstly demonstrated the presence of miRNA in the plasma of PCa patients [75]. Since then, a large number of miRNAs were shown to be deregulated in PCa patients; in particular, miR-21, miR-30c, miR-125b, miR-141, miR-143, miR-148a, miR-205, miR-221 and miR-375 [76]. Liu et al., in 2018, performed a RT-PCR analysis of plasma samples collected from a cohort of n = 229 PCa patients on active surveillance, identifying three miRNA (miR-24, miR-223, and miR-375) that were significantly expressed in tumor patients. The authors elaborated two multi-variable logistic regression models, integrating the 3-miR score, PSA, the percentage of tumor cells in diagnostic samples and clinical variables. They showed that the 3-miR score ability to predict reclassification was not related to clinical variables and increased in comparison with clinical outcomes.

The authors concluded that the 3-miR score combined with PSA may represent a non-invasive high negative predictive value tool to identify patients on active surveillance who have indolent PCa [53]. Alhasan et al. identified in circulating miRNAs (miR-200c, miR-605, miR-135a, miR-433, and miR-106a) a molecular signature to detect high-risk PCa [54]. In 2017, Ferreira de Souza et al. analyzing plasma mRNA and miRNA of 102 untreated patients with PCa and 50 healthy subjects, identified differentially expressed *OR51E2* (olfactory receptor, family 51, subfamily E, member 2) and *SIM2* (single-minded 2) mRNAa, miR-200b and miR-200c. In addition, they showed that the *OR51E2* and *SIM2* genes association with miR-200b and miR-200c could be a diagnostic marker able to discriminate PCa samples from healthy controls with a sensitivity of 67% and specificity of 75% [55].

2.3. CTC

Circulating tumor cells (CTCs) originating from primary tumor are detectable in blood or lymphatic fluid [77]. Nevertheless, the use of CTCs for diagnosis is limited by the rarity of this cell population in blood [78]. In 2020, Ried et al. tested 20 CTCs samples from PCa patients, obtained with ISET®-CTC methodology, using the Immuno-Cyto-Chemistry staining (ICC) with PSA and protein antibodies, showing a positive result in almost all of the patients (18/20). In addition, in 27 early-stage patients, CTCs were found in 25 cases and 20 out of them had ICC-PSA-positive markers. Thus, a 99% positive predictive value and a 97% negative predictive value have been highlighted for the ISET-CTC-ICC approach [56]. Over the years, the importance of CTCs detection has also acquired clinical relevance as a prognostic and predictive biomarker [79]. Prospective trials showed that patients with an increase in CTCs amount within four weeks after chemotherapy could not benefit from treatment [57]. In 2021, Scher et al. displayed that the identification of CTCs, through the Epic Sciences platform, represents a prognostic biomarker for the progression of metastatic castration-resistant PCa (mCRPC) starting a second-generation androgen receptor signaling inhibitor (ARSI) [80].

2.4. EVs

In cancer development, EVs play a pivotal role in the signaling pathway network between tumor cells and the microenvironment [81,82]. In metastatic PCa patients, EVs promote metastasis by establishing the pre-metastatic niche (PMN). In fact, exosomes containing miRNAs (miR-21 and miR-139) promote PMS modifications [83]. For these reasons, EVs can have diagnostic and prognostic value in PCa patients. Several studies demonstrated that exosomes are more numerous in PCa patients than in healthy individuals [58–60,84]. However, according to Gao et al., nowadays, there are no standard methods to collect and analyze samples, rendering clinical and preclinical data inconsistent [81].

3. Urine Biomarkers in the Detection of PCa

Urine may be considered a suitable integrating source of clinical biomarkers that could play a pivotal role in the diagnosis, prognosis and PCa patients management [85]. From urine samples, various analytes may be isolated and detected. Among them, ucfDNA/RNA, miRNA, circulating tumor cells (CTCs) and extracellular vesicles (EVs) play a promising role in the clinical management of urogenital malignancy patients [86]. Urine cell-free DNA (ucfDNA) has recently been investigated in order to identify a novel potential biological source of nucleic acids able to integrate circulating nucleic acids from plasma samples in urogenital malignancy patients [87].

Remarkably, molecular analysis of urine analytes is characterized by several advantages: non-invasive sampling, with high volume of reproducible samples available in all time points with respect to low compliant sampling preparation [88]. Urinary biomarkers useful to predict biopsy outcome are often unimodal; a single urine fraction (i.e., cell-free fractions or cell-pellet) or biological cancer characteristic are considered to evaluate PCa status. Although a single test shows the accuracy and promising clinical relevance, the integration of multiple types of information could display a higher predictive value. ExoGrail is a multivariable risk model that integrate information from different clinical parameters. ExoGrail combines the expression level evaluation of Engrailed-2 (EN2), a protein contained in vesicles actively secreted by PCa cells and detected in urine samples with data from urinary cell-free RNA measurement. ExoGrail could be useful to assess PCa risk-assessment prior to an invasive tissue biopsy [89].

3.1. ctDNA

Based on recent literature data on the ctDNA fragmentation index in solid tumor patients, Casadio et al. carried out a pilot study on a retrospective series of bladder and prostate tumor patients aimed to technically validate the implementation of ucfDNA fragmentation index as a screening tool in PCa cohort [90]. Overall, it has been shown that urine DNA integrity is capable of distinguishing between PCa patients and healthy individuals with an accuracy of about 80% [61]. Moreover, Salvi et al. compared ucfDNA fragmentation index between $n = 67$ prostate malignant lesions and $n = 64$ benign prostate lesions grading in illness severity. Molecular data were obtained from a qPCR analysis of three oncogenic sequences longer than 250 bp (*c-MYC*, *HER2* and *AR*). Results showed a lower clinical predictive value than PSA in terms of sensitivity (0.58 vs. 0.95) and specificity (0.44 vs. 0.69), respectively [62]. In this context, PCA3 represents the first urine long noncoding RNA biomarker identified and approved by Food and Drug Administration (FDA) that could improve the detection rate of PCa [91]. Despite an increasing specificity, the quite low sensitive rate highlighted the necessity to discover other targets [92]. The expression of aberrant RNA transcript (*TMPRSS2: ERG*) represents a pathogenic mechanism in the development and progression of PCa [93]. Several studies have elucidated the prognostic role of residual or persistent *TMPRSS2-ERG* gene fusion expression in patients with castration resistant PCa [93,94]. A qRT-PCR analysis performed to detect *TMPRSS2: ERG* gene rearrangement in a retrospective series of $n = 19$ PCa patients ($n = 11$ prebiopsy and $n = 8$ pre-radical prostatectomy samples, respectively) revealed that 8 out of 19 (42.0%) PCa patients showed a detectable *TMPRSS2: ERG* aberrant gene fusion expression. In addition, it has been calculated the qRT-PCR sensitivity for urine *TMPRSS2: ERG* rearrangement detection by performing a Fluorescent in situ Hybridization (FISH) assay on corresponding PCa specimens. In this setting, FISH detected *TMPRSS2: ERG* in three patients with high frequency detected mutation from urine samples, while also highlighting a positive result in two patients negative for *TMPRSS2: ERG* gene fusion detection in ucfRNA specimens [63]. Accordingly, the implementation of the urine-based biomarkers in clinical practice was optimized with the diffusion of commercially available tests (IntelliScore -Exosome Diagnostics, Waltham, MA, USA and SelectMDx- MDxHealth, Irvine, CA, USA) aimed to determinate PCa patients selected for required tissue biopsy. In the era of "multi-omics" analysis, the development and diffusion of ultra-deep highly sensitive platforms, allowing to measure low target concentration in scant starting samples, have revolutionized the testing strategies in the clinical practice of tumor patients [95–97]. In an ongoing clinical trial promoted by the American Society of Clinical Oncology Genitourinary (ASCO-GU) an NGS assay, able to cover hot spot mutations in $n = 152$ cancer-related genes (PredicineCARE™, Predicine, Hayward, CA, USA), was used on blood and urine-derived circulating nucleic acids from $n = 59$ treatment-naïve PCa patients. Molecular profiling was then compared with corresponding data obtained from gold standard tissue specimens. Preliminary data elucidated a similar mutation profile between urine and corresponding tissue specimens with a sensitivity of 86.7% [98].

3.2. ctRNA

Recently, novel small non-coding RNAs have been investigated as promising diagnostic biomarkers for PCa patients [99,100]. Small RNA harbored by extracellular vesicles (EVs) could be considered a valuable marker for PCa diagnosis. Mckiernan et al. collected urine specimens from $n = 1563$ subjects. After a validation study aimed to evaluate gene expression signature in three genes (*PCA3, ERG* and *SPDEF*) involved in PCa progression, they focused on $n = 255$ not biopsied PCa patients with PSA level >2. The exosomes-derived gene expression profile showed a higher predictive value than PSA (AUC 0.73; 95% CI, 0.68–0.77 vs. AUC 0.63; 95% CI, 0.58–0.68) in the identification of high-grade PCa patients with respect to intermediate positive and negative biopsy from PCa patients. In addition, gene expression signature from urine exosomes also demonstrated a reliable clinically relevant predictive role (NPV 91.0%) in the decision making of patients with negative histological results [64]. Interestingly, the EPI urine biomarker was significantly associated with low-risk disease, making it a good test to select patients for AS [101].

3.3. CTC

Another approach to improve the diagnostic stage in PCa patients is based on the evaluation of circulating tumor cells (CTCs). The unique technical strategy approved by FDA for the detection of CTCs in peripheral blood of advanced solid tumor patients is the CellSearch test, able to detect (≥ 2 CTCs in 57% of metastatic PCa patients). In addition, CTC isolation from biological fluids have been recently improved with the implementation of microfluidic technology [102,103]. This technology provides a high-throughput and low-cost analysis and allows accurate CTC separation by cell size in an inert matrix [65,104]. CTCs isolation, confirmed by fluorescent staining (GPC-1$^+$), was observed in 12 out of 14 patients (86.0%) while CTCs detection was negative in 11 out of 14 control group patients (79.0%). In the remaining cases, a weak GPC-1$^+$ positive signal showed <8 CTC correctly detected. In addition, a positive correlation between GPC-1$^+$ positive CTCs and PSA level was observed ($r = 0.27$) [105].

4. The Role of Liquid Biopsy in Follow-Up

PCa is commonly considered a "hormones-dependent disease", since androgen controls PCa initiation and progression. Androgen deprivation therapy (ADT) represents the first-line therapeutic choice. Although ADT is effective to block tumor growth, this strategy often fails. Monitoring treatment efficacy represents a relevant aspect; currently, serum PSA and imaging are applied to follow treatment efficacy in PCa. However, the evaluation of early bone metastasis using imaging methods remains challenging, and PSA levels may be affected by AR signaling inhibitors. PCa often gains androgen independence, known as castration-resistant PCa (CRPC), characterized by metastatic spreading, significant mutational burden and copy number alteration, poor prognosis and a low survival rate [106]. CRPC often spreads in multiple sites per patient. Nowadays, despite several treatment options being available with varied mechanisms of action suitable for CRPC, long-term complete regression of CRPC is a rare phenomenon [107]. CRPC could depend to the transcriptional activity reactivation of androgen receptor (AR), because of *AR* gene mutations or amplification, leading to antiandrogens or other steroids promiscuous binding, or *AR* splice variants constitutively activated [108,109]. Since some tumors exhibit acquired resistance to specific chemotherapy agents could be possible to maximize the therapeutic efficacy by characterizing the tumor signature throughout the treatment. In this scenario, liquid biopsy has an advantage over tumor biopsy to capture genomic events from distant clones that are driving tumor progression [110]. Liquid biopsy may be used to early detect and manage a chemoresistance before the treatment pressure selects the most aggressive subclone of the tumor making it prevalent in tumor tissue. It has been demonstrated that the exosome-RNA and CTC isolated by plasma samples could be used to detect the androgen receptor splicing variant 7 (AR-V7), a predictive variant of resistance to AR signaling inhibitors. Furthermore, Tagawa and coworkers showed that the absence of the same variants in mCRPC CTC patients may be associated with better taxane treatment outcomes [111–113]. In addition, liquid biopsy could be also used to predict resistance to PARP inhibitors (PARPi), which are approved for treatment or maintenance therapy for several malignancies, including PCa. Tumors with somatic or germline *BRCA* mutations may be responsive to PARPi and platinum chemotherapy; liquid biopsy in this case can detect an acquired *BRCA* reversion associated with a poor response to PARPi [114]. In conclusion, given the high mutational burden characterizing CRPC, liquid biopsy may be a useful tool for early detection of tumor driving mutation, which eventually leads to chemoresistance and tumor progression. In this scenario, the follow-up using longitudinal analysis with liquid biopsy approach allows both the quantitative tracking of tumor burden to monitor treatment response and the assessment of clonal evolution by comparing genomic profiles over time.

5. Perspectives, Limitations and Future Perspectives

Biomarkers development for precision, tailored medicine in PCa management could be accelerated by liquid biopsy. Moreover, liquid biopsy could implement genomic testing into routine clinical practice, providing signatures of metastatic sites. The CTC counts, circulating nucleic acids amount and fragmentation, the ctDNA methylation status, represent prognostic and response biomarkers that could potentially guide therapeutic decisions in clinical practice. However, it should be noticed that liquid biopsy assays require analytical validation and should be clinically qualified for endorsement in routine clinical use. In this context, further evaluation in clinical trials and wide prospective studies are required. In addition, high cost, technology access and wide heterogeneity in definitions and isolation platforms impact the introduction of these biomarkers in routine clinical testing. The EVs use in a clinical setting is promising, but the standardization of isolation and application methods is challenging. Although liquid biopsy shows the significant potential to track the PCa clonal evolution that could be helpful to design an adapt, tailored therapeutic strategy to overcome cancer recurrence and increase the patient lifespan, developing liquid biopsy biomarkers still faces considerable challenges that hinder their clinical application. Firstly, despite the accessibility of powerful and high throughput tests, there is not enough evidence to support the routine use of liquid biopsy for early-stage cancer, making treatment decisions, monitoring, predicting response or for cancer screening. Secondly, the wide use of liquid biopsy in the clinical practice is still hampered by the costs and the limited knowledge of this technology in secondary centers. Indeed, liquid biopsy is too expensive for small centers to be used as a routine laboratory technique, with costs associated with equipment, reagents and properly trained personnel. Furthermore, in order to obtain the best results from liquid biopsy, a synergic work between urologists, oncologists and biochemist/bioinformatics is required during all the processes of this technology. Lastly, the post-processing laboratory work and statistical analysis needed are much more complex and time-consuming than the conventional pathology. As a result, also in this case, all the processes related to the comparison, interpretation and delivery of results have higher associated costs and resources consumption [115,116]. Despite the promising future of ctDNA as a driver of cancer treatment, several challenges need to be faced. There is a strong need to decrease costs and analysis time and to ameliorate the diagnostic performance for early cancer and minimal residual disease (MRD) detection. The technical challenges of turnaround time and costs will probably be addressed soon. The main barrier remains the clinical validation of ctDNA for the use as MRD and cancer screening biomarker. Currently, the liquid biopsy role in PCa management does not exceed the simple prognostic assessment. Thus far, the main issue to incorporate this approach in clinical decision-making is the lack of interventional studies demonstrating a clear advantage for the metastatic PCa patients. Further larger and long-term studies are required to assess whether ctDNA evaluation can be used for treatment-decision making. The identification of targetable alterations and emerging resistance biomarkers represents an attractive feature of liquid biopsy, particularly in CRPC, and could implement the precision medicine therapeutics in PCa. In the next years, the improvements of our knowledge in liquid biopsy application in decision-making strategy for mCRPC patients promise to revolutionize the mCRPC and dramatically improve the survival rate and quality of life of these patients.

6. Conclusions

PCa represent a major public health burden, whose incidence progressively grows. Although several progresses have been placed into investigating novel diagnostic and prognostic biomarkers for PCa, considering the inability of current biomarkers to predict disease aggressiveness, new efforts are needed to paint the intriguing PCa picture. Therefore, the discovery of novel and effective tools for early diagnosis, follow-up and prognosis in PCa patients is claimed. In this scenario, the liquid biopsy field in PCa has advanced exponentially, developing prognostic and predictive biomarkers and holding promise for a minimally invasive approach of monitoring tumor evolution. In this review, we described urinary and circulating biomarkers based on CTC, RNA and DNA as novel tools to improve the characterization and the treatment of PCa patients. These liquid biopsy biomarkers show the potential to gain comprehensive information on PCa genetic landscape, and give information about the metastatic sites. Liquid biopsy could guide therapeutic decisions and accelerate the development of precision medicine in PCa. The recent advancement of molecular biology techniques available will bring to the development of new standardized liquid biopsy tests with high sensitivity and specificity, and lower cost that could promote the diffusion of liquid biopsy in routine clinical practice. Designing a dynamic therapeutic strategy based on tumor features detected in real-time through the liquid biopsy could significantly improve the survival rate and the quality of life of PCa patients. Remarkably, nucleic acids extracted from biological fluids play a crucial role in the clinical management of PCa patients. Among conventional body fluids, peripheral blood still remains the most suitable source of nucleic acids, because a wide series of literature data critically evaluate the preclinical and analytical issues for blood-derived nucleic acids. Conversely, little was known about the use of nucleic acids purified from urine samples. However, due to their close connection with prostatic glands, further studies should be performed to evaluate the clinical meaning of biomarkers from urine samples.

Author Contributions: Study design, B.B., F.C. and E.D.Z.; data curation, B.F.M., G.R., P.P., F.P., E.L.C., A.P. and A.R.; writing—original draft preparation, B.F.M., F.C., G.R., P.P. and E.L.C.; writing—review and editing, E.D.Z., D.T., U.M., G.T., A.P., C.B. and B.B.; project administration, F.C. All authors have read and agreed to the published version of the manuscript.

Funding: This research received no external funding.

Conflicts of Interest: P.P. has received personal fees as speaker bureau from Novartis, unrelated to the current work. A.R. reports advisory board role/consultancy for AstraZeneca, Novartis, Pfizer and MSD, unrelated to the current work. U.M. has received personal fees (as consultant and/or speaker bureau) from Boehringer Ingelheim, Roche, MSD, Amgen, Thermo Fisher Scientifics, Eli Lilly, Diaceutics, GSK, Merck and AstraZeneca, Janssen, Diatech, Novartis and Hedera unrelated to the current work. G.T. reports personal fees (as speaker bureau or advisor) from Roche, MSD, Pfizer, Boehringer Ingelheim, Eli Lilly, BMS, GSK, Menarini, AstraZeneca, Amgen and Bayer, unrelated to the current work. The authors declare that the research was conducted in the absence of any commercial or financial relationships that could be construed as a potential conflict of interest.

References

1. Sung, H.; Ferlay, J.; Siegel, R.L.; Laversanne, M.; Soerjomataram, I.; Jemal, A.; Bray, F. No Title. *CA Cancer J. Clin.* **2021**, *71*, 209–249. [CrossRef] [PubMed]
2. Rebello, R.J.; Oing, C.; Knudsen, K.E.; Loeb, S.; Johnson, D.C.; Reiter, R.E.; Gillessen, S.; Van der Kwast, T.; Bristow, R.G. Prostate cancer. *Nat. Rev. Dis Primers* **2021**, *7*, 9. [CrossRef] [PubMed]
3. Gandaglia, G.; Leni, R.; Bray, F.; Fleshner, N.; Freedland, S.J.; Kibel, A.; Stattin, P.; Van Poppel, H.; La Vecchia, C. Epidemiology and Prevention of Prostate Cancer. *Eur. Urol. Oncol.* **2021**, *4*, 877–892. [CrossRef] [PubMed]
4. Mazzone, E.; Preisser, F.; Nazzani, S.; Tian, Z.; Bandini, M.; Gandaglia, G.; Fossati, N.; Montorsi, F.; Graefen, M.; Shariat, S.F.; et al. The Effect of Lymph Node Dissection in Metastatic Prostate Cancer Patients Treated with Radical Prostatectomy: A Contemporary Analysis of Survival and Early Postoperative Outcomes. *Eur. Urol. Oncol.* **2019**, *5*, 541–548. [CrossRef] [PubMed]
5. Pernar, C.H.; Ebot, E.M.; Wilson, K.M.; Mucci, L.A. The Epidemiology of Prostate Cancer. *Cold Spring Harb. Perspect. Med.* **2018**, *8*, a030361. [CrossRef]
6. Shimizu, H.; Ross, R.K.; Bernstein, L.; Yatani, R.; Henderson, B.E.; Mack, T.M. Cancers of the prostate and breast among Japanese and white immigrants in Los Angeles County. *Br. J. Cancer* **1991**, *63*, 963–966. [CrossRef]
7. Yu, H.; Harris, R.E.; Gao, Y.T.; Gao, R.; Wynder, E.L. Comparative epidemiology of cancers of the colon, rectum, prostate and breast in Shanghai, China versus the United States. *Int. J. Epidemiol.* **1991**, *20*, 76–81. [CrossRef]
8. Siegel, R.L.; Miller, K.D.; Jemal, A. Cancer statistics. *CA Cancer J. Clin.* **2018**, *68*, 7–30. [CrossRef]
9. Sweeney, C.J.; Chen, Y.H.; Carducci, M.; Liu, G.; Jarrard, D.F.; Eisenberger, M.; Wong, Y.N.; Hahn, N.; Kohli, M.; Cooney, M.M.; et al. Chemohormonal Therapy in Metastatic Hormone-Sensitive Prostate Cancer. *N. Engl. J. Med.* **2015**, *373*, 737–746. [CrossRef]
10. Perdana, N.R.; Mochtar, C.A.; Umbas, R.; Hamid, A.R.A. The Risk Factors of Prostate Cancer and Its Prevention: A Literature Review. *Acta Med. Indones.* **2016**, *48*, 228–238.
11. Grozescu, T.; Popa, F. Prostate cancer between prognosis and adequate/proper therapy. *J. Med. Life* **2017**, *10*, 5–12. [PubMed]
12. Bancroft, E.K.; Raghallaigh, H.N.; Page, E.C.; Eeles, R.A. Updates in Prostate Cancer Research and Screening in Men at Genetically Higher Risk. *Curr. Genet. Med. Rep.* **2021**, *9*, 47–58. [CrossRef] [PubMed]
13. Vietri, M.T.; D'Elia, G.; Caliendo, G.; Resse, M.; Casamassimi, A.; Passariello, L.; Albanese, L.; Cioffi, M.; Molinari, A.M. Hereditary Prostate Cancer: Genes Related, Target Therapy and Prevention. *Int. J. Mol. Sci.* **2021**, *22*, 3753. [CrossRef]
14. Pritchard, C.C.; Mateo, J.; Walsh, M.F.; De Sarkar, N.; Abida, W.; Beltran, H.; Garofalo, A.; Gulati, R.; Carreira, S.; Eeles, R. Inherited DNA-Repair Gene Mutations in Men with Metastatic Prostate Cancer. *N. Engl. J. Med.* **2016**, *375*, 443–453. [CrossRef]
15. Brandão, A.; Paulo, P.; Teixeira, M.R. Hereditary Predisposition to Prostate Cancer: From Genetics to Clinical Implications. *Int. J. Mol. Sci.* **2020**, *21*, 5036. [CrossRef] [PubMed]
16. Vidal, A.C.; Oyekunle, T.; Howard, L.E.; De Hoedt, A.M.; Kane, C.J.; Terris, M.K.; Cooperberg, M.R.; Amling, C.L.; Klaassen, Z.; Freedland, S.J.; et al. Obesity, race, and long-term prostate cancer outcomes. *Cancer* **2020**, *126*, 3733–3741. [CrossRef] [PubMed]
17. Olivas, A.; Price, R.S. Obesity, Inflammation, and Advanced Prostate Cancer. *Nutr. Cancer* **2021**, *73*, 2232–2248. [CrossRef]

18. Crocetto, F.; Pandolfo, S.D.; Aveta, A.; Martino, R.; Trama, F.; Caputo, V.F.; Barone, B.; Abate, M.; Sicignano, E.; Cilio, S.; et al. A Comparative Study of the Triglycerides/HDL Ratio and Pseudocholinesterase Levels in Patients with Bladder Cancer. *Diagnostics* **2022**, *12*, 431. [CrossRef]
19. Tarantino, G.; Crocetto, F.; Di Vito, C.; Creta, M.; Martino, R.; Pandolfo, S.D.; Pesce, S.; Napolitano, L.; Capone, D.; Imbimbo, C. Association of NAFLD and Insulin Resistance with Non Metastatic Bladder Cancer Patients: A Cross-Sectional Retrospective Study. *J. Clin. Med.* **2021**, *10*, 346. [CrossRef]
20. Gacci, M.; Russo, G.I.; De Nunzio, C.; Sebastianelli, A.; Salvi, M.; Vignozzi, L.; Tubaro, A.; Morgia, G.; Serni, S. Meta-analysis of metabolic syndrome and prostate cancer. *Prostate Cancer Prostatic Dis.* **2017**, *20*, 146–155. [CrossRef]
21. La Civita, E.; Liotti, A.; Cennamo, M.; Crocetto, F.; Ferro, M.; Liguoro, P.; Cimmino, A.; Imbimbo, C.; Beguinot, F.; Formisano, P.; et al. Peri-Prostatic Adipocyte-Released TGFβ Enhances Prostate Cancer Cell Motility by Upregulation of Connective Tissue Growth Factor. *Biomedicines* **2021**, *9*, 1692. [CrossRef] [PubMed]
22. Liang, Z.; Xie, B.; Li, J.; Wang, X.; Wang, S.; Meng, S.; Ji, A.; Zhu, Y.; Xu, X.; Zheng, X.; et al. Hypertension and risk of prostate cancer: A systematic review and meta-analysis. *Sci. Rep.* **2016**, *6*, 31358. [CrossRef] [PubMed]
23. Nguyen-Nielsen, M.; Borre, M. Diagnostic and Therapeutic Strategies for Prostate Cancer. *Semin. Nucl. Med.* **2016**, *46*, 484–490. [CrossRef] [PubMed]
24. Ragsdale, J.W., 3rd; Halstater, B.; Martinez-Bianchi, V. Prostate cancer screening. *Prim. Care* **2014**, *41*, 355–370. [CrossRef]
25. Stamey, T.A.; Yang, N.; Hay, A.R.; McNeal, J.E.; Freiha, F.S.; Redwine, E. Prostate-specific antigen as a serum marker for adenocarcinoma of the prostate. *N. Engl. J. Med.* **1987**, *317*, 909–916. [CrossRef]
26. Semjonow, A.; Brandt, B.; Oberpenning, F.; Roth, S.; Hertle, L. Discordance of assay methods creates pitfalls for the interpretation of prostate-specific antigen values. *Prostate Suppl.* **1996**, *7*, 3–16. [CrossRef]
27. Ferro, M.; De Cobelli, O.; Lucarelli, G.; Porreca, A.; Busetto, G.M.; Cantiello, F.; Damiano, R.; Autorino, R.; Musi, G.; Vartolomei, M.D.; et al. Beyond PSA: The Role of Prostate Health Index (phi). *Int. J. Mol. Sci.* **2020**, *21*, 1184. [CrossRef]
28. Catalona, W.J.; Richie, J.P.; Ahmann, F.R.; Hudson, M.A.; Scardino, P.T.; Flanigan, R.C.; DeKernion, J.B.; Ratliff, T.L.; Kavoussi, L.R.; Dalkin, B.L.; et al. Comparison of digital rectal examination and serum prostate specific antigen in the early detection of prostate cancer: Results of a multicenter clinical trial of 6630 men. *J. Urol.* **1994**, *151*, 1283–1290. [CrossRef]
29. Ferro, M.; Lucarelli, G.; de Cobelli, O.; Del Giudice, F.; Musi, G.; Mistretta, F.A.; Luzzago, S.; Busetto, G.M.; Buonerba, C.; Sciarra, A.; et al. The emerging landscape of tumor marker panels for the identification of aggressive prostate cancer: The perspective through bibliometric analysis of an Italian translational working group in uro-oncology. *Minerva Urol. Nephrol.* **2021**, *73*, 442–451. [CrossRef]
30. Smeenge, M.; Barentsz, J.; Cosgrove, D.; de la Rosette, J.; de Reijke, T.; Eggener, S.; Frauscher, F.; Kovacs, G.; Matin, S.F.; Mischi, M.; et al. Role of transrectal ultrasonography (TRUS) in focal therapy of prostate cancer: Report from a Consensus Panel. *BJU Int.* **2012**, *110*, 942–948. [CrossRef]
31. Mottet, N.; van den Bergh, R.C.N.; Briers, E.; Van den Broeck, T.; Cumberbatch, M.G.; De Santis, M.; Fanti, S.; Fossati, N.; Gandaglia, G.; Gillessen, S.; et al. EAU-EANM-ESTRO-ESUR-SIOG Guidelines on Prostate Cancer-2020 Update. Part 1: Screening, Diagnosis, and Local Treatment with Curative Intent. *Eur. Urol.* **2021**, *79*, 243–262. [CrossRef] [PubMed]
32. Cornford, P.; van den Bergh, R.C.N.; Briers, E.; Van den Broeck, T.; Cumberbatch, M.G.; De Santis, M.; Fanti, S.; Fossati, N.; Gandaglia, G.; Gillessen, S.; et al. EAU-EANM-ESTRO-ESUR-SIOG Guidelines on Prostate Cancer. Part II-2020 Update: Treatment of Relapsing and Metastatic Prostate Cancer. *Eur. Urol.* **2021**, *79*, 263–282. [CrossRef] [PubMed]
33. Rapisarda, S.; Bada, M.; Crocetto, F.; Barone, B.; Arcaniolo, D.; Polara, A.; Imbimbo, C.; Grosso, G. The role of multiparametric resonance and biopsy in prostate cancer detection: Comparison with definitive histological report after laparoscopic/robotic radical prostatectomy. *Abdom. Radiol.* **2020**, *45*, 4178–4184. [CrossRef] [PubMed]
34. Derin, O.; Fonseca, L.; Sanchez-Salas, R.; Roberts, M.J. Infectious complications of prostate biopsy: Winning battles but not war. *World J. Urol.* **2020**, *38*, 2743–2753. [CrossRef]
35. Stefanova, V.; Buckley, R.; Flax, S.; Spevack, L.; Hajek, D.; Tunis, A.; Lai, E.; Loblaw, A.; Collaborators. Transperineal Prostate Biopsies Using Local Anesthesia: Experience with 1287 Patients. Prostate Cancer Detection Rate, Complications and Patient Tolerability. *J. Urol.* **2019**, *201*, 1121–1126. [CrossRef]
36. Ferro, M.; La Civita, E.; Liotti, A.; Cennamo, M.; Tortora, F.; Buonerba, C.; Crocetto, F.; Lucarelli, G.; Busetto, G.M.; Del Giudice, F. Liquid Biopsy Biomarkers in Urine: A Route towards Molecular Diagnosis and Personalized Medicine of Bladder Cancer. *J. Pers. Med.* **2021**, *11*, 237. [CrossRef]
37. Crocetto, F.; Barone, B.; Ferro, M.; Busetto, G.M.; La Civita, E.; Buonerba, C.; Di Lorenzo, G.; Terracciano, D.; Schalken, J.A. Liquid biopsy in bladder cancer: State of the art and future perspectives. *Crit. Rev. Oncol. Hematol.* **2022**, *170*, 103577. [CrossRef]
38. Serrano, M.J.; Garrido-Navas, M.C.; Diaz Mochon, J.J.; Cristofanilli, M.; Gil-Bazo, I.; Pauwels, P.; Malapelle, U.; Russo, A.; Lorente, J.A.; Ruiz-Rodriguez, A.J.; et al. Precision Prevention and Cancer Interception: The New Challenges of Liquid Biopsy. International Society of Liquid Biopsy. *Cancer Discov.* **2020**, *10*, 1635–1644. [CrossRef]
39. Crocetto, F.; Cimmino, A.; Ferro, M.; Terracciano, D. Circulating tumor cells in bladder cancer: A new horizon of liquid biopsy for precision medicine. *J. Basic Clin. Physiol. Pharmacol.* **2021**. [CrossRef]
40. Soda, N.; Rehm, B.H.A.; Sonar, P.; Nguyen, N.T.; Shiddiky, M.J.A. Advanced liquid biopsy technologies for circulating biomarker detection. *J. Mater. Chem. B* **2019**, *7*, 6670–6704. [CrossRef]

41. Geeurickx, E.; Hendrix, A. Targets, pitfalls and reference materials for liquid biopsy tests in cancer diagnostics. *Mol. Asp. Med.* **2020**, *72*, 100828. [CrossRef] [PubMed]
42. Marrugo-Ramírez, J.; Mir, M.; Samitier, J. Blood-Based Cancer Biomarkers in Liquid Biopsy: A Promising Non-Invasive Alternative to Tissue Biopsy. *Int. J. Mol. Sci.* **2018**, *19*, 2877. [CrossRef] [PubMed]
43. Jia, S.; Zhang, R.; Li, Z.; Li, J. Clinical and biological significance of circulating tumor cells, circulating tumor DNA, and exosomes as biomarkers in colorectal cancer. *Oncotarget* **2017**, *8*, 55632–55645. [CrossRef] [PubMed]
44. Crowley, E.; Di Nicolantonio, F.; Loupakis, F.; Bardelli, A. Liquid biopsy: Monitoring cancer-genetics in the blood. *Nat. Rev. Clin. Oncol.* **2013**, *10*, 472–484. [CrossRef]
45. Zhang, W.; Xia, W.; Lv, Z.; Ni, C.; Xin, Y.; Yang, L. Liquid Biopsy for Cancer: Circulating Tumor Cells, Circulating Free DNA or Exosomes? *Cell Physiol. Biochem.* **2017**, *41*, 755–768. [CrossRef]
46. Neumann, M.H.D.; Bender, S.; Krahn, T.; Schlange, T. ctDNA and CTCs in Liquid Biopsy—Current Status and Where We Need to Progress. *Comput. Struct. Biotechnol. J.* **2018**, *16*, 190–195. [CrossRef]
47. Chen, E.; Cario, C.L.; Leong, L.; Lopez, K.; Márquez, C.P.; Chu, C.; Li, P.S.; Oropeza, E.; Tenggara, I.; Cowan, J.; et al. Cell-free DNA concentration and fragment size as a biomarker for prostate cancer. *Sci. Rep.* **2021**, *11*, 5040. [CrossRef]
48. Corbetta, M.; Chiereghin, C.; De Simone, I.; Soldà, G.; Zuradelli, M.; Giunta, M.; Lughezzani, G.; Buffi, N.M.; Hurlem, R.; Saita, A.; et al. Post-Biopsy Cell-Free DNA from Blood: An Open Window on Primary Prostate Cancer Genetics and Biology. *Front. Oncol.* **2021**, *11*, 654140. [CrossRef]
49. Kwee, S.; Song, M.A.; Cheng, I.; Loo, L.; Tiirikainen, M. Measurement of circulating cell-free DNA in relation to 18F-fluorocholine PET/CT imaging in chemotherapy-treated advanced prostate cancer. *Clin. Transl. Sci.* **2012**, *5*, 65–70. [CrossRef]
50. Patsch, K.; Matasci, N.; Soundararajan, A.; Diaz, P.; Agus, D.B.; Ruderman, D.; Gross, M.E. Monitoring dynamic cytotoxic chemotherapy response in castration-resistant prostate cancer using plasma cell-free DNA (cfDNA). *BMC Res. Notes* **2019**, *12*, 275. [CrossRef]
51. Mehra, N.; Dolling, D.; Sumanasuriya, S.; Christova, R.; Pope, L.; Carreira, S.; Seed, G.; Yuan, W.; Goodall, J.; Hall, E.; et al. Plasma Cell-free DNA Concentration and Outcomes from Taxane Therapy in Metastatic Castration-resistant Prostate Cancer from Two Phase III Trials (FIRSTANA and PROSELICA). *Eur. Urol.* **2018**, *74*, 83–291. [CrossRef] [PubMed]
52. Wyatt, A.W.; Annala, M.; Aggarwal, R.; Beja, K.; Feng, F.; Youngren, J.; Foye, A.; Lloyd, P.; Nykter, M.; Beer, T.M.; et al. Concordance of Circulating Tumor DNA and Matched Metastatic Tissue Biopsy in Prostate Cancer. *J. Natl. Cancer Inst.* **2017**, *109*, djx118. [CrossRef] [PubMed]
53. Liu, R.S.C.; Olkhov-Mitsel, E.; Jeyapala, R.; Zhao, F.; Commisso, K.; Klotz, L.; Loblaw, A.; Liu, S.K.; Vesprini, D.; Fleshner, N.E.; et al. Assessment of Serum microRNA Biomarkers to Predict Reclassification of Prostate Cancer in Patients on Active Surveillance. *J. Urol.* **2018**, *6*, 1475–1481. [CrossRef] [PubMed]
54. Alhasan, A.H.; Scott, A.W.; Wu, J.J.; Feng, G.; Meeks, J.J.; Thaxton, C.S.; Mirkin, C.A. Circulating microRNA signature for the diagnosis of very high-risk prostate cancer. *Proc. Natl. Acad. Sci. USA* **2016**, *113*, 10655–10660. [CrossRef]
55. Souza, M.F.; Kuasne, H.; Barros-Filho, M.C.; Cilião, H.L.; Marchi, F.A.; Fuganti, P.E.; Paschoal, A.R.; Rogatto, S.R.; Cólus, I.M.S. Circulating mRNAs and miRNAs as candidate markers for the diagnosis and prognosis of prostate cancer. *PLoS ONE* **2017**, *12*, e0184094. [CrossRef]
56. Ried, K.; Tamanna, T.; Matthews, S.; Eng, P.; Sali, A. New Screening Test Improves Detection of Prostate Cancer Using Circulating Tumor Cells and Prostate-Specific Markers. *Front. Oncol.* **2020**, *10*, 582. [CrossRef]
57. Zapatero, A.; Gómez-Caamaño, A.; Cabeza Rodriguez, M.Á.; Muinelo-Romay, L.; Martin de Vidales, C.; Abalo, A.; Calvo Crespo, P.; Leon Mateos, L.; Olivier, C.; Vega Piris, L.V. Detection and dynamics of circulating tumor cells in patients with high-risk prostate cancer treated with radiotherapy and hormones: A prospective phase II study. *Radiat. Oncol.* **2020**, *15*, 137. [CrossRef]
58. Park, Y.H.; Shin, H.W.; Jung, A.R.; Kwon, O.S.; Choi, Y.J.; Park, J.; Lee, J.Y. Prostate-specific extracellular vesicles as a novel biomarker in human prostate cancer. *Sci. Rep.* **2016**, *6*, 30386. [CrossRef]
59. Tavoosidana, G.; Ronquist, G.; Darmanis, S.; Yan, J.; Carlsson, L.; Wu, D.; Conze, T.; Ek, P.; Semjonow, A.; Eltze, E.; et al. Multiple recognition assay reveals prostasomes as promising plasma biomarkers for prostate cancer. *Proc. Natl. Acad. Sci. USA* **2011**, *108*, 8809–8814. [CrossRef]
60. Biggs, C.N.; Siddiqui, K.M.; Al-Zahrani, A.A.; Pardhan, S.; Brett, S.I.; Guo, Q.Q.; Yang, J.; Wolf, P.; Power, N.E.; Durfee, P.N.; et al. Prostate extracellular vesicles in patient plasma as a liquid biopsy platform for prostate cancer using nanoscale flow cytometry. *Oncotarget* **2016**, *7*, 8839–8849. [CrossRef]
61. Casadio, V.; Calistri, D.; Salvi, S.; Gunelli, R.; Carretta, E.; Amadori, D.; Silvestrini, R.; Zoli, W. Urine cell-free DNA integrity as a marker for early prostate cancer diagnosis: A pilot study. *Biomed. Res. Int.* **2013**, *2013*, 270457. [CrossRef] [PubMed]
62. Salvi, S.; Gurioli, G.; Martignano, F.; Foca, F.; Gunelli, R.; Cicchetti, G.; De Giorgi, U.; Zoli, W.; Calistri, D.; Casadio, V. Urine Cell-Free DNA Integrity Analysis for Early Detection of Prostate Cancer Patients. *Dis. Mark.* **2015**, *2015*, 574120. [CrossRef] [PubMed]
63. Laxman, B.; Tomlins, S.A.; Mehra, R.; Morris, D.S.; Wang, L.; Helgeson, B.E.; Shah, R.B.; Rubin, M.A.; Wei, J.T.; Chinnaiyan, A.M. Noninvasive detection of TMPRSS2:ERG fusion transcripts in the urine of men with prostate cancer. *Neoplasia* **2006**, *8*, 885–888. [CrossRef] [PubMed]

64. McKiernan, J.; Donovan, M.J.; O'Neill, V.; Bentink, S.; Noerholm, M.; Belzer, S.; Skog, J.; Kattan, M.W.; Partin, A.; Andriole, G.; et al. A Novel Urine Exosome Gene Expression Assay to Predict High-grade Prostate Cancer at Initial Biopsy. *JAMA Oncol.* **2016**, *2*, 882–889. [CrossRef]
65. Campbell, D.H.; Lund, M.E.; Nocon, A.L.; Cozzi, P.J.; Frydenberg, M.; De Souza, P.; Schiller, B.; Beebe-Dimmer, J.L.; Ruterbusch, J.J.; Walsh, B.J. Detection of glypican-1 (GPC-1) expression in urine cell sediments in prostate cancer. *PLoS ONE* **2018**, *13*, e0196017. [CrossRef]
66. Snyder, M.W.; Kircher, M.; Hill, A.J.; Daza, R.M.; Shendure, J. Cell-free DNA Comprises an In Vivo Nucleosome Footprint that Informs Its Tissues-of-Origin. *Cell* **2016**, *164*, 57–68. [CrossRef]
67. Mayrhofer, M.; De Laere, B.; Whitington, T.; Van Oyen, P.; Ghysel, C.; Ampe, J.; Ost, P.; Demey, W.; Hoekx, L.; Schrijvers, D.; et al. Cell-free DNA profiling of metastatic prostate cancer reveals microsatellite instability, structural rearrangements and clonal hematopoiesis. *Genome Med.* **2018**, *10*, 85. [CrossRef]
68. Mouliere, F.; Chandrananda, D.; Piskorz, A.M.; Moore, E.K.; Morris, J.; Ahlborn, L.B.; Mair, R.; Goranova, T.; Marass, F.; Heider, K.; et al. Enhanced detection of circulating tumor DNA by fragment size analysis. *Sci. Transl. Med.* **2018**, *10*, eaat4921. [CrossRef]
69. Liu, H.; Gao, Y.; Vafaei, S.; Gu, X.; Zhong, X. The Prognostic Value of Plasma Cell-Free DNA Concentration in the Prostate Cancer: A Systematic Review and Meta-Analysis. *Front. Oncol.* **2021**, *11*, 599602. [CrossRef]
70. Vanaja, D.K.; Ehrich, M.; Van den Boom, D.; Cheville, J.C.; Karnes, R.J.; Tindall, D.J.; Cantor, C.R.; Young, C.Y. Hypermethylation of genes for diagnosis and risk stratification of prostate cancer. *Cancer Investig.* **2009**, *27*, 549–560. [CrossRef]
71. Chen, G.; Jia, G.; Chao, F.; Xie, F.; Zhang, Y.; Hou, C.; Huang, Y.; Tang, H.; Yu, J.; Zhang, J.; et al. Urine- and Blood-Based Molecular Profiling of Human Prostate Cancer. *Front. Oncol.* **2022**, *12*, 759791. [CrossRef] [PubMed]
72. Boerrigter, E.; Groen, L.N.; Van Erp, N.P.; Verhaegh, G.W.; Schalken, J.A. Clinical utility of emerging biomarkers in prostate cancer liquid biopsies. *Expert. Rev. Mol. Diagn.* **2020**, *20*, 219–230. [CrossRef] [PubMed]
73. Kim, W.T.; Kim, W.J. MicroRNAs in prostate cancer. *Prostate Int.* **2013**, *1*, 3–9. [CrossRef]
74. Zhang, Z.; Qin, Y.W.; Brewer, G.; Jing, Q. MicroRNA degradation and turnover: Regulating the regulators. *Wiley Interdisc. Rev. RNA* **2012**, *3*, 593–600. [CrossRef]
75. Mitchell, P.S.; Parkin, R.K.; Kroh, E.M.; Fritz, B.R.; Wyman, S.K.; Pogosova-Agadjanyan, E.L.; Peterson, A.; Noteboom, J.; O'Briant, K.C.; Allen, A.; et al. Circulating microRNAs as stable blood-based markers for cancer detection. *Proc. Natl. Acad. Sci. USA* **2008**, *105*, 10513–10518. [CrossRef] [PubMed]
76. Abramovic, I.; Ulamec, M.; Katusic Bojanac, A.; Bulic-Jakus, F.; Jezek, D.; Sincic, N. miRNA in prostate cancer: Challenges toward translation. *Epigenomics* **2020**, *12*, 543–558. [CrossRef]
77. Yu, M.; Stott, S.; Toner, M.; Maheswaran, S.; Haber, D.A. Circulating tumor cells: Approaches to isolation and characterization. *J. Cell Biol.* **2011**, *192*, 373–382. [CrossRef]
78. Balázs, K.; Antal, L.; Sáfrány, G.; Lumniczky, K. Blood-Derived Biomarkers of Diagnosis, Prognosis and Therapy Response in Prostate Cancer Patients. *J. Pers. Med.* **2021**, *11*, 296. [CrossRef]
79. Fehm, T.; Sagalowsky, A.; Clifford, E.; Beitsch, P.; Saboorian, H.; Euhus, D.; Meng, S.; Morrison, L.; Tucker, T.; Lane, N. Cytogenetic evidence that circulating epithelial cells in patients with carcinoma are malignant. *Clin. Cancer Res.* **2002**, *8*, 2073–2084.
80. Scher, H.I.; Armstrong, A.J.; Schonhoft, J.D.; Gill, A.; Zhao, J.L.; Barnett, E.; Carbone, E.; Lu, J.; Antonarakis, E.S.; Luo, J.; et al. Development and validation of circulating tumour cell enumeration (Epic Sciences) as a prognostic biomarker in men with metastatic castration-resistant prostate cancer. *Eur. J. Cancer* **2021**, *150*, 83–94. [CrossRef]
81. Gao, Z.; Pang, B.; Li, J.; Gao, N.; Fan, T.; Li, Y. Emerging Role of Exosomes in Liquid Biopsy for Monitoring Prostate Cancer Invasion and Metastasis. *Front. Cell Dev. Biol.* **2021**, *9*, 679527. [CrossRef] [PubMed]
82. Lorenc, T.; Klimczyk, K.; Michalczewska, I.; Słomka, M.; Kubiak-Tomaszewska, G.; Olejarz, W. Exosomes in Prostate Cancer Diagnosis, Prognosis and Therapy. *Int. J. Mol. Sci.* **2020**, *21*, 2118. [CrossRef] [PubMed]
83. Hu, G.; Xie, L.; Zhou, Y.; Cai, X.; Gao, P.; Xue, B. Roles and Clinical Application of Exosomes in Prostate Cancer. *Front. Urol.* **2022**, *2*, 4. [CrossRef]
84. Vlaeminck-Guillem, V. Extracellular Vesicles in Prostate Cancer Carcinogenesis, Diagnosis, and Management. *Front. Oncol.* **2018**, *8*, 222. [CrossRef] [PubMed]
85. Truong, M.; Yang, B.; Jarrard, D.F. Toward the detection of prostate cancer in urine: A critical analysis. *J. Urol.* **2013**, *189*, 422–429. [CrossRef]
86. Kim, W.T.; Kim, Y.H.; Jeong, P.; Seo, S.P.; Kang, H.W.; Kim, Y.J.; Yun, S.J.; Lee, S.C.; Moon, S.K.; Choi, Y.H.; et al. Urinary cell-free nucleic acid IQGAP3: A new non-invasive diagnostic marker for bladder cancer. *Oncotarget* **2018**, *9*, 14354–14365. [CrossRef]
87. Santos, V.; Freitas, C.; Fernandes, M.G.; Sousa, C.; Reboredo, C.; Cruz-Martins, N.; Mosquera, J.; Hespanhol, V.; Campelo, R. Liquid biopsy: The value of different bodily fluids. *Biomark. Med.* **2022**, *16*, 127–145. [CrossRef]
88. Lu, T.; Li, J. Clinical applications of urinary cell-free DNA in cancer: Current insights and promising future. *Am. J. Cancer Res.* **2017**, *7*, 2318–2332.
89. Connell, S.P.; Mills, R.; Pandha, H.; Morgan, R.; Cooper, C.S.; Clark, J.; Brewer, D.S. The Movember Gap Urine Biomarker Consortium. Integration of Urinary EN2 Protein & Cell-Free RNA Data in the Development of a Multivariable Risk Model for the Detection of Prostate Cancer Prior to Biopsy. *Cancers* **2021**, *13*, 2102.

90. Mathios, D.; Johansen, J.S.; Cristiano, S.; Medina, J.E.; Phallen, J.; Larsen, K.R.; Bruhm, D.C.; Niknafs, N.; Ferreira, L.; Adleff, V.; et al. Detection and characterization of lung cancer using cell-free DNA fragmentomes. *Nat. Commun.* **2021**, *12*, 5060. [CrossRef]
91. Birnbaum, J.K.; Feng, Z.; Gulati, R.; Fan, J.; Lotan, Y.; Wei, J.T.; Etzioni, R. Projecting Benefits and Harms of Novel Cancer Screening Biomarkers: A Study of PCA3 and Prostate Cancer. *Cancer Epidemiol. Biomark. Prev.* **2015**, *24*, 677–682. [CrossRef] [PubMed]
92. Loeb, S.; Partin, A.W. PCA3 Urinary Biomarker for Prostate Cancer. *Rev. Urol.* **2010**, *12*, e205-6. [PubMed]
93. Perner, S.; Demichelis, F.; Beroukhim, R.; Schmidt, F.H.; Mosquera, J.M.; Setlur, S.; Tchinda, J.; Tomlins, S.A.; Hofer, M.D.; Pienta, K.G. TMPRSS2:ERG fusion-associated deletions provide insight into the heterogeneity of prostate cancer. *Cancer Res.* **2006**, *66*, 8337–8341. [CrossRef] [PubMed]
94. Linja, M.J.; Savinainen, K.J.; Saramäki, O.R.; Tammela, T.L.; Vessella, R.L.; Visakorpi, T. Amplification and overexpression of androgen receptor gene in hormone-refractory prostate cancer. *Cancer Res.* **2001**, *61*, 3550–3555. [PubMed]
95. de Biase, D.; Fassan, M.; Malapelle, U. Next-Generation Sequencing in Tumor Diagnosis and Treatment. *Diagnostics* **2020**, *10*, 962. [CrossRef] [PubMed]
96. Pisapia, P.; Costa, J.L.; Pepe, F.; Russo, G.; Gragnano, G.; Russo, A.; Iaccarino, A.; de Miguel-Perez, D.; Serrano, M.J.; Denninghoff, V.; et al. Next generation sequencing for liquid biopsy based testing in non-small cell lung cancer in 2021. *Crit. Rev. Oncol. Hematol.* **2021**, *161*, 03311. [CrossRef]
97. Rolfo, C.; Cardona, A.F.; Cristofanilli, M.; Paz-Ares, L.; Diaz Mochon, J.J.; Duran, I.; Raez, L.E.; Russo, A.; Lorente, J.A.; Malapelle, U.; et al. Challenges and opportunities of cfDNA analysis implementation in clinical practice: Perspective of the International Society of Liquid Biopsy (ISLB). *Crit. Rev. Oncol. Hematol.* **2020**, *151*, 102978. [CrossRef]
98. Dong, X.; Zheng, T.; Zhang, M.; Dai, C.; Wang, L.; Wang, L.; Zhang, R.; Long, Y.; Wen, D.; Xie, F.; et al. Circulating Cell-Free DNA-Based Detection of Tumor Suppressor Gene Copy Number Loss and Its Clinical Implication in Metastatic Prostate Cancer. *Front. Oncol.* **2021**, *11*, 720727. [CrossRef]
99. Rönnau, C.G.; Verhaegh, G.W.; Luna-Velez, M.V.; Schalken, J.A. Noncoding RNAs as novel biomarkers in prostate cancer. *Biomed. Res. Int.* **2014**, *2014*, 591703. [CrossRef]
100. Alarcón-Zendejas, A.P.; Scavuzzo, A.; Jiménez-Ríos, M.A.; Álvarez-Gómez, R.M.; Montiel-Manríquez, R.; Castro-Hernández, C.; Jiménez-Dávila, M.A.; Pérez-Montiel, D.; González-Barrios, R.; Jiménez-Trejo, F.; et al. The promising role of new molecular biomarkers in prostate cancer: From coding and non-coding genes to artificial intelligence approaches. *Prostate Cancer Prostatic Dis.* **2022**, 1–13. [CrossRef]
101. Kretschmer, A.; Kajau, H.; Margolis, E.; Tutrone, R.; Grimm, T.; Trottmann, M.; Stief, C.; Stoll, G.; Fischer, C.A.; Flinspach, C. Validation of a CE-IVD, urine exosomal RNA expression assay for risk assessment of prostate cancer prior to biopsy. *Sci. Rep.* **2022**, *12*, 4777. [CrossRef] [PubMed]
102. Rafeie, M.; Zhang, J.; Asadnia, M.; Li, W.; Warkiani, M.E. Multiplexing slanted spiral microchannels for ultra-fast blood plasma separation. *Lab. Chip.* **2016**, *16*, 2791–2802. [CrossRef] [PubMed]
103. Kulasinghe, A.; Tran, T.H.; Blick, T.; O'Byrne, K.; Thompson, E.W.; Warkiani, M.E.; Nelson, C.; Kenny, L.; Punyadeera, C. Enrichment of circulating head and neck tumour cells using spiral microfluidic technology. *Sci. Rep.* **2017**, *7*, 42517. [CrossRef]
104. Wang, S.; Qiu, Y.; Bai, B. The Expression, Regulation, and Biomarker Potential of Glypican-1 in Cancer. *Front. Oncol.* **2019**, *9*, 614. [CrossRef] [PubMed]
105. Rzhevskiy, A.S.; Razavi Bazaz, S.; Ding, L.; Kapitannikova, A.; Sayyadi, N.; Campbell, D.; Walsh, B.; Gillatt, D.; Ebrahimi Warkiani, M.; Zvyagin, A.V. Rapid and Label-Free Isolation of Tumour Cells from the Urine of Patients with Localised Prostate Cancer Using Inertial Microfluidics. *Cancers* **2019**, *12*, 81. [CrossRef] [PubMed]
106. Robinson, D.; Van Allen, E.M.; Wu, Y.M.; Schultz, N.; Lonigro, R.J.; Mosquera, J.M.; Montgomery, B.; Taplin, M.E.; Pritchard, C.C.; Attard, G.; et al. Integrative Clinical Genomics of Advanced Prostate Cancer. *Cell* **2015**, *162*, 454. [CrossRef]
107. Yan, B.; Meng, X.; Wang, X.; Wei, P.; Qin, Z. Complete regression of advanced prostate cancer for ten years: A case report and review of the literature. *Oncol. Lett.* **2013**, *6*, 590–594. [CrossRef]
108. Rossi, V.; Di Zazzo, E.; Galasso, G.; De Rosa, C.; Abbondanza, C.; Sinisi, A.A.; Altucci, L.; Migliaccio, A.; Castoria, G. Estrogens Modulate Somatostatin Receptors Expression and Synergize with the Somatostatin Analog Pasireotide in Prostate Cells. *Front. Pharmacol.* **2019**, *10*, 28. [CrossRef]
109. Di Zazzo, E.; Galasso, G.; Giovannelli, P.; Di Donato, M.; Di Santi, A.; Cernera, G.; Rossi, V.; Abbondanza, C.; Moncharmont, B.; Sinisi, A.A.; et al. Prostate cancer stem cells: The role of androgen and estrogen receptors. *Oncotarget* **2016**, *7*, 193–208. [CrossRef]
110. Wan, J.C.M.; Massie, C.; Garcia-Corbacho, J.; Mouliere, F.; Brenton, J.D.; Caldas, C.; Pacey, S.; Baird, R.; Rosenfeld, N. Liquid biopsies come of age: Towards implementation of circulating tumour DNA. *Nat. Rev. Cancer* **2017**, *17*, 223–238. [CrossRef]
111. Tagawa, S.T.; Antonarakis, E.S.; Gjyrezi, A.; Galletti, G.; Kim, S.; Worroll, D.; Stewart, J.; Zaher, A.; Szatrowski, T.P.; Ballman, K.V.; et al. Expression of AR-V7 and ARv567es in Circulating Tumor Cells Correlates with Outcomes to Taxane Therapy in Men with Metastatic Prostate Cancer Treated in TAXYNERGY. *Clin. Cancer Res.* **2019**, *25*, 1880–1888. [CrossRef] [PubMed]
112. Wang, J.; Zhang, Y.; Wei, C.; Gao, X.; Yuan, P.; Gan, J.; Li, R.; Liu, Z.; Wang, T.; Wang, S.; et al. Prognostic Value of Androgen Receptor Splice Variant 7 in the Treatment of Metastatic Castration-Resistant Prostate Cancer: A Systematic Review and Meta-Analysis. *Front. Oncol.* **2020**, *10*, 562504. [CrossRef] [PubMed]

113. Liu, R.-J.; Hu, Q.; Li, S.-Y.; Mao, W.-P.; Xu, B.; Chen, M. The Role of Androgen Receptor Splicing Variant 7 in Predicting the Prognosis of Metastatic Castration-Resistant Prostate Cancer: Systematic Review and Meta-Analysis. *Technol. Cancer Res. Treat.* **2021**, *20*, 15330338211035260. [CrossRef] [PubMed]
114. Shroff, R.T.; Hendifar, A.; McWilliams, R.R.; Geva, R.; Epelbaum, R.; Rolfe, L.; Goble, S.; Lin, K.K.; Biankin, A.V.; Giordano, H.; et al. Rucaparib Monotherapy in Patients with Pancreatic Cancer and a Known Deleterious BRCA Mutation. *JCO Precis. Oncol.* **2018**, *2018*, PO.17.00316. [CrossRef] [PubMed]
115. Ignatiadis, M.; Sledge, G.W.; Jeffrey, S.S. Liquid biopsy enters the clinic—Implementation issues and future challenges. *Nat. Rev. Clin. Oncol.* **2021**, *18*, 297–312. [CrossRef] [PubMed]
116. Arneth, B. Update on the types and usage of liquid biopsies in the clinical setting: A systematic review. *BMC Cancer* **2018**, *18*, 527. [CrossRef] [PubMed]

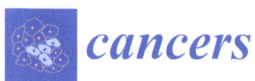

Review

BRCA Mutations in Ovarian and Prostate Cancer: Bench to Bedside

Stergios Boussios [1,2,3,*], Elie Rassy [4], Michele Moschetta [5], Aruni Ghose [1,6,7,8], Sola Adeleke [9,10,11], Elisabet Sanchez [1], Matin Sheriff [12], Cyrus Chargari [4] and Nicholas Pavlidis [13]

1. Department of Medical Oncology, Medway NHS Foundation Trust, Windmill Road, Gillingham ME7 5NY, UK
2. Faculty of Life Sciences & Medicine, School of Cancer & Pharmaceutical Sciences, King's College London, London SE1 9RT, UK
3. AELIA Organization, 9th Km Thessaloniki-Thermi, 57001 Thessaloniki, Greece
4. Department of Medical Oncology, Gustave Roussy Institut, 94805 Villejuif, France
5. Novartis Institutes for BioMedical Research, CH 4033 Basel, Switzerland
6. Department of Medical Oncology, Barts Cancer Centre, St. Bartholomew's Hospital, Barts Health NHS Trust, London E1 1BB, UK
7. Department of Medical Oncology, Mount Vernon Cancer Centre, East and North Hertfordshire NHS Trust, London KT1 2EE, UK
8. Centre for Education, Faculty of Life Sciences and Medicine, King's College London, London SE1 9RT, UK
9. High Dimensional Neurology Group, UCL Queen's Square Institute of Neurology, London WC1N 3BG, UK
10. Department of Oncology, Guy's and St Thomas' Hospital, London SE1 9RT, UK
11. School of Cancer & Pharmaceutical Sciences, King's College London, Strand, London WC2R 2LS, UK
12. Department of Urology, Medway NHS Foundation Trust, Windmill Road, Gillingham ME7 5NY, UK
13. Medical School, University of Ioannina, Stavros Niarchou Avenue, 45110 Ioannina, Greece
* Correspondence: stergiosboussios@gmail.com

Citation: Boussios, S.; Rassy, E.; Moschetta, M.; Ghose, A.; Adeleke, S.; Sanchez, E.; Sheriff, M.; Chargari, C.; Pavlidis, N. BRCA Mutations in Ovarian and Prostate Cancer: Bench to Bedside. *Cancers* 2022, *14*, 3888. https://doi.org/10.3390/cancers14163888

Academic Editors: Paula A. Oliveira, Ana Faustino and Lúcio Lara Santos

Received: 4 July 2022
Accepted: 10 August 2022
Published: 11 August 2022

Publisher's Note: MDPI stays neutral with regard to jurisdictional claims in published maps and institutional affiliations.

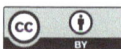

Copyright: © 2022 by the authors. Licensee MDPI, Basel, Switzerland. This article is an open access article distributed under the terms and conditions of the Creative Commons Attribution (CC BY) license (https://creativecommons.org/licenses/by/4.0/).

Simple Summary: DNA damage is one of the hallmarks of cancer. Epithelial ovarian cancer (EOC) —especially the high-grade serous subtype—harbors a defect in at least one DNA damage response (DDR) pathway. Defective DDR results from a variety of lesions affecting homologous recombination (HR) and nonhomologous end joining (NHEJ) for double strand breaks, base excision repair (BER), and nucleotide excision repair (NER) for single strand breaks and mismatch repair (MMR). Apart from the EOC, mutations in the DDR genes, such as *BRCA1* and *BRCA2*, are common in prostate cancer as well. Among them, *BRCA2* lesions are found in 12% of metastatic castration-resistant prostate cancers, but very rarely in primary prostate cancer. Better understanding of the DDR pathways is essential in order to optimize the therapeutic choices, and has led to the design of biomarker-driven clinical trials. Poly(ADP-ribose) polymerase (PARP) inhibitors are now a standard therapy for EOC patients, and more recently have been approved for the metastatic castration-resistant prostate cancer with alterations in DDR genes. They are particularly effective in tumours with HR deficiency.

Abstract: DNA damage repair (DDR) defects are common in different cancer types, and these alterations can be exploited therapeutically. Epithelial ovarian cancer (EOC) is among the tumours with the highest percentage of hereditary cases. *BRCA1* and *BRCA2* predisposing pathogenic variants (PVs) were the first to be associated with EOC, whereas additional genes comprising the homologous recombination (HR) pathway have been discovered with DNA sequencing technologies. The incidence of DDR alterations among patients with metastatic prostate cancer is much higher compared to those with localized disease. Genetic testing is playing an increasingly important role in the treatment of patients with ovarian and prostate cancer. The development of poly (ADP-ribose) polymerase (PARP) inhibitors offers a therapeutic strategy for patients with EOC. One of the mechanisms of PARP inhibitors exploits the concept of synthetic lethality. Tumours with *BRCA1* or *BRCA2* mutations are highly sensitive to PARP inhibitors. Moreover, the synthetic lethal interaction may be exploited beyond germline *BRCA* mutations in the context of HR deficiency, and this is an area of ongoing research. PARP inhibitors are in advanced stages of development as a treatment for metastatic castration-resistant prostate cancer. However, there is a major concern regarding the need to identify reliable biomarkers predictive of treatment response. In this review, we explore the mechanisms of DDR, the potential for genomic analysis of ovarian and prostate cancer, and therapeutics of PARP inhibitors, along with predictive biomarkers.

Keywords: DNA damage repair; homologous recombination; PARP inhibitors; ovarian cancer; prostate cancer

1. Introduction

Spontaneous DNA damage occurs on the order of 10^4–10^5 events per cell per day, and it is considered to have a causal role in aging. This includes spontaneous/endogenous genotoxic stress, as well as environmental/iatrogenic sources of genotoxic stress [1]. Endogenous sources of DNA damage and chromatin organization contribute to mutational processes that have been recorded in cancer genomes. Moreover, metabolism is a crucial cellular process that can become harmful for cells by leading to DNA damage. This can occur by an increase in oxidative stress or through the generation of toxic byproducts. In contrast, sources for exogenous DNA damage are rare and include ionizing and ultraviolet radiation, as well as various chemicals agents. Different mutational processes generate unique combinations of mutation types, termed "mutational signatures". In the past few years, large-scale analyses have revealed many mutational signatures across the spectrum of human cancer types [2,3]. Genomic instability can arise from a genetic or epigenetic mutation in a mutator gene such as in a DNA damage repair (DDR) gene [4]. Several mechanisms can be activated to repair damaged DNA, including homologous recombination (HR) repair, nonhomologous end joining (NHEJ), base excision repair (BER), nucleotide excision repair (NER), and mismatch repair (MMR) [5,6]. HR is the main mechanism for high-fidelity repair of double-strand DNA breaks (DSB) [7]. Mutations in genes related to this pathway may lead to HR deficiency. Among them, *BRCA1/2* mutations are the most frequent and lead to hereditary breast and epithelial ovarian cancer (EOC). Hereditary breast and ovarian cancer due to mutations in these genes is the most common cause of hereditary forms of both breast and ovarian cancer, accounting for 30–70% and approximately 90% of cases, respectively [8]. In individuals harboring mutations in *BRCA1/2* genes, the probability of developing breast cancer over a lifetime is around 85%, and that of EOC is about 20–40% [9]. *BRCA1* and *BRCA2* mutation carriers are mostly single heterozygous with only one mono-allelic deleterious mutation on one of these two genes. Excluding individuals of Ashkenazi descent, it is uncommon to identify carriers of two deleterious mutations either within the same gene (biallelic) or in both genes (trans-heterozygous). Trans-heterozygous mutations in both *BRCA1* and *BRCA2* genes are clinically correlated with an early age of onset and a severe disease compared to single heterozygous *BRCA* mutation carriers. Breast and ovarian cancer risks differ depending on the position and the type of *BRCA1* and *BRCA2* mutations. Importantly, two different mutations on the same allele may be associated with a distinctive phenotype, since each mutation is located in a different domain of the BRCA protein. Consequently, the interaction of BRCA with several other proteins could be disturbed. Therefore, these altered protein-protein interactions may impact on the phenotype. The *BRCA* mutation location also affects the EOC risk. *BRCA1* and *BRCA2* have been identified in the ovarian cancer cluster region in or near exon 11, and in the breast cancer cluster region in multiple regions other than exon 11 so far. In a recently published report, the authors presented the distribution of the age at diagnosis of EOC with *BRCA* mutation in detail, and analyzed the age by each common mutation type in a Japanese population [10]. The most common mutation in *BRCA1* was *L63X*, followed by *Q934 X*, *STOP799*, and *Y1853C*. Among them, *L63X* and *Y1853C* were located in the breast cancer cluster region, whereas *Q934 X* and *STOP799* were in the ovarian cancer cluster region. As far as the *BRCA2* mutations are concerned, the most common was *R2318X*, followed by *STOP1861*, *Q3026X*, *S1882X*, *P3039P*, *STOP613*, *S2835X*, and

STOP2868. Among them, *R2318X*, *STOP1861*, and *S1882X* were located in the ovarian cancer cluster region, whilst *S2835X* and *STOP2868* were located in the breast cancer cluster region. Finally, *Q3026X*, *P3039P*, and *STOP613* were not located in either the ovarian or breast cancer cluster regions. Moreover, the majority of serous papillary peritoneal carcinoma are high-grade tumours, and thus present *p53* and *BRCA* mutations [11]. A number of additional variants in genes beyond *BRCA1/2* have been identified and are suspected to play a significant role in ovarian carcinogenesis. Approximately 20% of castration-resistant prostate cancer patients harbour germline or somatic mutations in one of the DDR genes, which supports the mechanism of synthetic lethality [12]. The two main composite HR deficiency tests available in clinical practice apply next-generation sequencing (NGS) or microarray assays to simultaneously search for *BRCA* mutations and genomic scars.

From the therapeutic point of view, targeting the DDR pathway is a reasonable approach. Within this context, several poly (ADP-ribose) polymerase (PARP) inhibitors have been considered for the treatment of several malignancies, including EOC and prostate cancer. Based on the successful application of PARP inhibitors in BRCA-deficient breast cancer and EOC, PARP inhibitors are currently being investigated for the treatment of metastatic prostate cancer with promising results [13]. In this review, we discuss the current landscape of genetic testing and management of the hereditary risk for EOC and prostate cancer, and the application of PARP inhibitors in the precision treatment of these clinical entities. Furthermore, we highlight the importance of developing predictive biomarkers for the optimal selection of the patients who benefit from the PARP inhibitors.

2. Molecular Landscape

DNA damage is a frequent event during cell life and can be spontaneous or caused by cell metabolism or by environmental agents. There have been six primary pathways of DNA repair identified, which are variably used to address DSB and single-stranded DNA break (SSB) damage from a variety of mechanisms of injury. HR and NHEJ recombination are the two major pathways responsible for repairing DSB, whereas the primary mechanisms for resolving SSB are the BER, NER, MMR, and translesional synthesis [5,8]. The function of the primary DDR pathways begins with sensing DNA damage. The next step is the recruitment of proteins involved in building the repair complexes [12]. The potential absence, reduction, or dysfunction of these proteins may result in loss of function of proper DDR. HR pathways become active in the S/G2 phase due to the availability of a sister chromatid, whereas NHEJ repairs DSB throughout all cell cycle phases except the M phase. DSB end resection directs the pathway towards HR during the S/G2 phase. Apparently, only 30% of DSB undergo resection, and hence HR in the G2 phase. On the other hand, during the S phase, DSB are mainly repaired by HR, although two-ended DSB may still be repaired by NHEJ, unless the replication machinery encounters the DSB ends. In addition to cell cycle-dependent regulation, DSB end complexity is critical for directing preferential repair by HR. SSB normally do not compromise the integrity of DSB. However, if an SSB is left unrepaired and the lesion is encountered by DNA machinery that separates the DNA duplex into two component SSB, an SSB can be converted into a one-ended DSB [14]. SSB and DSB also arise during aberrant DNA topoisomerase reactions, spontaneously or upon exposure to specific inhibitors [15]. Break-induced replication (BIR) is one of the pathways that drives genome instability, as it results in a loss of heterozygosity, mutations, and nonreciprocal translocations [16]. In fact, DSB at collapsed forks are single ended, with no second end available for classical HR repair. These breaks can be processed by BIR, a conservative DNA synthesis mechanism described as an HR-based repair pathway for one-ended DNA DSB [17].

2.1. Homologous Recombination and Nonhomologous End Joining

DSB are one of the most common and cytotoxic types of DDR associated with significant genomic aberrations, which if left unrepaired or improperly repaired may lead to cell death. DSB are repaired by a number of repair pathways, the most important of which involve HR and NHEJ [8,13].

HR is restricted to the S and G2 phases of the cell cycle due to the cell cycle-dependent availability of sister chromatids. This is also correlated with the fact that cyclin-dependent kinases (CDKs) have a modulatory role on DSB components, including their influence on enzymes involved in HR [18]. NHEJ is an error-prone process that simply fuses the two broken ends together, whereas HR is error-free, using the genetically identical sister chromatid as a template for repair. This statement is largely based on the fact that the mechanism of HR requires the search for a homologous partner to repair DNA, in contrast to NHEJ. However, nowadays, that position has been reconsidered. The products of HR are gene conversion, associated or not with crossing-over. Such products can account for genetic diversity or instability arising through HR. Gene conversion may transfer genetic information in a non-reciprocal manner between two hetero-alleles, resulting in a loss of heterozygosity. It can also transfer one stop codon from a pseudogene to a related coding sequence, leading to its extinction. Mus81 and Yen1 endonucleases, as well as Slx4, promote replication template switching during BIR, thus participate in the generation of complex rearrangements when repeated sequences dispersed throughout the genome are involved [19]. NHEJ is faster than HR and mainly occurs in the G1 phase [20]. Nevertheless, there is recent evidence that NHEJ functions throughout the cell cycle. Beyond the already-known proteins, such as Ku70/80, DNA-PKcs, Artemis, DNA pol λ/μ, DNA ligase IV-XRCC4, and XLF, new proteins are involved in the NHEJ, namely PAXX, MRI/CYREN, TARDBP of TDP-43, IFFO1, ERCC6L2, and RNase H2. Among them, MRI/CYREN has dual role, as it stimulates NHEJ in the G1 phase of the cell cycle, while it inhibits the pathway in the S and G2 phases [21]. The extent of DNA end resection is the primary factor that determines whether repair is carried out via NHEJ or HR. 53BP1 and the cofactors PTIP or RIF1-shieldin protect the broken DNA end, inhibit long-range end resection, and thus promote NHEJ. The cell cycle, the chromatin environment, and the complexity of the DNA end break affect the DNA resection [22]. In HR repair, the nuclease meiotic recombination 11-like (MRE11) forms a complex with RAD50 and NBS1 (Nijmegen breakage syndrome 1)—MRN complex—which detects double-strand breaks (DSBs) and recruits and activates ATM at DNA ends [23,24]. Replication protein A (RPA) is the major protein that binds ssDNA with a high affinity. ATR interacts with a partner ATRIP and recognizes RPA-covered ssDNA (RPA-ssDNA). For the activation of the ATR, apart from the recruitment of the ATR-ATRIP complex (ATR-ATRIP) to RPA-ssDNA, checkpoint regulators—such as TopBP1 and ETAA1—participate as well. TopBP1 is recruited to sites of DNA damage or stalled replication forks and engage with the Rad9-Rad1-Hus1 complex at dsDNA-ssDNA junctions, leading to stimulation of the ATR-ATRIP kinase. Similarly, ETAA1 directly activates ATR-ATRIP. Thus, ATR-ATRIP is recruited by recognizing RPA-ssDNA and subsequently activated in a multiple-step process. In budding yeast, the Mec1-Ddc2 complex (Mec1-Ddc2) corresponds to ATR-ATRIP [25]. Single-stranded DNA generated by resection is coated by RPA, which recruits Ddc2 and the Mec1 checkpoint kinase [26]. That leads to the formation of nucleoprotein filaments in ssDNA, which are essential for the homology search in sister chromatid and strand exchange [27]. KAT5 is an acetyltransferase, participating—among others—in transcriptional regulation, chromatin remodeling, histone acetylation, and DNA repair. The ability of KAT5 to regulate chromatin structure at DSB is mediated through its interaction with a multifunctional remodeling complex (NuA4 complex), which is recruited to DSB. The NuA4-KAT5 complex acetylates histones H2AX and H4 at DSB, and modifies chromatin architecture to facilitate DSB repair. The phosphorylation of the c-terminal of the histone variant H2AX by ATM is crucial in DSB repair. H2AX is rapidly phosphorylated on chromatin domains surrounding the DSB. Then, the mdc1 scaffold protein binds directly to γH2AX and formulates a platform for the recruitment of other DNA repair proteins, including BRCA1 at the DSB [28].

A number of factors have been believed to stabilize the NHEJ complex at DSBs including Ku, the DNA-PK catalytic subunit (PKcs), and the kinase activity of DNA-PKcs.

This multi-unit complex recruits further proteins, such as Artemis and PNK, to repair it into a normal DNA structure. The biochemical activity of DNA ligases results in the sealing of breaks between 5′-phosphate and 3′-hydroxyl termini within a strand of DNA [29].

2.2. Synthetic Lethality

In 2005, the idea of synthetic lethality in the DDR pathway, via *BRCA1* mutation, was published by two groups [30,31]. The concept of synthetic lethality applies when two non-lethal defects combine and result in a lethal phenotype. Inactivation of one gene allele by mutation and inhibition is not toxic for cells. The synthetic lethality strategy requires gene pairs that, when simultaneously inactivated, cause cell death. Figure 1 demonstrates the genetic landscape of synthetic lethality. However, if *BRCA1* is mutated, PARP inhibition would prevent DDR and lead to tumour cell apoptosis. Therefore, inactivation of both demonstrates synthetic lethality. PARP inhibition specifically in *BRCA1/2* deficient tumour cells can result in up to a 1000-fold increased sensitivity as compared to BRCA wild-type tumour cells [30]. Synthetic lethality could also be used in tumours which share molecular features of *BRCA* mutated tumours—known as "BRCAness". Therefore, mutation of genes beyond *BRCA* in the HR pathway expands the indication of PARP inhibitors. The broader use of synthetic lethality targeting the HR pathway is still being investigated [32].

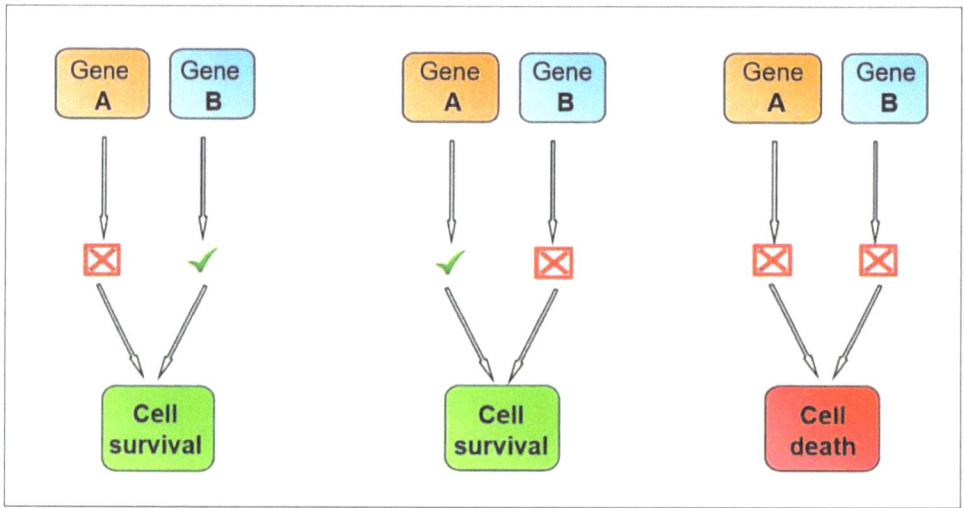

Figure 1. Schematic of synthetic lethality in cancer.

Inactivation of Rad52 in BRCA2-deficient cells results in synthetic lethality, which makes Rad52 a tumour-specific target for therapy in BRCA2-deficient tumours. As Rad52 is required for cellular proliferation in BRCA2-defective cells, silencing of Rad52 could cause BRCA2-defective tumour cells. Therefore, inactivation of Rad52 could be reasonable approach for the treatment of a BRCA-defective subset of tumours. Rad52 also represents a potential therapeutic target because no *Rad52* mutations or inactivation has been documented in tumours. Other synthetically lethal relationships have been reported for Rad52, with X-ray repair complementing defective repair in XRCC3 [33]. Recent studies showed that Rad52 is involved in multiple DDR pathways, including a BRCA-independent HR repair involving Rad51, single-strand annealing (SSA), BIR repair, RNA-templated DSB repair, and transcription-associated HR involving XPG. However, how Rad52 activity helps HR-deficient cancers to survive is unclear. A recently published study demonstrated that inhibition of RPA:RAD52 protein-protein interaction (PPI) appears to inhibit Rad52-mediated DNA repair, and that mitoxantrone may be a potent Rad52 inhibitor [34]. It has also been proposed that targeting of Rad52 with small molecule inhibitors will disrupt the Rad52-dependent HR sub-pathway in BRCA1- and BRCA2-deficient cells, causing their lethality. In a study, the selected inhibitors of two different chemotypes exhibited an inhibitory effect on tested BRCA1- and BRCA2-deficient cells [35]. More recently, synthetic lethal interactors of *BRCA1/2* have been identified, including DNA polymerase theta (*POLQ*), flap structure-specific endonuclease 1 (*FEN1*), and apurinic/apyrimidinic endodeoxyribonuclease 2 (*APE2*) [36]. The function of Rad52 in replication fork repair following stress is still not clear. Genotoxic stress results in cell cycle arrest, which is implemented by checkpoint kinases CHK1 and CHK2. CHK1 mainly responds to short replication stress, whereas CHK2 is activated during chronic stress leading to DSB formation. CHK1 activation occurs via phosphorylation by ATR. Active CHK1 targets Cdc25 A phosphatase, which upon phosphorylation undergoes proteasomal degradation. This leads to the reduction of Cdk2/Cyclin A complex activity, conferring checkpoint arrest. CHK1 protein also interacts with BRCA2 and Rad51 proteins, directly phosphorylating them for the formation of active Rad51 nucleofilament, especially during replication blockage. It has been shown that Rad52 overexpression in BRCA2 deficient cells leads to restoration of checkpoint arrest during replication stress and the mitigation of excess origin firing observed in BRCA2 deficient cells [37]. It is still unknown whether PALB2 participates in recruiting and regulating Rad52 in RAD51-mediated HR. The specific genetic interactions of BRCA1 and PALB2 with Rad52 have not yet been clarified; nevertheless, it is considered that BRCA1 and PALB2 are independent of Rad52, which would be compatible with a synthetically lethal relationship. However, it is also possible that Rad52-Rad51-driven HR could be dependent on BRCA1 or PALB2. Repair of DSB relies upon the BRCA1-PALB2-BRCA2 pathway, with Rad52 functioning in an alternative pathway that mediates Rad51-directed repair when deficiencies exist in BRCA1, PALB2, or BRCA2. Nevertheless, a cooperative role for Rad52 and BRCA2 in mediating RAD51 function cannot be definitively excluded [38].

Conversely, certain *Rad52* mutations rescue *BRCA2* mutations. *hRad52 S346X* is a mutation that codes for a Rad52 protein, with 17.2% of its amino acid sequence absent from its C terminus. In a study, this mutation was found to protect against the development of breast cancer in *BRCA1/2* mutation mutants [39]. *hRad52 S346X* also suppressed the elevated frequency of SSA caused by reducing the level of *BRCA2*. Therefore, *hRad52 S346X* may suppress tumourigenesis in BRCA2-deficient cells by suppressing the mutagenic effects of elevated SSA. Alternatively, the suppression of SSA by *hRad52 S346X* may block tumour formation in BRCA2-deficient cells, given the loss of two mechanisms of DSB repair. The observation that *Rad52 S346X* decreases the risk of cancer in BRCA mutants suggests that Rad52 inhibitors may also be a tool for the reduction of breast cancer risk in this subset of patients. However, the toxicity and impact of long-term use of such inhibitors should be further evaluated [40].

2.3. Mismatch Repair (MMR)

Base mismatches and insertion-deletion loops (IDLs) that occur during replication are repaired by the MMR pathway, demonstrated in Figure 2 [41]. MMR reduces DNA errors 100–1000 fold, and prevents them from becoming fixed mutations during cellular proliferation [42,43]. The role of MMR defects in the development of cancer was first established when mutation in *MSH2* was linked to hereditary nonpolyposis colorectal cancer, also known as Lynch syndrome [44]. Over time, the MMR genes *MLH1*, *MSH2*, *MSH6*, and *PMS2* were associated to an autosomal dominant, hereditary predisposition to colon cancer. These cancers were hallmarked by germline loss-of-function alterations. Given that prostate is not a Lynch-associated cancer, a focus on somatic mutations leading to the deficiencies in MMR prostate cancer phenotype is reasonable. There are eight MMR genes that have been investigated so far; *hMSH2*, *hMSH3*, *hMSH5*, *hMSH6*, *hMLH1*, *hPMS1* (*hMLH2*), *hMLH3*, and *hPMS2* (*hMLH4*). The prevalence of deficiencies in MMR in prostate cancer has been reported between 3% and 5%. Among the MMR genes, defects within the *MSH2* and *MSH6* gene have been the most frequently reported in patients with prostate cancer. In contrast to other cancers, complex structural rearrangements appear to be an important cause of deficiencies in MMR in prostate cancer. The product of the gene *hMSH2* is the principal corrective MSH protein. The MSH2/MSH6 and MSH2/MSH3 heterodimers function as sensors, recognizing mismatched DNA [45]. The predominance of the heterodimer MSH2/MSH6 is explained by the fact that MSH6 is expressed 10 times more than MSH3. The heterodimer MSH2/MSH6 initiates the repair of small IDLs, while MSH2/MSH3 repairs larger IDLs, up to 13 nt in size [46]. Patients with deficiencies in MMR are eligible for immune checkpoint inhibitor therapy in second-line treatment for metastatic castration-resistant prostate cancer [47].

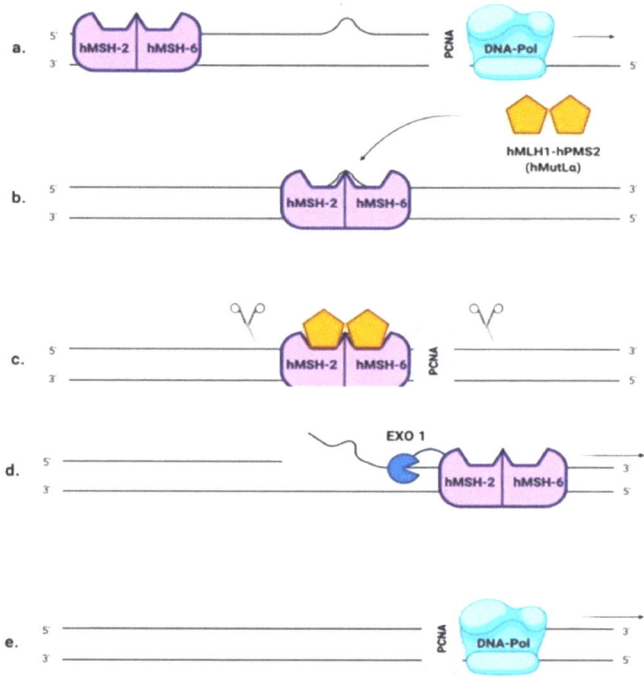

Figure 2. Schematic representation of the mismatch repair (MMR) system. (**a**) MMR enzymes scan the DNA and remove the wrongly incorporated bases from the newly synthesized, non-methylated strand by using the DNA polymerase. (**b**) In MMR, the incorrectly added base is detected after replication by hMutSα, which recruits hMutLα. (**c**) hMutLα detects this base and removes it from the newly synthesized strand. (**d**) hMutSα activates EXO1 and the entire segment of DNA is removed. (**e**) DNA polymerase participates on the replacement of the DNA by correctly paired nucleotides.

Specific mutational signatures have been identified in tumours with mutations in the exonuclease (proofreading) domain of polymerase epsilon (POLE), as well as tumours with mutations or epigenetic silencing of MMR genes. Initially, the position was that simultaneous loss of both POLE or polymerase delta (POLD1) proofreading and MMR function could not be tolerated by cells due to excessive accumulation of mutations. However, an analysis of tumours from children with biallelic germline MMR deficiency demonstrated a subset of tumours with remarkably high mutation burdens (>250 mutations/Mb) that also had a somatic mutation in POLE or POLD1 [48].

Malfunctioning of MMR proteins, due either to mutation or reduced expression, suggests the correlation of cancer development to the aberrations of all or the majority of MMR proteins. In EOC, MMR deficiency is the second common cause of hereditary ovarian cancer—only behind HR deficiency—accounting for 10–15% of hereditary ovarian carcinomas [42]. Apart from the inherited gene mutations, additional mechanisms of gene inactivation leading to loss of expression of one of the main MMR genes occurs in up to 29% of cases [42]. Furthermore, it has been reported that high mRNA levels of MSH6, MLH1, and PMS2 were associated with a prolonged overall survival (OS) in EOC. That supports the potential positive prognostic value of MMR genes in EOC patients treated with platinum-based chemotherapy [49]. Prostate cancer has high prevalence of DDR genes alterations. In the metastatic setting, the Prostate Cancer Foundation-Stand Up To Cancer (SU2C-PCF) team identified a high proportion of actionable mutations, including 23% with mutations and other alterations in DDR genes, such as *BRCA2* (13%), ATM (7.3%), and *BRCA1* (0.3%), along with mutations in MMR genes, such as MSH2 (2%) [50]. Recently, the first phase I dose-escalation study of the ATM inhibitor M3541 in combination with palliative radiotherapy in patients with advanced solid tumours was published [51]. M3541 had pharmacokinetic limitations that prevented an analysis of efficacy. Although the clinical development of M3541 was halted, the ATM pathway still represents an attractive therapeutic target. Indeed, the development of the second-generation ATM inhibitor M4076 is ongoing [52]. As far as the ovarian cancer is concerned, ATARI is the first clinical trial aiming to determine whether a synthetic lethal interaction between the tumour suppressor gene *ARID1A* and *ATR* translates into improved outcomes [53]. The inclusion of the olaparib combined with the ATR inhibitor ceralasertib will investigate whether the two classes of DDR inhibitors have the potential to provide clinical activity. The study trial will also aim to identify novel biomarkers of ATR inhibitor response and resistance.

3. Susceptibility to EOC

Around 20–25% of unselected EOC patients carry pathogenic variants (PVs) in a number of genes that mostly encode for proteins involved in DDR pathways [54]. Indeed, NGS revealed that beyond *BRCA1/2*, mutations in HR effectors, such as *PALB2*, *RAD51*, *ATM*, *BRIP1*, *BARD1*, and *CHEK2* occurs in up to a fifth of the patients with high-grade serous ovarian cancer [55]. PVs in each of these genes is associated with variable risk for EOC development. Moreover, mutated or downregulated *ARID1A* significantly compromises HR repair of DNA DSBs [56]. ARID1A is recruited to DSBs via its interaction with ATR. ATR inhibition in ARID1A defective cells thus increases large scale genomic rearrangements and ultimately causes cell death. Loss of function mutations in *ARID1A* leading to a loss of protein expression are a frequent observation in EOC of clear cell and endometroid histology. Finally, PVs genes involved in the MMR pathway account for 10–15% of hereditary EOC, typically in endometrioid or clear-cell histological subtypes [57].

3.1. BRCA1 and BRCA2 Genes in EOC

PVs in *BRCA1/2* genes are detected in 10–15% of unselected EOC patients, accounting for the majority of hereditary cases [58]. *BRCA1* and *BRCA2* PVs confer 44% and 17% lifetime risks for EOC diagnosis, respectively, whilst the relevant risk in the general population is approximately 1% [59]. The carriers of *BRCA1* and *BRCA2* PVs are specifically susceptible to develop high-grade serous ovarian cancer, with a median age of onset at about 51 and 61 years, respectively [60]. PVs in *BRCA1/2* in EOC are correlated with prolonged OS, visceral disease distribution, higher response rates to platinum-based chemotherapy, and sensitivity to PARP inhibitors.

The identification of *BRCA1* and *BRCA2* PVs is recommended as an effort of primary prevention for EOC. Cascade screening is the systematic identification and testing of relatives of a known mutation carrier. This strategy determines whether asymptomatic relatives also carry the known variant, in view of offering risk-reducing options to reduce the morbidity and mortality. On the other hand, all negatively tested family relatives have a lifetime EOC risk, compatible with the general population.

The proposed primary prevention strategy for EOC risk reduction among *BRCA1* and *BRCA2* carriers is bilateral salpingo-oophorectomy (BSO), which can reduce the risk for EOC diagnosis up to 96% [60]. *BRCA1* carriers are considered to undergo BSO after the age of 35 and before the age of 40 years, whereas in those with *BRCA2* mutations, BSO can be proposed after the age of 40 and before the age of 45 years, due to the lower penetrance and later onset of diagnosis [61]. The fallopian tube has been established as the origin of the majority of high-grade serous ovarian cancers. The serous tubal intraepithelial carcinoma (STIC) theory originated based on the observation of the presence of occult lesions on the fallopian tubes of women with *BRCA1/2* mutations following prophylactic surgery [62]. That led to the consideration of salpingectomy with ovarian retention until the age of natural menopause within the context of primary prevention [63].

3.2. Beyond BRCA1 and BRCA2 Genes in Ovarian Cancer

Besides RAD51 and its meiotic counterpart DMC1, five additional mammalian paralogs of bacterial RecA were discovered two decades ago. RAD51B, RAD51C, and RAD51D were discovered based on DNA sequence alignments, and XRCC2 and XRCC3 through functional complementation of the ionizing radiation sensitivity of Chinese hamster mutant cells. These proteins display limited sequence homology to each other and to RAD51, and are generally reported as classical RAD51 paralogs. Classical RAD51 paralogs were proposed to form two biochemically and functionally distinct subcomplexes, i.e., the RAD51B-RAD51C-RAD51D-XRCC2 complex (BCDX2) and the RAD51C-XRCC3 complex (CX3), showing common, but also distinct, biochemical properties (Figure 3). All human RAD51 paralogs were shown to associate with nascent DNA, but the mechanistic roles of these factors in replication were not investigated systematically. Chinese hamster ovary or DT40 cell lines carrying different mutations in individual genes displayed specific defects in replication fork progression and stability. The paralogs play roles at the early and late stages of HR. The inability of cell lines deficient in RAD51C, XRCC2, and XRCC3 to form damage-induced RAD51 nuclear foci suggests that these three proteins are important in the homology search and strand invasion phase of HR. Except for RAD51B, RAD51 paralog mutants have been isolated and characterized in Chinese hamster cells. In human cells, however, only XRCC3 ablated cells generated in the human colon carcinoma HCT116 cell line have been reported to date. RAD51 paralogs have been implicated in the prevention of aberrant mitoses and aneuploidy, RAD51B, RAD51C, and XRCC3 are implicated in cell cycle checkpoint, RAD51D and XRCC3 in telomere maintenance, and RAD51C, XRCC2, and XRCC3 in termination of gene conversion tracts.

While patients with biallelic mutations in RAD51 and its mediators have been identified in patients with Fanconi anaemia, monoallelic germline mutations in RAD51 mediators are correlated to predisposition to cancer. This is thought to be frequently caused by a somatic loss of heterozygosity (LOH) event, where the second functional copy of the gene is deleted, resulting in genomic instability. Both *RAD51C* and *RAD51D* are EOC susceptibility genes; nevertheless, hereditary ovarian cancer is most commonly caused by a mutation in *BRCA1/2* genes. The prevalence of *RAD51C* loss-of-function germline PVs varies between 0.3% and 1.1%. The lifetime risk of EOC among *RAD51C* carriers is approximately 5% [64]. Damaging *RAD51D* variants are marginally less frequent than *RAD51C* PVs among EOC patients, observed in approximately 0.2% of unselected cases [65]. The relevant percentage in those with strong family history is up to 0.9% [66]. According to the National Comprehensive Cancer Network (NCCN) guidelines, BSO may be considered in the scenario of PVs in any of these genes [67]. Furthermore, genetic defects in *RAD51C* and *RAD51D* genes can function as biomarkers for PARP sensitivity.

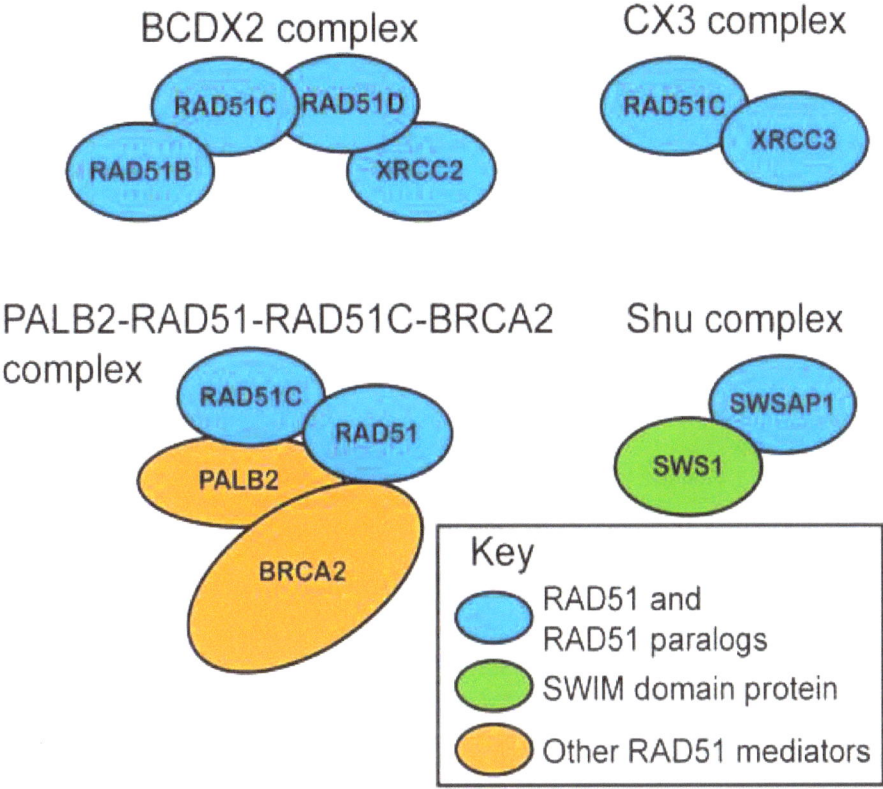

Figure 3. Schematic representation of the mammalian RAD51 paralog-containing complexes.

Several germline PVs in the so-called moderate- and low-penetrance genes have been associated with a moderate lifetime risk of EOC. The prevalence of *BRIP1* gPVs among familial EOC patients has been reported to be 0.7%, whilst the relevant cumulative lifetime risk among *BRIP* mutants has been estimated as 5–5.8%, predominantly following menopause [68,69]. The elevated risk for EOC diagnosis justifies recommendation for salpingo-oophorectomies among asymptomatic carriers, in line with family history and individual's preference.

PALB2 PVs are quite rare among EOC patients, identified in less than 0.5% of cases interrogated [65,68]. Biallelic mutations in PALB2 cause Fanconi anemia subtype FA-N, whereas monoallelic mutations predispose to breast, ovarian, and pancreatic familial cancers [70]. Clinical testing for *PALB2* in EOC is not currently recommended, but can be considered in cases with strong family history for ovarian cancer. The majority of studies reported relative risks between 0.9 and 5.5, but lacked statistical power [67]. It has been observed that *PALB2* associated tumours are sensitive to platinum-based chemotherapy and PARP inhibitors [71].

Furthermore, about 1% of all EOC cases can be attributed to PVs in MMR genes [72]. *MSH2* PVs seem to be associated with the higher risk of 10–24%, followed by *MLH1* PVs with a relevant risk of 5–20%, by the age of 70 years [73]. Finally, *MSH6* PVs confer much lower risks, ranging from 1–11%. In contrast, *PMS2* PVs are not associated with increased EOC risk [73]. Finally, in terms of the non-EOC, a subset of germ-cell tumours can acquire *KRAS*-activating mutations and other genetic alterations, such as *BRCA1/2*, *KIT*, and *MAPK*. However, the efficacy of targeted therapy and genomic features contributing to chemoresistance still remain to be elucidated [74]. Similarly, even though the rate of *BRCA1* and *BRCA2* mutations in ovarian carcinosarcomas is difficult to be determined, the genomic sequencing in some studies has demonstrated loss of function mutations in HR genes. As such, PARP inhibition may be effective even in ovarian carcinosarcomas [75].

3.3. Tumour Testing in Ovarian Cancer

Germline and somatic genetic alterations can be identified through tumour testing. On the other hand, germline analysis alone cannot detect somatic mutations. However, there are several factors that may impact the accuracy of tumour testing, meaning it cannot be considered as a gold standard for the potential identification of germline variant detection. Firstly, in most cases, the initial material for tumour testing is DNA extracted from formalin-fixed paraffin-embedded tissues, which can be technically challenging to amplify. Tumour microdissection is required to obtain tumour DNA. An additional concern is tumour heterogeneity and the actual percentage of tumour cells that are included in the tumour specimen from which DNA will be extracted.

If a mutation is identified, the sequencing of the normal cells is required to clarify whether the mutation is germline or somatic. The order by which the germline and somatic BRCA mutational analysis should be performed is an ongoing concern. Germline testing remains in the first place. When initial healthy cell sequencing discards germline PVs, tumour testing should be performed, since somatic mutations can influence treatment decisions. However, there are countries where somatic BRCA testing is performed first, as a screening tool. Patients found to have a mutation in the tumour are then referred to the Genetics team for germline genetic analysis. For those without identified mutations in the tumour, further germline BRCA testing is not recommended. The American Society of Clinical Oncology (ASCO) and the European Society for Medical Oncology (ESMO) guidelines suggest germline testing, followed by somatic tumour testing for the non-carriers of a germline PV. Although trials of EOC treatment stratify patients based on HR deficiency assays, ASCO guidelines do not recommend its routine use [76].

Enumeration of circulating tumour cells (CTC) in the blood may stratify the patients into high- and low-risk groups and serve as a prognostic biomarker for OS and progression-free survival (PFS) in several malignancies. Recent studies have also revealed that characterization of CTC could help predict treatment response. Whether CTC detection is associated with prognosis in EOC remains controversial. Within this context, the standardization of CTC detection techniques is of great importance. Many markers have been applied to the enrichment and screening of EOC CTC. The positive rate of CTC in EOC patients was 60% in advanced stage disease in a study using the CellSearch system targeting EpCAM+ [77]. The detection of CTC using immunomagnetic CTC enrichment targeting EpCAM and MUC1, followed by RT-PCR to detect EpCAM, MUC1, CA125, and ERCC1 positive cells has also been reported [78].

Recently, circulating tumour DNA (ctDNA), was found in plasma, and demonstrated a high correlation with EOC prognosis. PCR-based approaches have been successfully applied in ctDNA analysis, but are limited to detection of certain specific known mutations. NGS has been used for DNA mutation profiling and tumour mutation burden determination, whilst other approaches, such as whole-genome sequencing and cancer-personalized profiling by deep sequencing, have a broad range of applications, including evaluation of tumour mutation burden, detection of epigenetic changes, and diagnostics or identification of resistance mutations in EOC [79].

4. Susceptibility to Prostate Cancer

4.1. BRCA1 and BRCA2 Genes in Prostate Cancer

The incidence of prostate cancer is greater among *BRCA* mutation carriers; namely, 1.35-fold and 2.64-fold greater in BRCA1 and BRCA2 carriers, respectively [80]. In the case of functional loss of *BRCA1* and *BRCA2* genes, DDR occurs by non-conservative and potentially mutagenic mechanisms. This genomic instability is considered to be related to the cancer predisposition caused by deleterious mutations in *BRCA* genes.

The incidence for *BRCA2* mutations is 4.45 (95% confidence interval (CI) 2.99–6.61), which is higher as compared to *BRCA1* (2.35, 95% CI 1.43–3.88) [81]. Consequently, *BRCA2* germline mutations increase the risk of prostate cancer 8.6-fold by the age of 65 years [82]. The first analysis of the IMPACT trial concluded that patients with *BRCA2* PVs have elevated levels of serum prostate specific antigen (PSA) at diagnosis, predominantly high Gleason tumours, increased rates of nodal and distant metastases, and finally high recurrence rates [83]. Three oligonucleotide/oligosaccharide-binding domains (OB) folds (OB1, 2, and 3) have been revealed in the DNA-binding domain (DBD) of BRCA2 by structural studies. OB1 and OB2 are associated with the highest risk of prostate cancer [84]. In a study of 6500 patients with *BRCA1* and *BRCA2* PVs, c.756-c 1000 and c.7914p regions in BRCA2 were reported as negative biomarkers for high risk of Gleason 8b prostate cancer [85].

BRCA1 differentially regulates IGF-IR expression in androgen receptor (AR)-positive and AR-negative prostate cancer cells [86]. It has been reported that in a cohort of sporadic prostate cancer patients treated with radical prostatectomy, the higher probability of advanced tumour stage and the reduced disease-free survival were correlated with somatic *BRCA1* loss, which was due to hypermethylation or a deletion of the promoter [87].

Up to 8% of non-metastatic prostate cancer patients may respond to PARP inhibitors, irrespective of the fact that the HR deficiency is not derived from *BRCA* mutations [88]. This may be related to the *CDH1* gene loss (encodes cadherin 1) or inactivation of the *SPOP* gene (encodes Speckle-type POZ protein), which represent early events in carcinogenesis [89].

Strict separation of somatic and germline variants is not regularly performed; nevertheless, somatic *BRCA* mutations are more frequent in late stages of prostate cancer. Based on that, a new solid or liquid biopsy is highly recommended for an updated snapshot of the tumour.

4.2. Beyond BRCA

Prostate cancer is enriched for genomic alterations in DDR pathways [90]. In 2015, the Cancer Genome Atlas (TCGA) analyzed 333 primary prostate cancers. Alterations in DDR genes were common, affecting about one fifth of samples through mutations or deletions in *BRCA1/2, CDK12, ATM, FANCD2*, or *RAD51C* [91]. In terms of the metastatic setting, the study by the International Stand Up to Cancer-Prostate Cancer Foundation team (SU2C-PCF) evaluated 150 specimens and identified 8% with germline DDR mutations and 23% with somatic DDR alterations [50]. *BRCA2* was the most frequently mutated gene (13%), followed by *ATM* (7.3%), *MSH2* (2%) and *BRCA1, FANCA, MLH1, RAD51B* and *RAD51C* (0.3% for all). Similarly, in the large phase III PROfound study, among 28% of the analyzed samples were detected alterations in 15 DDR genes. The highest prevalence was found in *BRCA2* (8.7%), followed by *CDK12* (6.3%), *ATM* (5.9%), *CHEK2* (1.2%), and *BRCA1* (1%). The frequency of the DDR gene alterations between metastatic sites and primary disease was similar (32% vs. 27%, respectively) [92]. Co-occurring aberrations in two or more DDR genes were revealed in 2.2% of cases.

PROREPAIR-B is the first prospective multicenter cohort study evaluating the prevalence and effect of germline DDR mutations on metastatic castration-resistant prostate cancer outcomes [93]. Patients were screened for 107 DDR mutations. Among them, 16.2% were found to be DDR carriers, including 6.2% who carried mutations in *BRCA2, ATM*, or *BRCA1*.

The BRCAness phenotype may be induced pharmacologically or due to genetic alterations in HR genes other than *BRCA1/2*, including *ATM, ATR, CHEK1, RAD51*, the Fanconi anaemia complementation group family of genes and others. HR gene alterations were investigated in the TRITON2 study. The objective response rate (ORR) was 44% for patients with *BRCA* genes, but only 9.5% for *ATM* and 0% for *CDK12, CHEK2,* and other DDR genes [94]. Due to the doubts concerning BRCAness, experimental biomarkers have been proposed. Among them are included HR gene alteration, functional assays of HR capacity, as well as transcriptomic and mutational signatures [95].

4.3. Tumour Testing in Prostate Cancer

NGS implications are widely available for the detection of germline or somatic HR repair mutations, along with copy-number changes and genomic instability in prostate cancer [96]. The choice of the optimal material for genetic testing is challenging. Given the heterogeneity and instability of the tumour genome, metastatic sites may be better sources for identification of genetic alterations than the primary prostate tumour [97]. Brain and visceral metastases have the highest frequency of mutations among HR deficiency genes.

In the case of disease progression, it is recommended to repeat somatic mutation tests [98]. However, germline testing using NGS does not detect somatic mutations, which represent approximately 50% of *BRCA* mutations in metastatic castration-resistant prostate cancer [50]. For the detection of somatic HR repair mutations, CTC and ctDNA testing are highly recommended [99]. ctDNA plasma tests may be used in the absence of tissue or when re-biopsy is undesirable. However, the sensitivity of ctDNA plasma tests may be lower as compared to tumour tissue testing [100]. Ideally, a multiplex testing approach using different biological sample types can be implemented in order to increase the number of patients who undergo genomic analysis for actionable mutations.

From the screening programmes point of view, the previously reported IMPACT study facilitated annual PSA screening in families with germline *BRCA1/2* mutations [83,101]. The interim analysis of the study has reported that after 3 years of PSA screening in men with germline *BRCA1/2* mutations, those with a *BRCA2* mutation had increased incidence of prostate cancer, younger age at diagnosis, and higher risk of developing clinically significant tumours [83]. The study suggested that PSA testing in men with germline *BRCA1/2* mutations, with a threshold of 3ng/mL for biopsy, may be highly specific for the detection of early-stage disease [101]; nevertheless, this is not yet incorporated in compendium guidelines.

The NCCN guidelines (version 2.2021, July 2022) propose consideration of tumour testing for HR repair mutations (*BRCA1/2, ATM, CHEK2, PALB2, FANCA, RAD51D,* and *CDK12*), as well as microsatellite instability or MMR status (*MLH1, MSH2, MSH6,* and *PMS2*) in patients with regional, high-risk localised or metastatic prostate cancer [102]. The recommendation for germline testing also includes families with a history of cancer, and specific populations with high risk of prostate cancer, such as Ashkenazi Jews [102].

5. PARP Inhibitors Development across Tumour Types

There is an urgent need to better understand how the genomic and epigenomic heterogeneity intrinsic to EOC is reflected at the protein level, and how this information could potentially lead to prolonged survival [103]. The PARP inhibitors are a family of enzymes capable of catalyzing the transfer of ADP-ribose to target proteins. Among the 17 identified members of the PARP family, PARP-1 is the best characterized. It is responsible for approximately 90% of PARylation activity, whereas PARP-2 and to a lesser extent PARP-3 function in fewer, but overlapping, DNA repair processes [104]. With the binding of PARP to damaged sites, its catalytic activity and eventual release from DNA potentiate the response of a cancer cell to DNA breaks induced by chemotherapeutics and radiation [105]. The approved PARP inhibitors inhibit both PARP-1, -2, and -3. AZD5305 is a novel agent, designed as a highly potent and selective inhibitor of PARP-1 with DNA-trapping activity. The phase I/II PETRA trial evaluated AZD5305 as monotherapy in patients with advanced metastatic breast, pancreatic, or prostate cancer with germline *BRCA1, BRCA2, PALB2,* or *RAD51C* mutations [106]. There was preliminary evidence of early circulating tumour DNA responses. AZD5305 significantly improved pharmacokinetics and exposure to a target compared with the already approved first-generation PARP inhibitors, and thus represents a major advance over them.

Several PARP inhibitors in clinical development have different potencies as PARP-1 catalytic inhibitors and as PARP-'trappers'. PARP inhibitors differ in terms of their metabolism; olaparib and rucaparib are metabolized by cytochrome P450 enzymes, whilst niraparib by carboxylesterase-catalyzed amide hydrolysis [107]. The potent antitumour effects of PARP inhibitors were originally observed in tumours harboring germline *BRCA1/2* mutations, such as familial breast and ovarian cancer. Among evaluated PARP inhibitors, olaparib, niraparib, and rucaparib are approximately 100-fold more potent than veliparib, while talazoparib has the most enhanced trapping potency [108]. The most common adverse events induced by PARP inhibitors are gastro-intestinal manifestations, myelosuppression, and fatigue. Nausea is the most prevalent gastro-intestinal adverse event. Symptoms are mainly mild and daily prokinetic, and antihistamine drugs are therapeutically recommended. Recalcitrant nausea or vomiting can be successfully controlled with a variety of antiemetic drugs, such as metoclopramide, prochlor-perazine, phenothiazine, dexamethasone, olanzapine, haloperidol, or lorazepam. Of note, the neurokinin-1 receptor antagonist aprepitant is contraindicated with olaparib, since it is a strong CYP3A4 inhibitor and may derange olaparib's plasma concentrations. Other frequent gastrointestinal symptoms are constipation, vomiting, and diarrhoea, but grade 3 or 4 toxicities occur in less than 4% of patients. The treatment of choice is senna or polyethylene glycol 3350 for constipation, or loperamide for diarrhoea. Haematological toxicities tend to occur early after treatment initiation, with recovery after a few months. Among them, anaemia is the most common, related to PARP2 inhibition and erythrogenesis. In patients treated with niraparib, haematological adverse events represent the majority of grade 3 and 4 events, followed by rucaparib and olaparib. Haematological toxicities are the most common cause of dose modification, interruption, and discontinuation. The indications for transfusions include the symptomatic anaemia and the haemoglobin values of less than 7 g/dL. Thrombocytopenia of any grade is also more pronounced with niraparib. The cause of thrombocytopenia has been shown to be associated with a reversible decrease in megakaryocyte proliferation and maturation. Finally, fatigue is common for all PARP inhibitors and seems to be a class effect. Approximately 60–70% of patients experience fatigue of any grade with the three approved PARP inhibitors. The recommended management includes non-pharmacological approaches, such as exercise, massage therapy, and cognitive behavioural therapy, whilst pharmacological interventions with psychostimulants, such as methylphenidate and ginseng, may be considered in more symptomatic patients. The synthetic lethality may act against severe PARP inhibitor-mediated toxicity.

The successful story of PARP inhibitors in BRCA-deficient advanced breast and ovarian cancer has led to further investigation of their efficacy in prostate cancer, pancreatic and biliary tract malignancies, glioblastoma, and lung cancer. PARP inhibitors may also be effective in malignancies involving somatic mutations in DDR genes beyond *BRCA1/2*. They could also potentiate immunotherapeutic activity in many ways. Indeed, they increase neoantigen burden through DNA damage. Presence of HR deficiencies such as *BRCA1/2* mutations cause amplification of tumour mutational burden and contribute to immune checkpoint inhibitor sensitivity. Furthermore, PARP inhibitor-induced DNA damage could promote recruitment of T cells via the stimulator of interferon genes (STING) pathway and type I interferons. Finally, PARP inhibitors can lead to acute inflammation, remodeling of the tumour microenvironment, and thus enhancement of immune response [109].

5.1. Development of PARP Inhibitors in EOC

The standard treatment for ovarian cancer consists of cytoreductive surgery, followed by postoperative platinum-based chemotherapy. Neoadjuvant chemotherapy is an alternative option for selected patients, which offers the opportunity to test upfront chemosensitivity and to identify patients at higher risk of relapse [110]. Nevertheless, disease recurrence is a common phenomenon. Bevacizumab—a humanized monoclonal IgG antibody that targets vascular endothelial growth factor (VEGF) receptor—was the first antiangiogenic agent to show clear therapeutic activity in recurrent disease in combination with chemotherapy, based on the results of two randomized controlled phase III trials [111]. Clinical trials of PARP inhibitors have assessed their efficacy and tolerance in the treatment of EOC. Three PARP inhibitors have been approved for the management of EOC in different settings; olaparib, rucaparib, and niraparib.

Chronologically, in 2014, the EMA approved olaparib in maintenance setting for patients with recurrent high grade serous EOC and *BRCA1/2* mutations. The initial study enrolled 19 patients with platinum-sensitive relapse. This study demonstrated improved PFS vs. placebo (8.4 vs. 4.8 months, hazard ratio (HR) 0.35), which was more pronounced in the subset with germline/somatic *BRCA1/2* mutations (11.2 vs. 4.3 months, HR 0.18) [112]. In the same year, the FDA approved olaparib as the first-in-class PARP inhibitor for germline BRCA-mutated patients, previously treated with at least three lines of chemotherapy [113]. In 2018, the approval was expanded to all platinum-sensitive patients, regardless of *BRCA1/2* status. The confirmatory phase III SOLO-2 trial demonstrated median PFS of 19.1 vs. 5.5 months for olaparib and placebo, respectively, in germline BRCA1/2 mutants [114].

Rucaparib was approved by FDA and EMA in December 2016 and May 2018, respectively, for those previously treated with two or more lines of platinum-based chemotherapy, who cannot tolerate further platinum. The phase II ARIEL2 study confirmed that rucaparib prolonged PFS in patients with platinum-sensitive recurrence [115]. BRCA1/2-mutant cancers had improved response (80% vs. 10%) and prolonged PFS compared to the LOH low subgroup (HR 0.27, $p < 0.0001$). A subsequent post hoc analysis concluded that a cut off of 16% compared to 14% for the LOH assay may represent a better predictor of PFS [116].

Finally, the FDA and EMA approved niraparib in maintenance setting in March and November 2017, respectively, based on the phase III NOVA trial [117]. Patients with platinum-sensitive disease were enrolled, regardless of either germline BRCA1/2 or HR deficiency status, while results were stratified to investigate the potential predictive role of HR deficiency biomarkers. Definition of HR deficiency was determined by the myChoice HRD test, which incorporates LOH, telomeric allelic imbalance (TAI), and large-scale state transitions (LST). Median PFS for the non-germline BRCA carriers but signature-positive patients favoured niraparib (12.9 vs. 3.8 months, $p < 0.001$). Even patients without the HR-related signature achieved longer median PFS (6.9 vs. 3.8, $p = 0.02$). These data support that overall platinum-sensitivity status is correlated with PARP inhibitor sensitivity, although more benefit is seen in patients with canonical HR defects. A recently published meta-analysis explored the diversity of efficacy and safety of different PARP inhibitors in patients with EOC [118]. The results showed that either olaparib, niraparib, or rucaparib could prolong PFS over a placebo, whereas their long-term benefit was not limited to *BRCA* mutation status. Nevertheless, the analysis indicated that there was no difference in OS between olaparib and niraparib vs. the placebo. Finally, olaparib had the fewest grade 3 or higher adverse events, whereas no difference was identified between niraparib and rucaparib. However, we must be careful when considering those interpretations due to the methodological heterogeneity of the analysis.

Registration studies that led to approvals of PARP inhibitors for treatment of EOC are resumed in Table 1.

Table 1. Clinical trials of PARP inhibitors in ovarian cancer.

Study	Phase	Population	Treatment Arms	Outcome	P	Ref
STUDY 19	II	(1) Platinum-sensitive, advanced HGSOC (2) At least two prior lines of platinum-based CTH (3) Unselected for BRCA status	(A) Olaparib 400 mg BID (B) Placebo	(A): Median PFS 1. Overall population: 8.4 vs. 4.8 m 2. BRCA mutants: 11.2 vs. 4.3 m 3. BRCA wild type: 7.4 vs. 5.5 m (B): OS 1. Overall population: 29.8 vs. 27.8 m 2. BRCA mutants: 34.9 vs. 31.9 m 3. BRCA wild type: 24.5 vs. 26.2 m (C): ORR 12% vs. 4%	(A1): <0.001 (A2): <0.0001 (A3): 0.0075 (B1): 0.44 (B2): 0.19 (B3): 0.96 (C): 0.12	[112]
STUDY 42	II	(1) Platinum-resistant, advanced HGSOC (2) BRCA mutations	Olaparib 400 mg BID	(1) ORR: 34% (2) MDR: 7.9 m (3) PFS: 7 m (4) OS: 16.6 m		[113]
SOLO 2	III	(1) Platinum-sensitive, advanced HGSOC or HGEOC (2) At least two prior lines of platinum-based CTH (3) BRCA mutations	(A) Olaparib 300 mg BID (B) Placebo	Median PFS: 19.1 vs. 5.5 m	<0.0001	[114]
ARIEL2	II	Platinum-sensitive, advanced HGSOC or HGEOC	Rucaparib 600 mg BID	(A): Median PFS 1. BRCA mutants: 12.8 m 2. BRCA wild type LOH high: 5.7 m 3. BRCA wild type LOH low: 5.2 m (B): ORR 1. BRCA mutants: 80% 2. BRCA wild type LOH high: 39% 3. BRCA wild type LOH low: 13%	(A1): <0.0001 (A2): 0.011 (A3): 0.011	[115]
NOVA	III	(1) Platinum-sensitive, advanced HGSOC (2) At least two prior lines of platinum-based CTH (3) Stratification by gBRCAmut	(A) Niraparib 300 mg BID (B) Placebo	Median PFS (1) gBRCA mutants: 21 vs. 5.5 m (2) BRCA wild type HRD (+): 12.9 vs. 3.8 m (3) Overall non-gBRCA mutants: 9.3 vs. 3.9 m	(1): <0.0001 (2): <0.00001 (3): <0.0001	[117]
STUDY 10	I/II	(1) Platinum-sensitive, advanced HGSOC or HGEOC; (2) gBRCAmut (phase II PART 2A)	Rucaparib 600 mg BID	(1) ORR: 59.5% (2) MDR: 7.8 m		[119]
SOLO 1	III	(1) Platinum-sensitive, advanced HGSOC (2) BRCA mutations	(A) Olaparib 300 mg BID (B) Placebo	Median PFS: NR vs. 13.8 m 3-year PFS: 69% vs. 35%	<0.001 <0.001	[120]
SOLO 3	III	Recurrent gBRCAm EOC	(A) Olaparib (B) CTH	Median PFS: 13.4 vs. 9.2 m	0.013	[121]

Table 1. Cont.

Study	Phase	Population	Treatment Arms	Outcome	P	Ref
PRIMA	III	Newly diagnosed advanced EOC with response to platinum-based CTH	(A) Niraparib 300 mg BID (B) Placebo	Median PFS (1) HRD (+): 21.9 vs. 10.4 m (2) Overall population: 13.8 vs. 8.2 m	(1): <0.001 (2): <0.001	[122]
QUADRA	II	(1) Platinum-sensitive, advanced HGSOC (2) HRD (+)	Niraparib 300 mg BID	(1) ORR 27.5% (2) DCR 68.6%		[123]
ARIEL3	III	Recurrent EOC after response to platinum-based CTH	(A) Rucaparib 600 mg BID (B) Placebo	Median PFS (1) BRCA mutants: 16.6 vs. 5.4 m (2) HRD (+): 13.6 vs. 5.4 m (3) ITT population: 10.8 vs. 5.4 m	(1): <0.0001 (2): <0.0001 (3): <0.001	[124]
PAOLA-1	III	Newly diagnosed, advanced, high-grade ovarian cancer with response after first-line platinum-taxane CTH plus bevacizumab	(A) Bevacizumab + olaparib maintenance (B) Bevacizumab + placebo	Median PFS (1) Overall population: 22.1 vs. 16.6 m (2) HRD (+): 37.2 vs. 17.7 m (3) HRD without BRCA mutations: 28.1 vs. 16.6 m	(1): <0.001	[125]

Abbreviations: PARP: poly(ADP-ribose) polymerase; Ref: reference; HGSOC: high-grade serous ovarian cancer; HGEOC: high-grade endometrioid cancer; gBRCAmut: germline BRCA mutation; BID: twice a day (bis in die); ORR: overall response rate; MDR: median duration of response; m: months; CTH: chemotherapy; PFS: progression-free survival; OS: overall survival; NR: not reached; EOC: epithelial ovarian cancer; HRD: homologous recombination deficiency; DCR, disease control rate; LOH: loss of heterozygosis; ITT: intent-to-treat.

5.2. Development of PARP Inhibitors in Prostate Cancer

Until 2010, patients with metastatic castration-resistant prostate cancer have been treated with chemotherapy, which can be combined with androgen deprivation therapy (ADT). The addition of ADT to localised prostate radiotherapy improves survival as it sensitises prostate cancer to radiotherapy-induced cell death [126]. Technological advancements in the past two decades revealed that residual androgens, ADT-induced AR splice variants, and AR mutations are common mechanisms of metastatic castration-resistant prostate cancer. Within this context, AR signaling inhibitors are included among the agents that have been approved for the treatment of metastatic castration-resistant prostate cancer [127]. AR is a critical regulator of DDR in prostate cancer, through regulation of the expression and activity of DNAPK. This is an enzyme that is key for the process of repairing DSB through NHEJ and also serves as a transcriptional modulator. AR-induced DNAPK activation promotes transcriptional networks that lead to cell migration and metastasis, thus linking the AR-DNA repair axis to tumour progression [128]. The combination of PARP inhibition and AR signaling inhibitors could represent an example of synthetic lethality. AR is a ligand-inducible transcription factor, whereas AR signaling inhibitors cause HR deficit. ADT results in the state of BRCAness, leading to sensitivity of prostate cancer to PARP inhibition in combination with AR signaling inhibitors [129]. Multiple clinical trials are studying PARP inhibitors as either monotherapy or combined therapy for prostate cancer. Among them, olaparib was the first PARP inhibitor showing efficacy in metastatic castration-resistant prostate cancer patients with prior progression to standard treatment. The combination of rucaparib with AR has been approved to guide therapy based on paclitaxel harmful *BRCA* mutations in patients with metastatic castration-resistant prostate cancer. This is the rationale behind the clinical trials of veliparib and talazoparib as well. Key clinical trial data for these four PARP inhibitors in prostate are depicted in Table 2.

Table 2. Clinical trials of PARP inhibitors in prostate cancer.

Clinical Trial ID	Phase	PARP Inhibitor	Population	PSA Response Rate	Primary Endpoint	Ref
NCT01682772	II	Olaparib	mCRPC patients previously treated with abiraterone or enzalutamide, and cabazitaxel	33% of patients (95%, 20–48)	RR, PSA, CTC	[130]
NCT01682772	II	Olaparib	mCRPC patients: (1) previously treated with one or two taxanes (2) DDR gene mutations	PSA levels decrease by ≥ 50%: 100% of BRCA2 and FANCA mutated mCRPC patients	RR, PSA, CTC	[131]
NCT02987543	III	Olaparib	mCRPC patients: (1) disease progression whilst on enzalutamide or abiraterone (2) ≥1 HRR gene mutation	Olaparib group: 30% of patients Control group: 10% of patients	rPFS	[132]
NCT02952534	II	Rucaparib	mCRPC patients: germline or somatic alteration in ≥1 prespecified HRR gene	47.8% of BRCA-mutated patients (95%, 26.8–69.4)	ORR	[133]
NCT04455750	III	Rucaparib	mCRPC patients, resistant to testosterone-deprivation therapy	Not completed	rPFS, OS	[134]
NCT02854436	II	Niraparib	mCRPC patients: (1) DDR gene mutations (2) disease progression on taxane and AR-targeted therapy	57% of patients (95% CI, 34–77)	ORR	[135]
NCT03148795	II	Talazoparib	mCRPC patients: (1) DDR-mutated (2) disease progression on taxane or AR-targeted therapy	Not completed	ORR	[136]
NCT04821622	III	Talazoparib	mCSPC patients with DDR gene mutations	Not completed	rPFS	[137]

Abbreviations: PARP: poly(ADP-ribose) polymerase; Ref: reference; mCRPC: metastatic castration-resistant prostate cancer; RR: response rate; PSA: prostate specific antigen; CTC: circulating tumour cells; DDR: DNA damage repair; HRR: homologous recombination repair; rPFS: radiographic progression-free survival; ORR: objective response rate; OS: overall survival; AR: androgen receptor; mCSPC: metastatic castration-sensitive prostate cancer.

The United Kingdom (UK)-based TOPARP (Trial of PARP inhibition in prostate cancer) phase II trial was conducted in two stages. TOPARP-A assessed anti-tumour activity of olaparib in a sporadic metastatic castration-resistant prostate cancer population, whilst TOPARP-B was conducted in a subset with known genomic background, specifically *BRCA2* or *ATM* mutations [130,131]. In the TOPARP-A study, olaparib led to a response rate of 33% (95% CI 20–48), reduction in CTC of 29%, and 50% decrease in PSA levels of 22% over the whole cohort [130]. However, when TOPARP-B patients were stratified based on NGS results, 88% responded to olaparib; namely, 80% of those with *ATM* mutations and all BRCA2 mutants. On the other hand, only 2 of 33 biomarker-negative patients (6%) had a response to olaparib (sensitivity of 88% and specificity of 94%) [131]. These studies concluded that olaparib is primarily effective in metastatic castration-resistant prostate cancer patients with HR deficiency. Tumours with *BRCA1* or *BRCA2* alterations were more sensitive to olaparib as compared to those with alterations in any other DDR gene.

In the phase III biomarker-driven PROfound trial, the patients were divided into two cohorts. Cohort A assigned patients with *BRCA1*, *BRCA2*, and *ATM* mutations, and cohort B comprised those with mutations in one of the remaining 12 DDR genes [132]. The patients were given olaparib 300 mg twice daily and second line AR signaling inhibitors in a 2:1 ratio. In cohort A, the median radiographic PFS was 7.4 and 3.5 months in favour of olaparib, whilst the median OS was 18.5 and 15.1 months, respectively (HR 0.64, $p = 0.02$). The study met the primary endpoint for radiographic PFS. Based on the positive results of the PROfound trial, the FDA approved olaparib in January 2020 for the treatment of metastatic castration-resistant prostate cancer in patients with deleterious DDR gene mutations, followed by new hormone therapy. Even though it is an approved modality in the United States of America and Europe, this is not the case in the UK.

The TRITON2 and GALAHAD phase II trials investigated the potential therapeutic benefit of rucaparib and niraparib, respectively, in metastatic castration-resistant prostate cancer patients with DDR mutations and disease progression after AR signalling inhibitor or chemotherapy [133,135]. The TRITON2 trial enrolled 190 metastatic castration-resistant prostate cancer patients to be treated with rupacarib 600 mg twice daily. Among them, 52% had a *BRCA1/2* mutation, and the remaining had *ATM* (30%), *CDK12* (7%), *CHEK2* (4%), and other mutated genes (7%). The ORR was 44% for patients with *BRCA* mutations, but only 9.5% for *ATM*, and 0% for the remaining DDR genes [133]. These positive preliminary findings led to the FDA approval of rucaparib in May 2020 for *BRCA1/2* mutated metastatic castration-resistant prostate cancer patients who progressed after one to two lines of AR-directed therapy and one taxane-based chemotherapy. However, the TRITON2 study has not detected accurate biomarkers in non-*BRCA*-mutated tumours.

The GALAHAD trial enrolled 165 metastatic castration-resistant prostate cancer patients with germline pathogenic or somatic biallelic pathogenic alterations in *BRCA1* or *BRCA2* (BRCA cohort), or in other prespecified DDR genes (non-BRCA cohort), who were treated with niraparib 300 mg twice daily. The composite response rate—defined as ORR, conversion of CTC to <5/7.5 mL blood or ≥50% decline in PSA—was 63% in the BRCA and 17% in the non-BRCA cohort, respectively [135]. Similar to olaparib, rucaparib was approved by the FDA—but not by the EMA—for the treatment of metastatic castration-resistant prostate cancer patients with germline and/or somatic *BRCA1/2* mutations, who progressed on AR signaling inhibitor or taxane. Of note, the GALAHAD study stratified patients with biallelic mutations, whilst the TRITON2 and PROfound trials evaluated mono- and biallelic mutations in tumour tissue or plasma and tumour tissue, respectively. Whether the origin and type of *BRCA1/2* mutation (monoallelic vs. biallelic, somatic vs. germline) may potentially affect therapeutic response to PARP inhibitors requires further investigation.

6. Developing Predictive Biomarkers for PARP Inhibitors

The first clinical biomarker for the evaluation of response to PARP inhibitors was platinum sensitivity. The platinum-free interval is correlated with the clinical benefit rate of olaparib in *BRCA1/2* mutated EOC patients. The reported—in a phase I study—clinical benefit rate for the olaparib were 69.2% and 45.8% for the platinum-sensitive and platinum-resistant groups, respectively [138]. The subset of patients with germline *BRCA1/2*-mutated, platinum-sensitive disease achieved the best response to olaparib. On the other hand, the response to platinum-based chemotherapy is not always compatible with the response to PARP inhibitors. This is based on the fact that platinum sensitivity may result from defects in other DDR mechanisms, including NER [139]. Moreover, the secondary restoration of the function of *BRCA1/2* or other HR genes may lead to resistance to PARP inhibition, rather than to platinum resistance [140].

Multiplexed NGS panels investigate the mutation status of multiple genomic regions of interest, either through amplification or capture-based technologies. Multiplexed panels are successfully implemented in clinical practice, based on their lower cost and burden of bioinformatics requirements for the analysis of the data.

Molecular signatures, such as the HR deficiency scores, are crucial for therapeutic decisions. Most of the evidence on the predictive value of such signatures was obtained from the randomized trials of PARP inhibitors rucaparib and niraparib in EOC. HR deficiency is involved in the tumourigenesis of approximately 50% of high-grade serous ovarian carcinoma, whilst about 20% are caused by mutations in HR genes beyond *BRCA1/2* [141].

Several FDA-approved companion diagnostic tests for PARP inhibitors are currently available. BRACAnalysis CDx consists of two in vitro assays for germline *BRCA1/2* mutational identification; the BRACAnalysis CDx Sanger sequencing and the BRACAnalysis CDx Large Rearrangement Test (BART®). They are used for sequence variants and large rearrangements, respectively. Potential limitations of BRACAnalysis CDx are the detection of deletions > 5 bp, insertions > 2 bp, RNA transcript processing errors, and differentiation between gene duplication and triplication [142]. An additional critical limitation of these signatures is that the mutational/LOH patterns do not revert when a tumour has recovered HR function. As such, they may not be able to accurately predict PARP inhibitors' sensitivity in the subset of patients who have been previously treated and progressed on DNA damaging chemotherapy. Myriad's myChoice HR deficiency is an enhancement of BRACAnalysis CDx that identifies both germline and somatic *BRCA1/2* mutations, along with HR deficiency [143]. The created genomic scarring composite score represents a sum of LOH, TAI, and LST.

The RAD51 assay is also a promising candidate for predicting responses to PARP inhibition. RAD51 is an important protein in the HR repair pathway that can be easily detected with an immunofluorescence assay [144]. The induction of RAD51 foci formation after DNA damage has been associated with HR repair proficiency [139]. RAD51 can accurately identify all *PALB2*-mutated tumours as HR-deficient in clinical breast samples [145]. The RAD51 foci assay has also successfully been used as an in vitro predictive biomarker for PARP inhibition in cultures from the ascitic fluid of patients with EOC [146].

As far as prostate cancer is concerned, it has been reported that 30% of patients with metastatic castration-resistant prostate cancer respond to treatment with PARP inhibitors [131]. The first successful prostate cancer biomarker study was the previously mentioned PROfound study, which demonstrated that patients with *BRCA1*, *BRCA2*, and *ATM* alterations responded better to PARP inhibitors and achieved a longer radiographic PFS and OS. In contrast, patients with long-tail DDR alterations did not experience clinical benefit [92]. Moreover, prostate cancer with *BRCA2* had better outcome as compared to those with *BRCA1* mutations, after treatment with PARP inhibitors [147]. Furthermore, Lotan et al., reported that in a three-cohort study, patients with primary prostate cancer and germline *BRCA2* mutations had the highest genomic scarring composite score, followed by the *ATM* and *CHEK2* alterations [148]. Apparently, those with *BRCA2* mutations respond better to PARP inhibitors as compared to the prostate cancer patients with *ATM* and *CHEK2* alterations [132]; nevertheless, the same correlation with higher genomic scarring composite scores has been revealed in the respective DDR gene mutations [148]. The implication of PARP inhibitors beyond *BRCA1/2* mutation—in cases of the 'BRCAness' phenotype—highlights the importance of future trials investigating predictive biomarkers beyond BRCA [149].

The activity of PARP1 is believed to be a new biomarker for sensitivity to PARP inhibitor, as it has been reported that increased PARP1 activity correlates positively with disease progression in prostate cancer. PARP1 enhances E2F1-related mechanisms of HR [150]. E2F1 is a transcription factor that regulates the cell cycle and activates cell proliferation. Therefore, the inhibition of PARP1 results in BRCAness, due to decreased expression of DDR genes.

Finally, a recent study used CRISPR-Cas9 screens for the potential identification of PARP inhibitors' sensitivity marker. Interestingly, it has been revealed that alterations in the genes encoding the RNase H2 enzyme complex (RNASEH2A, RNASEH2B, and RNASEH2C) may cause PARP inhibitor sensitivity through impaired ribonucleotide excision repair [151].

7. BRCA Mutations and Radiation Response

Mutations in genes implied in response to DNA damage were shown to impact on radiation response in various preclinical models. Indeed, the NHEJ and HR are two major mechanisms required for repair of radiation-induced DSBs [152]. In vitro and in vivo experiments demonstrated increased sensitivity to ionizing radiation in ovarian cancer cells carrying defective BRCA1, with data suggesting a role of BRCA1 in Foxp3 mediated radiation resistance [152]. There are therefore theoretical concerns on potential increased radiation sensitivity of normal tissue among *BRCA1* mutation carriers, but also potential increased effectiveness against tumours. Despite this preclinical background, clinical data, mainly obtained in breast cancer patients, did not provide a clear signal that there would be differences in prognosis after adjuvant radiotherapy in patients with BRCA-associated breast cancer or sporadic breast cancer [153]. The place of radiotherapy for ovarian cancers is now quite limited, though the survival benefit afforded by molecular targeted agents leads to long-term survivors, with new indications for stereotactic body radiotherapy in oligoprogressive or oligopersistent disease. For prostate cancer, radiation therapy has a more substantial role, especially in curative strategies. There is a strong rationale to associate radiotherapy with PARP inhibitors, and preclinical data confirmed the potential of such association, leading to more frequent DNA damages, but also to immunogenic effects (e.g., enhanced infiltration of cytotoxic T lymphocytes into the tumour bed, increased expression of PD-1/PDL-1) [154]. To date, only few early phase clinical trials tested PARP inhibitors with radiotherapy, showing the feasibility of such association [155]. Howeve, it remains uncertain whether such an association would lead to different efficacy or safety profiles among patients with *BRCA1/2* mutations. The possibility to reverse systemic resistance to immunotherapy or to PARP inhibitors through irradiation of selected metastatic sites is another area of research [156].

8. Conclusions and Future Directions

Copy number variations (CNVs) which include deletions, duplications, inversions, translocations, and other forms of chromosomal re-arrangements are common to human cancers [157–160]. Apart from the local chromosomal architecture, CNVs are driven by the internal cellular or nuclear physiology of each cancer tissue [161]. A recently published study proposed GraphChrom—a novel graph neural network-based framework—for predicting cancer from chromosomal rearrangement endpoints [162]. Approximately half of all cancers have somatic integrations of retrotransposons. A study analyzed the patterns and mechanisms of cancer retrotransposition on a multidimensional scale, across 2954 cancer genomes, integrated with rearrangement, and transcriptomic and copy number data [163]. Major restructuring of cancer genomes may emerge from aberrant L1 retrotransposition events in tumours with high retrotransposition rates. L1-mediated deletions can promote the loss of megabase-scale regions of a chromosome, which may involve centromeres and telomeres. The majority of such genomic rearrangements would be harmful for a cancer clone. However, L1-mediated deletions may promote cancer-driving rearrangements that involve the loss of tumour-suppressor genes and/or the amplification of oncogenes. Through that mechanism, cancer clones acquire new mutations that help them to survive.

BRCA1 and *BRCA2* genes encode proteins required to restore broken DNA by HR. If mutations inactivate either the *BRCA1* or *BRCA2* gene, then the broken DNA can become pathogenic. Pieces of DNA get lost or reattach at the wrong positions on the original or different chromosomes. In *BRCA1* or *BRCA2* mutants, these errors lead to chromosomal re-arrangements and shifts typical of hereditary breast cancers. Chromosomal re-arrangements may be critical events leading to hereditary breast cancers, but our knowledge of what causes these events is limited. Immune deficits in *BRCA1* and *BRCA2* mutants may allow the reactivation of latent EBV infections or new herpes viral infections [164]. DNA breaks induced by exogenous human herpesvirus 4 (EBV) nucleases may then become pathogenic. The availability of breast cancer genomic sequences allows testing of the possibility that EBV contributes to the incorrect reattachment of broken chromosomes in hereditary breast cancer. The relationship between breast cancer chromosome breaks and viruses may become actionable.

Based on the available evidence on germline and tumour testing for EOC patients, germline genetic testing should be offered to all women diagnosed with EOC. The analysis should be able to detect damaging variants in all genes associated to ovarian cancer susceptibility, rather than just *BRCA1/2* genes. Tumour testing, at least for *BRCA1/2* genes, is recommended for all women testing negative for germline PVs. PARP inhibitors have attracted great attention and illustrate a paradigm of bench-to-bedside medicine. HR deficiency remains a strong predictor of clinical benefit from these agents. The current state of HR deficiency testing can identify patients with EOC who will most likely benefit from PARP inhibitors. Precise biomarkers for negative response prediction are pivotal. Better understanding of BRCA and its role in the development and outcomes of EOC provides a great potential to prevent many cases through improved access to genetic screening, and also to revolutionize the long-term treatment.

Equally, prostate cancer germline and somatic mutations have been found especially in the *BRCA* genes, and subsequently, germline and somatic testing is recommended. This has changed the molecular classification of prostate cancer and expands the available therapeutic options. The evaluation of the safety and efficacy of multiple PARP inhibitors has led to encouraging results. This is crucial as prostate cancer was devoid of predictive therapeutic biomarkers in the past. PARP inhibitors were initially thought to be relevant for DDR mutations, but their therapeutic implication has been expanded, as they may be combined with AR signaling and immune checkpoint inhibitors. The assessment of this strategy with potential for an increased targeted population represents an ongoing effort. The clinical outcome can be affected by several parameters including tumour vs. liquid biopsy, somatic vs. germline mutations, and programmed death-ligand 1 (PD-L1) positivity on tumour cells vs. immune cells. Finally, it is prudent to explore the resistance mechanisms to PARP inhibitors by utilizing non-invasive tools such as cfDNA, as this would help the development of subsequent treatment strategies.

Author Contributions: Conceptualization, S.B. and N.P.; methodology, E.R.; software, M.M.; validation, A.G., S.A. and E.S.; formal analysis, M.S.; investigation, C.C.; resources, E.S.; data curation, E.R.; writing—original draft preparation, S.B.; writing—review and editing, E.R., M.M. and C.C.; visualization, A.G.; supervision, N.P.; project administration, S.A.; funding acquisition, S.B. All authors have read and agreed to the published version of the manuscript.

Funding: This research received no external funding.

Conflicts of Interest: The authors declare no conflict of interest.

References

1. Yousefzadeh, M.; Henpita, C.; Vyas, R.; Soto-Palma, C.; Robbins, P.; Niedernhofer, L. DNA damage-how and why we age? *eLife* **2021**, *10*, e62852. [CrossRef] [PubMed]
2. ICGC/TCGA Pan-Cancer Analysis of Whole Genomes Consortium. Pan-cancer analysis of whole genomes. *Nature* **2020**, *578*, 82–93. [CrossRef] [PubMed]
3. Alexandrov, L.B.; Kim, J.; Haradhvala, N.J.; Huang, M.N.; Tian Ng, A.W.; Wu, Y.; Boot, A.; Covington, K.R.; Gordenin, D.A.; Bergstrom, E.N.; et al. The repertoire of mutational signatures in human cancer. *Nature* **2020**, *578*, 94–101. [CrossRef] [PubMed]
4. Ghose, A.; Moschetta, M.; Pappas-Gogos, G.; Sheriff, M.; Boussios, S. Genetic Aberrations of DNA Repair Pathways in Prostate Cancer: Translation to the Clinic. *Int. J. Mol. Sci.* **2021**, *22*, 9783. [CrossRef] [PubMed]
5. Boussios, S.; Moschetta, M.; Karihtala, P.; Samartzis, E.P.; Sheriff, M.; Pappas-Gogos, G.; Ozturk, M.A.; Uccello, M.; Karathanasi, A.; Tringos, M.; et al. Development of new poly(ADP-ribose) polymerase (PARP) inhibitors in ovarian cancer: Quo Vadis? *Ann. Transl. Med.* **2020**, *8*, 1706. [CrossRef]
6. Revythis, A.; Limbu, A.; Mikropoulos, C.; Ghose, A.; Sanchez, E.; Sheriff, M.; Boussios, S. Recent Insights into PARP and Immuno-Checkpoint Inhibitors in Epithelial Ovarian Cancer. *Int. J. Environ. Res. Public Health* **2022**, *19*, 8577. [CrossRef]
7. Heyer, W.D.; Ehmsen, K.T.; Liu, J. Regulation of homologous recombination in eukaryotes. *Annu. Rev. Genet.* **2010**, *44*, 113–139. [CrossRef]
8. Boussios, S.; Mikropoulos, C.; Samartzis, E.; Karihtala, P.; Moschetta, M.; Sheriff, M.; Karathanasi, A.; Sadauskaite, A.; Rassy, E.; Pavlidis, N. Wise Management of Ovarian Cancer: On the Cutting Edge. *J. Pers. Med.* **2020**, *10*, 41. [CrossRef]

9. Yamauchi, H.; Takei, J. Management of hereditary breast and ovarian cancer. *Int. J. Clin. Oncol.* **2018**, *23*, 45–51. [CrossRef]
10. Sekine, M.; Enomoto, T.; Arai, M.; Den, H.; Nomura, H.; Ikeuchi, T.; Nakamura, S.; Registration Committee of the Japanese Organization of Hereditary Breast and Ovarian Cancer. Differences in age at diagnosis of ovarian cancer for each BRCA mutation type in Japan: Optimal timing to carry out risk-reducing salpingo-oophorectomy. *J. Gynecol. Oncol.* **2022**, *33*, e46. [CrossRef]
11. Pavlidis, N.; Rassy, E.; Vermorken, J.B.; Assi, T.; Kattan, J.; Boussios, S.; Smith-Gagen, J. The outcome of patients with serous papillary peritoneal cancer, fallopian tube cancer, and epithelial ovarian cancer by treatment eras: 27 years data from the SEER registry. *Cancer Epidemiol.* **2021**, *75*, 102045. [CrossRef]
12. Shah, S.; Rachmat, R.; Enyioma, S.; Ghose, A.; Revythis, A.; Boussios, S. BRCA Mutations in Prostate Cancer: Assessment, Implications and Treatment Considerations. *Int. J. Mol. Sci.* **2021**, *22*, 12628. [CrossRef]
13. Boussios, S.; Rassy, E.; Shah, S.; Ioannidou, E.; Sheriff, M.; Pavlidis, N. Aberrations of DNA repair pathways in prostate cancer: A cornerstone of precision oncology. *Expert. Opin. Ther. Targets* **2021**, *25*, 329–333. [CrossRef]
14. Katsuki, Y.; Jeggo, P.A.; Uchihara, Y.; Takata, M.; Shibata, A. DNA double-strand break end resection: A critical relay point for determining the pathway of repair and signaling. *Genome Instab. Dis.* **2020**, *1*, 155–171. [CrossRef]
15. Ranjha, L.; Howard, S.M.; Cejka, P. Main steps in DNA double-strand break repair: An introduction to homologous recombination and related processes. *Chromosoma* **2018**, *127*, 187–214. [CrossRef]
16. Sakofsky, C.J.; Malkova, A. Break induced replication in eukaryotes: Mechanisms, functions, and consequences. *Crit. Rev. Biochem. Mol. Biol.* **2017**, *52*, 395–413. [CrossRef]
17. Llorente, B.; Smith, C.E.; Symington, L.S. Break-induced replication: What is it and what is it for? *Cell Cycle* **2008**, *7*, 859–864. [CrossRef]
18. Kciuk, M.; Gielecińska, A.; Mujwar, S.; Mojzych, M.; Kontek, R. Cyclin-dependent kinases in DNA damage response. *Biochim. Biophys. Acta Rev. Cancer* **2022**, *1877*, 188716. [CrossRef]
19. Guirouilh-Barbat, J.; Lambert, S.; Bertrand, P.; Lopez, B.S. Is homologous recombination really an error-free process? *Front. Genet.* **2014**, *5*, 175. [CrossRef]
20. Bhattacharjee, S.; Nandi, S. Choices have consequences: The nexus between DNA repair pathways and genomic instability in cancer. *Clin. Transl. Med.* **2016**, *5*, 45. [CrossRef]
21. Ghosh, D.; Raghavan, S.C. Nonhomologous end joining: New accessory factors fine tune the machinery. *Trends Genet.* **2021**, *37*, 582–599. [CrossRef]
22. Xu, Y.; Xu, D. Repair pathway choice for double-strand breaks. *Essays Biochem.* **2020**, *64*, 765–777. [CrossRef]
23. Ma, Y.; Pannicke, U.; Schwarz, K.; Lieber, M.R. Hairpin opening and overhang processing by an Artemis/DNA-dependent protein kinase complex in nonhomologous end joining and V(D)J recombination. *Cell* **2002**, *108*, 781–794. [CrossRef]
24. Zang, Y.; Pascal, L.E.; Zhou, Y.; Qiu, X.; Wei, L.; Ai, J.; Nelson, J.B.; Zhong, M.; Xue, B.; Wang, S.; et al. ELL2 regulates DNA non-homologous end joining (NHEJ) repair in prostate cancer cells. *Cancer Lett.* **2018**, *415*, 198–207. [CrossRef]
25. Biswas, H.; Goto, G.; Wang, W.; Sung, P.; Sugimoto, K. Ddc2ATRIP promotes Mec1ATR activation at RPA-ssDNA tracts. *PLoS Genet.* **2019**, *15*, e1008294. [CrossRef]
26. Koch, C.A.; Agyei, R.; Galicia, S.; Metalnikov, P.; O'Donnell, P.; Starostine, A.; Weinfeld, M.; Durocher, D. Xrcc4 physically links DNA end processing by polynucleotide kinase to DNA ligation by DNA ligase IV. *EMBO J.* **2004**, *23*, 3874–3885. [CrossRef]
27. Stracker, T.H.; Petrini, J.H. The MRE11 complex: Starting from the ends. *Nat. Rev. Mol. Cell Biol.* **2011**, *12*, 90–103. [CrossRef]
28. Sun, Y.; Jiang, X.; Price, B.D. Tip60: Connecting chromatin to DNA damage signaling. *Cell Cycle* **2010**, *9*, 930–936. [CrossRef]
29. Liu, D.; Keijzers, G.; Rasmussen, L.J. DNA mismatch repair and its many roles in eukaryotic cells. *Mutat. Res. Rev. Mutat. Res.* **2017**, *773*, 174–187. [CrossRef]
30. Farmer, H.; McCabe, N.; Lord, C.J.; Tutt, A.N.; Johnson, D.A.; Richardson, T.B.; Santarosa, M.; Dillon, K.J.; Hickson, I.; Knights, C.; et al. Targeting the DNA repair defect in BRCA mutant cells as a therapeutic strategy. *Nature* **2005**, *434*, 917–921. [CrossRef]
31. Bryant, H.E.; Schultz, N.; Thomas, H.D.; Parker, K.M.; Flower, D.; Lopez, E.; Kyle, S.; Meuth, M.; Curtin, N.J.; Helleday, T. Specific killing of BRCA2-deficient tumours with inhibitors of poly(ADP-ribose) polymerase. *Nature* **2005**, *434*, 913–917. [CrossRef] [PubMed]
32. Boussios, S.; Karihtala, P.; Moschetta, M.; Abson, C.; Karathanasi, A.; Zakynthinakis-Kyriakou, N.; Ryan, J.E.; Sheriff, M.; Rassy, E.; Pavlidis, N. Veliparib in ovarian cancer: A new synthetically lethal therapeutic approach. *Investig. New Drugs.* **2020**, *38*, 181–193. [CrossRef] [PubMed]
33. Feng, Z.; Scott, S.P.; Bussen, W.; Sharma, G.G.; Guo, G.; Pandita, T.K.; Powell, S.N. Rad52 inactivation is synthetically lethal with BRCA2 deficiency. *Proc. Natl. Acad. Sci. USA* **2011**, *108*, 686–691. [CrossRef] [PubMed]
34. Al-Mugotir, M.; Lovelace, J.J.; George, J.; Bessho, M.; Pal, D.; Struble, L.; Kolar, C.; Rana, S.; Natarajan, A.; Bessho, T.; et al. Selective killing of homologous recombination-deficient cancer cell lines by inhibitors of the RPA:RAD52 protein-protein interaction. *PLoS ONE* **2021**, *16*, e0248941. [CrossRef] [PubMed]
35. Huang, F.; Goyal, N.; Sullivan, K.; Hanamshet, K.; Patel, M.; Mazina, O.M.; Wang, C.X.; An, W.F.; Spoonamore, J.; Metkar, S.; et al. Targeting BRCA1- and BRCA2-deficient cells with RAD52 small molecule inhibitors. *Nucleic Acids. Res.* **2016**, *44*, 4189–4199. [CrossRef]
36. Patel, P.S.; Algouneh, A.; Hakem, R. Exploiting synthetic lethality to target BRCA1/2-deficient tumors: Where we stand. *Oncogene* **2021**, *40*, 3001–3014. [CrossRef]

37. Mahajan, S.; Raina, K.; Verma, S.; Rao, B.J. Human RAD52 protein regulates homologous recombination and checkpoint function in BRCA2 deficient cells. *Int. J. Biochem. Cell Biol.* **2019**, *107*, 128–139. [CrossRef]
38. Lok, B.H.; Carley, A.C.; Tchang, B.; Powell, S.N. RAD52 inactivation is synthetically lethal with deficiencies in BRCA1 and PALB2 in addition to BRCA2 through RAD51-mediated homologous recombination. *Oncogene* **2013**, *32*, 3552–3558. [CrossRef]
39. Adamson, A.W.; Ding, Y.C.; Mendez-Dorantes, C.; Bailis, A.M.; Stark, J.M.; Neuhausen, S.L. The RAD52 S346X variant reduces risk of developing breast cancer in carriers of pathogenic germline BRCA2 mutations. *Mol. Oncol.* **2020**, *14*, 1124–1133. [CrossRef]
40. Biswas, K.; Sharan, S.K. RAD52 S346X variant reduces breast cancer risk in BRCA2 mutation carriers. *Mol. Oncol.* **2020**, *14*, 1121–1123. [CrossRef]
41. Jiricny, J. Postreplicative mismatch repair. *Cold Spring Harb. Perspect. Biol.* **2013**, *5*, a012633. [CrossRef]
42. Xiao, X.; Melton, D.W.; Gourley, C. Mismatch repair deficiency in ovarian cancer—Molecular characteristics and clinical implications. *Gynecol. Oncol.* **2014**, *132*, 506–512. [CrossRef]
43. Boussios, S.; Ozturk, M.A.; Moschetta, M.; Karathanasi, A.; Zakynthinakis-Kyriakou, N.; Katsanos, K.H.; Christodoulou, D.K.; Pavlidis, N. The Developing Story of Predictive Biomarkers in Colorectal Cancer. *J. Pers. Med.* **2019**, *9*, 12. [CrossRef]
44. Adeleke, S.; Haslam, A.; Choy, A.; Diaz-Cano, S.; Galante, J.R.; Mikropoulos, C.; Boussios, S. Microsatellite instability testing in colorectal patients with Lynch syndrome: Lessons learned from a case report and how to avoid such pitfalls. *Per. Med.* **2022**, *19*, 277–286. [CrossRef]
45. Reyes, G.X.; Schmidt, T.T.; Kolodner, R.D.; Hombauer, H. New insights into the mechanism of DNA mismatch repair. *Chromosoma* **2015**, *124*, 443–462. [CrossRef]
46. Kumar, C.; Piacente, S.C.; Sibert, J.; Bukata, A.R.; O'Connor, J.; Alani, E.; Surtees, J.A. Multiple factors insulate Msh2-Msh6 mismatch repair activity from defects in Msh2 domain I. *J. Mol. Biol.* **2011**, *411*, 765–780. [CrossRef]
47. Sokolova, A.O.; Cheng, H.H. Genetic Testing in Prostate Cancer. *Curr. Oncol. Rep.* **2020**, *22*, 5. [CrossRef]
48. Shlien, A.; Campbell, B.B.; de Borja, R.; Alexandrov, L.B.; Merico, D.; Wedge, D.; Van Loo, P.; Tarpey, P.S.; Coupland, P.; Behjati, S.; et al. Combined hereditary and somatic mutations of replication error repair genes result in rapid onset of ultra-hypermutated cancers. *Nat. Genet.* **2015**, *47*, 257–262. [CrossRef]
49. Zhao, C.; Li, S.; Zhao, M.; Zhu, H.; Zhu, X. Prognostic values of DNA mismatch repair genes in ovarian cancer patients treated with platinum-based chemotherapy. *Arch. Gynecol. Obstet.* **2018**, *297*, 153–159. [CrossRef]
50. Robinson, D.; Van Allen, E.M.; Wu, Y.M.; Schultz, N.; Lonigro, R.J.; Mosquera, J.M.; Montgomery, B.; Taplin, M.E.; Pritchard, C.C.; Attard, G.; et al. Integrative clinical genomics of advanced prostate cancer. *Cell* **2015**, *161*, 1215–1228. [CrossRef]
51. Waqar, S.N.; Robinson, C.; Olszanski, A.J.; Spira, A.; Hackmaster, M.; Lucas, L.; Sponton, L.; Jin, H.; Hering, U.; Cronier, D.; et al. Phase I trial of ATM inhibitor M3541 in combination with palliative radiotherapy in patients with solid tumors. *Investig. New Drugs* **2022**, *40*, 596–605. [CrossRef]
52. Fuchss, T.; Graedler, U.; Schiemann, K.; Kuhn, D.; Kubas, H.; Dahmen, H.; Zimmermann, A.; Zenke, F.; Blaukat, A. Highly potent and selective ATM kinase inhibitor M4076: A clinical candidate drug with strong anti-tumor activity in combination therapies [abstract]. In Proceedings of the American Association for Cancer Research Annual Meeting 2019 (AACR), Atlanta, GA, USA, 29 March–3 April 2019.
53. Banerjee, S.; Stewart, J.; Porta, N.; Toms, C.; Leary, A.; Lheureux, S.; Khalique, S.; Tai, J.; Attygalle, A.; Vroobel, K.; et al. ATARI trial: ATR inhibitor in combination with olaparib in gynecological cancers with ARID1A loss or no loss (ENGOT/GYN1/NCRI). *Int. J. Gynecol. Cancer* **2021**, *31*, 1471–1475. [CrossRef]
54. Walsh, T.; Casadei, S.; Lee, M.K.; Pennil, C.C.; Nord, A.S.; Thornton, A.M.; Roeb, W.; Agnew, K.J.; Stray, S.M.; Wickramanayake, A.; et al. Mutations in 12 genes for inherited ovarian, fallopian tube, and peritoneal carcinoma identified by massively parallel sequencing. *Proc. Natl. Acad. Sci. USA* **2011**, *108*, 18032–18037. [CrossRef]
55. Boussios, S.; Karihtala, P.; Moschetta, M.; Karathanasi, A.; Sadauskaite, A.; Rassy, E.; Pavlidis, N. Combined Strategies with Poly (ADP-Ribose) Polymerase (PARP) Inhibitors for the Treatment of Ovarian Cancer: A Literature Review. *Diagnostics* **2019**, *9*, 87. [CrossRef]
56. Shah, S.; Cheung, A.; Kutka, M.; Sheriff, M.; Boussios, S. Epithelial Ovarian Cancer: Providing Evidence of Predisposition Genes. *Int. J. Environ. Res. Public Health* **2022**, *19*, 8113. [CrossRef]
57. Lheureux, S.; Gourley, C.; Vergote, I.; Oza, A.M. Epithelial ovarian cancer. *Lancet* **2019**, *393*, 1240–1253. [CrossRef]
58. Song, H.; Cicek, M.S.; Dicks, E.; Harrington, P.; Ramus, S.J.; Cunningham, J.M.; Fridley, B.L.; Tyrer, J.P.; Alsop, J.; Jimenez-Linan, M.; et al. The contribution of deleterious germline mutations in BRCA1, BRCA2 and the mismatch repair genes to ovarian cancer in the population. *Hum. Mol. Genet.* **2014**, *23*, 4703–4709. [CrossRef]
59. Kuchenbaecker, K.B.; Hopper, J.L.; Barnes, D.R.; Phillips, K.A.; Mooij, T.M.; Roos-Blom, M.J.; Jervis, S.; van Leeuwen, F.E.; Milne, R.L.; Andrieu, N.; et al. Risks of Breast, Ovarian, and Contralateral Breast Cancer for BRCA1 and BRCA2 Mutation Carriers. *JAMA* **2017**, *317*, 2402–2416. [CrossRef]
60. Kotsopoulos, J.; Gronwald, J.; Karlan, B.; Rosen, B.; Huzarski, T.; Moller, P.; Lynch, H.T.; Singer, C.F.; Senter, L.; Neuhausen, S.L.; et al. Age-specific ovarian cancer risks among women with a BRCA1 or BRCA2 mutation. *Gynecol. Oncol.* **2018**, *150*, 85–91. [CrossRef]
61. Finch, A.P.; Lubinski, J.; Møller, P.; Singer, C.F.; Karlan, B.; Senter, L.; Rosen, B.; Maehle, L.; Ghadirian, P.; Cybulski, C.; et al. Impact of oophorectomy on cancer incidence and mortality in women with a BRCA1 or BRCA2 mutation. *J. Clin. Oncol.* **2014**, *32*, 1547–1553. [CrossRef]

62. Piek, J.M.; Verheijen, R.H.; Kenemans, P.; Massuger, L.F.; Bulten, H.; van Diest, P.J. BRCA1/2-related ovarian cancers are of tubal origin: A hypothesis. *Gynecol. Oncol.* **2003**, *90*, 491. [CrossRef]
63. Daly, M.B.; Dresher, C.W.; Yates, M.S.; Jeter, J.M.; Karlan, B.Y.; Alberts, D.S.; Lu, K.H. Salpingectomy as a means to reduce ovarian cancer risk. *Cancer Prev. Res.* **2015**, *8*, 342–348. [CrossRef] [PubMed]
64. Loveday, C.; Turnbull, C.; Ruark, E.; Xicola, R.M.; Ramsay, E.; Hughes, D.; Warren-Perry, M.; Snape, K.; Eccles, D.; Evans, D.G.; et al. Germline RAD51C mutations confer susceptibility to ovarian cancer. *Nat. Genet.* **2012**, *44*, 475–476. [CrossRef] [PubMed]
65. Lilyquist, J.; LaDuca, H.; Polley, E.; Davis, B.T.; Shimelis, H.; Hu, C.; Hart, S.N.; Dolinsky, J.S.; Couch, F.J.; Goldgar, D.E. Frequency of mutations in a large series of clinically ascertained ovarian cancer cases tested on multi-gene panels compared to reference controls. *Gynecol. Oncol.* **2017**, *147*, 375–380. [CrossRef]
66. Loveday, C.; Turnbull, C.; Ramsay, E.; Hughes, D.; Ruark, E.; Frankum, J.R.; Bowden, G.; Kalmyrzaev, B.; Warren-Perry, M.; Snape, K.; et al. Germline mutations in RAD51D confer susceptibility to ovarian cancer. *Nat. Genet.* **2011**, *43*, 879–882. [CrossRef]
67. Daly, M.B.; Pal, T.; Berry, M.P.; Buys, S.S.; Dickson, P.; Domchek, S.M.; Elkhanany, A.; Friedman, S.; Goggins, M.; Hutton, M.L.; et al. Genetic/Familial High-Risk Assessment: Breast, Ovarian, and Pancreatic, Version 2.2021, NCCN Clinical Practice Guidelines in Oncology. *J. Natl. Compr. Cancer Netw.* **2021**, *19*, 77–102. [CrossRef]
68. Ramus, S.J.; Song, H.; Dicks, E.; Tyrer, J.P.; Rosenthal, A.N.; Intermaggio, M.P.; Fraser, L.; Gentry-Maharaj, A.; Hayward, J.; Philpott, S.; et al. Germline Mutations in the BRIP1, BARD1, PALB2, and NBN Genes in Women With Ovarian Cancer. *J. Natl. Cancer Inst.* **2015**, *107*, djv214. [CrossRef]
69. Seal, S.; Thompson, D.; Renwick, A.; Elliott, A.; Kelly, P.; Barfoot, R.; Chagtai, T.; Jayatilake, H.; Ahmed, M.; Spanova, K.; et al. Truncating mutations in the Fanconi anemia J gene BRIP1 are low-penetrance breast cancer susceptibility alleles. *Nat. Genet.* **2006**, *38*, 1239–1241. [CrossRef]
70. Ducy, M.; Sesma-Sanz, L.; Guitton-Sert, L.; Lashgari, A.; Gao, Y.; Brahiti, N.; Rodrigue, A.; Margaillan, G.; Caron, M.C.; Côté, J.; et al. The Tumor Suppressor PALB2: Inside Out. *Trends Biochem. Sci.* **2019**, *44*, 226–240. [CrossRef]
71. Polak, P.; Kim, J.; Braunstein, L.Z.; Karlic, R.; Haradhavala, N.J.; Tiao, G.; Rosebrock, D.; Livitz, D.; Kübler, K.; Mouw, K.W.; et al. A mutational signature reveals alterations underlying deficient homologous recombination repair in breast cancer. *Nat. Genet.* **2017**, *49*, 1476–1486. [CrossRef]
72. Mills, A.M.; Longacre, T.A. Lynch Syndrome Screening in the Gynecologic Tract: Current State of the Art. *Am. J. Surg. Pathol.* **2016**, *40*, e35–e44. [CrossRef]
73. Møller, P.; Seppälä, T.; Bernstein, I.; Holinski-Feder, E.; Sala, P.; Evans, D.G.; Lindblom, A.; Macrae, F.; Blanco, I.; Sijmons, R.; et al. Cancer incidence and survival in Lynch syndrome patients receiving colonoscopic and gynaecological surveillance: First report from the prospective Lynch syndrome database. *Gut* **2017**, *66*, 464–472. [CrossRef]
74. Cheung, A.; Shah, S.; Parker, J.; Soor, P.; Limbu, A.; Sheriff, M.; Boussios, S. Non-Epithelial Ovarian Cancers: How Much Do We Really Know? *Int. J. Environ. Res. Public Health* **2022**, *19*, 1106. [CrossRef]
75. Boussios, S.; Karathanasi, A.; Zakynthinakis-Kyriakou, N.; Tsiouris, A.K.; Chatziantoniou, A.A.; Kanellos, F.S.; Tatsi, K. Ovarian carcinosarcoma: Current developments and future perspectives. *Crit. Rev. Oncol. Hematol.* **2019**, *134*, 46–55. [CrossRef]
76. Konstantinopoulos, P.A.; Norquist, B.; Lacchetti, C.; Armstrong, D.; Grisham, R.N.; Goodfellow, P.J.; Kohn, E.C.; Levine, D.A.; Liu, J.F.; Lu, K.H.; et al. Germline and Somatic Tumor Testing in Epithelial Ovarian Cancer: ASCO Guideline. *J. Clin. Oncol.* **2020**, *38*, 1222–1245. [CrossRef]
77. Lou, E.; Vogel, R.I.; Teoh, D.; Hoostal, S.; Grad, A.; Gerber, M.; Monu, M.; Lukaszewski, T.; Deshpande, J.; Linden, M.A.; et al. Assessment of Circulating Tumor Cells as a Predictive Biomarker of Histology in Women With Suspected Ovarian Cancer. *Lab. Med.* **2018**, *49*, 134–139. [CrossRef]
78. Kuhlmann, J.D.; Wimberger, P.; Bankfalvi, A.; Keller, T.; Schöler, S.; Aktas, B.; Buderath, P.; Hauch, S.; Otterbach, F.; Kimmig, R.; et al. ERCC1-positive circulating tumor cells in the blood of ovarian cancer patients as a predictive biomarker for platinum resistance. *Clin. Chem.* **2014**, *60*, 1282–1289. [CrossRef]
79. Yang, F.; Tang, J.; Zhao, Z.; Zhao, C.; Xiang, Y. Circulating tumor DNA: A noninvasive biomarker for tracking ovarian cancer. *Reprod. Biol. Endocrinol.* **2021**, *19*, 178. [CrossRef]
80. Oh, M.; Alkhushaym, N.; Fallatah, S.; Althagafi, A.; Aljadeed, R.; Alsowaida, Y.; Jeter, J.; Martin, J.R.; Babiker, H.M.; McBride, A.; et al. The association of BRCA1 and BRCA2 mutations with prostate cancer risk, frequency, and mortality: A meta-analysis. *Prostate* **2019**, *79*, 880–895. [CrossRef]
81. Nyberg, T.; Frost, D.; Barrowdale, D.; Evans, D.G.; Bancroft, E.; Adlard, J.; Ahmed, M.; Barwell, J.; Brady, A.F.; Brewer, C.; et al. Prostate Cancer Risks for Male BRCA1 and BRCA2 Mutation Carriers: A Prospective Cohort Study. *Eur. Urol.* **2020**, *77*, 24–35. [CrossRef]
82. Kote-Jarai, Z.; Leongamornlert, D.; Saunders, E.; Tymrakiewicz, M.; Castro, E.; Mahmud, N.; Guy, M.; Edwards, S.; O'Brien, L.; Sawyer, E.; et al. BRCA2 is a moderate penetrance gene contributing to young-onset prostate cancer: Implications for genetic testing in prostate cancer patients. *Br. J. Cancer* **2011**, *105*, 1230–1234. [CrossRef]
83. Page, E.C.; Bancroft, E.K.; Brook, M.N.; Assel, M.; Hassan Al Battat, M.; Thomas, S.; Taylor, N.; Chamberlain, A.; Pope, J.; Raghallaigh, H.N.; et al. Interim Results from the IMPACT Study: Evidence for Prostate-specific Antigen Screening in BRCA2 Mutation Carriers. *Eur. Urol.* **2019**, *76*, 831–842. [CrossRef]

84. Patel, V.L.; Busch, E.L.; Friebel, T.M.; Cronin, A.; Leslie, G.; McGuffog, L.; Adlard, J.; Agata, S.; Agnarsson, B.A.; Ahmed, M.; et al. Association of Genomic Domains in BRCA1 and BRCA2 with Prostate Cancer Risk and Aggressiveness. *Cancer Res.* **2020**, *80*, 624–638. [CrossRef]
85. Giri, V.N.; Knudsen, K.E.; Kelly, W.K.; Abida, W.; Andriole, G.L.; Bangma, C.H.; Bekelman, J.E.; Benson, M.C.; Blanco, A.; Burnett, A.; et al. Role of Genetic Testing for Inherited Prostate Cancer Risk: Philadelphia Prostate Cancer Consensus Conference 2017. *J. Clin. Oncol.* **2018**, *36*, 414–424. [CrossRef] [PubMed]
86. Schayek, H.; Haugk, K.; Sun, S.; True, L.D.; Plymate, S.R.; Werner, H. Tumor suppressor BRCA1 is expressed in prostate cancer and controls insulin-like growth factor I receptor (IGF-IR) gene transcription in an androgen receptor-dependent manner. *Clin. Cancer Res.* **2009**, *15*, 1558–1565. [CrossRef] [PubMed]
87. Bednarz, N.; Eltze, E.; Semjonow, A.; Rink, M.; Andreas, A.; Mulder, L.; Hannemann, J.; Fisch, M.; Pantel, K.; Weier, H.U.; et al. BRCA1 loss preexisting in small subpopulations of prostate cancer is associated with advanced disease and metastatic spread to lymph nodes and peripheral blood. *Clin. Cancer Res.* **2010**, *16*, 3340–3348. [CrossRef] [PubMed]
88. Sigorski, D.; Iżycka-Świeszewska, E.; Bodnar, L. Poly(ADP-Ribose) Polymerase Inhibitors in Prostate Cancer: Molecular Mechanisms, and Preclinical and Clinical Data. *Target. Oncol.* **2020**, *15*, 709–722. [CrossRef] [PubMed]
89. Testa, U.; Castelli, G.; Pelosi, E. Cellular and Molecular Mechanisms Underlying Prostate Cancer Development: Therapeutic Implications. *Medicines* **2019**, *6*, 82. [CrossRef]
90. Saxby, H.; Mikropoulos, C.; Boussios, S. An Update on the Prognostic and Predictive Serum Biomarkers in Metastatic Prostate Cancer. *Diagnostics* **2020**, *10*, 549. [CrossRef]
91. Cancer Genome Atlas Research Network. The Molecular Taxonomy of Primary Prostate Cancer. *Cell* **2015**, *163*, 1011–1025. [CrossRef]
92. Hussain, M.; Mateo, J.; Fizazi, K.; Saad, F.; Shore, N.; Sandhu, S.; Chi, K.N.; Sartor, O.; Agarwal, N.; Olmos, D.; et al. Survival with Olaparib in Metastatic Castration-Resistant Prostate Cancer. *N. Engl. J. Med.* **2020**, *383*, 2345–2357. [CrossRef]
93. Castro, E.; Romero-Laorden, N.; Del Pozo, A.; Lozano, R.; Medina, A.; Puente, J.; Piulats, J.M.; Lorente, D.; Saez, M.I.; Morales-Barrera, R.; et al. PROREPAIR-B: A Prospective Cohort Study of the Impact of Germline DNA Repair Mutations on the Outcomes of Patients With Metastatic Castration-Resistant Prostate Cancer. *J. Clin. Oncol.* **2019**, *37*, 490–503. [CrossRef]
94. Abida, W.; Campbell, D.; Patnaik, A.; Shapiro, J.D.; Sautois, B.; Vogelzang, N.J.; Voog, E.G.; Bryce, A.H.; McDermott, R.; Ricci, F.; et al. Non-BRCA DNA Damage Repair Gene Alterations and Response to the PARP Inhibitor Rucaparib in Metastatic Castration-Resistant Prostate Cancer: Analysis From the Phase II TRITON2 Study. *Clin. Cancer Res.* **2020**, *26*, 2487–2496. [CrossRef]
95. Lord, C.J.; Ashworth, A. BRCAness revisited. *Nat. Rev. Cancer* **2016**, *16*, 110–120. [CrossRef]
96. Mohler, J.L.; Antonarakis, E.S. NCCN Guidelines Updates: Management of Prostate Cancer. *J. Natl. Compr. Cancer Netw.* **2019**, *17*, 583–586.
97. Mateo, J.; Seed, G.; Bertan, C.; Rescigno, P.; Dolling, D.; Figueiredo, I.; Miranda, S.; Nava Rodrigues, D.; Gurel, B.; Clarke, M.; et al. Genomics of lethal prostate cancer at diagnosis and castration resistance. *J. Clin. Investig.* **2020**, *130*, 1743–1751. [CrossRef]
98. Dall'Era, M.A.; McPherson, J.D.; Gao, A.C.; DeVere White, R.W.; Gregg, J.P.; Lara, P.N., Jr. Germline and somatic DNA repair gene alterations in prostate cancer. *Cancer* **2020**, *126*, 2980–2985. [CrossRef]
99. Moreno, J.G.; Gomella, L.G. Evolution of the Liquid Biopsy in Metastatic Prostate Cancer. *Urology* **2019**, *132*, 1–9. [CrossRef]
100. Merker, J.D.; Oxnard, G.R.; Compton, C.; Diehn, M.; Hurley, P.; Lazar, A.J.; Lindeman, N.; Lockwood, C.M.; Rai, A.J.; Schilsky, R.L.; et al. Circulating Tumor DNA Analysis in Patients with Cancer: American Society of Clinical Oncology and College of American Pathologists Joint Review. *J. Clin. Oncol.* **2018**, *36*, 1631–1641. [CrossRef]
101. Bancroft, E.K.; Page, E.C.; Castro, E.; Lilja, H.; Vickers, A.; Sjoberg, D.; Assel, M.; Foster, C.S.; Mitchell, G.; Drew, K.; et al. Targeted prostate cancer screening in BRCA1 and BRCA2 mutation carriers: Results from the initial screening round of the IMPACT study. *Eur. Urol.* **2014**, *66*, 489–499. [CrossRef]
102. National Comprehensive Cancer Network. Prostate Cancer Early Detection. National Comprehensive Cancer Network. Version 2.2021—14 July 2021. Available online: https://www.nccn.org/professionals/physician_gls/pdf/prostate_detection.pdf (accessed on 3 June 2022).
103. Ghose, A.; Gullapalli, S.V.N.; Chohan, N.; Bolina, A.; Moschetta, M.; Rassy, E.; Boussios, S. Applications of Proteomics in Ovarian Cancer: Dawn of a New Era. *Proteomes* **2022**, *10*, 16. [CrossRef]
104. Langelier, M.F.; Riccio, A.A.; Pascal, J.M. PARP-2 and PARP-3 are selectively activated by 5′ phosphorylated DNA breaks through an allosteric regulatory mechanism shared with PARP-1. *Nucleic. Acids. Res.* **2014**, *42*, 7762–7775. [CrossRef]
105. Lord, C.J.; Ashworth, A. PARP inhibitors: Synthetic lethality in the clinic. *Science* **2017**, *355*, 1152–1158. [CrossRef]
106. Yap, T.A.; Im, S.A.; Schram, A.M.; Sharp, A.; Balmana, J.; Baird, R.D.; Brown, J.S.; Schwaederle, M.; Pilling, E.A.; Moorthy, G.; et al. PETRA: First in class, first in human trial of the next generation PARP1-selective inhibitor AZD5305 in patients with BRCA1/2, PALB2, or RAD51C/D mutations. *Cancer Res.* **2022**, *82*, CT007. [CrossRef]
107. Boussios, S.; Karathanasi, A.; Cooke, D.; Neille, C.; Sadauskaite, A.; Moschetta, M.; Zakynthinakis-Kyriakou, N.; Pavlidis, N. PARP Inhibitors in Ovarian Cancer: The Route to "Ithaca". *Diagnostics* **2019**, *9*, 55. [CrossRef]
108. Boussios, S.; Abson, C.; Moschetta, M.; Rassy, E.; Karathanasi, A.; Bhat, T.; Ghumman, F.; Sheriff, M.; Pavlidis, N. Poly (ADP-Ribose) Polymerase Inhibitors: Talazoparib in Ovarian Cancer and Beyond. *Drugs R D* **2020**, *20*, 55–73. [CrossRef]

109. Demircan, N.C.; Boussios, S.; Tasci, T.; Öztürk, M.A. Current and future immunotherapy approaches in ovarian cancer. *Ann. Transl. Med.* **2020**, *8*, 1714. [CrossRef]
110. Moschetta, M.; Boussios, S.; Rassy, E.; Samartzis, E.P.; Funingana, G.; Uccello, M. Neoadjuvant treatment for newly diagnosed advanced ovarian cancer: Where do we stand and where are we going? *Ann. Transl. Med.* **2020**, *8*, 1710. [CrossRef]
111. Perren, T.J.; Swart, A.M.; Pfisterer, J.; Ledermann, J.A.; Pujade-Lauraine, E.; Kristensen, G.; Carey, M.S.; Beale, P.; Cervantes, A.; Kurzeder, C.; et al. A phase 3 trial of bevacizumab in ovarian cancer. *N. Engl. J. Med.* **2011**, *365*, 2484–2496. [CrossRef]
112. Ledermann, J.; Harter, P.; Gourley, C.; Friedlander, M.; Vergote, I.; Rustin, G.; Scott, C.L.; Meier, W.; Shapira-Frommer, R.; Safra, T.; et al. Olaparib maintenance therapy in patients with platinum-sensitive relapsed serous ovarian cancer: A preplanned retrospective analysis of outcomes by BRCA status in a randomised phase 2 trial. *Lancet Oncol.* **2014**, *15*, 852–861. [CrossRef]
113. Kaufman, B.; Shapira-Frommer, R.; Schmutzler, R.K.; Audeh, M.W.; Friedlander, M.; Balmaña, J.; Mitchell, G.; Fried, G.; Stemmer, S.M.; Hubert, A.; et al. Olaparib monotherapy in patients with advanced cancer and a germline BRCA1/2 mutation. *J. Clin. Oncol.* **2015**, *33*, 244–250. [CrossRef] [PubMed]
114. Pujade-Lauraine, E.; Ledermann, J.A.; Selle, F.; Gebski, V.; Penson, R.T.; Oza, A.M.; Korach, J.; Huzarski, T.; Poveda, A.; Pignata, S.; et al. Olaparib tablets as maintenance therapy in patients with platinum-sensitive, relapsed ovarian cancer and a BRCA1/2 mutation (SOLO2/ENGOT-Ov21): A double-blind, randomised, placebo-controlled, phase 3 trial. *Lancet Oncol.* **2017**, *18*, 1274–1284. [CrossRef]
115. Swisher, E.M.; Lin, K.K.; Oza, A.M.; Scott, C.L.; Giordano, H.; Sun, J.; Konecny, G.E.; Coleman, R.L.; Tinker, A.V.; O'Malley, D.M.; et al. Rucaparib in relapsed, platinum-sensitive high-grade ovarian carcinoma (ARIEL2 Part 1): An international, multicentre, open-label, phase 2 trial. *Lancet Oncol.* **2017**, *18*, 75–87. [CrossRef]
116. Coleman, R.L.; Swisher, E.M.; Oza, A.M.; Scott, C.L.; Giordano, H.; Lin, K.K.; Konecny, G.E.; Tinker, A.; O'Malley, D.M.; Kristeleit, R.S.; et al. Refinement of prespecified cutoff for genomic loss of heterozygosity (LOH) in ARIEL2 part 1: A phase II study of rucaparib in patients (PTS) with high grade ovarian carcinoma (HGOC). *J. Clin. Oncol.* **2016**, *34*, 5540. [CrossRef]
117. Mirza, M.R.; Monk, B.J.; Herrstedt, J.; Oza, A.M.; Mahner, S.; Redondo, A.; Fabbro, M.; Ledermann, J.A.; Lorusso, D.; Vergote, I.; et al. Niraparib Maintenance Therapy in Platinum-Sensitive, Recurrent Ovarian Cancer. *N. Engl. J. Med.* **2016**, *375*, 2154–2164. [CrossRef]
118. Luo, J.; Ou, S.; Wei, H.; Qin, X.; Jiang, Q. Comparative Efficacy and Safety of Poly (ADP-Ribose) Polymerase Inhibitors in Patients with Ovarian Cancer: A Systematic Review and Network Meta-Analysis. *Front. Oncol.* **2022**, *12*, 815265. [CrossRef]
119. Kristeleit, R.; Shapiro, G.I.; Burris, H.A.; Oza, A.M.; LoRusso, P.; Patel, M.R.; Domchek, S.M.; Balmaña, J.; Drew, Y.; Chen, L.M.; et al. A Phase I-II Study of the Oral PARP Inhibitor Rucaparib in Patients with Germline BRCA1/2-Mutated Ovarian Carcinoma or Other Solid Tumors. *Clin. Cancer Res.* **2017**, *23*, 4095–4106. [CrossRef]
120. Moore, K.; Colombo, N.; Scambia, G.; Kim, B.G.; Oaknin, A.; Friedlander, M.; Lisyanskaya, A.; Floquet, A.; Leary, A.; Sonke, G.S.; et al. Maintenance Olaparib in Patients with Newly Diagnosed Advanced Ovarian Cancer. *N. Engl. J. Med.* **2018**, *379*, 2495–2505. [CrossRef]
121. Penson, R.T.; Valencia, R.V.; Cibula, D.; Colombo, N.; Leath, C.A., 3rd; Bidziński, M.; Kim, J.W.; Nam, J.H.; Madry, R.; Hernández, C.; et al. Olaparib Versus Nonplatinum Chemotherapy in Patients with Platinum-Sensitive Relapsed Ovarian Cancer and a Germline BRCA1/2 Mutation (SOLO3): A Randomized Phase III Trial. *J. Clin. Oncol.* **2020**, *38*, 1164–1174. [CrossRef]
122. González-Martín, A.; Pothuri, B.; Vergote, I.; DePont Christensen, R.; Graybill, W.; Mirza, M.R.; McCormick, C.; Lorusso, D.; Hoskins, P.; Freyer, G.; et al. Niraparib in Patients with Newly Diagnosed Advanced Ovarian Cancer. *N. Engl. J. Med.* **2019**, *381*, 2391–2402. [CrossRef]
123. Moore, K.N.; Secord, A.A.; Geller, M.A.; Miller, D.S.; Cloven, N.; Fleming, G.F.; Wahner Hendrickson, A.E.; Azodi, M.; DiSilvestro, P.; Oza, A.M.; et al. Niraparib monotherapy for late-line treatment of ovarian cancer (QUADRA): A multicentre, open-label, single-arm, phase 2 trial. *Lancet Oncol.* **2019**, *20*, 636–648. [CrossRef]
124. Coleman, R.L.; Oza, A.M.; Lorusso, D.; Aghajanian, C.; Oaknin, A.; Dean, A.; Colombo, N.; Weberpals, J.I.; Clamp, A.; Scambia, G.; et al. Rucaparib maintenance treatment for recurrent ovarian carcinoma after response to platinum therapy (ARIEL3): A randomised, double-blind, placebo-controlled, phase 3 trial. *Lancet* **2017**, *390*, 1949–1961. [CrossRef]
125. Ray-Coquard, I.; Pautier, P.; Pignata, S.; Pérol, D.; González-Martín, A.; Berger, R.; Fujiwara, K.; Vergote, I.; Colombo, N.; Mäenpää, J.; et al. Olaparib plus Bevacizumab as First-Line Maintenance in Ovarian Cancer. *N. Engl. J. Med.* **2019**, *381*, 2416–2428. [CrossRef]
126. Saxby, H.; Boussios, S.; Mikropoulos, C. Androgen Receptor Gene Pathway Upregulation and Radiation Resistance in Oligometastatic Prostate Cancer. *Int. J. Mol. Sci.* **2022**, *23*, 4786. [CrossRef]
127. Attard, G.; Murphy, L.; Clarke, N.W.; Cross, W.; Jones, R.J.; Parker, C.C.; Gillessen, S.; Cook, A.; Brawley, C.; Amos, C.L.; et al. Abiraterone acetate and prednisolone with or without enzalutamide for high-risk non-metastatic prostate cancer: A meta-analysis of primary results from two randomised controlled phase 3 trials of the STAMPEDE platform protocol. *Lancet* **2022**, *399*, 447–460. [CrossRef]
128. Knudsen, K.E. The AR-DNA repair axis: Insights into prostate cancer aggressiveness. *Can. J. Urol.* **2019**, *26*, 22–23.
129. Virtanen, V.; Paunu, K.; Ahlskog, J.K.; Varnai, R.; Sipeky, C.; Sundvall, M. PARP Inhibitors in Prostate Cancer—The Preclinical Rationale and Current Clinical Development. *Genes* **2019**, *10*, 565. [CrossRef]

130. Mateo, J.; Carreira, S.; Sandhu, S.; Miranda, S.; Mossop, H.; Perez-Lopez, R.; Nava Rodrigues, D.; Robinson, D.; Omlin, A.; Tunariu, N.; et al. DNA-Repair Defects and Olaparib in Metastatic Prostate Cancer. *N. Engl. J. Med.* **2015**, *373*, 1697–1708. [CrossRef]
131. Mateo, J.; Porta, N.; Bianchini, D.; McGovern, U.; Elliott, T.; Jones, R.; Syndikus, I.; Ralph, C.; Jain, S.; Varughese, M.; et al. Olaparib in patients with metastatic castration-resistant prostate cancer with DNA repair gene aberrations (TOPARP-B): A multicentre, open-label, randomised, phase 2 trial. *Lancet Oncol.* **2020**, *21*, 162–174. [CrossRef]
132. De Bono, J.; Mateo, J.; Fizazi, K.; Saad, F.; Shore, N.; Sandhu, S.; Chi, K.N.; Sartor, O.; Agarwal, N.; Olmos, D.; et al. Olaparib for Metastatic Castration-Resistant Prostate Cancer. *N. Engl. J. Med.* **2020**, *382*, 2091–2102. [CrossRef]
133. Abida, W.; Patnaik, A.; Campbell, D.; Shapiro, J.; Bryce, A.H.; McDermott, R.; Sautois, B.; Vogelzang, N.J.; Bambury, R.M.; Voog, E.; et al. Rucaparib in Men With Metastatic Castration-Resistant Prostate Cancer Harboring a BRCA1 or BRCA2 Gene Alteration. *J. Clin. Oncol.* **2020**, *38*, 3763–3772. [CrossRef] [PubMed]
134. Rao, A.; Heller, G.; Ryan, C.J.; VanderWeele, D.J.; Lewis, L.D.; Tan, A.; Watt, C.; Chen, R.C.; Kohli, M.; Barata, P.C.; et al. Alliance A031902 (CASPAR): A randomized, phase (ph) 3 trial of enzalutamide with rucaparib/placebo as novel therapy in first-line metastatic castration-resistant prostate cancer (mCRPC). *J. Clin. Oncol.* **2022**, *40*, TPS194. [CrossRef]
135. Smith, M.R.; Scher, H.I.; Sandhu, S.; Efstathiou, E.; Lara, P.N., Jr.; Yu, E.Y.; George, D.J.; Chi, K.N.; Saad, F.; Ståhl, O.; et al. Niraparib in patients with metastatic castration-resistant prostate cancer and DNA repair gene defects (GALAHAD): A multicentre, open-label, phase 2 trial. *Lancet Oncol.* **2022**, *23*, 362–373. [CrossRef]
136. De Bono, J.S.; Mehra, N.; Scagliotti, G.V.; Castro, E.; Dorff, T.; Stirling, A.; Stenzl, A.; Fleming, M.T.; Higano, C.S.; Saad, F.; et al. Talazoparib monotherapy in metastatic castration-resistant prostate cancer with DNA repair alterations (TALAPRO-1): An open-label, phase 2 trial. *Lancet Oncol.* **2021**, *22*, 1250–1264. [CrossRef]
137. Agarwal, N.; Azad, A.; Fizazi, K.; Mateo, J.; Matsubara, N.; Shore, N.D.; Chakrabarti, J.; Chen, H.-C.; Lanzalone, S.; Niyazov, A.; et al. Talapro-3: A phase 3, double-blind, randomized study of enzalutamide (ENZA) plus talazoparib (TALA) versus placebo plus enza in patients with DDR gene mutated metastatic castration-sensitive prostate cancer (mCSPC). *J. Clin. Oncol.* **2022**, *40*, TPS221. [CrossRef]
138. Fong, P.C.; Yap, T.A.; Boss, D.S.; Carden, C.P.; Mergui-Roelvink, M.; Gourley, C.; De Greve, J.; Lubinski, J.; Shanley, S.; Messiou, C.; et al. Poly(ADP-ribose) polymerase inhibition: Frequent durable responses in BRCA carrier ovarian cancer correlating with platinum-free interval. *J. Clin. Oncol.* **2010**, *28*, 2512–2519. [CrossRef]
139. Jiang, X.; Li, X.; Li, W.; Bai, H.; Zhang, Z. PARP inhibitors in ovarian cancer: Sensitivity prediction and resistance mechanisms. *J. Cell Mol. Med.* **2019**, *23*, 2303–2313. [CrossRef]
140. Norquist, B.; Wurz, K.A.; Pennil, C.C.; Garcia, R.; Gross, J.; Sakai, W.; Karlan, B.Y.; Taniguchi, T.; Swisher, E.M. Secondary somatic mutations restoring BRCA1/2 predict chemotherapy resistance in hereditary ovarian carcinomas. *J. Clin. Oncol.* **2011**, *29*, 3008–3015. [CrossRef]
141. Bitler, B.G.; Watson, Z.L.; Wheeler, L.J.; Behbakht, K. PARP inhibitors: Clinical utility and possibilities of overcoming resistance. *Gynecol. Oncol.* **2017**, *147*, 695–704. [CrossRef]
142. Gunderson, C.C.; Moore, K.N. BRACAnalysis CDx as a companion diagnostic tool for Lynparza. *Expert Rev. Mol. Diagn.* **2015**, *15*, 1111–1116. [CrossRef]
143. Myriad. Tumor BRACAnalysis CDxTM. Available online: http://myriadgenetics.eu/products/tumor-bracanalysis-cdx-2/?lang=gb (accessed on 3 June 2022).
144. Ohmoto, A.; Yachida, S. Current status of poly(ADP-ribose) polymerase inhibitors and future directions. *Onco Targets Ther.* **2017**, *10*, 5195–5208. [CrossRef]
145. Castroviejo-Bermejo, M.; Cruz, C.; Llop-Guevara, A.; Gutiérrez-Enríquez, S.; Ducy, M.; Ibrahim, Y.H.; Gris-Oliver, A.; Pellegrino, B.; Bruna, A.; Guzmán, M.; et al. A RAD51 assay feasible in routine tumor samples calls PARP inhibitor response beyond BRCA mutation. *EMBO Mol. Med.* **2018**, *10*, e9172. [CrossRef]
146. Mukhopadhyay, A.; Plummer, E.R.; Elattar, A.; Soohoo, S.; Uzir, B.; Quinn, J.E.; McCluggage, W.G.; Maxwell, P.; Aneke, H.; Curtin, N.J.; et al. Clinicopathological features of homologous recombination-deficient epithelial ovarian cancers: Sensitivity to PARP inhibitors, platinum, and survival. *Cancer Res.* **2012**, *72*, 5675–5682. [CrossRef]
147. Markowski, M.C.; Antonarakis, E.S. BRCA1 Versus BRCA2 and PARP Inhibitor Sensitivity in Prostate Cancer: More Different Than Alike? *J. Clin. Oncol.* **2020**, *38*, 3735–3739. [CrossRef]
148. Lotan, T.L.; Kaur, H.B.; Salles, D.C.; Murali, S.; Schaeffer, E.M.; Lanchbury, J.S.; Isaacs, W.B.; Brown, R.; Richardson, A.L.; Cussenot, O.; et al. Homologous recombination deficiency (HRD) score in germline BRCA2- versus ATM-altered prostate cancer. *Mod. Pathol.* **2021**, *34*, 1185–1193. [CrossRef]
149. Stopsack, K.H. Efficacy of PARP Inhibition in Metastatic Castration-resistant Prostate Cancer is Very Different with Non-BRCA DNA Repair Alterations: Reconstructing Prespecified Endpoints for Cohort B from the Phase 3 PROfound Trial of Olaparib. *Eur. Urol.* **2021**, *79*, 442–445. [CrossRef]
150. Schiewer, M.J.; Mandigo, A.C.; Gordon, N.; Huang, F.; Gaur, S.; de Leeuw, R.; Zhao, S.G.; Evans, J.; Han, S.; Parsons, T.; et al. PARP-1 regulates DNA repair factor availability. *EMBO Mol. Med.* **2018**, *10*, e8816. [CrossRef]
151. Zimmermann, M.; Murina, O.; Reijns, M.A.M.; Agathanggelou, A.; Challis, R.; Tarnauskaitė, Ž.; Muir, M.; Fluteau, A.; Aregger, M.; McEwan, A.; et al. CRISPR screens identify genomic ribonucleotides as a source of PARP-trapping lesions. *Nature* **2018**, *559*, 285–289. [CrossRef]

152. Kan, C.; Zhang, J. BRCA1 Mutation: A Predictive Marker for Radiation Therapy? *Int. J. Radiat. Oncol. Biol. Phys.* **2015**, *93*, 281–293. [CrossRef]
153. Vallard, A.; Magné, N.; Guy, J.B.; Espenel, S.; Rancoule, C.; Diao, P.; Deutsch, E.; Rivera, S.; Chargari, C. Is breast-conserving therapy adequate in BRCA 1/2 mutation carriers? The radiation oncologist's point of view. *Br. J. Radiol.* **2019**, *92*, 20170657. [CrossRef]
154. Césaire, M.; Thariat, J.; Candéias, S.M.; Stefan, D.; Saintigny, Y.; Chevalier, F. Combining PARP inhibition, radiation, and immunotherapy: A possible strategy to improve the treatment of cancer? *Int. J. Mol. Sci.* **2018**, *19*, 3793. [CrossRef]
155. Barcellini, A.; Loap, P.; Murata, K.; Villa, R.; Kirova, Y.; Okonogi, N.; Orlandi, E. PARP Inhibitors in Combination with Radiotherapy: To Do or Not to Do? *Cancers* **2021**, *13*, 5380. [CrossRef]
156. Chargari, C.; Levy, A.; Paoletti, X.; Soria, J.C.; Massard, C.; Weichselbaum, R.R.; Deutsch, E. Methodological Development of Combination Drug and Radiotherapy in Basic and Clinical Research. *Clin. Cancer Res.* **2020**, *26*, 4723–4736. [CrossRef]
157. Schneider, G.; Schmidt-Supprian, M.; Rad, R.; Saur, D. Tissue-specific tumorigenesis: Context matters. *Nat. Rev. Cancer* **2017**, *17*, 239–253. [CrossRef]
158. Martin, S.A.; Hewish, M.; Lord, C.J.; Ashworth, A. Genomic instability and the selection of treatments for cancer. *J. Pathol.* **2010**, *220*, 281–289. [CrossRef]
159. Du, Q.; Bert, S.A.; Armstrong, N.J.; Caldon, C.E.; Song, J.Z.; Nair, S.S.; Gould, C.M.; Luu, P.L.; Peters, T.; Khoury, A.; et al. Replication timing and epigenome remodelling are associated with the nature of chromosomal rearrangements in cancer. *Nat. Commun.* **2019**, *10*, 416. [CrossRef]
160. Yi, K.; Ju, Y.S. Patterns and mechanisms of structural variations in human cancer. *Exp. Mol. Med.* **2018**, *50*, 1–11. [CrossRef]
161. Mirzaei, G.; Petreaca, R.C. Distribution of copy number variations and rearrangement endpoints in human cancers with a review of literature. *Mutat. Res.* **2022**, *824*, 111773. [CrossRef]
162. Mirzaei, G. GraphChrom: A Novel Graph-Based Framework for Cancer Classification Using Chromosomal Rearrangement Endpoints. *Cancers* **2022**, *14*, 3060. [CrossRef]
163. Rodriguez-Martin, B.; Alvarez, E.G.; Baez-Ortega, A.; Zamora, J.; Supek, F.; Demeulemeester, J.; Santamarina, M.; Ju, Y.S.; Temes, J.; Garcia-Souto, D.; et al. Pan-cancer analysis of whole genomes identifies driver rearrangements promoted by LINE-1 retrotransposition. *Nat. Genet.* **2020**, *52*, 306–319. [CrossRef]
164. Polansky, H.; Schwab, H. How latent viruses cause breast cancer: An explanation based on the microcompetition model. *Bosn. J. Basic Med. Sci.* **2019**, *19*, 221–226. [CrossRef] [PubMed]

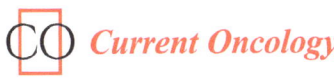

Article

High Neuroticism Is Related to More Overall Functional Problems and Lower Function Scores in Men Who Had Surgery for Non-Relapsing Prostate Cancer

Alv A. Dahl [1,*] and Sophie D. Fosså [1,2]

1. Department of Oncology, National Resource Center for Late Effects after Cancer Treatment, Oslo University Hospital, N-0424 Oslo, Norway
2. Faculty of Medicine, University of Oslo, N-0318 Oslo, Norway
* Correspondence: alvdah@ous-hf.no; Tel.: +47-22-934-909; Fax: +47-22-934-553

Abstract: The personality trait of neuroticism is associated with adverse health outcomes after cancer treatment, but few studies concern men treated for prostate cancer. We examined men with high and low neuroticism treated with radical prostatectomy for curable prostate cancer without relapse. We compared overall problems and domain summary scores (DSSs) between these groups, and if high neuroticism at pre-treatment was a significant predictor of overall problems and DSSs at follow-up. A sample of 462 relapse-free Norwegian men self-rated neuroticism, overall problems, and DSSs by the EPIC-26 before surgery and at three years' follow-up. Twenty-one percent of the sample had high neuroticism. Patients with high neuroticism reported significantly more overall problems and DSSs at pre-treatment. At follow-up, only overall bowel problems and urinary irritation/obstruction and bowel DSSs were different. High neuroticism was a significant predictor of overall bowel problems and bowel and irritation/obstruction DSSs at follow-up. High neuroticism at pre-treatment was significantly associated with a higher rate of overall problems both at pre-treatment and follow-up and had some significant predictions concerning bowel problems and urinary obstruction at follow-up. Screening for neuroticism at pre-treatment could identify patients in need of more counseling concerning later adverse health outcomes.

Keywords: prostate cancer; neuroticism; radical prostatectomy; overall problems; prospective study; generalized estimation equations

1. Introduction

After cancer therapy, patient-reported outcome measures (PROMs) of dysfunctions and associated problems (bother), often combined as adverse health outcomes (AHOs), have become increasingly popular as a supplement to doctors' evaluations. Concerning PROMs for men with prostate cancer (PCa), two international working groups have recommended the use of the Expanded Prostate Cancer Index Composite 26-question Short Form (EPIC-26) [1,2].

PROMs cover the personal subjective health experiences of the patients. These experiences are influenced by their daily health-related activities and their current mental functioning. Personality represents a major element of such functioning, regularly defined as "enduring patterns of perceiving, relating to, and thinking about the environment and oneself" [3]. Personality traits are prominent aspects of personality, and after being established in adolescence, they remain relatively stable over time and various life situations as characteristic patterns of coping and interpersonal functioning [3]. Modern personality theory defines five basic personality traits, which are established during childhood and adolescence and remain stable during the rest of life. However, recent research implies that basic traits may be modified by interventions or traumas like cancer [4,5]. Neuroticism is the most important basic trait concerning health and disease and is defined as follows:

"Neuroticism is the propensity to experience negative emotions, including anxiety, fear sadness, anger, guilt, disgust, irritability, loneliness, worry, self-consciousness, dissatisfaction, hostility, embarrassment, reduced self-confidence, and feelings of vulnerability, in reaction to various types of stress" [6]. Neuroticism has a skewed distribution in the general population, with 11 to 20% of males having high neuroticism depending on the cut-off level applied [7].

In the general population, a high neuroticism score predisposes to many somatic diseases, mental disorders, and premature death [8–10]. High neuroticism is also a predictor of emotional distress in cancer patients a year after diagnosis, but none of these studies concerned PCa patients [11].

Despite its obvious relevance for PCa patients, the relation between neuroticism and AHOs after surgery is covered by few studies. One prospective study by our research group showed that some neuroticism versus no neuroticism at pre-treatment predicted increased sexual bother (problems) one year after radical prostatectomy (RP) [12]. Another of our prospective studies concerned men treated with robot-assisted prostatectomy (RALP) or radiotherapy. At follow-up 24 months post-treatment, multivariate analyses showed that higher neuroticism at pre-treatment was significantly associated with urinary bother, a trend for significance with sexual bother, and no significant association with bowel bother [13].

No prospective studies known to us of PCa patients treated with RP have examined the impact of pre-treatment high neuroticism on patient-rated overall problems or domain summary scores (DSSs) at pre-treatment and at several years' follow-up. To fill this gap available pre-treatment and three years' post-treatment EPIC-26 overall problem ratings and DSSs were analyzed related to high and low levels of neuroticism at pre-treatment. We asked the following research questions: (1) Do men with high versus low neuroticism report more overall problems or significantly lower (worse) DSSs at both time points? (2) Is high neuroticism at pre-treatment a significant predictor of overall problems and DSSs three years after RP?

2. Material and Methods

2.1. Design

This multicenter study had a longitudinal design and attempted to evaluate AHOs prospectively after RP and radiotherapy. Between November 2008 and December 2009, PCa patients with planned RP were included in the Norwegian Urinary Cancer Group (NUCG) VII study for PCa [12]. Men aged ≤80 years at diagnosis and with no adjuvant treatment were eligible. We had no data on the type of RP performed in the individual patients, but most of them had been operated with an open approach without attempts at nerve sparing.

Neuroticism at pre-treatment and the AHOs at several time points were based on responses to a questionnaire. The questionnaire was completed before RP (pre-treatment), and patients completed mailed questionnaires one and three years after RP. In order to study the long-term effects, we only present findings from the pre-treatment and from the three years' follow-up evaluations.

2.2. Scales

The EPIC-26 is a PROM for rating PCa-related AHOs of the *last four weeks* covering urinary, bowel, sexual, and hormonal functional domains with four to six items each [14,15], but the last domain was omitted due to lack of hormone treatment of the sample. The EPIC-26 covers different degrees of dysfunction but also contains three items by which the patients rate their overall urinary, bowel, and sexual problems (Q5, Q7, and Q12). The overall problems and 20 other EPIC-26 items (Q1-Q13e) measuring dysfunctions had five scoring alternatives that are from zero to 100 points: "None" (100), "Very Small" (75), "Small" (50), "Moderate" (25), and "Big" (0). These ratings were dichotomized as "Hardly any problem" (scores 100 and 75, defined as reference) and "Problem present" (scores 50 to 0). Three EPIC-26 items (Q2, Q3, and Q9) had four scoring alternatives:

"No dysfunction/no pad use" (100), "Occasional dysfunction/one pad per day" (67), "Frequent dysfunction/two pads per day" (33), and "Always dysfunction/three or more pads" (0), which were dichotomized as "Hardly any problem/dysfunction" (scores 100 and 67, reference) and "Problem" (scores 33 and 0).

We also calculated the DSSs of the urinary incontinence and irritation/obstruction, bowel, and sexual domains at pre-treatment and follow-up. Lower DSSs imply more dysfunction.

Neuroticism was measured by the patients' responses to an abbreviated version of the Eysenck Personality Questionnaire (EPQ-18) using six items with responses of "yes" (1) and "no" (0) [16]. (See Supplementary Materials). Based on the right-skewed distribution of the sum score, we defined "high neuroticism" by scores 2–6 and "low neuroticism" by scores 0–1. This resulted in a group of 97 patients (21%) with high neuroticism and 365 (79%) with low neuroticism (reference). Cronbach's coefficient alpha for neuroticism was 0.72.

2.3. Other Variables

The patients rated their *level of education* [≤12 years (short) versus >12 years (long, reference)], *relationship status* (paired (reference) versus non-paired), *work status* (paid work versus pensioned), and *co-morbidity* classified as zero (reference), one, or two or more coexisting somatic disease(s) among those listed in the EPIC-50 [17]. Based on data from the patients' medical records, three *risk groups* were defined, and low risk was referenced [18]. *Nerve sparing* of unilateral or bilateral neurovascular bundles was identified, and no nerve sparing was referenced.

2.4. Statistics

Descriptive statistics: Continuous variables were analyzed with *t*-tests and Mann–Whitney tests in case of skewed distributions. Categorical variables were analyzed with Fisher's exact tests.

Generalized estimation equations (GEEs) were used to identify independent pre-treatment variables that were significant predictors of the rates of overall problems and the DSSs. The GEE is a multivariate binary logistic (overall problems present/absent) or linear regression (DSSs) model of dependent variables at follow-up, examining associations with independent variables assessed at pre-treatment [19]. Independent variables examined in the GEE were significantly associated with overall problems or DSSs at follow-up: age at pre-treatment, D'Amico risk groups, nerve sparing, neuroticism, not living with partner, co-morbidity, and EPIC-26 overall problem rates and DSSs at pre-treatment. Since age at diagnosis correlated highly with work status, the latter variable was not included in the GEE analyses. The strength of associations in the GEE analyses was expressed by beta coefficients with 95%CIs [19].

The level of significance was set to *p*-values < 0.05, and all tests were two-sided. The data were analyzed with SPSS for PC version 26 (IBM, Armonk, NY, USA).

3. Results

3.1. Patients

In all, 688 patients had RP, and among them, 675 completed the neuroticism part of the questionnaire at pre-treatment. At three years' follow-up, 13 patients were deceased, and 551 (83%) delivered new questionnaires. Since biochemical relapse (having two or more PSA-values of >0.2 µg/L after RP) [20] implied additional treatment with radiotherapy and/or hormones, 89 (16%) men who relapsed before follow-up were omitted from the analyses. The sample examined therefore consisted of 462 men.

3.2. Rate of High Neuroticism

According to our definition 97 men had high neuroticism (21.0%, 95%, CI 17.3–24.7%), and 365 men had low neuroticism.

3.3. Cross-Sectional Comparisons between the Neuroticism Groups

Table 1 (left part) displays the differences between the high and low neuroticism groups at pre-treatment. No significant between-group differences were observed for PCa-related, socio-demographic, or health-related variables, and the same was observed at follow-up (Table 1, right part).

Table 1. Characteristics of the high and low neuroticism groups at pre-treatment and follow-up (N = 462).

Variables	Pre-Treatment			Follow-Up		
	High Neuroticism N = 97	Low Neuroticism N = 365	p	High Neuroticism N = 97	Low Neuroticism N = 365	p
Age at diagnosis, mean (SD)	62.3 (5.2)	62.9 (5.4)	0.29			
Age at survey, mean (SD)				65.4 (5.1)	66.0 (5.4)	0.30
Follow-up time, mean (SD)				3.1 (0.3)	3.1 (0.4)	0.87
D'Amico categories, N (%)			0.46			
Low risk	15 (15)	73 (20)				
Intermediate risk	59 (61)	198 (54)				
High risk	23 (24)	94 (26)				
Nerve sparing			0.10			
None	36 (37)	166 (46)				
Unilateral	34 (35)	89 (24)				
Bilateral	27 (28)	108 (30)				
>12 years' education, N (%)	51 (53)	196 (54)	0.25			
Living with partner, N (%)	82 (85)	320 (91)	0.08			
Work status, N (%)			0.75			
Paid work	59 (62)	213 (60)				
Pensioned	37 (38)	144 (40)				
Co-morbidity, N (%)			0.48			0.56
None	59 (62)	245 (68)		79 (81)	300 (82)	
1 disease	30 (32)	92 (25)		14 (14)	57 (16)	
≥2 diseases	6 (6)	25 (7)		4 (5)	8 (2)	

At pre-treatment, the high neuroticism group had significantly higher rates of overall urinary and sexual problems, but not overall bowel problem compared to the low neuroticism group (Table 2, left part). All DSSs were also significantly lower in the high neuroticism group. The high neuroticism patients reported significantly more dysfunction problems on most of the urinary and sexual items and some of the bowel items than men in the low neuroticism group.

At follow-up, patients of the high neuroticism group reported significantly higher rates of overall bowel problems and more problems on most bowel items compared to the low neuroticism group (Table 2, right part). Overall urinary and sexual problems did not show significant between-group differences with few significant differences in the problems on the single items scores of these domains. The irritation/obstruction and bowel DSSs were significantly lower at follow-up in the high neuroticism group, while no significant differences were observed concerning the DSSS of urinary leakage or sexual domain.

Table 2. EPIC-26 rates of problems and DSSs of the high and low neuroticism groups at pre-treatment and follow-up (N = 462).

Variables	Pre-Treatment			Follow-Up		
EPIC-26 Problems, N (%)	High Neuroticism N = 97	Low Neuroticism N = 365	p	High Neuroticism N = 97	Low Neuroticism N = 365	p
Urinary domain						
Leakage (Q1)	15 (16)	18 (5)	<0.001	45 (47)	138 (39)	0.134
Lack of control (Q2)	1 (1)	5 (1)	0.791	11 (12)	29 (8)	0.300
Pad use (Q3)	3 (3)	0 (0)	0.009	17 (18)	53 (15)	0.479
Dripping (Q4a)	11 (12)	15 (4)	0.008	34 (36)	101 (29)	0.166
Pain (Q4b)	8 (8)	9 (3)	0.009	9 (10)	10 (3)	0.004
Bleeding (Q4c)	1 (1)	3 (1)	0.860	6 (6)	12 (3)	0.195
Weak stream (Q4d)	41 (44)	104 (30)	0.012	22 (23)	54 (15)	0.066
Frequent need (Q4e)	51 (53)	135 (38)	0.009	44 (46)	115 (32)	0.012
Urinary problem (Q5)	38 (40)	88 (25)	0.004	32 (34)	103 (29)	0.378
Bowel domain						
Urgency (Q6a)	7 (7)	11 (3)	0.061	8 (8)	7 (2)	0.002
Increased frequency (Q6b)	13 (14)	17 (5)	0.002	7 (7)	13 (4)	0.129
Loss of control (Q6c)	3 (3)	4 (1)	0.161	7 (7)	4 (1)	0.001
Bloody stools (Q6d)	1 (1)	5 (1)	0.779	4 (4)	3 (1)	0.020
Pain (Q6e)	15 (16)	22 (6)	0.003	16 (17)	13 (4)	<0.001
Bowel problem (Q7)	12 (12)	24 (7)	0.062	13 (14)	22 (6)	0.015
Sexual domain						
Erectile problem (Q8a)	59 (63)	178 (49)	0.018	80 (85)	303 (89)	0.359
Orgasmic problem (Q8b)	57 (61)	149 (41)	0.001	72 (77)	248 (73)	0.428
Poor quality erections (Q9)	18 (19)	42 (12)	0.068	61 (65)	190 (56)	0.105
Infrequent erections (Q10)	37 (39)	83 (23)	0.002	72 (77)	244 (71)	0.313
Poor sexual function (Q11)	70 (75)	227 (62)	0.028	87 (93)	304 (89)	0.301
Sexual problem (Q12)	48 (51)	130 (36)	0.008	66 (70)	248 (70)	0.889
EPIC-26 DSSs (SD)						
Urinary leakage	82.0 (16.4)	86.1 (9.8)	<0.001	68.8 (26.8)	73.5 (27.0)	0.067
Urinary irritation/obstruct	77.6 (17.1)	84.0 (15.3)	<0.001	82.8 (16.1)	89.2 (13.8)	<0.001
Bowel domain	92.9 (12.1)	96.0 (8.1)	0.018	92.3 (14.3)	96.8 (7.1)	0.003
Sexual domain	57.9 (27.4)	69.7 (29.7)	0.001	28.0 (30.2)	32.3 (29.3)	0.214

3.4. Predictors for Overall Problem Rates and Mean Scores at Follow-Up

For both overall urinary, bowel, and sexual problems at follow-up, corresponding problems at pre-treatment were the strongest significant positive predictors (Table 3). In addition, at follow-up, high neuroticism predicted more bowel problems and bilateral nerve sparing less sexual problems with no nerve sparing as reference.

Concerning all DSSs at follow-up, the corresponding DSSs at pre-treatment again were the strongest significant positive predictors (Table 4). High neuroticism was a significant predictor of lower urinary irritation/obstruction and bowel DSSs at follow-up. Younger age was a significant predictor of lower urinary leakage DSSs/High D'Amico risk group and bilateral nerve sparing were significant predictors of better sexual DSSs compared to their references at follow-up. Younger age at diagnosis was a significant predictor of less severe urinary leakage and sexual DSSs.

Table 3. General estimating equations (GEEs) estimates of predictors of overall problem present at 3-year follow-up.

Variables	Overall Urinary Problem Present B 95%CI Wald p	Overall Bowel Problem Present B 95%CI Wald p	Overall Sexual Problem Present B 95%CI Wald p
D'Amico risk groups			
Low (reference)	0.0	0.0	0.0
Intermediate	0.17 −0.42–0.75 0.58	−0.43 −1.38–0.51 0.37	0.20 −0.34–0.73 0.47
High	0.43 −0.24–1.09 0.21	−1.03 −2.20–0.15 0.09	−0.10 −0.73–0.53 0.76
Nerve sparing			
None (reference)	0.0	0.0	0.0
Unilateral	−0.40 −0.94–0.15 0.15	0.16 −0.72–1.04 0.72	−0.17 −0.68–0.35 0.53
Bilateral	0.32 −0.19–0.83 0.21	−0.14 −1.08–0.80 0.77	−0.68 −1.20–−0.16 0.01
Non-paired relation	0.31 −0.38–0.99 0.38	0.44 −0.76–1.64 0.47	−0.34 −1.00–0.32 0.32
Short education	−0.04 −0.49–0.42 0.87	−0.60 −1.43–0.24 0.16	−0.13 −0.57–0.30 0.55
Age at diagnosis	0.01 −0.03–0.05 0.60	0.05 −0.03–0.12 0.19	0.01 −0.04–0.05 0.77
High neuroticism	0.12 −0.40–0.64 0.65	0.87 0.05–1.69 0.04	−0.14 −0.68–0.40 0.61
Co-morbidity			
None (reference)	0.0	0.0	0.0
1 disease	−0.39 −0.90–0.13 0.14	−0.14 −0.98–0.70 0.74	0.44 −0.07–0.94 0.09
≥2 diseases	−0.50 −1.36–0.37 0.26	−0.11 −1.17–0.95 0.84	−0.04 −0.92–2.81 0.93
Problem at pre-treatment	0.64 0.16–1.11 0.009	2.63 1.64–3.62 <0.001	1.01 0.52–1.50 <0.001

Table 4. General estimating equations (GEEs) estimates of predictors of domain summary scores (DSSs) at 3-year follow-up.

Variables	Urinary Leakage Symptom Domain Score B 95%CI Wald p	Urinary Irritation/Obstruction Symptom Domain Score B 95%CI Wald p	Bowel Symptom Domain Score B 95%CI Wald p	Sexual Symptom Domain Score B 95%CI Wald p
D'Amico risk groups				
Low (reference)	0.0	0.0	0.0	0.0
Intermediate	−1.81 −8.58–4.97 0.60	−0.70 −3.88–2.50 0.67	1.49 −0.51–3.50 0.15	−2.58 −11.47–2.16 0.18
High	−1.25 −9.16–6.66 0.76	−1.11 −4.60–2.38 0.53	1.75 −0.42–3.93 0.11	−9.13 −16.91–1.36 0.02
Nerve sparing				
None	0.0	0.0	0.0	0.0
Unilateral	0.86 −5.13–6.85 0.78	−1.08 −4.14–1.97 0.49	1.09 −0.86–3.30 0.28	−5.63 −11.60–0.33 0.06
Bilateral	−4.55 −11.04–1.94 0.17	−1.39 −4.73–1.96 0.42	0.87 −0.79–2.52 0.30	−6.64 −12.52–−0.77 0.03
Non-paired relation	−6.05 −15.14–3.04 0.19	−5.32 −9.87–−0.76 0.022	−1.94 −5.76–1.88 0.32	−2.23 −10.36–5.89 0.59
Short education	0.53 −4.69–5.74 0.84	−2.23 −4.89–0.44 0.10	1.15 −0.41–2.70 0.15	−1.44 −6.50–3.62 0.58
Age at diagnosis	−0.63 −1.12–−0.15 0.01	−0.01 −0.24–0.2 0.90	−0.04 −0.16–0.08 0.56	−0.95 −1.46–−0.44 <0.001
High neuroticism	−2.61 −8.37–3.14 0.37	−4.16 −7.74–0.58 0.023	−2.88 −5.07–−0.69 0.01	1.37 −4.95–7.70 0.67
Co-morbidity				
None (reference)	0.0	0.0	0.0	0.0
1 disease	3.69 −2.26–9.64 0.22	2.33 −0.75–5.41 0.14	−0.98 −2.71–0.75 0.27	−2.99 −11.50–5.52 0.49
≥2 diseases	6.00 −1.86–13.86 0.14	−2.87 −7.70–1.95 0.24	−3.20 −6.53–0.13 0.06	−0.41 −8.46–7.64 0.92
DSS at pre-treatment	0.39 0.12–0.66 0.005	0.23 0.12–0.34 <0.001	0.50 0.35–0.66 <0.001	0.45 0.36–0.55 <0.001

4. Discussion

In our sample, 21% of the men who had RP for PCa reported high neuroticism at pre-treatment. Related to our research questions we first observed that men with high neuroticism at pre-treatment reported significantly higher rates of overall urinary and sexual problems, while the difference for bowel problems was close to significant ($p = 0.06$). Significant between-group differences were found for most urinary and sexual items, and for some bowel items. All pre-treatment DSSs were significantly lower (worse) in the high neuroticism group.

At follow-up, those with high neuroticism had significantly more overall bowel problems, while the differences were non-significant for overall urinary and sexual problems and their corresponding items. The high neuroticism group also had lower bowel and urinary irritation/obstruction DSSs. For all overall problems and all DSSs at follow-up, the corresponding measures at pre-treatment were significant positive predictors. High neuroticism at pre-treatment predicted more overall bowel problems and worse bowel and irritation/obstruction DSSs at follow-up.

The predictive power of pre-treatment sexual function, age, and nerve sparing for erectile function two years after RP has been demonstrated previously [21]. Pre-treatment overall sexual problems significantly predicted the same measure after more than a year of follow-up in men who had RP [22]. As to the number of patients with overall urinary and bowel problems and urinary- and bowel-related DSSs after RP, we found no predictive studies of the corresponding pre-treatment measurements. However, in combined samples of patients treated with RP or radiotherapy, pre-treatment overall problems and DSSs were predictive of these variables two years later [13,23]. We confirmed that older age at diagnosis was a significant predictor of worse urinary leakage and worse sexuality after RP [24].

Compared to our previous prospective study of neuroticism in men treated with RP and radiotherapy at 24 months' follow-up for localized PCA [13], the present study supplements at three years' follow-up that overall problems and DSSs at pre-treatment were significant predictors of these variables at three years' follow-up. In another previous paper presenting findings from the NUCG VII study, our group reported that "any neuroticism" at pre-treatment was a significant predictor of overall sexual problems (bother) at one-year follow-up [12], and a similar prediction was not observed by the current study at three years' follow-up. However, that study used a cut-off ≥ 1 for "any neuroticism", giving a prevalence of 41%, while we used a cut-off ≥ 2 with a prevalence of 21% for "high neuroticism". Use of different statistical methods for predictor analyses in that paper and the present study could also explain why the findings differ.

An interesting finding is that overall sexual problems and most functional sexual issues are significantly more common at pre-treatment in the high neuroticism versus the low neuroticism group. However, at follow-up, these group differences are non-significant. Our tentative explanation is that sexual problems and functions at pre-treatment are mostly determined by psychological factors, i.e., neuroticism and corresponding anxiety and depression [10]. After RP, anatomical factors become much stronger, and therefore, the between-group differences become non-significant at follow-up. We presume that the same explanation also can be applied to the findings concerning urinary problems and functions.

In contrast, the rate of overall bowel problems remained associated with high neuroticism, which then can be viewed as a significant predictor of such problems. The explanation could be that the bowel system hardly is affected by the anatomical changes of RP leaving more influence on high neuroticism. Another explanation could be the fact that bowel function is strongly influenced by mental factors through the so-called "bladder–gut–brain" axis [25]. However, the proportions of men with overall bowel problems are <8% of the sample both at pre-treatment and follow-up, casting doubt on the validity of this finding.

Other studies of neuroticism in PCa patients have cross-sectional designs. Perry et al. [26] demonstrated that emotional distress, depression, and suicidal ideation were significantly associated with high neuroticism in a heterogeneous PCa sample. Gerhart et al. [27] found that men with PCa and high neuroticism showed more depression, anxiety, and worry compared to men with low neuroticism. However, none of these studies included analyses of overall problems (bother). As to pre-treatment findings on the EPIC-26 in men with PCa, a recent German study only reported on dysfunctional AOHs and not on overall problems [28].

Personality traits such as neuroticism, are rated as "how you *usually* behave, feel, or act" in contrast to transient states represented by anxiety and depression based on scores of the last 1–2 weeks. Personality traits are stable cognitive and emotional reaction patterns finally set during childhood and adolescence but somewhat modified later in life [4]. Recently, neuroticism and other basic personality traits are considered as more modifiable through psychological and pharmacological interventions and systematic training [5]. These findings give more optimism concerning modifications of high neuroticism and warrant referral of motivated patients to such interventions.

Since high neuroticism is significantly associated with overall problems and DSSs both at pre-treatment and follow-up, clinicians responsible for men after RP should be attentive to high neuroticism as a risk factor for increased problem experience. Eventually, urologists should consider if completion of a short screening PROM for neuroticism (see Supplementary Materials) should be part of the pre-operative evaluation procedure as a supplement to the EPIC-26. However, our findings also support the statement that having any overall problems or low DSSs at pre-treatment implies an increased risk for similar problems and DSSs three years later. This fact and identification of high neuroticism should be themes during the pre-treatment counseling of men with PCa.

Our study had a considerable sample size, and we also considered the prospective design, use of established PROMs with documented psychometric properties, and use of the GEE statistics as strengths of our study.

A limitation of our study was that the participants only rated neuroticism at pre-treatment and not at follow-up. Another limitation was that the psychological data were based on questionnaire responses rather than on psychological evaluation performed by interviews.

In conclusion, the current study only weakly supported high neuroticism as a predictor of overall bowel problems and bowel DSS at three years' follow-up. However, high neuroticism was significantly associated with higher overall problem rates and lower DSSs both at pre-treatment and follow-up. Screening for neuroticism could therefore be helpful for the clinicians in their pre-treatment counseling of PCa patients regarding overall problems and low DSSs after RP.

Supplementary Materials: The following supporting information can be downloaded at: https://www.mdpi.com/article/10.3390/curroncol29080459/s1, See Supplementary Materials File.

Author Contributions: S.D.F. designed the NUCG VII study, and she contributed significantly to the data collection and quality assurance at different time points. She also contributed significantly to the interpretation of data, and to drafting of the manuscript. A.A.D. analyzed and interpreted the data, and he drafted the different versions of the manuscript. All authors have read and agreed to the published version of the manuscript.

Funding: The NUCG VII study was funded by the South-Eastern Health Board of Norway, the Norwegian Cancer Society, and the Legacies of The Norwegian Radium Hospital foundation and the Norwegian Cancer Society.

Institutional Review Board Statement: The study was approved by the Regional Ethics Committee of Southern Norway (Reference No. 13605).

Informed Consent Statement: All participants gave written informed consent.

Data Availability Statement: According to Norwegian data legislation, the data of this study cannot be made generally available. Requests should be sent to the corresponding author.

Acknowledgments: The authors gratefully acknowledge the skillful support from the local collaborators at the 14 urological units.

Conflicts of Interest: The authors declare no conflict of interest.

References

1. Martin, N.E.; Masey, L.; Stowell, C.; Bangma, C.; Briganti, A.; Bill-Axelson, A.; Blute, M.; Catto, J.; Chen, R.C.; D'Amico, A.V.; et al. Defining a standard set of patient-centred outcomes for men with localized prostate cancer. *Eur. Urol.* **2015**, *67*, 460–467. [CrossRef] [PubMed]
2. Morgans, A.K.; van Bommel, A.C.; Stowell, C.; Abraham, J.A.; Basch, E.; Bekelman, J.E.; Berry, D.L.; Bossi, A.; Davis, I.D.; De Reijke, T.M.; et al. Development of a standardized set of patient-cantered outcomes for advanced prostate cancer: An international effort for a unified approach. *Eur. Urol.* **2015**, *68*, 891–898. [CrossRef] [PubMed]
3. American Psychiatric Association. *Diagnostic and Statistical Manual of Mental Disorders*, 5th ed.; American Psychiatric: Washington, DC, USA, 2013.
4. Roberts, B.W.; Yoon, H.J. Personality psychology. *Annu. Rev. Psychol.* **2022**, *73*, 489–516. [CrossRef] [PubMed]
5. Bleidorn, W.; Hill, P.L.; Hennecke, M.; Denissen, J.J.A.; Jokela, M.; Hopwood, C.J.; Jokela, M.; Kandler, C.; Lucas, R.E.; Luhmann, M.; et al. The policy relevance of personality traits. *Am. Psychol.* **2019**, *74*, 1056–1067. [CrossRef]
6. Jeronimus, B.F.; Kotov, R.; Riese, H.; Ormel, J. Neuroticism's prospective association with mental disorders halves after adjustment for baseline symptoms and psychiatric history, but the adjusted association hardly decay with time: A meta-analysis on 59 longitudinal/prospective studies with 443 313 participants. *Psychol. Med.* **2016**, *46*, 2883–2906.
7. Lahey, B.B. Public significance of neuroticism. *Am. Psychol.* **2009**, *64*, 241–256. [CrossRef]
8. Graham, E.K.; Rutsohn, J.P.; Turiano, N.A.; Bendayan, R.; Batterham, P.J.; Gerstorf, D.; Katz, M.J.; Reynolds, C.A.; Sharp, E.S.; Yoneda, T.B.; et al. Personality predicts mortality risk: An integrative data analysis of 15 international longitudinal studies. *J. Res. Pers.* **2017**, *70*, 174–186. [CrossRef]
9. Dahl, A.A. The link between personality problems and cancer. *Future Oncol.* **2010**, *6*, 691–707. [CrossRef]
10. Ormel, J.; Jeronimus, B.F.; Kotov, R.; Riese, H.; Bos, E.H.; Hankin, B.; Rosmalen, J.G.M.; Oldehinkel, A.J. Neuroticism and common mental disorders: Meaning and utility of a complex relationship. *Clin. Psychol. Rev.* **2013**, *33*, 686–697. [CrossRef]
11. Cook, S.A.; Salmon, P.; Hayes, G.; Byrne, A.; Fisher, P.L. Predictors of emotional distress a year or more after diagnosis of cancer: A systematic review of the literature. *Psycho-Oncology* **2018**, *27*, 791–801. [CrossRef]
12. Steinsvik, E.A.S.; Axcrona, K.; Dahl, A.A.; Eri, L.M.; Stensvold, A.; Fosså, S.D. Can sexual bother after radical prostatectomy be predicted preoperatively? Findings from a prospective national study of the relation between sexual function, activity, and bother. *BJU Int.* **2011**, *109*, 1366–1374. [CrossRef] [PubMed]
13. Stensvold, A.; Dahl, A.A.; Brennhovd, B.; Småstuen, M.C.; Fosså, S.D.; Lilleby, W.; Steinsvik, A.; Axcrona, K.; Smeland, S. Bother problems in prostate cancer patients after curative treatment. *Urol. Oncol.* **2013**, *31*, 1067–1078. [CrossRef] [PubMed]
14. Szymanski, K.M.; Wei, J.T.; Dunn, R.L. Development and validation of an abbreviated version of the Expanded Prostate Cancer Index Composite instrument for measuring health-related quality of life among prostate cancer survivors. *Urology* **2010**, *76*, 1245–1250. [CrossRef] [PubMed]
15. Axcrona, K.; Nilsson, R.; Brennhovd, B.; Sørebø, Ø.; Fosså, S.D.; Dahl, A.A. Psychometric properties of the Expanded Prostate Cancer Index Composite-26 instrument in a cohort of radical prostatectomy patients: Theoretical and practical examinations. *BMC Urol.* **2017**, *17*, 111. [CrossRef]
16. Grav, S.; Stordal, E.; Romild, U.K.; Hellzen, O. The relationship between neuroticism, extraversion, and depression in the HUNT study: In relation to age and gender. *Issues Ment. Health Nurs.* **2012**, *33*, 777–785. [CrossRef]
17. Wei, J.T.; Dunn, R.L.; Litwin, M.S. Development and validation of the Expanded Prostate Cancer Index Composite (EPIC) for comprehensive assessment of health-related quality of life in men with prostate cancer. *Urology* **2000**, *36*, 899–905. [CrossRef]
18. D'Amico, A.V.; Whittington, R.; Malkowicz, S.B.; Schultz, D.; Blank, K.; Broderick, G.A.; Tomaszewski, J.E.; Renshaw, A.A.; Kaplan, I.; Beard, C.J.; et al. Biochemical outcome after radical prostatectomy, external beam radiation therapy, or interstitial radiation therapy for clinically localized prostate cancer. *JAMA* **1998**, *280*, 969–974. [CrossRef]
19. Wang, M. Generalized estimating equations in longitudinal data analyses: A review and recent developments. *Adv. Stat.* **2014**, *2014*, 303728. [CrossRef]
20. Mottet, N.; Bellmunt, J.; Bolla, M.; Briers, E.; Cumberbatch, M.G.; De Santis, M.; Fossati, N.; Gross, T.; Henry, A.M.; Joniau, S.; et al. EAU-ESTRO-SIOG guidelines on prostate cancer. Part 1: Screening, diagnosis, and local treatment with curative intent. *Eur. Urol.* **2017**, *71*, 618–629. [CrossRef]
21. Alemozaffar, M.; Regan, M.M.; Cooperberg, M.R.; Wei, J.T.; Michalski, J.M.; Sandler, H.M.; Hembroff, L.; Sadetsky, N.; Saigal, C.S.; Litwin, M.S.; et al. Prediction of erectile function following treatment for prostate cancer. *JAMA* **2011**, *306*, 1205–1214. [CrossRef]
22. Kimura, M.; Banez, L.L.; Polascik, T.J.; Bernal, R.M.; Gerber, L.; Robertson, C.N.; Donatucci, C.F.; Moul, J.W. Sexual bother and function after radical prostatectomy: Predictors of sexual bother recovery in men despite persistent post-operative sexual dysfunction. *Andrology* **2013**, *1*, 256–1261. [CrossRef] [PubMed]
23. Stensvold, A.; Dahl, A.A.; Brennhovd, B.; Cvancarova, M.; Fosså, S.D.; Lilleby, W.; Axcrona, K.; Smeland, S. Methods for prospective studies of adverse effects as applied to prostate cancer patients treated with surgery or radiotherapy without hormones. *Prostate* **2012**, *72*, 668–676. [CrossRef] [PubMed]

24. Li, X.; Zhang, H.; Jia, H.; Wang, Y.; Song, Y.; Liao, L.; Zhang, X. Urinary continence outcomes of four years of follow-up and predictors of four years follow-up of early and late urinary continence in continence of patients undergoing robot-assisted radical prostatectomy. *BMC Urol.* **2020**, *20*, 29. [CrossRef] [PubMed]
25. Leue, C.; Kruimel, J.; Vrijens, D.; Masclee, A.; van Os, J.; van Koeveringe, C. Functional urological disorders: A sensitized defence response in the bladder-gut-brain axis. *Nat. Rev. Urol.* **2017**, *14*, 153–163. [CrossRef] [PubMed]
26. Perry, L.M.; Hoerger, M.; Silberstein, J. Understanding the distressed prostate cancer patient: Role of personality. *Psycho-Oncology* **2018**, *27*, 810–816. [CrossRef]
27. Gerhart, J.; Schmidt, E.; Lillis, T.; O'Mahony, S.; Duberstein, P.; Hoerger, M. Anger proneness and prognostic pessimism in men with prostate cancer. *Am. J. Hosp. Palliat. Med.* **2017**, *34*, 497–504. [CrossRef]
28. Roth, R.; Dieng, S.; Oesterle, A.; Feick, G.; Carl, G.; Hinkel, A.; Steiner, T.; Kaftan, B.T.; Kunath, F.; Hadaschik, B.; et al. Determinants of self-reported functional status (EPIC-26) in patients prior to treatment. *World J. Urol.* **2021**, *39*, 27–36. [CrossRef]

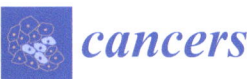

Review

A Treatment Paradigm Shift: Targeted Radionuclide Therapies for Metastatic Castrate Resistant Prostate Cancer

Ephraim E. Parent [1,*] and Adam M. Kase [2]

1. Department of Radiology, Mayo Clinic, 4500 San Pablo Road, Jacksonville, FL 32224, USA
2. Division of Hematology Oncology, Mayo Clinic, Jacksonville, FL 32224, USA
* Correspondence: parent.ephraim@mayo.edu

Simple Summary: Metastatic prostate cancer has traditionally been treated with a combination of hormonal and chemotherapy regimens. With the recent FDA approval of targeted radionuclide therapeutics, there is now a new class of therapy that is routinely available to patients and clinicians. This review explores the most commonly studied therapeutic radiopharmaceuticals and their appropriate use and contraindications. Additionally, we detail how these therapeutic radiopharmaceuticals can fit into the common medical oncology practice and future directions of this field of medicine.

Abstract: The recent approval of ^{177}Lu PSMA-617 (Pluvicto®) by the United States Food and Drug Administration (FDA) is the culmination of decades of work in advancing the field of targeted radionuclide therapy for metastatic prostate cancer. ^{177}Lu PSMA-617, along with the bone specific radiotherapeutic agent, ^{223}RaCl$_2$ (Xofigo®), are now commonly used in routine clinical care as a tertiary line of therapy for men with metastatic castrate resistant prostate cancer and for osseus metastatic disease respectively. While these radiopharmaceuticals are changing how metastatic prostate cancer is classified and treated, there is relatively little guidance to the practitioner and patient as to how best utilize these therapies, especially in conjunction with other more well-established regimens including hormonal, immunologic, and chemotherapeutic agents. This review article will go into detail about the mechanism and effectiveness of these radiopharmaceuticals and less well-known classes of targeted radionuclide radiopharmaceuticals including alpha emitting prostate specific membrane antigen (PSMA)-, gastrin-releasing peptide receptor (GRPR)-, and somatostatin targeted radionuclide therapeutics. Additionally, a thorough discussion of the clinical approach of these agents is included and required futures studies.

Keywords: prostate cancer; radionuclide therapy; bone; PSMA; GRPR; somatostatin

Citation: Parent, E.E.; Kase, A.M. A Treatment Paradigm Shift: Targeted Radionuclide Therapies for Metastatic Castrate Resistant Prostate Cancer. *Cancers* 2022, *14*, 4276. https://doi.org/10.3390/cancers14174276

Academic Editors: Paula A. Oliveira, Ana Faustino and Lúcio Lara Santos

Received: 1 August 2022
Accepted: 30 August 2022
Published: 1 September 2022

Publisher's Note: MDPI stays neutral with regard to jurisdictional claims in published maps and institutional affiliations.

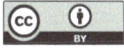

Copyright: © 2022 by the authors. Licensee MDPI, Basel, Switzerland. This article is an open access article distributed under the terms and conditions of the Creative Commons Attribution (CC BY) license (https://creativecommons.org/licenses/by/4.0/).

1. Introduction

Prostate cancer (PCa) is the second most common cancer among men in the United States, with one out of eight men diagnosed during their lifetime [1]. When identified early, patients with PCa can undergo highly curative therapy with definitive radical prostatectomy or radiotherapy. However, up to 30% of patients with PCa will eventually develop metastatic castration-resistant prostate cancer (mCRPC), as prostate cancer becomes androgen independent [2,3]. Despite androgen independence, androgen deprivation therapy remains the backbone of treatment, in addition to, bone modifying agents and cancer-directed therapy. Metastatic disease to the bone poses great morbidity with skeletal-related events and pain, overall, negatively impacting quality of life. Bone modifying agents such as bisphosphonates (zoledronic acid) and receptor activator of nuclear factor κ B ligand (RANKL) inhibitor (denosumab) are necessary in CRPC patients with bone metastases to prevent SREs which are known to increase the risk of death and reduce quality of life [4,5]. There are multiple cancer directed therapeutic options available that improve overall survival (OS) in mCRPC which include androgen signaling inhibitors (abiraterone, enalutamide), chemotherapy (docetaxel, cabazitaxel), autologous cellular immunotherapy (sipuleucel-T) and poly-ADP-ribose polymerase inhibitors (olaparib, rucaparib); however, despite these systemic therapies, mCRPC remains incurable [6]. Advances in the field of targeted radionuclide therapy for mCRPC has led to the widespread adoption of bone specific radionuclide therapy (^{223}Ra dichloride; Xofigo®) and prostate-specific membrane antigen (PSMA) targeted radiotherapy (^{177}Lu PSMA-617; Pluvicto®) (Table 1). In this review, we will discuss these United States Food and Drug Administration (FDA) approved radiotherapeutics for mCRPC and discuss other radionuclide therapies in development including alpha (α) emitting PSMA radiopharmaceuticals, gastrin-releasing peptide receptor (GRPC) targeted α/β emitting radiopharmaceuticals, and somatostatin targeted radionuclide therapy (^{177}Lu DOTATATE, Lutathera®).

Table 1. Pivotal Phase II/III studies leading to FDA approval of ^{223}RaCl$_2$ and ^{177}Lu PSMA-617.

^{223}RaCl$_2$			
Alpha Emitter Radium-223 and Survival in Metastatic Prostate Cancer (ALSYMPCA) [7]	^{223}RaCl$_2$ vs. placebo in mCRPC with bone metastasis	Phase III	^{223}RaCl$_2$ improved overall survival vs. placebo (median, 14.0 months vs. 11.2 months).
Addition of radium-223 to abiraterone acetate and prednisone or prednisolone in patients with castration-resistant prostate cancer and bone metastases (ERA 223) [8]	Abiraterone acetate + prednisone/prednisolone with ^{223}RaCl$_2$ vs. placebo	Phase III	Addition of ^{223}RaCl$_2$ did not improve symptomatic skeletal event-free survival and was associated with increasing frequency of fractures (9% vs. 3%).
Prospective Evaluation of Bone Metabolic Markers as Surrogate Markers of Response to Radium-223 Therapy in Metastatic Castration-resistant Prostate Cancer [9,10]	Enzalutamide + ^{223}RaCl$_2$ vs. enzalutamide alone	Phase II	Combination Enzalutamide + ^{223}RaCl$_2$ did not show increase in fractures or other adverse events and showed improved bone metabolic markers.
Radium-223 Safety, Efficacy, and Concurrent Use with Abiraterone or Enzalutamide: First U.S. Experience from an Expanded Access Program [11]	^{223}RaCl$_2$ + concurrent abiraterone acetate or enzalutamide	Phase II	Patients with less advanced disease (<3 prior therapies) were more likely to benefit from ^{223}RaCl$_2$
^{177}Lu PSMA-617			
Lutetium-177–PSMA-617 for Metastatic Castration-Resistant Prostate Cancer [12]	^{177}Lu PSMA-617 +SOC vs. SOC alone	Phase III	^{177}Lu PSMA-617 +SOC (compared to SOC alone) improved rPFS (median, 8.7 vs. 3.4 months) and OS (median, 15.3 vs. 11.3 months).
[^{177}Lu]Lu-PSMA-617 versus cabazitaxel in patients with metastatic castration-resistant prostate cancer (TheraP): a randomized, open-label, phase 2 trial [13].	^{177}Lu PSMA-617 vs. cabazitaxel	Phase III	^{177}Lu PSMA-617 arm had greater PSA response (65%) vs. cabazitaxel (37%) Grade 3–4 adverse events occurred in (33%) of 98 men in the ^{177}Lu PSMA-617 v 45 (53%) of 85 men in the cabazitaxel group.

2. Bone Specific Radiotherapeutics

Nearly 90% of patients with mCRPC will ultimately develop osseous metastatic disease leading to pain and negatively impacting quality of life [14]. There have been several alpha-(α) and beta-(β) emitting bone specific therapeutic radiopharmaceuticals for men with mCRPC in development over the years with ^{223}Radium dichloride (^{223}RaCl$_2$; Xofigo®) becoming the first FDA approved agent in prostate cancer in 2013. Compared to other radiopharmaceutical agents analogous to ^{223}RaCl$_2$, ^{223}RaCl$_2$ has an advantage due to its short half-life of 11.4 days and decay predominately through α-emission, allowing for high linear energy transfer (LET) and high amounts of double-stranded DNA breaks when in the decay pathway. Other previously utilized bone targeted radionuclides (phosphorus-32, samarium-153, strontium-89) decayed through β-emission which results in a lower LET and fewer DNA breaks [15]. ^{223}RaCl$_2$ physiologically behaves like calcium and forms complexes with bone matrix hydroxyapatite, preferentially being incorporated into areas of high bone turnover which is typically seen in osteoblastic bone metastases, the predominant form of osseous disease in patients with mCRPC [15]. ^{223}RaCl$_2$ is rapidly cleared from the blood with only 20% of the injected dose remaining in the blood 15 min after injection, and at 4 h 61% is localized to the skeleton with the remaining 39% in the bowel for subsequent fecal elimination. Given the fecal route of elimination, dose adjustments for patients with hepatic or renal dysfunction are not necessary. ^{223}RaCl$_2$ is administered intravenously at 55 KBq/kg every 4 weeks for 6 cycles. As ^{223}RaCl$_2$ decays via α particles, which have a negligible path length in air, patients can be immediately released to go home after administration.

The Alpharadin in Symptomatic Prostate Cancer Patients (ALSYMPCA) trial was a phase III randomized double-blind placebo-controlled trial with 921 patients who had symptomatic mCRPC with two or more bone metastases detected with skeletal scintigraphy and without evidence of visceral metastatic disease. Patients were enrolled to receive either ^{223}RaCl$_2$ every 4 weeks for 6 cycles or placebo, the study met the primary endpoint of an improved OS of 14.9 mo vs. 11.3 mo (Hazard ratio (HR) 0.70; 95% CI, 0.58 to 0.83; $p < 0.001$) [7]. Secondary endpoints including time to first symptomatic skeletal event (SSE), time to rise in alkaline phosphatase, and prostate specific antigen (PSA) progression were also improved in the ^{223}RaCl$_2$ arm and there were no significant differences in adverse events between the two groups. Perhaps more importantly, the quality of life was improved in the ^{223}RaCl$_2$ group based on validated instruments: EuroQol 5-dimentsion 5- level (EQ-5D) and Functional Assessment of Cancer Therapy-Prostate (FACT-P) [16]. A secondary reanalysis also found that patients on the ^{223}RaCl$_2$ arm also had fewer hospitalization days per patient (4.44 vs. 6.68; $p = 0.004$) in the first year after treatment and improvement in pain compared to the placebo group [17].

The FDA approved ^{223}RaCl$_2$ for the use in patients with mCRPC who have symptomatic bone metastases and no visceral disease. While this remains the primary indication for treatment with ^{223}RaCl$_2$, there have been several studies demonstrating that ^{223}RaCl$_2$ may also benefit men with asymptomatic bone disease. In a single arm prospective study with 708 patients, asymptomatic (n = 135, 19%) patients were more likely to complete therapy with ^{223}RaCl$_2$ compared to symptomatic (n = 548, 77%) patients; in addition, overall survival (HR 0.486), time to progression (HR 0.722), and time to first SSE (HR 0.328) were better in asymptomatic patients compared to symptomatic patients [18]. There have also been efforts to incorporate the use of ^{223}RaCl$_2$ in mCRPC patients with visceral metastases, given that most patients with mCRPC have a large component of bony disease regardless of their visceral involvement [14]. Assessing treatment response to ^{223}RaCl$_2$ with molecular imaging remains a challenge with commonly utilized bone specific radiopharmaceuticals (e.g., ^{99m}Tc methylene diphosphonate (MDP) as both benign healing and metastatic disease can have a similar presentation (Figure 1). Increases in PSA levels, which often portend progression of disease, are often seen with ^{223}RaCl$_2$ treatment and should not be relied upon in the decision to stop ^{223}RaCl$_2$ [19]. Additionally, while treatment with ^{223}RaCl$_2$ has been shown to lead to drops in alkaline phosphatase and lactate dehydrogenase levels, these markers are also not dependable to determine the effectiveness of ^{223}RaCl$_2$ [20]. As ^{223}RaCl$_2$ localizes to the bone marrow, blood counts should be monitored to ensure the absolute neutrophil count (ANC) is $\geq 1 \times 10^9$/L and platelets are $\geq 50 \times 10^9$/L before each treatment with ^{223}RaCl$_2$. If hematologic values do not recover 6–8 weeks after the last ^{223}RaCl$_2$ treatment, ^{223}RaCl$_2$ should be discontinued.

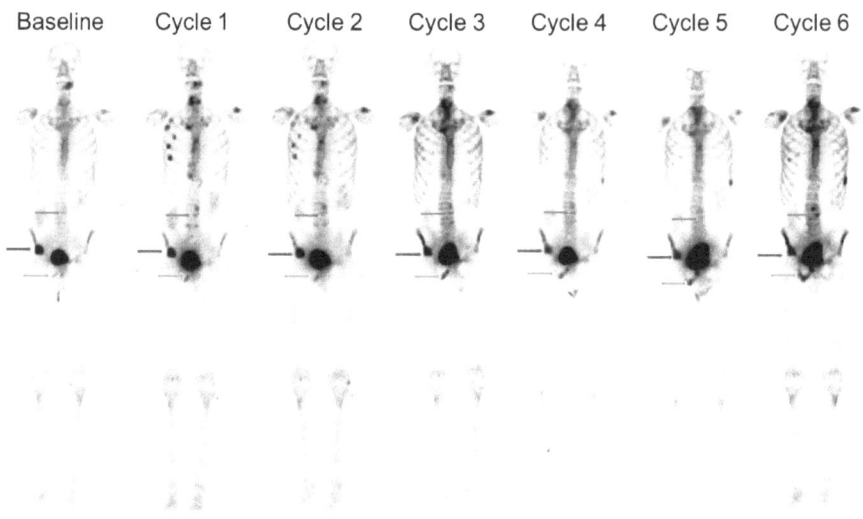

Figure 1. ^{99m}Tc MDP bone scintigraphy evaluation of ^{223}RaCl$_2$ therapy. Gleason score 4 + 3 = 7 prostate cancer undergoing serial ^{99m}Tc methylene diphosphonate (MDP) bone scans and with known osseous metastatic deposits (arrows) during treatment with 6 cycles of ^{223}RaCl. Patient is concurrently maintained on Lupron, and bone protective therapy with abiraterone and prednisone. At baseline prior to ^{223}RaCl$_2$, he was treated with oxycodone for pain control and had a baseline PSA of 10.9 ng/mL. Lack of quantitative measurements limits the standard planar evaluation of response to therapy. Serial MDP bone scintigraphy demonstrated some improvement in the right iliac metastatic deposit (red arrow) with ^{223}RaCl therapy but progressive disease in the right inferior pubic ramus (green arrow) and lumbar spine (blue arrow). Note right sided post traumatic rib fractures at cycle 1 and cycle 2.

3. Beta Emitting PSMA Targeted Radiotherapeutics

PSMA is a transmembrane glutamate carboxypeptidase that is highly expressed in prostate cancer and has become a leading target in diagnostic imaging and a powerful new therapeutic target. PSMA is expressed in more than 90% of metastatic PCa lesions and demonstrates higher expression with greater Gleason scores [21,22]. Given the differential expression of PSMA between PCa and normal tissues, small molecule PSMA targeted radiotherapeutics have been developed for prostate cancer, such as the FDA approved ^{177}Lu PSMA-617 (Pluvicto®) and the promising non-FDA approved ^{177}Lu PSMA I&T. The benefit of this targeted molecular therapy is based on the binding, internalization, and retention of the PSMA ligands within tumor cells [23].

^{177}Lu PSMA-617 was FDA approved on 23 March 2022 for the treatment of patients with PSMA-positive mCRPC and who have been treated with an androgen receptor (AR) pathway inhibitor and taxane-based chemotherapy [24]. PSMA PET is essential to identify patients with mCRPC who will benefit PSMA-targeted radioligand therapy (RLT) [25], with beta (e.g., Lu-177) or alpha (Ac-225) PSMA radiotherapeutics [26,27] (Figure 2). There are currently two FDA approved PSMA PET radiopharmaceuticals for patients with suspected prostate cancer metastasis who are candidates for initial definitive therapy or suspected recurrence based on elevated PSA levels: ^{68}Ga PSMA-11 (Ga 68 gozezotide, Illuccix®, Locametz®) and ^{18}F DCFPyL (Piflufolastat F 18, Pylarify®). The FDA package insert for ^{177}Lu PSMA-617 (Pluvicto®) specifies that patients selected for treatment must use the FDA approved PSMA PET radiopharmaceutical ^{68}Ga PSMA-11 (Illuccix®, Locametz®) to confirm the presence of PSMA-positive disease [24]. However, of note, NCCN guidelines state that PET imaging with either ^{68}Ga PSMA-11 or ^{18}F DCFPyL can be used to determine eligibility for ^{177}Lu PSMA-617 therapy [28]. Additionally, Novartis has announced a strategic collaboration with Lantheus to include ^{18}F DCFPyL in clinical trials with Lu PSMA-617 RLT, suggesting ^{18}F DCFPyL PET may be acceptable in the future prior to ^{177}Lu PSMA-617 RLT [29].

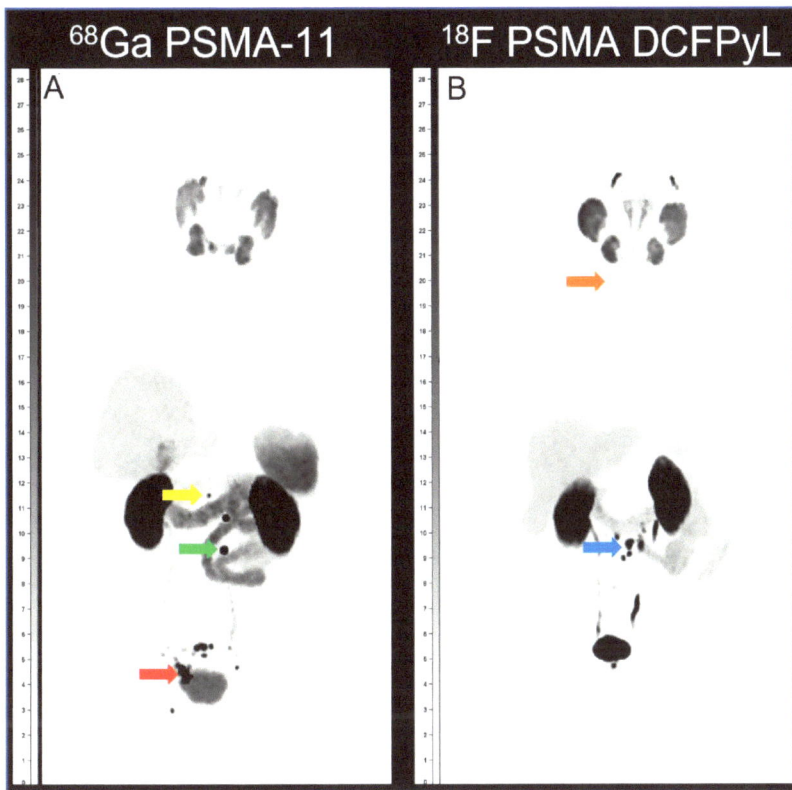

Figure 2. ^{68}Ga PSMA-11 and ^{18}F PSMA DCFPyL PET evaluation of mCRPC prior to ^{177}Lu PMSA-617 RLT. Two patients with mCRPC undergoing PSMA PET prior to ^{177}Lu PMSA-617 therapy. Patient A with Gleason score 3 + 4 = 7 prostate cancer status post prostatectomy, salvage radiation- and cryotherapy. PSA of 0.42 ng/mL at time of ^{68}Ga PSMA-11 PET/CT for evaluation prior to ^{177}Lu PSMA-617 therapy. Anterior view of ^{68}Ga PSMA-11 PET maximum intensity projection (MIP) (**A**) demonstrates intense PSMA uptake along the prostatectomy bed and rectum (red arrow) retroperitoneal and pelvic lymph nodes (green arrow) and osseous metastatic deposit involving the L1 vertebral body (yellow arrow). Patient B with Gleason 4 + 5 = 9 prostate cancer status post radiation therapy and androgen deprivation therapy, and PSA of 3 ng/mL. Anterior view MIP (**B**) demonstrates intense PSMA uptake along retroperitoneal lymph nodes (blue arrow). Incidental note of symmetric PSMA uptake along benign celiac ganglia (orange arrow).

Two major multicenter clinical trials, VISION (USA and Canada) and TheraP (Australia), investigated the outcome of patients with mCRPC after ablation with ^{177}Lu PSMA-617 [12,13]. The phase III VISION trial evaluated ^{177}Lu PSMA-617 in 831 patients with mCRPC and was the principal justification for FDA approval of ^{177}Lu PSMA-617 RLT. Primary outcomes measured radiographic progression-free survival (rPFS) and OS between ^{177}Lu PSMA-617 RLT plus SOC versus standard of care (SOC) alone. When compared to SOC alone, ^{177}Lu PSMA-617 plus SOC significantly prolonged rPFS (median, 8.7 vs. 3.4 months; HR for progression or death 0.40; 99.2% CI, 0.29 to 0.57) and median OS (15.3 vs. 11.3 months; HR for death, 0.62; 95% CI, 0.52 to 0.74; $p < 0.001$). The phase II TheraP trial, compared ^{177}Lu PSMA-617 to cabazitaxel in 200 men with mCRPC. The primary endpoint was PSA response defined by a reduction of PSA ≥ 50% from baseline. In contrast to the VISION trial, TheraP set PSMA SUVmax requirements of at least one lesion on ^{68}Ga-PSMA-11 PET with $SUV_{max} > 20$, and the remaining metastatic lesions $SUV_{max} > 10$, and no discordant hypermetabolic disease. PSA responses were more frequent among men in the ^{177}Lu PSMA-617 group versus the cabazitaxel group (66% vs. 37%, respectively).

The TheraP trial outcomes are considered superior to the VISION trial, likely as the result of exclusion of mCRPC patients with discordant hypermetabolic lesions. While the VISION trial used conventional imaging to exclude patients with discordant lesions (positive lesions on CT and negative on PSMA PET), the TheraP trial used functional techniques including ^{18}F-fludeoxyglucose (FDG) PET/CT in conjunction with PSMA PET/CT, and patients with at least one discordant hypermetabolic lesion, PSMA (−)/FDG (+), were excluded. Patients with mCRPC and with discordant hypermetabolic lesions have been shown to have worse outcomes and discordant hypermetabolic disease is often seen in a sizable minority of patients with mCRPC [30,31]. In a study of 56 patients, Chen et al. found that 23.2% had at least one PSMA (−)/FDG (+) lesion, and that PSA and Gleason score were both higher in these patients with discordant hypermetabolic disease [32]. A sub-analysis of a single center phase II trial of ^{177}Lu PSMA-617 RLT similarly found that 16/50 patients had at least one PSMA (−)/FDG (+) lesion and were deemed ineligible for ^{177}Lu PSMA-617 therapy. The OS of these patients with discordant hypermetabolic disease was 2.6 months (compared to 13.5 months for patients that received ^{177}Lu PSMA-617) [33].

While the FDA package insert for ^{177}Lu PSMA-617 does not specify any contraindications to therapy, the EANM guidelines have published contraindications for PSMA-RLT [26]. For the most part, these guidelines have mirrored the inclusions and exclusion criteria of large phase II/III trials such as VISION [12] and TheraP [13] with some minor variations. These contraindications include: (1) Life expectancy is less than 6 months and ECOG performance status > 2. (2) Unacceptable medical or radiation safety risk. (3) Unmanageable urinary tract obstruction or hydronephrosis. (4) Inadequate organ function (GFR < 30 mL/min or creatinine > 2-fold upper limit of normal (ULN); liver enzymes > 5-fold ULN). (5) Inadequate marrow function (with total white cell count less than 2.5×10^9/L or platelet count less than 75×10^9/L). (6) Conditions (e.g., spinal cord compression and unstable fractures) which require timely interventions (e.g., radiation therapy and surgery) and in which PSMA-RLT might be performed afterwards depending upon the patient's condition.

General radiation safety precautions should be followed with ^{177}Lu-PSMA RLT, with local and national guidelines dictating specific clinical practice. Radiation safety precautions may be modeled after ^{177}Lu-DOTATATE therapy for neuroendocrine tumors given a shared radionuclide [26,34]. A recent meta-analysis of ^{177}Lu PSMA-617 dosimetry found that the lacrimal and salivary glands are the critical organs with the kidneys also receiving a significant radiation dose [35]. The calculated radiation absorbed doses to the lacrimal and salivary glands after 4 cycles of ^{177}Lu PSMA-617 is near the tolerated dose limit whereas the dose to the kidneys is far below the dose tolerance limits. ^{177}Lu PSMA-617 has been shown to have a low, but significant, rate of adverse events (AE) in several clinical studies. In the phase III VISION study, 52.7% of patients experienced a grade 3 or higher AE, as compared to 38.0% of patients with similar events in the control group. Anemia was the most common grade ≥3 AE, observed in 12.9% of subjects. Additionally, a recently published meta-analysis of 250 studies with a total of 1192 patients similarly found that while grade 3 and 4 toxicities were uncommon, anemia was the highest reported adverse event for both ^{177}Lu PSMA-617 (0.19 [0.06–0.15]) and ^{177}Lu PSMA—I&T (0.09 [0.05–0.16]) [36]. Greater than 35% of patients in the treatment group of the VISION trial experienced fatigue, dry mouth, or nausea, though almost entirely grade ≤ 2 AE [12]. Adverse event incidence was similar to smaller early phase studies that preceded the VISION study [13,37–39].

4. Dosimetry and Future Developments of PSMA Targeted Radiotherapeutics

Utilizing dosimetry to tailor dosing to a patient's particular biology has potential to potentiate the benefits of ^{177}Lu PSMA-617 RLT. While the large TheraP [13] and VISION [12] trials employed a fixed dosing of 200 mCi (7.4 GBq), a small study demonstrated safety of dosing of up to 250 mCi (9.3 GBq) in selected cohorts [40]. In principle, a patient-centered dosing scheme can calculate a safe maximum tolerated activity and maximize radiation dose to tumors [41,42]. This need to augment ^{177}Lu PSMA-617 dosage is underscored by a study that showed that patients receiving less than 10 Gy to tumors were unlikely to achieve a PSA response ($\geq$50% PSA decline in pretreatment PSA) [43]. Additionally, recent studies have demonstrated a "tumor sink" effect, where patients with particularly high burden disease demonstrated reduced delivery of ^{68}Ga-PSMA-11 [44] or ^{177}Lu PSMA-617 [45] to target tissues. Unfortunately, the ability of the treating physician to prescribe a tailored dose of ^{177}Lu PSMA-617 to patients is currently almost non-existent in the United States, given the one-size-fits-all approach Novartis has employed of providing a fixed dose of 200 mCi per cycle of ^{177}Lu PSMA-617.

There are several open questions and innovations that promise to further extend the role of ^{177}Lu PSMA-617 in PCa. For example, the synergistic effects from combination therapies as well as the appropriate sequencing of the treatment in the disease course remain uncertain. Both VISION and TheraP were deployed late in mCRPC disease when patients have limited therapeutic options remaining. Both trials demonstrate ^{177}Lu-PSMA-617 RLT to be effective at improving clinical outcomes; however, patients may also benefit if therapy is employed earlier in their disease course. Several trials are currently underway in hopes of answering this question. The UpFrontPSMA and PSMAddition trials seek to determine the efficacy and safety of ^{177}Lu PSMA-617 in men with metastatic hormone-sensitive prostate cancer. Other trials are assessing ^{177}Lu PSMA-617 as first-line therapy for mCRPC or in the neoadjuvant setting for localized PCa.

5. Alpha Emitting PSMA Targeted Radiotherapeutics

Another area of emerging interest is the use of α emitting radioisotopes for PSMA targeted radiotherapy. Actinium-225 is an α emitting radioisotope that has been chelated to several PSMA chemical ligands, including PSMA-617 [46]. Kratochwil et al. [47] reported two patients who had complete responses to ^{225}Ac PSMA-617, including one who had previously progressed after ^{177}Lu PSMA-617 treatment. This initial report has been confirmed in several small case series [46,48]. Pooling 10 small studies together, a recent meta-analysis found a 62.8% PSA50 (decrease in PSA $\geq$50% compared to baseline) response rate for ^{225}Ac PSMA-617 [49]. Particular attention to evaluating ^{225}Ac PSMA-617 in mCRPC patients that have failed previous lines of therapy, including ^{177}Lu PSMA-617, is ongoing. The high LET and different microdosimetry in tumors exposed to α particles is seen to overcome cellular defences when resistance to β emitters (e.g., Lu-177) is found [50,51]. A retrospective analysis of 26 men with progressive mCRPC that had undergone several previous therapies, including ^{177}Lu PSMA-617, found that ^{225}Ac PSMA-617 resulted in a $\geq$50% PSA drop in 65% of patients [52], but with greater hemotoxicity and permanent xerostomia [46] than in patients with less advanced disease [53]. Of note, the short path length of α particles is especially valuable in the treatment of patients with extensive skeletal metastatic disease, with the goal of protecting the normal bone marrow from the AE seen with ^{177}Lu PSMA-617 as previously discussed [54]. In a retrospective study of patients treated with ^{225}Ac PSMA-617, 106 patients were found to have either multifocal ($\geq$20) skeletal metastases (n = 72, 67.9%), or a diffuse pattern of axial skeletal involvement with or without appendicular skeletal involvement (i.e., superscan pattern) on ^{68}Ga PSMA-11. Eighty-five of the 106 patients (80.2%) treated with ^{225}Ac PSMA-617 achieved a PSA response of $\geq$50% and had only rare hematologic toxicity with renal dysfunction being a significant risk factor [55]. As ^{225}Ac/ ^{177}Lu-PSMA radiopharmaceuticals have different benefits and risks, small trials have also incorporated a "tandem" therapy strategy with small doses of ^{225}Ac-PSMA being administered together with ^{177}Lu-PSMA and with promising results [56].

One major challenge in the clinical use of ^{225}Ac-PSMA beyond the scope of small research studies is the limited availability of the isotope itself, but there are many ongoing efforts to increase the global supply of ^{225}Ac and other α-emitting radioisotopes.

6. Gastrin-Releasing Peptide Receptor (GRPR) Targeted Radiotherapeutics

While efforts towards clinical applications of gastrin-releasing peptide receptor (GRPR) targeted radionuclide therapy are behind those of PSMA targeted radiopharmaceuticals, GRPR is a prime target for radionuclide therapy in men with mCRPC who may have failed β/α PSMA therapy. GRPR (also known as bombesin receptor 2 (BB2)) is a transmembrane receptor expressed on the surface of many cancers and is overexpressed in most PCa [57,58]. Bombesin is a 14-amino acid peptide agonist that binds with high affinity to GRPR and has been shown to increase the motility and metastatic potential of prostate cancer cells [59]. Many diagnostic and therapeutic radiopharmaceuticals have been developed using bombesin as the pharmaceutical core for targeted diagnostic and radiotherapeutic pairs for PCa [60–64]. The bombesin agonist ^{177}Lu AMBA demonstrated potential therapeutic effectiveness in several preclinical prostate cancer tumor models [65], but a phase I dose escalation study in patients with mCRPC was stopped due to severe adverse effects due to GRPR stimulation at the therapeutic levels of administered ^{177}Lu AMBA [66] and most other GRPR targeted radiotherapeutic agonists have encountered similar safety problems. Conversely, GRPR antagonists do not appear to cause any adverse side effects and most recent efforts have concentrated on GRPR antagonists. The GRPR antagonist ^{177}Lu RM2 has been evaluated in mCRPC patients with high uptake in prostate cancer cells and demonstrates rapid clearance from physiologic GRPR expressing tissues, such as the pancreas [67]. An additional highly potent GRPR antagonist, NeoBOMB1, is being evaluated in a multicenter study as a combined diagnostic/therapeutic drug with ^{68}Ga/^{177}Lu, respectively, [68]. One major problem with the bombesin-derived diagnostic and therapeutic radiopharmaceuticals is the rapid proteolytic degradation due to peptidases [69,70] with several biochemical modifications being explored in bombesin analogs including unnatural residues and peptidase inhibitors. As with PSMA, GRPR expression is modified by several hormonal and immunomodulators and the effectiveness of ^{177}Lu RM2 was found to be potentiated with the addition of the mTOR inhibitor rapamycin in preclinical trials [71]. Combination GRPR targeted radionuclide therapy and immunotherapy with ^{177}Lu RM26 and trastuzumab, respectively, lead to the synergistic therapy of prostate cancer in mice models [72].

7. Somatostatin Targeted Radiotherapeutics

Although a de novo clinical presentation of small cell neuroendocrine carcinoma of the prostate is rare, a subset of patients previously diagnosed with prostate adenocarcinoma may develop neuroendocrine features in later stages of mCRPC progression [73]. Neuroendocrine prostate cancer (NePC) is an aggressive variant of prostate cancer that most frequently retains early PCa genomic alterations and acquires new molecular changes making them resistant to traditional mCRPC therapies and AR targeted therapies have little effect [74]. Some of the difficulty in treating patients with mCRPC may be due to neuroendocrine differentiation [75]. Of particular importance, NePC is notorious for having little to no PSMA expression, resulting in no appreciable role for either PSMA PET imaging or ^{177}Lu/^{225}Ac PSMA targeted radionuclide therapy. Somatostatin, a neuropeptide that suppresses prostate growth and neovascularization by inducing cell-cycle arrest and apoptosis, is highly expressed in NePC cells (Figure 3) [76,77]. Somatostatin receptors have also been shown to be upregulated in prostate adenocarcinoma [78,79]. Preliminary case reports suggest that ^{68}Ga-DOTA labeled somatostatin analogs may have high sensitivity in identifying sites of mCRPC in addition to NePC [80–83]. In a recent study involving 12 patients with mCRPC, all patients had at least 1 blastic neuroendocrine metastasis with increased ^{68}Ga-DOTA uptake [84]. The large degree of somatostatin expression in NePC and mCRPC, suggests that ^{177}Lu-DOTATATE (Lutathera) may be an alternative to β/α PSMA therapy PSMA, either if having failed PSMA targeted radiotherapy or in the cases with no or little PSMA expression on PSMA PET. While ^{177}Lu-DOTATATE is used extensively for neuroendocrine carcinoma, there are only a couple of case reports of patients with NePC that have been treated with ^{177}Lu-DOTATATE with initial success [85]. This area requires further attention to demonstrate if it is a viable target for directed radionuclide therapy.

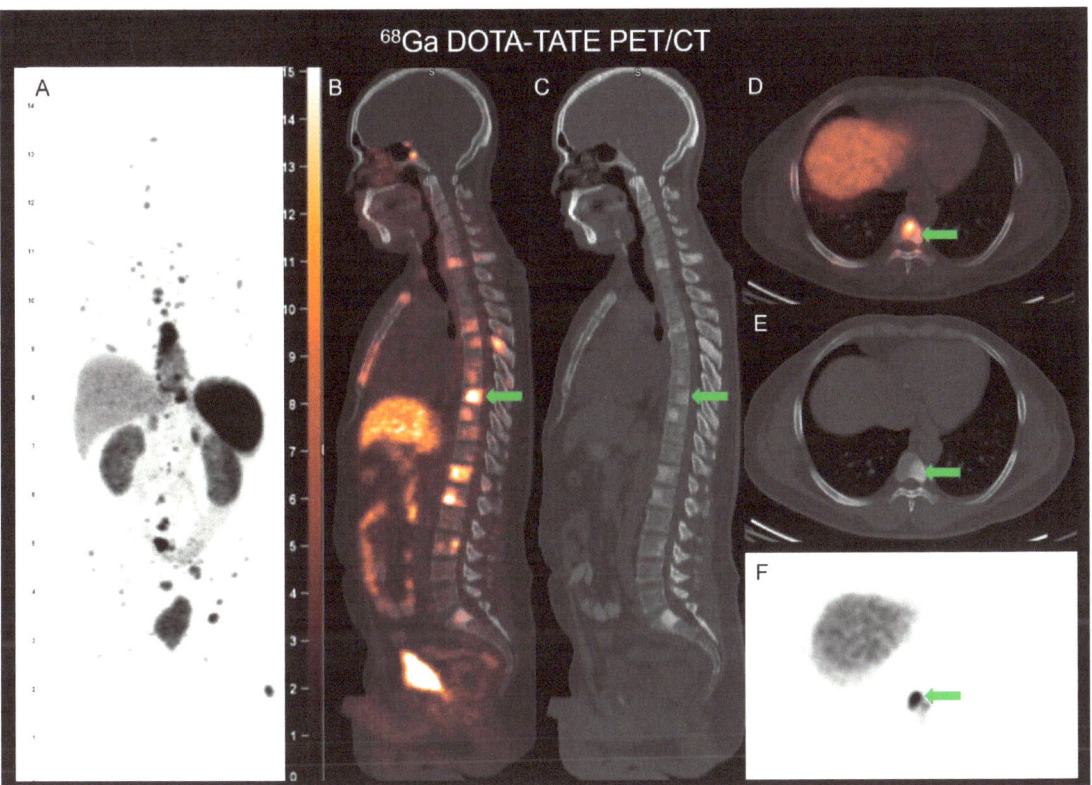

Figure 3. ^{68}Ga DOTATATE PET/CT evaluation of small cell neuroendocrine prostate carcinoma. Patient with Gleason score 5 + 4 = 9 mixed prostate small cell neuroendocrine carcinoma and acinar adenocarcinoma. Patient was started on ADT and cisplatin/etoposide prior to ^{68}Ga DOTATATE PET/CT. Anterior view of ^{68}Ga DOTATATE PET MIP (**A**) demonstrates multiple ^{68}Ga DOTATATE osseous and nodal metastatic deposits. Selected sagittal fused ^{68}Ga DOTATATE PET/CT (**B**) and CT (**C**) images show marked ^{68}Ga DOTATATE uptake greater than liver (SUVmax of 14.4) in several osseous lesions. Transaxial fused ^{68}Ga DOTATATE PET/CT (**D**) and CT (**E**) and PET (**F**) images show marked ^{68}Ga DOTATATE in the most avid T8 lesion having a SUVmax of 20.1 (green arrow). Patient did not demonstrate a PSA response to therapy and passed away 4 months after ^{68}Ga DOTATATE PET/CT.

8. Discussion and Clinician's Perspective

Understanding how to incorporate the two FDA approved radiopharmaceutical therapies, ^{223}RaCl$_2$ (Xofigo®) and ^{177}Lu-PSMA-617 (Pluvicto®) into the treatment paradigm of mCRPC is essential to maximize their therapeutic potential. While all FDA approved agents for mCRPC offer an absolute overall survival benefit, compared to their control arm, this incremental benefit only approaches 5 months for each therapy. Therefore, allowing the patients the opportunity to receive as many therapies as possible is paramount to derive the maximum survival benefit. The optimal sequence of these therapies is lacking, either in the literature or routine clinical practice; however, when selecting treatment, the clinician should consider the disease burden, tempo of disease, location of metastases, prior therapies utilized and anticipated therapies. The chosen sequence often depends on the provider's philosophy on treatment which could be aimed at aggressive approaches upfront to achieve timely disease control while the patient is fit enough to receive therapy, or a clinician may meet the tempo of disease with therapies that offer control of the disease with the least toxicity. These aspects of cancer care delivery should be considered when incorporating ^{223}RaCl$_2$ or ^{177}Lu-PSMA-617. The FDA approved label for ^{223}RaCl$_2$ allows for the treatment of symptomatic mCRPC patients with bone metastases, detected with conventional skeletal scintigraphy, without evidence of visceral metastatic disease. While all patients were symptomatic in the ALSYMPCA trial, symptomatic pain was broadly defined and opioid pain control was not required, and 44% of patients had only mild pain with nonopioid therapy at baseline and these patients also achieved a survival benefit when compared to placebo [86]. Therefore, ^{223}RaCl$_2$ should be considered earlier in the disease course when quality of life is still preserved. To further investigate the efficacy of ^{223}RaCl$_2$ surrounding chemotherapy, a prespecified subgroup analysis showed survival benefit was maintained regardless of prior docetaxel use [87]. This survival benefit is important to note because many patients that could benefit from ^{223}RaCl$_2$ are not candidates for chemotherapy or may decline chemotherapy. It is reported that 20–40% of patients with CRPC may not receive chemotherapy [7]; therefore, this targeted radionuclide therapy remains a possibility for patients who have not been exposed to chemotherapy, especially as the current indication for ^{177}Lu-PSMA-617 requires previous chemotherapy exposure. With triple therapy on the horizon (i.e., chemotherapy plus androgen receptor pathway inhibitor and ADT), understanding that a benefit can be achieved with ^{223}RaCl$_2$ after chemotherapy remains applicable to future patient populations who might receive chemotherapy in the metastatic hormone-sensitive setting. To further optimize ^{223}RaCl$_2$ efficacy, combination therapy is being investigated. In the ERA-223 trial, abiraterone acetate/prednisone was combined with ^{223}RaCl$_2$; however, the trial was unblinded early after more fractures and deaths were observed within the combination group [8]. The use of bone protective agents (BPA) was low in this cohort at 40% which led to the mandatory incorporation of BPA in the ongoing phase III EORTC-1333-GUGG trial (PEACE III trial) with enzalutamide plus ^{223}RaCl$_2$. The phase III trial is being investigated since the phase II trial with enzalutamide plus ^{223}RaCl$_2$ met its primary endpoint of decreasing bone metabolic markers and was associated with improved outcomes [9]. While not sufficiently powered to determine a true significant difference, the phase II secondary endpoints of OS, rPFS, and time to next treatment were longer in the combination group, 30.8 months vs. 20.6 months (p = 0.73), 11.5 months vs. 7.35 months (p = 0.96), and 15.9 months vs. 3.47 months (p = 0.067), respectively [10]. This suggests a potential role of combination therapy with ^{223}RaCl$_2$ plus enzalutamide which will be further determine based on the PEACE III results. As ^{223}RaCl$_2$ is designed for bone predominant disease, combination therapy with enzalutamide would allow for incorporating ^{223}RaCl$_2$ in patients who have both bone and lymph node disease to potentially acquire the survival benefits that both therapies offer. In a phase II open-label single arm study, as part of an expanded access program analysis, ^{223}RaCl$_2$ was determined to be safe regardless of concurrent androgen signaling inhibitor. In addition, ^{223}RaCl$_2$ survival was longer for patients who received less than 3 anticancer therapies [11]. In conclusion, ^{223}RaCl$_2$ remains a therapeutic option for symptomatic bone predominant disease with or without previous docetaxel exposure and should be incorporated earlier in the sequence of therapy to achieve the largest benefit. In addition, the clinician could consider concurrent therapy with enzalutamide to not only target bone disease, but also non-osseous lesions.

^{177}Lu-PSMA-617 is FDA approved for mCRPC patients previously treated with an androgen receptor pathway inhibitor (ARPI) and taxane-based chemotherapy. This radiopharmaceutical therapy is dependent on the presence of PSMA-positive lesions seen on ^{68}Ga-PSMA-11 PET imaging [88]. With the approval of ^{177}Lu-PSMA-617, clinicians now have a low toxicity therapeutic option for heavily pre-treated patients. In contrast to ^{223}RaCl$_2$ which does not result in radiologic responses, in patients with measurable or non-measurable disease at baseline who received ^{177}Lu-PSMA-617, the objective response rate (ORR) was 29.8% (vs. 1.7% control arm) and a complete response (CR) was achieved in 18 patients (5.6%). These complete responses are remarkable given ^{177}Lu-PSMA-617 was given in at least the third-line setting. These responses were based on RECIST v1.1 [12,13] and OS, with radiologic progression or response based on CT, MRI, or bone scintigraphy. Additionally, disease control was achieved in 89.0% of patients. Therefore, clinicians could consider assessing treatment response based on conventional imaging, rather than with PSMA PET as this imaging modality could be cost prohibitive.

In regard to PSA response, 46% of patients in the ^{177}Lu-PSMA-617 arm had a PSA response of $\geq$50% compared to the SOC alone arm of only 7.1% [88]. In the VISION trial, SOC predominately included gonadotropin-releasing hormone analogues, ARPI, bone protective agents and glucocorticoids. In the ^{177}Lu-PSMA-617 arm, 54.7% of patients received concurrent abiraterone or enzalutamide as part of their standard of care and 77.5% of patients in the standard of care alone arm received abiraterone or enzalutamide. A survival subgroup analysis was performed on patients based on presence of concurrent ARPI therapy with ^{177}Lu-PSMA-617. In patients who received ^{177}Lu-PSMA-617 plus ARPI the hazard ratio for death was 0.55 (95%, 0.43–0.70) and patients who received ^{177}Lu-PSMA-617 without ARPI the hazard ratio for death was 0.70 (0.53–0.93) [89]. Therefore, survival benefit was achieved regardless of the addition of an ARPI; however, uncertainty remains whether concurrent therapy could increase the efficacy further.

Clinical and pre-clinical studies have shown that ARPI, such as enzalutamide, can enhance PSMA expression with possible potentiation of the effect of ^{177}Lu-PSMA-617 therapy [90,91]. Further studies (ENZA-p) are ongoing to investigate the added benefit of concurrent therapy (^{177}Lu-PSMA-617 plus enzalutamide vs. enzalutamide alone), therefore, clinicians should consider financial toxicity and added adverse effects when considering concurrent RLT plus ARPI vs. RLT alone. The next consideration is how to incorporate ^{177}Lu-PSMA-617 into the current treatment sequence. Prior to ^{177}Lu-PSMA-617 FDA approval, cabazitaxel was established as the next therapeutic option after progressing on an ARPI and docetaxel based on the CARD trial. In this trial, cabazitaxel resulted in a mOS of 13.6 months vs. 11.0 months (HR 0.64; 95% CI, 0.46 to 0.89; p = 0.008) in patients treated with an ARPI not previously used (abiraterone or enzalutamide) [92]. The TheraP trial investigated the activity and safety of cabazitaxel vs. ^{177}Lu-PSMA-617 in patients with metastatic CRPC and who received prior docetaxel treatment. The ^{177}Lu-PSMA-617 treatment group achieved higher PSA responses compared to cabazitaxel, 66% vs. 37% ($p \leq$ 0.0001), respectively and had less grade 3–4 adverse events, 33% vs. 53%. After a median follow-up of 3 years, there was no survival difference between groups (19.1 months vs. 19.6 months; restricted mean survival team of 3 years). Since survival appears to be similar between these two agents it is important to contrast again the eligibility criteria used in the VISION and TheraP trial. In the VISION trial patients were required to have $\geq$ one PSMA-positive lesion and no PSMA-negative soft tissue-or visceral lesions $\geq$ 1 cm or PSMA-negative lymph nodes $\geq$ 2.5 cm; in the TheraP trial, patients underwent both FDG-PET and PSMA-PET imaging and patients were excluded if there were discordance (PSMA negative/FDG positive) since these patients have a poor survival with a median OS of 2.5 months [33]. While the majority of patients will meet these criteria for exclusively PSMA avid disease, clinicians should be aware of these conditions and consider chemotherapy with cabazitaxel or platinum-based chemotherapy if patients have significant visceral disease or non-PSMA lesions as outlined above and consider ^{177}Lu-PSMA-617 plus ARPI if no other treatment strategies are available.

Since ^{177}Lu-PSMA-617 is approved after ARPI and taxane-based therapy and without other contraindication, ^{177}Lu-PSMA-617 has the potential to be used after ^{223}RaCl$_2$ posing concern for myelotoxicity. As mentioned earlier adequate bone marrow function is a prerequisite for treatment with ^{177}Lu-PSMA-617, therefore, it was hypothesized that previous chemotherapy or radiation (i.e., ^{223}RaCl$_2$) could impact candidacy for ^{177}Lu-PSMA-617

RLT. A retrospective study was performed of 28 patients who received ^{177}Lu-PSMA-617 within 8- weeks after the last ^{223}RaCl$_2$ administration. Grade ≥ 3 hematologic toxicity was seen in 6 patients with anemia (17.9%), leukopenia (14.3%), and thrombocytopenia (21.4%) which appears similar to hematologic toxicity seen in the VISION trial. Regardless, adequate bone marrow function at the start of ^{177}Lu-PSMA-617 is necessary. Given the overall survival benefit and complete radiographic responses seen with ^{177}Lu-PSMA-617, this therapeutic option should be prioritized after progression on ARPI and taxane-based therapy. However, as discussed in this review, there is still much work that needs to be accomplished to evaluate these radionuclide therapeutics in earlier stages of disease and there are multiple ongoing clinical trials investigating the role of targeted radionuclide therapeutics for prostate cancer in conjunction with hormonal, chemotherapeutic, and immunologic treatments as stand along therapies (Table 2).

Table 2. Current ongoing targeted radionuclide clinical trials for prostate cancer [93].

ClinicalTrials.gov Identifier	Name of Study	Study Sponsor	Trials Phase	Location
PSMA				
NCT04443062	Lutetium-177-PSMA-617 in Oligo-metastatic Hormone Sensitive Prostate Cancer (Bullseye)	Radboud University Medical Center	Phase 2	The Netherlands
NCT05114746	Study of ^{177}Lu-PSMA-617 In Metastatic Castrate-Resistant Prostate Cancer in Japan	Novartis Pharmaceuticals	Phase 2	Japan
NCT05079698	A Study of Stereotactic Body Radiotherapy and ^{177}Lu-PSMA-617 for the Treatment of Prostate Cancer	Memorial Sloan Kettering Cancer Center	Phase 1	New York, USA
NCT03454750	Radiometabolic Therapy (RMT) With ^{177}Lu PSMA 617 in Advanced Castration Resistant Prostate Cancer (CRPC) (LU-PSMA)	Istituto Scientifico Romagnolo per lo Studio e la cura dei Tumori	Phase 2	Italy
NCT05219500	Targeted Alpha Therapy With ^{225}Actinium-PSMA-I&T of Castration-resISTant Prostate Cancer (TATCI5T)	Excel Diagnostics and Nuclear Oncology Center	Phase 2	Texas, USA
NCT04343885	In Men With Metastatic Prostate Cancer, What is the Safety and Benefit of Lutetium-^{177}PSMA Radionuclide Treatment in Addition to Chemotherapy (UpFrontPSMA)	Peter MacCallum Cancer Centre	Phase 2	Australia
NCT04419402	Enzalutamide With Lu PSMA-617 Versus Enzalutamide Alone in Men With Metastatic Castration-resistant Prostate Cancer (ENZA-p)	Australian and New Zealand Urogenital and Prostate Cancer Trials Group	Phase 2	Australia
NCT03780075	^{177}Lu-EB-PSMA617 Radionuclide Treatment in Patients With Metastatic Castration-resistant Prostate Cancer	Peking Union Medical College Hospital	Phase 1	China
NCT03874884	^{177}Lu-PSMA-617 Therapy and Olaparib in Patients With Metastatic Castration Resistant Prostate Cancer (LuPARP)	Peter MacCallum Cancer Centre	Phase 1	Australia
NCT05162573	EBRT + Lu-PSMA for N1M0 Prostate Cancer (PROQURE-1)	The Netherlands Cancer Institute	Phase 1	The Netherlands

Table 2. *Cont.*

ClinicalTrials.gov Identifier	Name of Study	Study Sponsor	Trials Phase	Location
NCT04769817	ProsTIC Registry of Men Treated With PSMA Theranostics	Peter MacCallum Cancer Centre	Observational	Australia
NCT04689828	^{177}Lu-PSMA-617 vs. Androgen Receptor-directed Therapy in the Treatment of Progressive Metastatic Castrate Resistant Prostate Cancer (PSMAfore)	Novartis Pharmaceuticals	Phase 3	Multinational
NCT04597411	Study of ^{225}Ac-PSMA-617 in Men With PSMA-positive Prostate Cancer	Endocyte	Phase 1	Australia
NCT04886986	^{225}Ac-J591 Plus ^{177}Lu-PSMA-I&T for mCRPC	Weill Medical College of Cornell University	Phase 1/2	New York, USA
NCT05340374	Cabazitaxel in Combination With ^{177}Lu-PSMA-617 in Metastatic Castration-resistant Prostate Cancer (LuCAB)	Peter MacCallum Cancer Centre	Phase 1/2	Australia
NCT05204927	Lu-177-PSMA-I&T for Metastatic Castration-Resistant Prostate Cancer	Curium US LLC	Phase 3	USA
NCT04647526	Study Evaluating mCRPC Treatment Using PSMA [Lu-177]-PNT2002 Therapy After Second-line Hormonal Treatment (SPLASH)	POINT Biopharma	Phase 3	Multinational
NCT04996602	Therapeutic Efficiency and Response to 2.0 GBq (55mCi) ^{177}Lu-EB-PSMA in Patients With mCRPC	Peking Union Medical College Hospital	Phase 1	China
NCT04720157	An International Prospective Open-label, Randomized, Phase III Study Comparing ^{177}Lu-PSMA-617 in Combination With SOC, Versus SOC Alone, in Adult Male Patients With mHSPC (PSMAddition)	Novartis Pharmaceuticals	Phase 3	Multinational
NCT05113537	Abemaciclib Before ^{177}Lu-PSMA-617 for the Treatment of Metastatic Castrate Resistant Prostate Cancer (UPLIFT)	Vadim S Koshkin	Phase 1	California, USA
NCT04946370	Maximizing Responses to Anti-PD1 Immunotherapy With PSMA-targeted Alpha Therapy in mCRPC	Weill Medical College of Cornell University	Phase 1/2	New York, USA
NCT04868604	^{64}Cu-SAR-bisPSMA and ^{67}Cu-SAR-bisPSMA for Identification and Treatment of PSMA-expressing Metastatic Castrate Resistant Prostate Cancer (SECuRE)	Clarity Pharmaceuticals Ltd.	Phase 1/2	USA
NCT05230251	Radioligand fOr locAl raDiorecurrent proStaTe cancER (ROADSTER)	Glenn Bauman, Lawson Health Research Institute	Phase 2	Canada
NCT04576871	Re-treatment ^{225}Ac-J591 for mCRPC	Weill Medical College of Cornell University	Phase 1	New York, USA
NCT04726033	^{64}Cu-TLX592 Phase I Safety, PK, Biodistribution and Dosimetry Study (CUPID Study) (CUPID)	Telix International Pty Ltd.	Phase 1	Australia
NCT04506567	Fractionated and Multiple Dose ^{225}Ac-J591 for Progressive mCRPC	Weill Medical College of Cornell University	Phase 1/2	New York, USA

Table 2. *Cont.*

ClinicalTrials.gov Identifier	Name of Study	Study Sponsor	Trials Phase	Location
NCT05150236	EVOLUTION: ^{177}Lu-PSMA Therapy Versus ^{177}Lu-PSMA in Combination With Ipilimumab and Nivolumab for Men With mCRPC (ANZUP2001)	Australian and New Zealand Urogenital and Prostate Cancer Trials Group	Phase 2	Australia
NCT05413850	Anti-tumour Activity of (^{177}Lu) rhPSMA-10.1 Injection	Blue Earth Therapeutics Ltd.	Phase 1/2	Maryland, USA
NCT04509557	[^{177}Lu]Ludotadipep Treatment in Patients With Metastatic Castration-resistant Prostate Cancer.	FutureChem	Phase 1	Republic of Korea
^{223}RaCl2				
NCT04521361	A Study to Assess How Radium-223 Distributes in the Body of Patients With Prostate Cancer Which Spread to the Bones	Bayer	Phase 1	Multinational
NCT04037358	RAdium-223 and SABR Versus SABR for Oligometastatic Prostate Cancers (RAVENS)	Sidney Kimmel Comprehensive Cancer Center at Johns Hopkins	Phase 2	Maryland, USA
NCT03574571	A Study to Test Radium-223 With Docetaxel in Patients With Prostate Cancer	Memorial Sloan Kettering Cancer Center	Phase 3	Multinational
NCT05133440	A Study of Stereotactic Body Radiation Therapy and Radium (Ra-223) Dichloride in Prostate Cancer That Has Spread to the Bones	Memorial Sloan Kettering Cancer Center	Phase 2	USA
NCT03737370	Fractionated Docetaxel and Radium 223 in Metastatic Castration-Resistant Prostate Cancer	Tufts Medical Center	Phase 1	USA
NCT04109729	Study of Nivolumab in Combination w Radium-223 in Men w Metastatic Castration Resistant Prostate Cancer (Rad2Nivo)	University of Utah	Phase 1/2	Utah, USA
NCT04206319	Radium-223 in Biochemically Recurrent Prostate Cancer	National Cancer Institute (NCI)	Phase 2	Maryland, USA
NCT04597125	Investigation of Radium-223 Dichloride (Xofigo), a Treatment That Gives Off Radiation That Helps Kill Cancer Cells, Compared to a Treatment That Inactivates Hormones (New Antihormonal Therapy, NAH) in Patients With Prostate Cancer That Has Spread to the Bone Getting Worse on or After Earlier NAH	Bayer	Phase 4	Multinational
NCT03432949	Radium-223 Combined With Dexamethasone as First-line Therapy in Patients With M+CRPC (TRANCE)	Bayer	Phase 4	Canada
NCT04071236	Radiation Medication (Radium-223 Dichloride) Versus Radium-223 Dichloride Plus Radiation Enhancing Medication (M3814) Versus Radium-223 Dichloride Plus M3814 Plus Avelumab (a Type of Immunotherapy) for Advanced Prostate Cancer Not Responsive to Hormonal Therapy	National Cancer Institute (NCI)	Phase 1/2	USA

Table 2. Cont.

ClinicalTrials.gov Identifier	Name of Study	Study Sponsor	Trials Phase	Location
NCT04704505	Bipolar Androgen Therapy (BAT) and Radium-223 (RAD) in Metastatic Castration-resistant Prostate Cancer (mCRPC) (BAT-RAD)	Sidney Kimmel Comprehensive Cancer Center at Johns Hopkins	Phase 2	Multinational
NCT03361735	Radium Ra 223 Dichloride, Hormone Therapy and Stereotactic Body Radiation Therapy in Treating Patients With Metastatic Prostate Cancer	City of Hope Medical Center	Phase 2	California, USA
NCT02194842	Phase III Radium 223 mCRPC-PEACE III (PEACE III)	European Organisation for Research and Treatment of Cancer—EORTC	Phase 3	Multinational
NCT04704505	Bipolar Androgen Therapy (BAT) and Radium-223 (RAD) in Metastatic Castration-resistant Prostate Cancer (mCRPC) (BAT-RAD)	Sidney Kimmel Comprehensive Cancer Center at Johns Hopkins	Phase 2	Multinational
GRPR				
NCT05283330	Safety and Tolerability of ^{212}Pb-DOTAM-GRPR1 ^{212}Pb-DOTAM-GRPR1 in Adult Subjects with Recurrent or Metastatic GRPR-expressing Tumors	Orano Med LLC	Phase 1	Not yet recruiting

9. Conclusions

With the introduction of multiple radiopharmaceuticals into clinical practice, there is a shift in the treatment paradigm for patients with advanced prostate cancer and clinicians are faced with determining how best to sequence these therapies. Given the success of ^{223}RaCl$_2$ and ^{177}Lu PSMA-617, targeted radionuclide therapeutics are now seen as a viable and important adjunct to the therapeutic algorithm that clinicians utilize. Several other classes of promising targeted radionuclide radiopharmaceuticals, both alpha and beta emitters, are also being explored and posed to complement existing treatment algorithms for prostate cancer.

Author Contributions: Both authors were involved with all aspects of this article. All authors have read and agreed to the published version of the manuscript.

Funding: This research received no external funding.

Conflicts of Interest: The authors declare no conflict of interest.

References

1. Siegel, R.L.; Miller, K.D.; Fuchs, H.E.; Jemal, A. Cancer statistics, 2022. *CA Cancer J. Clin.* **2022**, *72*, 7–33. [CrossRef] [PubMed]
2. Sung, H.; Ferlay, J.; Siegel, R.L.; Laversanne, M.; Soerjomataram, I.; Jemal, A.; Bray, F. Global Cancer Statistics 2020: GLOBOCAN Estimates of Incidence and Mortality Worldwide for 36 Cancers in 185 Countries. *CA Cancer J. Clin.* **2021**, *71*, 209–249. [CrossRef] [PubMed]
3. Mollica, V.; Rizzo, A.; Rosellini, M.; Marchetti, A.; Ricci, A.D.; Cimadamore, A.; Scarpelli, M.; Bonucci, C.; Andrini, E.; Errani, C.; et al. Bone Targeting Agents in Patients with Metastatic Prostate Cancer: State of the Art. *Cancers* **2021**, *13*, 546. [CrossRef] [PubMed]
4. So, A.; Chin, J.; Fleshner, N.; Saad, F. Management of skeletal-related events in patients with advanced prostate cancer and bone metastases: Incorporating new agents into clinical practice. *Can. Urol. Assoc. J.* **2012**, *6*, 465–470. [CrossRef]
5. Rizzo, A.; Mollica, V.; Cimadamore, A.; Santoni, M.; Scarpelli, M.; Giunchi, F.; Cheng, L.; Lopez-Beltran, A.; Fiorentino, M.; Montironi, R.; et al. Is There a Role for Immunotherapy in Prostate Cancer? *Cells* **2020**, *9*, 2051. [CrossRef]

6. Thompson, I.M., Jr.; Goodman, P.J.; Tangen, C.M.; Parnes, H.L.; Minasian, L.M.; Godley, P.A.; Lucia, M.S.; Ford, L.G. Long-term survival of participants in the prostate cancer prevention trial. *N. Engl. J. Med.* **2013**, *369*, 603–610. [CrossRef]
7. Parker, C.; Nilsson, S.; Heinrich, D.; Helle, S.I.; O'Sullivan, J.M.; Fossa, S.D.; Chodacki, A.; Wiechno, P.; Logue, J.; Seke, M.; et al. Alpha emitter radium-223 and survival in metastatic prostate cancer. *N. Engl. J. Med.* **2013**, *369*, 213–223. [CrossRef]
8. Smith, M.; Parker, C.; Saad, F.; Miller, K.; Tombal, B.; Ng, Q.S.; Boegemann, M.; Matveev, V.; Piulats, J.M.; Zucca, L.E.; et al. Addition of radium-223 to abiraterone acetate and prednisone or prednisolone in patients with castration-resistant prostate cancer and bone metastases (ERA 223): A randomised, double-blind, placebo-controlled, phase 3 trial. *Lancet. Oncol.* **2019**, *20*, 408–419. [CrossRef]
9. Agarwal, N.; Nussenzveig, R.; Hahn, A.W.; Hoffman, J.M.; Morton, K.; Gupta, S.; Batten, J.; Thorley, J.; Hawks, J.; Santos, V.S.; et al. Prospective Evaluation of Bone Metabolic Markers as Surrogate Markers of Response to Radium-223 Therapy in Metastatic Castration-resistant Prostate Cancer. *Clin. Cancer Res.* **2020**, *26*, 2104–2110. [CrossRef]
10. Maughan, B.L.; Kessel, A.; McFarland, T.R.; Sayegh, N.; Nussenzveig, R.; Hahn, A.W.; Hoffman, J.M.; Morton, K.; Sirohi, D.; Kohli, M.; et al. Radium-223 plus Enzalutamide Versus Enzalutamide in Metastatic Castration-Refractory Prostate Cancer: Final Safety and Efficacy Results. *Oncologist* **2021**, *26*, 1006-e2129. [CrossRef]
11. Sartor, O.; Vogelzang, N.J.; Sweeney, C.; Fernandez, D.C.; Almeida, F.; Iagaru, A.; Brown, A., Jr.; Smith, M.R.; Agrawal, M.; Dicker, A.P.; et al. Radium-223 Safety, Efficacy, and Concurrent Use with Abiraterone or Enzalutamide: First U.S. Experience from an Expanded Access Program. *Oncologist* **2017**, *23*, 193–202. [CrossRef] [PubMed]
12. Sartor, O.; de Bono, J.; Chi, K.N.; Fizazi, K.; Herrmann, K.; Rahbar, K.; Tagawa, S.T.; Nordquist, L.T.; Vaishampayan, N.; El-Haddad, G.; et al. Lutetium-177-PSMA-617 for Metastatic Castration-Resistant Prostate Cancer. *N. Engl. J. Med.* **2021**, *385*, 1091–1103. [CrossRef] [PubMed]
13. Hofman, M.S.; Emmett, L.; Sandhu, S.; Iravani, A.; Joshua, A.M.; Goh, J.C.; Pattison, D.A.; Tan, T.H.; Kirkwood, I.D.; Ng, S.; et al. [(177)Lu]Lu-PSMA-617 versus cabazitaxel in patients with metastatic castration-resistant prostate cancer (TheraP): A randomised, open-label, phase 2 trial. *Lancet* **2021**, *397*, 797–804. [CrossRef] [PubMed]
14. Den, R.B.; George, D.; Pieczonka, C.; McNamara, M. Ra-223 Treatment for Bone Metastases in Castrate-Resistant Prostate Cancer: Practical Management Issues for Patient Selection. *Am. J. Clin. Oncol.* **2019**, *42*, 399–406. [CrossRef]
15. Smith, A.W.; Greenberger, B.A.; Den, R.B.; Stock, R.G. Radiopharmaceuticals for Bone Metastases. *Semin. Radiat. Oncol.* **2021**, *31*, 45–59. [CrossRef]
16. Nilsson, S.; Cislo, P.; Sartor, O.; Vogelzang, N.J.; Coleman, R.E.; O'Sullivan, J.M.; Reuning-Scherer, J.; Shan, M.; Zhan, L.; Parker, C. Patient-reported quality-of-life analysis of radium-223 dichloride from the phase III ALSYMPCA study. *Ann. Oncol.* **2016**, *27*, 868–874. [CrossRef]
17. Parker, C.; Zhan, L.; Cislo, P.; Reuning-Scherer, J.; Vogelzang, N.J.; Nilsson, S.; Sartor, O.; O'Sullivan, J.M.; Coleman, R.E. Effect of radium-223 dichloride (Ra-223) on hospitalisation: An analysis from the phase 3 randomised Alpharadin in Symptomatic Prostate Cancer Patients (ALSYMPCA) trial. *Eur. J. Cancer* **2017**, *71*, 1–6. [CrossRef]
18. Heidenreich, A.; Gillessen, S.; Heinrich, D.; Keizman, D.; O'Sullivan, J.M.; Carles, J.; Wirth, M.; Miller, K.; Reeves, J.; Seger, M.; et al. Radium-223 in asymptomatic patients with castration-resistant prostate cancer and bone metastases treated in an international early access program. *BMC Cancer* **2019**, *19*, 12. [CrossRef]
19. Parker, C.; Heidenreich, A.; Nilsson, S.; Shore, N. Current approaches to incorporation of radium-223 in clinical practice. *Prostate Cancer Prostatic Dis.* **2018**, *21*, 37–47. [CrossRef]
20. Sartor, O.; Coleman, R.E.; Nilsson, S.; Heinrich, D.; Helle, S.I.; O'Sullivan, J.M.; Vogelzang, N.J.; Bruland, O.; Kobina, S.; Wilhelm, S.; et al. An exploratory analysis of alkaline phosphatase, lactate dehydrogenase, and prostate-specific antigen dynamics in the phase 3 ALSYMPCA trial with radium-223. *Ann. Oncol.* **2017**, *28*, 1090–1097. [CrossRef]
21. Sonni, I.; Eiber, M.; Fendler, W.P.; Alano, R.M.; Vangala, S.S.; Kishan, A.U.; Nickols, N.; Rettig, M.B.; Reiter, R.E.; Czernin, J.; et al. Impact of (68)Ga-PSMA-11 PET/CT on Staging and Management of Prostate Cancer Patients in Various Clinical Settings: A Prospective Single-Center Study. *J. Nucl. Med.* **2020**, *61*, 1153–1160. [CrossRef] [PubMed]
22. Tateishi, U. Prostate-specific membrane antigen (PSMA)-ligand positron emission tomography and radioligand therapy (RLT) of prostate cancer. *Jpn. J. Clin. Oncol.* **2020**, *50*, 349–356. [CrossRef] [PubMed]
23. Weineisen, M.; Schottelius, M.; Simecek, J.; Baum, R.P.; Yildiz, A.; Beykan, S.; Kulkarni, H.R.; Lassmann, M.; Klette, I.; Eiber, M.; et al. 68Ga- and 177Lu-Labeled PSMA I&T: Optimization of a PSMA-Targeted Theranostic Concept and First Proof-of-Concept Human Studies. *J. Nucl. Med.* **2015**, *56*, 1169–1176. [CrossRef]
24. PLUVICTOTM (Lutetium Lu 177 Vipivotide Tetraxetan) Injection, for Intravenous Use [Package Insert]. U.S. Food and Drug Administration. Available online: https://www.accessdata.fda.gov/drugsatfda_docs/label/2022/215833s000lbl.pdf (accessed on 2 August 2022).
25. Mokoala, K.; Lawal, I.; Lengana, T.; Kgatle, M.; Giesel, F.L.; Vorster, M.; Sathekge, M. PSMA Theranostics: Science and Practice. *Cancers* **2021**, *13*, 3904. [CrossRef]
26. Kratochwil, C.; Fendler, W.P.; Eiber, M.; Baum, R.; Bozkurt, M.F.; Czernin, J.; Delgado Bolton, R.C.; Ezziddin, S.; Forrer, F.; Hicks, R.J.; et al. EANM procedure guidelines for radionuclide therapy with (177)Lu-labelled PSMA-ligands ((177)Lu-PSMA-RLT). *Eur. J. Nucl. Med. Mol. Imaging* **2019**, *46*, 2536–2544. [CrossRef] [PubMed]
27. Ferdinandus, J.; Violet, J.; Sandhu, S.; Hofman, M.S. Prostate-specific membrane antigen theranostics: Therapy with lutetium-177. *Curr. Opin. Urol.* **2018**, *28*, 197–204. [CrossRef] [PubMed]

28. NCCN. NCCN Guidelines Version 4.2022 Prostate Cancer. Available online: https://www.nccn.org/professionals/physician_gls/pdf/prostate.pdf (accessed on 30 July 2022).
29. Lantheus. Available online: https://investor.lantheus.com/node/13566/pdf (accessed on 30 July 2022).
30. Michalski, K.; Ruf, J.; Goetz, C.; Seitz, A.K.; Buck, A.K.; Lapa, C.; Hartrampf, P.E. Prognostic implications of dual tracer PET/CT: PSMA ligand and [(18)F]FDG PET/CT in patients undergoing [(177)Lu]PSMA radioligand therapy. *Eur. J. Nucl. Med. Mol. Imaging* **2021**, *48*, 2024–2030. [CrossRef] [PubMed]
31. Hotta, M.; Gafita, A.; Czernin, J.; Calais, J. Outcome of patients with PSMA-PET/CT screen failure by VISION criteria and treated with ^{177}Lu-PSMA therapy: A multicenter retrospective analysis. *J. Nucl. Med.* **2022**. [CrossRef]
32. Chen, R.; Wang, Y.; Zhu, Y.; Shi, Y.; Xu, L.; Huang, G.; Liu, J. The Added Value of (18)F-FDG PET/CT Compared with (68)Ga-PSMA PET/CT in Patients with Castration-Resistant Prostate Cancer. *J. Nucl. Med.* **2022**, *63*, 69–75. [CrossRef]
33. Thang, S.P.; Violet, J.; Sandhu, S.; Iravani, A.; Akhurst, T.; Kong, G.; Ravi Kumar, A.; Murphy, D.G.; Williams, S.G.; Hicks, R.J.; et al. Poor Outcomes for Patients with Metastatic Castration-resistant Prostate Cancer with Low Prostate-specific Membrane Antigen (PSMA) Expression Deemed Ineligible for (177)Lu-labelled PSMA Radioligand Therapy. *Eur. Urol. Oncol.* **2019**, *2*, 670–676. [CrossRef]
34. Hope, T.A.; Abbott, A.; Colucci, K.; Bushnell, D.L.; Gardner, L.; Graham, W.S.; Lindsay, S.; Metz, D.C.; Pryma, D.A.; Stabin, M.G.; et al. NANETS/SNMMI Procedure Standard for Somatostatin Receptor-Based Peptide Receptor Radionuclide Therapy with (177)Lu-DOTATATE. *J. Nucl. Med.* **2019**, *60*, 937–943. [CrossRef] [PubMed]
35. Nautiyal, A.; Jha, A.K.; Mithun, S.; Rangarajan, V. Dosimetry in Lu-177-PSMA-617 prostate-specific membrane antigen targeted radioligand therapy: A systematic review. *Nucl. Med. Commun.* **2022**, *43*, 369–377. [CrossRef] [PubMed]
36. Sadaghiani, M.S.; Sheikhbahaei, S.; Werner, R.A.; Pienta, K.J.; Pomper, M.G.; Solnes, L.B.; Gorin, M.A.; Wang, N.Y.; Rowe, S.P. A Systematic Review and Meta-analysis of the Effectiveness and Toxicities of Lutetium-177-labeled Prostate-specific Membrane Antigen-targeted Radioligand Therapy in Metastatic Castration-Resistant Prostate Cancer. *Eur. Urol.* **2021**, *80*, 82–94. [CrossRef] [PubMed]
37. Rahbar, K.; Ahmadzadehfar, H.; Kratochwil, C.; Haberkorn, U.; Schäfers, M.; Essler, M.; Baum, R.P.; Kulkarni, H.R.; Schmidt, M.; Drzezga, A.; et al. German Multicenter Study Investigating 177Lu-PSMA-617 Radioligand Therapy in Advanced Prostate Cancer Patients. *J. Nucl. Med.* **2017**, *58*, 85–90. [CrossRef]
38. Hofman, M.S.; Violet, J.; Hicks, R.J.; Ferdinandus, J.; Thang, S.P.; Akhurst, T.; Iravani, A.; Kong, G.; Ravi Kumar, A.; Murphy, D.G.; et al. [(177)Lu]-PSMA-617 radionuclide treatment in patients with metastatic castration-resistant prostate cancer (LuPSMA trial): A single-centre, single-arm, phase 2 study. *Lancet Oncol.* **2018**, *19*, 825–833. [CrossRef]
39. Violet, J.; Sandhu, S.; Iravani, A.; Ferdinandus, J.; Thang, S.P.; Kong, G.; Kumar, A.R.; Akhurst, T.; Pattison, D.A.; Beaulieu, A.; et al. Long-Term Follow-up and Outcomes of Retreatment in an Expanded 50-Patient Single-Center Phase II Prospective Trial of (177)Lu-PSMA-617 Theranostics in Metastatic Castration-Resistant Prostate Cancer. *J. Nucl. Med.* **2020**, *61*, 857–865. [CrossRef]
40. Rathke, H.; Giesel, F.L.; Flechsig, P.; Kopka, K.; Mier, W.; Hohenfellner, M.; Haberkorn, U.; Kratochwil, C. Repeated ^{177}Lu-Labeled PSMA-617 Radioligand Therapy Using Treatment Activities of up to 9.3 GBq. *J. Nucl. Med.* **2018**, *59*, 459–465. [CrossRef]
41. Jackson, P.; Hofman, M.; McIntosh, L.; Buteau, J.P.; Kumar, A.R. Radiation Dosimetry in 177Lu-PSMA-617 Therapy. *Semin. Nucl. Med.* **2021**, *52*, 243–254. [CrossRef]
42. Lawhn-Heath, C.; Hope, T.A.; Martinez, J.; Fung, E.K.; Shin, J.; Seo, Y.; Flavell, R.R. Dosimetry in radionuclide therapy: The clinical role of measuring radiation dose. *Lancet Oncol.* **2022**, *23*, e75–e87. [CrossRef]
43. Violet, J.; Jackson, P.; Ferdinandus, J.; Sandhu, S.; Akhurst, T.; Iravani, A.; Kong, G.; Kumar, A.R.; Thang, S.P.; Eu, P. Dosimetry of 177Lu-PSMA-617 in metastatic castration-resistant prostate cancer: Correlations between pretherapeutic imaging and whole-body tumor dosimetry with treatment outcomes. *J. Nucl. Med.* **2019**, *60*, 517–523. [CrossRef]
44. Gafita, A.; Wang, H.; Robertson, A.; Armstrong, W.R.; Zaum, R.; Weber, M.; Yagubbayli, F.; Kratochwil, C.; Grogan, T.R.; Nguyen, K.; et al. Tumor Sink Effect in (68)Ga-PSMA-11 PET: Myth or Reality? *J. Nucl. Med.* **2022**, *63*, 226–232. [CrossRef] [PubMed]
45. Filss, C.; Heinzel, A.; Müller, B.; Vogg, A.T.J.; Langen, K.J.; Mottaghy, F.M. Relevant tumor sink effect in prostate cancer patients receiving 177Lu-PSMA-617 radioligand therapy. *Nuklearmedizin* **2018**, *57*, 19–25. [CrossRef] [PubMed]
46. Sathekge, M.; Bruchertseifer, F.; Knoesen, O.; Reyneke, F.; Lawal, I.; Lengana, T.; Davis, C.; Mahapane, J.; Corbett, C.; Vorster, M.; et al. (225)Ac-PSMA-617 in chemotherapy-naive patients with advanced prostate cancer: A pilot study. *Eur. J. Nucl. Med. Mol. Imaging* **2019**, *46*, 129–138. [CrossRef] [PubMed]
47. Kratochwil, C.; Bruchertseifer, F.; Giesel, F.L.; Weis, M.; Verburg, F.A.; Mottaghy, F.; Kopka, K.; Apostolidis, C.; Haberkorn, U.; Morgenstern, A. 225Ac-PSMA-617 for PSMA-Targeted α-Radiation Therapy of Metastatic Castration-Resistant Prostate Cancer. *J. Nucl. Med.* **2016**, *57*, 1941–1944. [CrossRef] [PubMed]
48. Van der Doelen, M.J.; Mehra, N.; van Oort, I.M.; Looijen-Salamon, M.G.; Janssen, M.J.R.; Custers, J.A.E.; Slootbeek, P.H.J.; Kroeze, L.I.; Bruchertseifer, F.; Morgenstern, A.; et al. Clinical outcomes and molecular profiling of advanced metastatic castration-resistant prostate cancer patients treated with (225)Ac-PSMA-617 targeted alpha-radiation therapy. *Urol. Oncol.* **2021**, *39*, e727–e729. [CrossRef]
49. Satapathy, S.; Sood, A.; Das, C.K.; Mittal, B.R. Evolving role of 225Ac-PSMA radioligand therapy in metastatic castration-resistant prostate cancer—a systematic review and meta-analysis. *Prostate Cancer Prostatic Dis.* **2021**, *24*, 880–890. [CrossRef]

50. Kratochwil, C.; Giesel, F.L.; Bruchertseifer, F.; Mier, W.; Apostolidis, C.; Boll, R.; Murphy, K.; Haberkorn, U.; Morgenstern, A. (2)(1)(3)Bi-DOTATOC receptor-targeted alpha-radionuclide therapy induces remission in neuroendocrine tumours refractory to beta radiation: A first-in-human experience. *Eur. J. Nucl. Med. Mol. Imaging* **2014**, *41*, 2106–2119. [CrossRef]
51. Kratochwil, C.; Bruchertseifer, F.; Rathke, H.; Bronzel, M.; Apostolidis, C.; Weichert, W.; Haberkorn, U.; Giesel, F.L.; Morgenstern, A. Targeted alpha-Therapy of Metastatic Castration-Resistant Prostate Cancer with (225)Ac-PSMA-617: Dosimetry Estimate and Empiric Dose Finding. *J. Nucl. Med.* **2017**, *58*, 1624–1631. [CrossRef]
52. Feuerecker, B.; Tauber, R.; Knorr, K.; Heck, M.; Beheshti, A.; Seidl, C.; Bruchertseifer, F.; Pickhard, A.; Gafita, A.; Kratochwil, C.; et al. Activity and Adverse Events of Actinium-225-PSMA-617 in Advanced Metastatic Castration-resistant Prostate Cancer After Failure of Lutetium-177-PSMA. *Eur. Urol.* **2021**, *79*, 343–350. [CrossRef]
53. Kratochwil, C.; Bruchertseifer, F.; Rathke, H.; Hohenfellner, M.; Giesel, F.L.; Haberkorn, U.; Morgenstern, A. Targeted alpha-Therapy of Metastatic Castration-Resistant Prostate Cancer with (225)Ac-PSMA-617: Swimmer-Plot Analysis Suggests Efficacy Regarding Duration of Tumor Control. *J. Nucl. Med.* **2018**, *59*, 795–802. [CrossRef]
54. Haberkorn, U.; Giesel, F.; Morgenstern, A.; Kratochwil, C. The Future of Radioligand Therapy: Alpha, beta, or Both? *J. Nucl. Med.* **2017**, *58*, 1017–1018. [CrossRef] [PubMed]
55. Lawal, I.O.; Morgenstern, A.; Vorster, M.; Knoesen, O.; Mahapane, J.; Hlongwa, K.N.; Maserumule, L.C.; Ndlovu, H.; Reed, J.D.; Popoola, G.O.; et al. Hematologic toxicity profile and efficacy of [(225)Ac]Ac-PSMA-617 alpha-radioligand therapy of patients with extensive skeletal metastases of castration-resistant prostate cancer. *Eur. J. Nucl. Med. Mol. Imaging* **2022**, *49*, 3581–3592. [CrossRef] [PubMed]
56. Khreish, F.; Ebert, N.; Ries, M.; Maus, S.; Rosar, F.; Bohnenberger, H.; Stemler, T.; Saar, M.; Bartholomä, M.; Ezziddin, S. (225)Ac-PSMA-617/(177)Lu-PSMA-617 tandem therapy of metastatic castration-resistant prostate cancer: Pilot experience. *Eur. J. Nucl. Med. Mol. Imaging* **2020**, *47*, 721–728. [CrossRef] [PubMed]
57. Pujatti, P.B.; Foster, J.M.; Finucane, C.; Hudson, C.D.; Burnet, J.C.; Pasqualoto, K.F.M.; Mengatti, J.; Mather, S.J.; de Araujo, E.B.; Sosabowski, J.K. Evaluation and comparison of a new DOTA and DTPA-bombesin agonist in vitro and in vivo in low and high GRPR expressing prostate and breast tumor models. *Appl. Radiat. Isot.* **2015**, *96*, 91–101. [CrossRef]
58. Mansi, R.; Fleischmann, A.; Macke, H.R.; Reubi, J.C. Targeting GRPR in urological cancers–from basic research to clinical application. *Nat. Rev. Urol.* **2013**, *10*, 235–244. [CrossRef]
59. Aprikian, A.G.; Tremblay, L.; Han, K.; Chevalier, S. Bombesin stimulates the motility of human prostate-carcinoma cells through tyrosine phosphorylation of focal adhesion kinase and of integrin-associated proteins. *Int. J. Cancer* **1997**, *72*, 498–504. [CrossRef]
60. Dalm, S.U.; Bakker, I.L.; de Blois, E.; Doeswijk, G.N.; Konijnenberg, M.W.; Orlandi, F.; Barbato, D.; Tedesco, M.; Maina, T.; Nock, B.A.; et al. 68Ga/177Lu-NeoBOMB1, a Novel Radiolabeled GRPR Antagonist for Theranostic Use in Oncology. *J. Nucl. Med.* **2017**, *58*, 293–299. [CrossRef]
61. Gourni, E.; Del Pozzo, L.; Kheirallah, E.; Smerling, C.; Waser, B.; Reubi, J.C.; Paterson, B.M.; Donnelly, P.S.; Meyer, P.T.; Maecke, H.R. Copper-64 Labeled Macrobicyclic Sarcophagine Coupled to a GRP Receptor Antagonist Shows Great Promise for PET Imaging of Prostate Cancer. *Mol. Pharm.* **2015**, *12*, 2781–2790. [CrossRef]
62. Liu, F.; Zhu, H.; Yu, J.; Han, X.; Xie, Q.; Liu, T.; Xia, C.; Li, N.; Yang, Z. (68)Ga/(177)Lu-labeled DOTA-TATE shows similar imaging and biodistribution in neuroendocrine tumor model. *Tumour Biol.* **2017**, *39*, 1010428317705519. [CrossRef]
63. Huynh, T.T.; van Dam, E.M.; Sreekumar, S.; Mpoy, C.; Blyth, B.J.; Muntz, F.; Harris, M.J.; Rogers, B.E. Copper-67-Labeled Bombesin Peptide for Targeted Radionuclide Therapy of Prostate Cancer. *Pharmaceuticals* **2022**, *15*, 728. [CrossRef]
64. Bakker, I.L.; Froberg, A.C.; Busstra, M.B.; Verzijlbergen, J.F.; Konijnenberg, M.; van Leenders, G.; Schoots, I.G.; de Blois, E.; van Weerden, W.M.; Dalm, S.U.; et al. GRPr Antagonist (68)Ga-SB3 PET/CT Imaging of Primary Prostate Cancer in Therapy-Naive Patients. *J. Nucl. Med.* **2021**, *62*, 1517–1523. [CrossRef] [PubMed]
65. Maddalena, M.E.; Fox, J.; Chen, J.; Feng, W.; Cagnolini, A.; Linder, K.E.; Tweedle, M.F.; Nunn, A.D.; Lantry, L.E. 177Lu-AMBA biodistribution, radiotherapeutic efficacy, imaging, and autoradiography in prostate cancer models with low GRP-R expression. *J. Nucl. Med.* **2009**, *50*, 2017–2024. [CrossRef] [PubMed]
66. Bodei, L.; Ferrari, M.; Nunn, A.; Llull, J.; Cremonesi, M.; Martano, L.; Laurora, G.; Scardino, E.; Tiberini, S.; Bufi, G.; et al. Lu-177-AMBA Bombesin analogue in hormone refractory prostate cancer patients: A phase I escalation study with single-cycle administrations. *Eur. J. Nucl. Med. Mol. Imaging* **2007**, *34*, S221.
67. Kurth, J.; Krause, B.J.; Schwarzenbock, S.M.; Bergner, C.; Hakenberg, O.W.; Heuschkel, M. First-in-human dosimetry of gastrin-releasing peptide receptor antagonist [(177)Lu]Lu-RM2: A radiopharmaceutical for the treatment of metastatic castration-resistant prostate cancer. *Eur. J. Nucl. Med. Mol. Imaging* **2020**, *47*, 123–135. [CrossRef] [PubMed]
68. Djaileb, L.; Morgat, C.; van der Veldt, A.; Virgolini, I.; Cortes, F.; Demange, A.; Orlandi, F.; Wegener, A. Preliminary diagnostic performance of [Ga-68]-NeoBOMB1 in patients with gastrin-releasing peptide receptor-positive breast, prostate, colorectal or lung tumors (NeoFIND). *J. Nucl. Med.* **2020**, *61*, 346.
69. Chatalic, K.L.; Kwekkeboom, D.J.; de Jong, M. Radiopeptides for Imaging and Therapy: A Radiant Future. *J. Nucl. Med.* **2015**, *56*, 1809–1812. [CrossRef]
70. Linder, K.E.; Metcalfe, E.; Arunachalam, T.; Chen, J.; Eaton, S.M.; Feng, W.; Fan, H.; Raju, N.; Cagnolini, A.; Lantry, L.E.; et al. In vitro and in vivo metabolism of Lu-AMBA, a GRP-receptor binding compound, and the synthesis and characterization of its metabolites. *Bioconjug Chem.* **2009**, *20*, 1171–1178. [CrossRef]

71. Dumont, R.A.; Tamma, M.; Braun, F.; Borkowski, S.; Reubi, J.C.; Maecke, H.; Weber, W.A.; Mansi, R. Targeted radiotherapy of prostate cancer with a gastrin-releasing peptide receptor antagonist is effective as monotherapy and in combination with rapamycin. *J. Nucl. Med.* **2013**, *54*, 762–769. [CrossRef]
72. Mitran, B.; Rinne, S.S.; Konijnenberg, M.W.; Maina, T.; Nock, B.A.; Altai, M.; Vorobyeva, A.; Larhed, M.; Tolmachev, V.; de Jong, M.; et al. Trastuzumab cotreatment improves survival of mice with PC-3 prostate cancer xenografts treated with the GRPR antagonist (177) Lu-DOTAGA-PEG2 -RM26. *Int. J. Cancer* **2019**, *145*, 3347–3358. [CrossRef]
73. Jimenez, R.E.; Nandy, D.; Qin, R.; Carlson, R.; Tan, W.; Kohli, M. Neuroendocrine differentiation patterns in metastases from advanced prostate cancer. *J. Clin. Oncol.* **2014**, *32*, 5085. [CrossRef]
74. Santoni, M.; Scarpelli, M.; Mazzucchelli, R.; Lopez-Beltran, A.; Cheng, L.; Cascinu, S.; Montironi, R. Targeting prostate-specific membrane antigen for personalized therapies in prostate cancer: Morphologic and molecular backgrounds and future promises. *J. Biol. Regul. Homeost Agents* **2014**, *28*, 555–563. [PubMed]
75. Parimi, V.; Goyal, R.; Poropatich, K.; Yang, X.J. Neuroendocrine differentiation of prostate cancer: A review. *Am. J. Clin. Exp. Urol.* **2014**, *2*, 273–285. [PubMed]
76. Nelson, E.C.; Cambio, A.J.; Yang, J.C.; Ok, J.H.; Lara, P.N., Jr.; Evans, C.P. Clinical implications of neuroendocrine differentiation in prostate cancer. *Prostate Cancer Prostatic Dis.* **2007**, *10*, 6–14. [CrossRef] [PubMed]
77. Borre, M.; Nerstrom, B.; Overgaard, J. Association between immunohistochemical expression of vascular endothelial growth factor (VEGF), VEGF-expressing neuroendocrine-differentiated tumor cells, and outcome in prostate cancer patients subjected to watchful waiting. *Clin. Cancer Res.* **2000**, *6*, 1882–1890. [PubMed]
78. Morichetti, D.; Mazzucchelli, R.; Santinelli, A.; Stramazzotti, D.; Lopez-Beltran, A.; Scarpelli, M.; Bono, A.V.; Cheng, L.; Montironi, R. Immunohistochemical expression and localization of somatostatin receptor subtypes in prostate cancer with neuroendocrine differentiation. *Int. J. Immunopathol. Pharm.* **2010**, *23*, 511–522. [CrossRef] [PubMed]
79. Montironi, R.; Cheng, L.; Mazzucchelli, R.; Morichetti, D.; Stramazzotti, D.; Santinelli, A.; Moroncini, G.; Galosi, A.B.; Muzzonigro, G.; Comeri, G.; et al. Immunohistochemical detection and localization of somatostatin receptor subtypes in prostate tissue from patients with bladder outlet obstruction. *Cell Oncol.* **2008**, *30*, 473–482. [CrossRef]
80. Gabriel, M.; Decristoforo, C.; Kendler, D.; Dobrozemsky, G.; Heute, D.; Uprimny, C.; Kovacs, P.; Von Guggenberg, E.; Bale, R.; Virgolini, I.J. 68Ga-DOTA-Tyr3-octreotide PET in neuroendocrine tumors: Comparison with somatostatin receptor scintigraphy and CT. *J. Nucl. Med.* **2007**, *48*, 508–518. [CrossRef]
81. Alonso, O.; Gambini, J.P.; Lago, G.; Gaudiano, J.; Quagliata, A.; Engler, H. In vivo visualization of somatostatin receptor expression with Ga-68-DOTA-TATE PET/CT in advanced metastatic prostate cancer. *Clin. Nucl. Med.* **2011**, *36*, 1063–1064. [CrossRef]
82. Chen, S.; Cheung, S.K.; Wong, K.N.; Wong, K.K.; Ho, C.L. 68Ga-DOTATOC and 68Ga-PSMA PET/CT Unmasked a Case of Prostate Cancer With Neuroendocrine Differentiation. *Clin. Nucl. Med.* **2016**, *41*, 959–960. [CrossRef]
83. Todorovic-Tirnanic, M.V.; Gajic, M.M.; Obradovic, V.B.; Baum, R.P. Gallium-68 DOTATOC PET/CT in vivo characterization of somatostatin receptor expression in the prostate. *Cancer Biother. Radiopharm.* **2014**, *29*, 108–115. [CrossRef]
84. Gofrit, O.N.; Frank, S.; Meirovitz, A.; Nechushtan, H.; Orevi, M. PET/CT With 68Ga-DOTA-TATE for Diagnosis of Neuroendocrine: Differentiation in Patients With Castrate-Resistant Prostate Cancer. *Clin. Nucl. Med.* **2017**, *42*, 1–6. [CrossRef]
85. Nesari Javan, F.; Aryana, K.; Askari, E. Prostate Cancer With Neuroendocrine Differentiation Recurring After Treatment With 177Lu-PSMA: A Chance for 177Lu-DOTATATE Therapy? *Clin. Nucl. Med.* **2021**, *46*, e480–e482. [CrossRef] [PubMed]
86. Parker, C.; Finkelstein, S.E.; Michalski, J.M.; O'Sullivan, J.M.; Bruland, Ø.; Vogelzang, N.J.; Coleman, R.E.; Nilsson, S.; Sartor, O.; Li, R.; et al. Efficacy and Safety of Radium-223 Dichloride in Symptomatic Castration-resistant Prostate Cancer Patients With or Without Baseline Opioid Use From the Phase 3 ALSYMPCA Trial. *Eur. Urol.* **2016**, *70*, 875–883. [CrossRef] [PubMed]
87. Hoskin, P.; Sartor, O.; O'Sullivan, J.M.; Johannessen, D.C.; Helle, S.I.; Logue, J.; Bottomley, D.; Nilsson, S.; Vogelzang, N.J.; Fang, F.; et al. Efficacy and safety of radium-223 dichloride in patients with castration-resistant prostate cancer and symptomatic bone metastases, with or without previous docetaxel use: A prespecified subgroup analysis from the randomised, double-blind, phase 3 ALSYMPCA trial. *Lancet Oncol.* **2014**, *15*, 1397–1406. [CrossRef]
88. Sartor, A.O.; la Fougère, C.; Essler, M.; Ezziddin, S.; Kramer, G.; Elllinger, J.; Nordquist, L.; Sylvester, J.; Paganelli, G.; Peer, A.; et al. Lutetium-177–prostate-specific membrane antigen ligand following radium-223 treatment in men with bone-metastatic castration-resistant prostate cancer: Real-world clinical experience. *J. Nucl. Med.* **2021**. [CrossRef]
89. Vaishampayan, N.; Morris, M.J.; Krause, B.J.; Vogelzang, N.J.; Kendi, A.T.; Nordquist, L.T.; Calais, J.; Nagarajah, J.; Beer, T.M.; El-Haddad, G.; et al. [177Lu]Lu-PSMA-617 in PSMA-positive metastatic castration-resistant prostate cancer: Prior and concomitant treatment subgroup analyses of the VISION trial. *J. Clin. Oncol.* **2022**, *40*, 5001. [CrossRef]
90. Hope, T.A.; Truillet, C.; Ehman, E.C.; Afshar-Oromieh, A.; Aggarwal, R.; Ryan, C.J.; Carroll, P.R.; Small, E.J.; Evans, M.J. 68Ga-PSMA-11 PET Imaging of Response to Androgen Receptor Inhibition: First Human Experience. *J. Nucl. Med.* **2017**, *58*, 81–84. [CrossRef] [PubMed]
91. Vaz, S.; Hadaschik, B.; Gabriel, M.; Herrmann, K.; Eiber, M.; Costa, D. Influence of androgen deprivation therapy on PSMA expression and PSMA-ligand PET imaging of prostate cancer patients. *Eur. J. Nucl. Med. Mol. Imaging* **2020**, *47*, 9–15. [CrossRef] [PubMed]
92. De Wit, R.; de Bono, J.; Sternberg, C.N.; Fizazi, K.; Tombal, B.; Wülfing, C.; Kramer, G.; Eymard, J.-C.; Bamias, A.; Carles, J.; et al. Cabazitaxel versus Abiraterone or Enzalutamide in Metastatic Prostate Cancer. *N. Engl. J. Med.* **2019**, *381*, 2506–2518. [CrossRef]
93. National Library of Medicine (NLM). Available online: https://www.ClinicalTrials.gov (accessed on 28 August 2022).

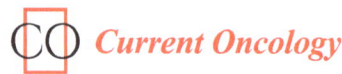 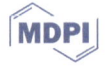

Article

The Diagnostic Value of PI-RADS v2.1 in Patients with a History of Transurethral Resection of the Prostate (TURP)

Jiazhou Liu [1,†], Shihang Pan [2,†], Liang Dong [1,†], Guangyu Wu [2], Jiayi Wang [1], Yan Wang [1], Hongyang Qian [1], Baijun Dong [1], Jiahua Pan [1], Yinjie Zhu [1,*] and Wei Xue [1,*]

1. Department of Urology, Ren Ji Hospital, School of Medicine, Shanghai Jiao Tong University, Shanghai 200127, China
2. Department of Imaging, Ren Ji Hospital, School of Medicine, Shanghai Jiao Tong University, Shanghai 200127, China
* Correspondence: zhuyinjie@renji.com (Y.Z.); xuewei@renji.com (W.X.); Tel.: +86-21-68383757 (Y.Z. & W.X.); Fax: +86-21-58394262 (Y.Z. & W.X.)
† These authors equally contributed to the study.

Abstract: To explore the diagnostic value of the Prostate Imaging–Reporting and Data System version 2.1 (PI-RADS v2.1) for clinically significant prostate cancer (CSPCa) in patients with a history of transurethral resection of the prostate (TURP), we conducted a retrospective study of 102 patients who underwent systematic prostate biopsies with TURP history. ROC analyses and logistic regression analyses were performed to demonstrate the diagnostic value of PI-RADS v2.1 and other clinical characteristics, including PSA and free/total PSA (F/T PSA). Of 102 patients, 43 were diagnosed with CSPCa. In ROC analysis, PSA, F/T PSA, and PI-RADS v2.1 demonstrated significant diagnostic value in detecting CSPCa in our cohort (AUC 0.710 (95%CI 0.608–0.812), AUC 0.768 (95%CI 0.676–0.860), AUC 0.777 (95%CI 0.688–0.867), respectively). Further, PI-RADS v2.1 scores of the peripheral and transitional zones were analyzed separately. In ROC analysis, PI-RADS v2.1 remained valuable in identifying peripheral-zone CSPCa (AUC 0.780 (95%CI 0.665–0.854); $p < 0.001$)) while having limited capability in distinguishing transitional zone lesions (AUC 0.533 (95%CI 0.410–0.557); $p = 0.594$)). PSA and F/T PSA retain significant diagnostic value for CSPCa in patients with TURP history. PI-RADS v2.1 is reliable for detecting peripheral-zone CSPCa but has limited diagnostic value when assessing transitional zone lesions.

Keywords: prostate cancer; transurethral resection of the prostate; multiparametric magnetic resonance imaging; prostate-specific antigen

1. Introduction

Prostate cancer (PCa) is one of the most common malignancies among men worldwide, leading to numerous cancer-related deaths [1,2]. To actively cope with this aggressive global health problem, efforts have been made in the past decades to improve the clinical detection of PCa.

PSA alone as a diagnostic biomarker is insufficient to distinguish PCa from benign prostatic diseases [3]. Studies have shown that at a total PSA level of 4.0 to 10.0 ng/mL, applying the marker of the free/total PSA ratio (F/T PSA) enhances the specificity of PSA testing [4,5]. Advances in imaging techniques have improved the diagnosis of PCa. Multiparametric magnetic resonance imaging (mpMRI) has become an effective noninvasive tool in the assessment of PCa and has demonstrated high value in the detection of clinically significant prostate cancer (CSPCa), defined as Gleason score ≥ 7 (including 3 + 4 with a prominent but not predominant Gleason 4 component) and/or volume ≥ 0.5 cc and/or extraprostatic extension (EPE) [6]. To standardize the diagnostic criteria of mpMRI, the Prostate Imaging–Reporting and Data System (PI-RADS) was drafted and lately renewed to version 2.1 [7,8]. A definitive diagnosis of PCa is based on a prostate biopsy. In practice, risk

Citation: Liu, J.; Pan, S.; Dong, L.; Wu, G.; Wang, J.; Wang, Y.; Qian, H.; Dong, B.; Pan, J.; Zhu, Y.; et al. The Diagnostic Value of PI-RADS v2.1 in Patients with a History of Transurethral Resection of the Prostate (TURP). *Curr. Oncol.* **2022**, *29*, 6373–6382. https://doi.org/10.3390/curroncol29090502

Received: 28 July 2022
Accepted: 1 September 2022
Published: 5 September 2022

Publisher's Note: MDPI stays neutral with regard to jurisdictional claims in published maps and institutional affiliations.

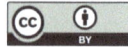

Copyright: © 2022 by the authors. Licensee MDPI, Basel, Switzerland. This article is an open access article distributed under the terms and conditions of the Creative Commons Attribution (CC BY) license (https://creativecommons.org/licenses/by/4.0/).

stratification beforehand by serum markers and imaging evaluation has greatly improved cancer detection rates and reduced unnecessary biopsies [9–11].

Benign prostatic hyperplasia (BPH) is a progressive disease commonly seen in elderly men and is often addressed by a transurethral resection of the prostate (TURP). We came to notice a certain group of patients in clinical practice who had a surgical history of TURP due to BPH and were suspected of PCa during follow-up visits. On account of the removal of transitional zone tissue during the TURP and possible adenoma regrowth during the follow-up period, serum PSA or F/T PSA testing may be influenced by surgical history. Moreover, with no consensus established yet, whether mpMRI retains diagnostic value also remains uncertain, and patients are, in this case, assigned to prostate biopsies based mainly on clinicians' judgment, leading to a certain number of unnecessary invasive procedures or delayed diagnoses. Given this situation, we hypothesize that PI-RADS v2.1 may be an effective tool in identifying patients suspected of PCa who require an immediate biopsy.

Therefore, in this present study, we aim to investigate the diagnostic values of PI-RADS v2.1 scores for CSPCa in a cohort of patients with a history of TURP.

2. Materials and Methods

2.1. Patients

In this retrospective study, consecutive patients who had undergone a 12-core transrectal ultrasound (TRUS)-guided prostate biopsy with previous TURP history at our department between October 2014 and August 2020 were recruited. PSA is reported to drop significantly within 3–6 months after TURP [12,13], while hemorrhage, edema, and early fibrosis at the surgical site after TURP may create biases for mpMRI examinations [14,15]. Therefore, patients who received TURP less than 1 year ago were excluded from the study. The total cohort size was 102. Informed consent was provided by all the participants, and the research was approved by the Institutional Ethical Committee. All patients had a history of receiving a conventional TURP procedure to treat lower urinary tract symptoms due to BPH and had negative pathological results on the removed tissues. Biopsy indication was PSA level > 4 ng/mL or suspected digital rectal exam results. Exclusion criteria consisted of patients with previous local treatment of the prostate other than TURP and patients with positive pathological reports prior to our procedure. Each patient drew blood for serum PSA and F/T PSA and underwent an mpMRI examination before the biopsy.

2.2. MRI and Reporting Protocol

All mpMRI included T2W, DW, and DCE imaging sequences. Two experienced genitourinary radiologists blinded to the clinical details reviewed and reported readouts following the standards of PI-RADS v2.1 [7,8]. Since the assessment of the transitional zone (TZ) and peripheral zone (PZ) relies on different key sequences of imaging, PI-RADS scores were proposed for each prostate zone separately for each patient. A single PI-RADS score of a patient represents the PI-RADS score of the dominant lesion in the whole gland, while PI-RADS TZ and PI-RADS PZ scores represent the PI-RADS score of the dominant lesion in the TZ and PZ, respectively.

2.3. Biopsy Protocol

All patients underwent a 12-core transrectal ultrasound (TRUS)-guided transperineal prostate biopsy. The well-designed biopsy template covers the bilateral anterior TZ, posterior TZ, anterior horn of PZ, anterior lateral PZ, posterior lateral PZ, and posterior medial PZ. The biopsy template is shown in Figure S1. Cores No. 1–8 are targeted to the PZ of the prostate, while Cores No. 9–12 are targeted to the TZ. Slight adjustments were made to adapt to the tissue defect caused by TURP and to cover all suspected lesions found in the imaging. All biopsies were performed by a single experienced urologist, and all samples were reviewed by a single specialized uropathologist to conclude the definitive diagnosis. Clinically significant cancer was defined following the PI-RADS V2.1 guidelines [7,8] as PCa with a histologic Gleason score ≥7 (including 3 + 4 with a prominent but not predominant Gleason 4 component) and/or volume ≥0.5 cc and/or extraprostatic extension (EPE).

2.4. Statistical Analysis

Statistical analyses were performed using SPSS version 26.0. Statistical significance was set as $p < 0.05$. We used the Mann–Whitney rank sum test for nonparametric variables and Fisher's exact chi-square test for categorical variables. Receiver operating characteristic (ROC) analyses were performed using biopsy results as the gold standard to reflect the diagnostic performance of PSA, F/T PSA, and PI-RADS v2.1. ROC curves were compared using the DeLong test. The area under the curve (AUC) and Youden's index were calculated. Logistic regression analyses were conducted to explore the predictive values of the variables, and the odds ratios (ORs) were computed to quantify the predictive ability of the factors.

3. Results

A total of 102 patients were included in the study. The median age was 73.5 years (interquartile range; IQR 68–78 years), the median time after TURP was 8 years (IQR 4–10.25 years), the median PSA level was 12.3 ng/mL (IQR 7.41–19.26 ng/mL), and the median F/T PSA was 0.15 (IQR 0.11–0.20). In all, 56 patients were diagnosed with PCa, among which 43 patients had CSPCa, while a Gleason score of 3 + 3 = 6 was present in the remaining 13. Table 1 shows the characteristics of patients with CSPCa and non-CSPCa or negative biopsy. While no significant difference was found in time after TURP between the two groups, patients presenting with CSPCa exhibited significantly older age ($p = 0.000$), higher PSA levels ($p = 0.006$), and lower F/T PSA ($p = 0.000$).

Table 1. Patient characteristics in different biopsy results.

	CSPCa	Non-CSPCa or Negative Biopsy	*p*-Value
Age (yrs), median (IQR)	77 (72–80)	70 (66–75)	0.000
Time after TURP (yrs), median (IQR)	6 (3–12)	8 (5–10)	0.557
PSA (ng/mL), median (IQR)	14.73 (10.97–36.00)	10.91 (6.19–15.89)	0.000
F/T PSA, median (IQR)	0.12 (0.09–0.15)	0.18 (0.13–0.23)	0.000
PI-RADS V2.1 n (%)			0.000
2	1 (2.3)	15 (25.4)	
3	4 (9.3)	19 (32.2)	
4	24 (55.8)	21 (35.6)	
5	14 (32.6)	4 (6.8)	

ROC curves were constructed to determine the diagnostic value of PSA, F/T PSA, and PI-RADS v2.1 in our cohort (Figure 1). The area-under-the-curve (AUC) value of PSA, F/T PSA, and PI-RADS v2.1 for predicting CSPCa was 0.710 (95 CI% 0.608–0.812), 0.768 (95 CI% 0.676–0.860), and 0.777 (95 CI% 0.688–0.867), respectively. A comparison of the three ROC curves showed no statistically significant differences. Setting the threshold at 23.81 ng/mL, PSA showed the best Youden's index score of 0.338, with the sensitivity, specificity, PPV, and NPV of 37.2%, 96.6%, 88.9%, and 67.9%, respectively, in differentiating CSPCa from this cohort. At a cutoff value of 10 ng/mL, PSA showed a sensitivity value of 76.7% (but a specificity of only 45.8%) and a PPV and NPV of 76.7% and 73.7% in differentiating CSPCa from this cohort. The best cutoff value for F/T PSA was obtained at 0.135. At this level, Youden's index, sensitivity, specificity, PPV, and NPV for F/T PSA were 0.467, 72.1%, 74.6%, 67.4%, and 78.6%. For PI-RADS v2.1, when the cutoff value is set as ≥4, the best Youden's index, sensitivity, specificity, PPV, and NPV were 0.460, 88.4%, 57.6%, 60.3%, and 87.2%, respectively. If the cutoff value is set as ≥3, the sensitivity, specificity, PPV, and NPV were 97.7%, 25.4%, 48.8%, and 93.8%, respectively.

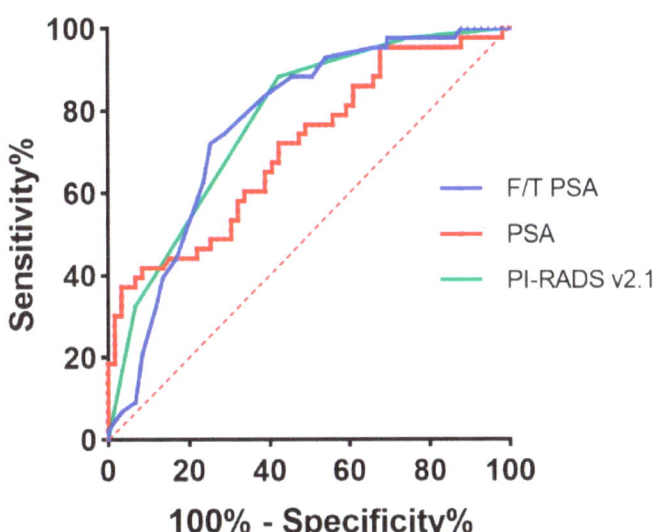

Figure 1. ROC curves of PSA, F/T PSA, and PI-RADS v2.1 in predicting CSPCa.

In univariate logistic regression analysis, age, PSA, F/T PSA (<0.135 vs. ≥0.135), and PI-RADS v2.1(≥3 vs. <3) showed significant associations with the biopsy results. However, in multivariate logistic regression analysis, only age, F/T PSA, and PI-RADS v2.1 remained independent predictors for CSPCa (Table S1).

Among the 43 patients with CSPCa biopsy results, 31 had CSPCa detected from both PZ and TZ cores, 11 had CSPCa detected only in the PZ, and 1 had CSPCa detected only in the TZ. The PI-RADS v2.1 TZ score and the PI-RADS v2.1 PZ score were proposed and analyzed (Table 2). There was a significant difference in PI-RADS v2.1 scores between patients with or without peripheral-zone CSPCa. Such a difference was not observed in the TZ subgroup, indicating PI-RADS v2.1 may not be an effective tool to diagnose CSPCa in the TZ in this cohort. Figure 2 shows the biopsy results by PI-RADS v2.1 TZ and PZ scores. For PI-RADS PZ scores of 2, 3, 4, and 5 in the peripheral zone, the CSPCa detection rates were 14.3%, 22.2%, 54.5%, and 83.3%, respectively.

Table 2. PI-RADS v2.1 scores for the peripheral zone and the transitional zone.

	CSPCa	Non-CSPCa/Negative Biopsy	*p*-Value
PI-RADS v2.1 PZ n (%)			
2	4 (9.5%)	24 (40.0%)	0.000
3	4 (9.5%)	14 (23.3%)	
4	24 (57.1%)	20 (33.3%)	
5	10 (23.8%)	2 (3.3%)	
PI-RADS v2.1 TZ n (%)			
No Suspected Lesions	11 (34.4%)	18 (25.7%)	0.167
2	7 (21.9%)	17 (24.3%)	
3	7 (21.9%)	24 (34.3%)	
4	6 (18.8%)	4 (5.7%)	
5	1 (3.1%)	7 (10.0%)	

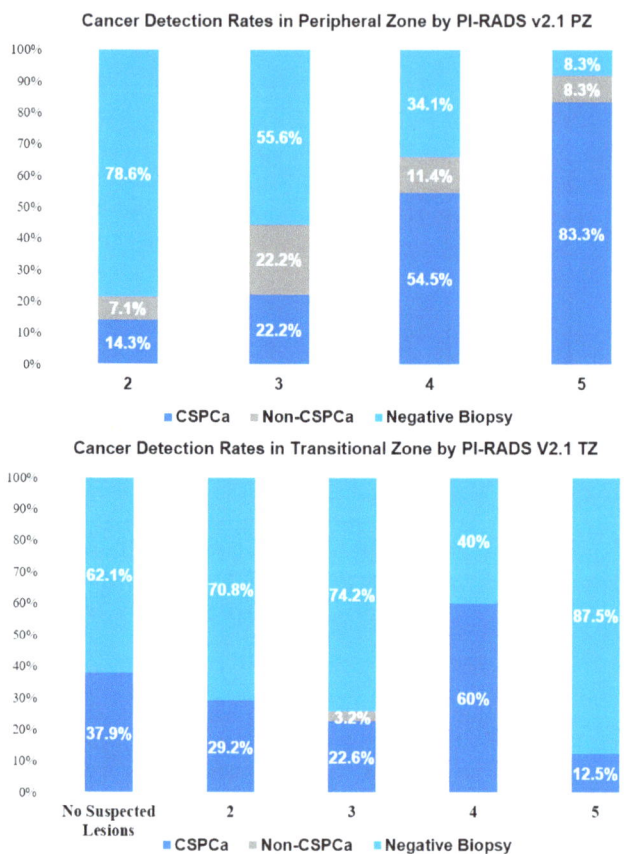

Figure 2. CSPCa detection rates by PI-RADS v2.1 scores.

In ROC analysis (Figure 3), PI-RADS v2.1 PZ obtained significant diagnostic value in the peripheral zone (AUC 0.780 (95%CI 0.665–0.854; $p < 0.001$)). At a cutoff value of ≥ 3, PI-RADS v2.1 PZ had the sensitivity, specificity, PPV, and NPV of 90.5%, 40.0%, 51.3%, and 85.7%, respectively. However, in the transitional zone, PI-RADS v2.1 TZ demonstrated no diagnostic value for CSPCa (AUC 0.533 (95%CI 0.410–0.557; $p = 0.594$)).

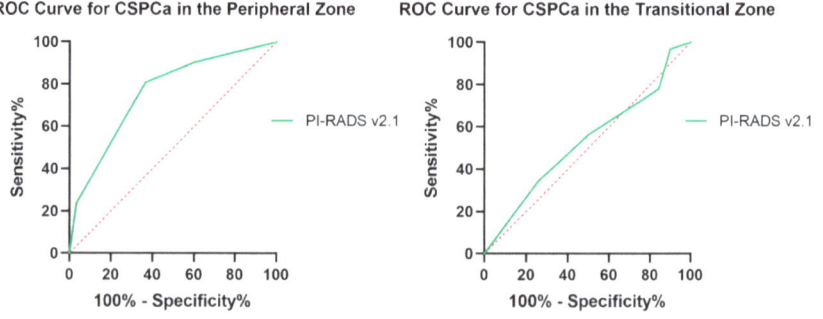

Figure 3. ROC curves of PI-RADS v2.1 in predicting CSPCa in the peripheral zone and the transitional zone.

In univariate logistic regression analysis (Table S2), compared to PI-RADS PZ score 2, the odds ratio was 7.200 (95%CI 2.140–24.230) for patients with a PI-RADS PZ score of 4 and 30.000 (95%CI 4.714–190.939) for patients with a PI-RADS PZ score of 5. PI-RADS PZ score ≥3 was an independent predictor for CSPCa (OR = 6.333, 95%CI 2.000–20.052, p = 0.002). As for the transitional zone, PI-RADS TZ scores of 2, 3, 4, and 5 showed no significant odds ratio compared to no suspected lesions by PI-RADS v2.1. PI-RADS TZ score ≥3 showed limited significance for predicting CSPCa (OR = 0.778, 95%CI 0.335–1.803, p = 0.558).

Figure 4 shows the mpMRI results of two patients. For both patients, the PI-RADS v2.1 scoring system demonstrated unsatisfactory diagnostic value in the transitional zone.

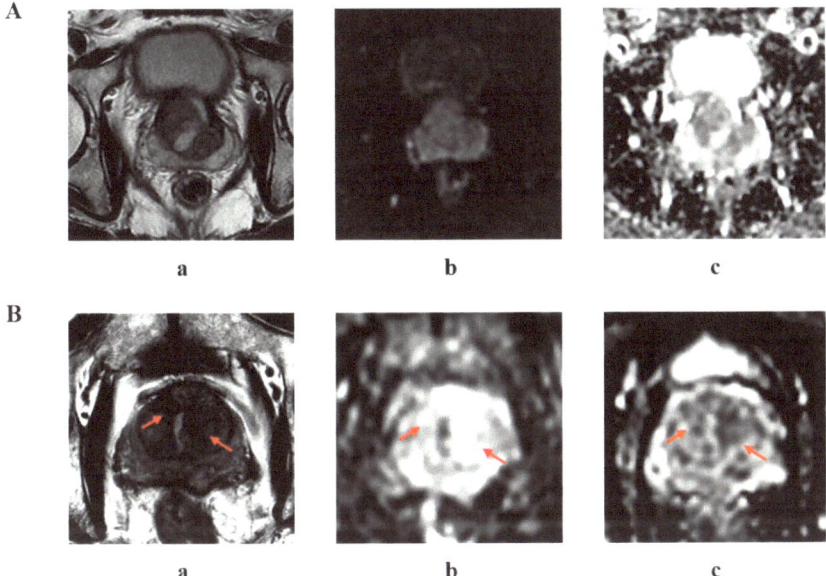

Figure 4. mpMRI results of two biopsy patients with TURP history. (**A**) A 63-year-old patient previously received TURP; no lesions with PI-RADS score ≥ 3 were found in TZ. Biopsy results showed CSPCa with a Gleason score of 4 + 3 = 7 in the TZ. (**B**) A 74-year-old patient previously received TURP; two lesions classified as PI-RADS score 4 were found in the bilateral TZ (arrow). Biopsy results were negative in the TZ. (a) T2-weighted image; (b) DWI with b-value of 1500 s/mm^2; (c) ADC map.

4. Discussion

Benign prostatic hyperplasia (BPH) is a condition with high prevalence among aged men; 50% of men with BPH develop LUTS that require medical intervention [16]. Transurethral resection of the prostate (TURP) has remained the cornerstone of BPH surgical treatment for decades. The TURP operation removes tissue from the TZ of the gland to address BPH-related obstruction, during which the PZ of the gland is not resected. It is reported that a secondary TURP is required to address the re-developed prostatic obstruction for 2.9%, 5.8%, and 7.4% of patients in 1, 5, and 8 years after primary TURP [17], which indicates a significant proportion of patients may experience adenoma regrowth in the resected TZ of the prostate after a TURP procedure. Therefore, patients are still at risk of PCa in both the PZ and the TZ of the gland after receiving a TURP. Although patients with a history of TURP are commonly seen in a urology clinic, few studies have addressed the clinical characteristics of this cohort. Clinical studies regarding diagnostic tests for PCa commonly set patients with prostatic surgery history into the exclusion criteria, leading to the scarcity of evidence for the diagnostic value of PSA, F/T PSA, or mpMRI results in this cohort.

We noticed the lack of references for patients suspected of PCa who also have a history of TURP, leading to our study being the first to look into this issue.

PSA levels can be affected by prostate volume or the presence of BPH or prostatitis. Aus et al. [13] reported that in 190 patients who underwent TURP due to BPH, the mean PSA levels were reduced by 70%, from 6.0 to 1.9 ng/mL 3–4 months after TURP, while the mean prostate volume was reduced by 58%, from 63.3 to 26.5 cc. Furuya et al. [18] found that the removal of 1 g of BPH tissue reduced serum PSA levels by an average of 0.18 ng/mL, revealing the correlation between serum PSA levels and the TZ volume. A TURP procedure removes BPH tissue from the TZ, resulting in a significant decrease in PSA, while the possible regrowth of adenoma at the surgery site may lead to an increase in PSA levels in the long term after surgery. Taken together, the baseline PSA levels appear uncertain in this cohort. Our study revealed positive results in the diagnostic value of the absolute PSA level in CSPCa in this cohort. Setting the cutoff value at 10 ng/mL, PSA shows high sensitivity (76.7%) but poor specificity (45.8%).

Catalona et al. [5] reported that at a 25% cutoff, F/T PSA detected 95% of cancers while avoiding 20% of unnecessary biopsies for patients with a PSA level of 4.0 to 10.0 ng/mL. The reasons for the changes in F/T PSA in PCa are not fully understood [19]. Recker et al. [20] explored the changes in serum total and free PSA in TURP patients and revealed that despite a decline in t-PSA by 72% post-TURP, F/T PSA remained stable (median 24.9% pre-op vs. 26.6% post-op), indicating the potential of F/T PSA in PCa detection after TURP. Consistent with their results, our study revealed the high diagnostic value of F/T PSA in CSPCa. At a cutoff value of 13.5%, the sensitivity and specificity in the cohort were 72.1% and 74.6%, respectively, and an F/T PSA under 13.5% indicated a nearly 9-fold higher risk for CSPCa.

PI-RADS v2.1 is a structured reporting system for standardizing the mpMRI results for detecting PCa. Our study revealed that PI-RADS v2.1 is a reliable tool for CSPCa detection in patients with a history of TURP. A cutoff at PI-RADS score ≥ 4 resulted in 88.4% of CSPCa cases found and 57.6% of unnecessary biopsies avoided. To further explore the value of PI-RADS V2.1, we reviewed the imaging scores of two prostatic zones separately. The results showed that PI-RADS V2.1 remains reliable in identifying CSPCa in the PZ. Rudolph et al. [21] reported CSPCa detection rates of 13.0%, 10.0%, 42.9%, and 68.3% for PI-RADS v2.1 scores of 2, 3, 4, and 5, respectively, in the PZ. The detection rates in the PZ of our patients are consistent with earlier studies of PI-RADS in the whole patient population [22–26], indicating that the PZ CSPCa lesions were not affected by the excision or regrowth of prostatic tissue. Therefore, when managing patients with a history of TURP, mpMRI can provide important references for PZ lesions, and a high PI-RADS PZ score should be an indication for biopsy.

Concerning the TZ, the performance of CSPCa detection was limited with PI-RADS v2.1 scores. For lesions with a PI-RADS v2.1 score of 2, 3, 4, and 5, CSPCa detection rates were reported to be 7.4%, 8.3%, 40.0%, and 61.7%, respectively, in the general biopsy patient population [21], which differ significantly from our findings in patients with TURP history. This result might be due to the tissue composition changes secondary to TURP, such as inflammatory tissue reactions consisting of mononuclear cells and giant cells [27] or a mixture of scar tissue, glandular tissue, and stromal tissue, which are commonly presented as areas with hypointensity in T2WI. In this instance, corresponding changes in T2W signals can easily mimic the diagnostic criteria for PI-RADS 4, which creates challenges for accurate imaging assessment [8]. From our results, mpMRI should not be referenced when assessing transitional zone lesions, and PI-RADS TZ scores should not be decisive factors when considering a biopsy.

To our knowledge, our study is the first study to probe into the diagnostic tests for CSPCa in patients with TURP history. This study has some limitations. First, it is a retrospective, single-center study with a relatively small sample size. Clinical characteristics of our cohort show great heterogeneity, especially in the time after TURP and PSA levels, which may reduce the representativeness of our study cohort. The small sample size limited the reliability of subgroup analysis. Studies [28,29] have suggested the monitoring of PSA dynamic changes or PSA velocity as a predictor for PCa in post-TURP patients. Pre-TURP PSA levels may provide reference cutoff values for our study. Unfortunately, due to the long interval since TURP and the lack of follow-up data in our patient cohort, such information was not available. PSA-density, as well as MRI-estimated lesion volume, has been reported to provide additional predictive value to the detection of CSPCa in the whole patient population [30–32]. However, impaired anatomy at the previous TURP site created difficulties for prostate and lesion volume measurements. The clinical implications of our findings remain inconclusive. Further large-sample prospective studies are needed to conclude the characteristics of such a cohort and explore optimal diagnostic procedures and treatment strategies.

5. Conclusions

Our study reveals that PSA and F/T PSA retain significant diagnostic value for CSPCa in patients with TURP history. PI-RADS v2.1 is reliable for detecting CSPCa in the PZ but has limited diagnostic value when assessing TZ lesions.

Supplementary Materials: The following supporting information can be downloaded at: https://www.mdpi.com/article/10.3390/curroncol29090502/s1, Figure S1: 12-core transrectal ultrasound (TRUS)-guided transperineal prostate biopsy template; Table S1: Univariate and multivariate logistic regression analysis for CSPCa; Table S2: Logistic regression analysis of PI-RADS v2.1 in the peripheral and transitional zones.

Author Contributions: Y.Z. and W.X.: conceptualization and supervision. J.L., G.W. and L.D.: investigation and writing—original draft preparation. J.W., Y.W. and H.Q.: resources. S.P., B.D. and J.P.: writing—review and editing. All authors have read and agreed to the published version of the manuscript.

Funding: This study was supported by the National Natural Science Foundation of China (81572536, 81672850, 81772742, 81702840, 81702542, 81972578, 81902863, 82002710, 82072847, 82003148, 82103485), the Shanghai Shen Kang Hospital Development Center (SHDC2020CR3014A), the Shanghai Sailing Program (20YF1425300), and the Incubating Program for Clinical Research and Innovation of Ren Ji Hospital Shanghai Jiao Tong University School of Medicine (PYZY 16-008, PYXJS16-015, RJZZ19-17, PYI20-04).

Institutional Review Board Statement: The study was conducted according to the guidelines of the Declaration of Helsinki and approved by the Shanghai Jiao Tong University School of Medicine, Ren Ji Hospital Ethics Committee (approval number SK2020-027, approved on 27 August 2020).

Informed Consent Statement: Informed consent was obtained from all subjects involved in the study.

Data Availability Statement: The data presented in this study are available upon request from the corresponding author. The data are not publicly available due to the privacy of patients.

Conflicts of Interest: The authors declare no conflict of interest.

References

1. Chen, R.; Ren, S.; Chinese Prostate Cancer, C.; Yiu, M.K.; Fai, N.C.; Cheng, W.S.; Ian, L.H.; Naito, S.; Matsuda, T.; Kehinde, E.; et al. Prostate cancer in Asia: A collaborative report. *Asian J. Urol.* **2014**, *1*, 15–29. [CrossRef] [PubMed]
2. Siegel, R.L.; Miller, K.D.; Jemal, A. Cancer statistics, 2020. *CA Cancer J. Clin.* **2020**, *70*, 7–30. [CrossRef] [PubMed]
3. Etzioni, R.; Penson, D.F.; Legler, J.M.; di Tommaso, D.; Boer, R.; Gann, P.H.; Feuer, E.J. Overdiagnosis due to prostate-specific antigen screening: Lessons from U.S. prostate cancer incidence trends. *J. Natl. Cancer Inst.* **2002**, *94*, 981–990. [CrossRef] [PubMed]
4. Huang, Y.; Li, Z.Z.; Huang, Y.L.; Song, H.J.; Wang, Y.J. Value of free/total prostate-specific antigen (f/t PSA) ratios for prostate cancer detection in patients with total serum prostate-specific antigen between 4 and 10 ng/mL: A meta-analysis. *Medicine* **2018**, *97*, e0249. [CrossRef]
5. Catalona, W.J.; Partin, A.W.; Slawin, K.M.; Brawer, M.K.; Flanigan, R.C.; Patel, A.; Richie, J.P.; deKernion, J.B.; Walsh, P.C.; Scardino, P.T.; et al. Use of the Percentage of Free Prostate-Specific Antigen to Enhance Differentiation of Prostate Cancer from Benign Prostatic Disease A Prospective Multicenter Clinical Trial. *JAMA* **1998**, *279*, 1542–1547. [CrossRef]
6. Bratan, F.; Niaf, E.; Melodelima, C.; Chesnais, A.L.; Souchon, R.; Mège-Lechevallier, F.; Colombel, M.; Rouvière, O. Influence of imaging and histological factors on prostate cancer detection and localisation on multiparametric MRI: A prospective study. *Eur. Radiol.* **2013**, *23*, 2019–2029. [CrossRef]

7. Turkbey, B.; Rosenkrantz, A.B.; Haider, M.A.; Padhani, A.R.; Villeirs, G.; Macura, K.J.; Tempany, C.M.; Choyke, P.L.; Cornud, F.; Margolis, D.J.; et al. Prostate Imaging Reporting and Data System Version 2.1: 2019 Update of Prostate Imaging Reporting and Data System Version 2. *Eur. Urol.* **2019**, *76*, 340–351. [CrossRef]
8. Weinreb, J.C.; Barentsz, J.O.; Choyke, P.L.; Cornud, F.; Haider, M.A.; Macura, K.J.; Margolis, D.; Schnall, M.D.; Shtern, F.; Tempany, C.M.; et al. PI-RADS Prostate Imaging—Reporting and Data System: 2015, Version 2. *Eur. Urol.* **2016**, *69*, 16–40. [CrossRef]
9. Thakur, V.; Singh, P.P.; Talwar, M.; Mukherjee, U. Utility of free/total prostate specific antigen (f/t PSA) ratio in diagnosis of prostate carcinoma. *Dis. Markers* **2003**, *19*, 287–292. [CrossRef]
10. Roobol, M.J.; Steyerberg, E.W.; Kranse, R.; Wolters, T.; van den Bergh, R.C.; Bangma, C.H.; Schröder, F.H. A risk-based strategy improves prostate-specific antigen-driven detection of prostate cancer. *Eur. Urol.* **2010**, *57*, 79–85. [CrossRef]
11. Wang, R.; Wang, H.; Zhao, C.; Hu, J.; Jiang, Y.; Tong, Y.; Liu, T.; Huang, R.; Wang, X. Evaluation of Multiparametric Magnetic Resonance Imaging in Detection and Prediction of Prostate Cancer. *PLoS ONE* **2015**, *10*, e0130207. [CrossRef] [PubMed]
12. Marks, L.S.; Dorey, F.J.; Rhodes, T.; Shery, E.D.; Rittenhouse, H.; Partin, A.W.; deKernion, J.B. Serum prostate specific antigen levels after transurethral resection of prostate: A longitudinal characterization in men with benign prostatic hyperplasia. *J. Urol.* **1996**, *156*, 1035–1039. [CrossRef]
13. Aus, G.; Bergdahl, S.; Frösing, R.; Lodding, P.; Pileblad, E.; Hugosson, J. Reference range of prostate-specific antigen after transurethral resection of the prostate. *Urology* **1996**, *47*, 529–531. [CrossRef]
14. Koopman, A.; Jenniskens, S.F.M.; Fütterer, J.J. Magnetic Resonance Imaging Assessment After Therapy in Prostate Cancer. *Top. Magn. Reson. Imaging* **2020**, *29*, 47–58. [CrossRef] [PubMed]
15. Potretzke, T.A.; Froemming, A.T.; Gupta, R.T. Post-treatment prostate MRI. *Abdom. Radiol.* **2020**, *45*, 2184–2197. [CrossRef]
16. Egan, K.B. The Epidemiology of Benign Prostatic Hyperplasia Associated with Lower Urinary Tract Symptoms: Prevalence and Incident Rates. *Urol. Clin. N. Am.* **2016**, *43*, 289–297. [CrossRef] [PubMed]
17. Madersbacher, S.; Lackner, J.; Brössner, C.; Röhlich, M.; Stancik, I.; Willinger, M.; Schatzl, G. Reoperation, myocardial infarction and mortality after transurethral and open prostatectomy: A nation-wide, long-term analysis of 23,123 cases. *Eur. Urol.* **2005**, *47*, 499–504. [CrossRef]
18. Furuya, Y.; Akakura, K.; Tobe, T.; Ichikawa, T.; Igarashi, T.; Ito, H. Changes in serum prostate-specific antigen following prostatectomy in patients with benign prostate hyperplasia. *Int. J. Urol.* **2000**, *7*, 447–451. [CrossRef] [PubMed]
19. Mikolajczyk, S.D.; Marks, L.S.; Partin, A.W.; Rittenhouse, H.G. Free prostate-specific antigen in serum is becoming more complex. *Urology* **2002**, *59*, 797–802. [CrossRef]
20. Recker, F.; Kwiatkowski, M.K.; Pettersson, K.; Piironen, T.; Lümmen, G.; Huber, A.; Tscholl, R. Enhanced expression of prostate-specific antigen in the transition zone of the prostate. A characterization following prostatectomy for benign hyperplasia. *Eur. Urol.* **1998**, *33*, 549–555. [CrossRef]
21. Rudolph, M.M.; Baur, A.D.J.; Cash, H.; Haas, M.; Mahjoub, S.; Hartenstein, A.; Hamm, C.A.; Beetz, N.L.; Konietschke, F.; Hamm, B.; et al. Diagnostic performance of PI-RADS version 2.1 compared to version 2.0 for detection of peripheral and transition zone prostate cancer. *Sci. Rep.* **2020**, *10*, 15982. [CrossRef] [PubMed]
22. Ahmed, H.U.; El-Shater Bosaily, A.; Brown, L.C.; Gabe, R.; Kaplan, R.; Parmar, M.K.; Collaco-Moraes, Y.; Ward, K.; Hindley, R.G.; Freeman, A.; et al. Diagnostic accuracy of multi-parametric MRI and TRUS biopsy in prostate cancer (PROMIS): A paired validating confirmatory study. *Lancet* **2017**, *389*, 815–822. [CrossRef]
23. Rouvière, O.; Puech, P.; Renard-Penna, R.; Claudon, M.; Roy, C.; Mège-Lechevallier, F.; Decaussin-Petrucci, M.; Dubreuil-Chambardel, M.; Magaud, L.; Remontet, L.; et al. Use of prostate systematic and targeted biopsy on the basis of multiparametric MRI in biopsy-naive patients (MRI-FIRST): A prospective, multicentre, paired diagnostic study. *Lancet Oncol.* **2019**, *20*, 100–109. [CrossRef]
24. Gross, M.D.; Marks, L.S.; Sonn, G.A.; Green, D.A.; Wang, G.J.; Shoag, J.E.; Cabezon, E.; Margolis, D.J.; Robinson, B.D.; Hu, J.C. Variation in Magnetic Resonance Imaging-Ultrasound Fusion Targeted Biopsy Outcomes in Asian American Men: A Multicenter Study. *J. Urol.* **2020**, *203*, 530–536. [CrossRef] [PubMed]
25. Alberts, A.R.; Roobol, M.J.; Verbeek, J.F.M.; Schoots, I.G.; Chiu, P.K.; Osses, D.F.; Tijsterman, J.D.; Beerlage, H.P.; Mannaerts, C.K.; Schimmöller, L.; et al. Prediction of High-grade Prostate Cancer Following Multiparametric Magnetic Resonance Imaging: Improving the Rotterdam European Randomized Study of Screening for Prostate Cancer Risk Calculators. *Eur. Urol.* **2019**, *75*, 310–318. [CrossRef]
26. Washino, S.; Okochi, T.; Saito, K.; Konishi, T.; Hirai, M.; Kobayashi, Y.; Miyagawa, T. Combination of prostate imaging reporting and data system (PI-RADS) score and prostate-specific antigen (PSA) density predicts biopsy outcome in prostate biopsy naïve patients. *BJU Int.* **2017**, *119*, 225–233. [CrossRef]
27. Sheu, M.H.; Chiang, H.; Wang, J.H.; Chang, Y.H.; Chang, C.Y. Transurethral resection of the prostate-related changes in the prostate gland: Correlation of MRI and histopathology. *J. Comput. Assist. Tomogr.* **2000**, *24*, 596–599. [CrossRef]
28. Wolff, J.M.; Boekels, O.; Borchers, H.; Jakse, G.; Rohde, D. Altered prostate specific antigen reference range after transurethral resection of the prostate. *Anticancer Res.* **2000**, *20*, 4977–4980.
29. Helfand, B.T.; Anderson, C.B.; Fought, A.; Kim, D.Y.; Vyas, A.; McVary, K.T. Postoperative PSA and PSA Velocity Identify Presence of Prostate Cancer After Various Surgical Interventions for Benign Prostatic Hyperplasia. *Urology* **2009**, *74*, 177–183. [CrossRef]

30. Deniffel, D.; Healy, G.M.; Dong, X.; Ghai, S.; Salinas-Miranda, E.; Fleshner, N.; Hamilton, R.; Kulkarni, G.; Toi, A.; van der Kwast, T.; et al. Avoiding Unnecessary Biopsy: MRI-based Risk Models versus a PI-RADS and PSA Density Strategy for Clinically Significant Prostate Cancer. *Radiology* **2021**, *300*, 369–379. [CrossRef]
31. Martorana, E.; Aisa, M.C.; Grisanti, R.; Santini, N.; Pirola, G.M.; Datti, A.; Gerli, S.; Bonora, A.; Burani, A.; Scalera, G.B.; et al. Lesion Volume in a Bi- or Multivariate Prediction Model for the Management of PI-RADS v2.1 Score 3 Category Lesions. *Turk. J. Urol.* **2022**, *48*, 268–277. [CrossRef] [PubMed]
32. Martorana, E.; Pirola, G.M.; Scialpi, M.; Micali, S.; Iseppi, A.; Bonetti, L.R.; Kaleci, S.; Torricelli, P.; Bianchi, G. Lesion volume predicts prostate cancer risk and aggressiveness: Validation of its value alone and matched with prostate imaging reporting and data system score. *BJU Int.* **2017**, *120*, 92–103. [CrossRef] [PubMed]

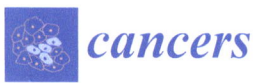

Article

Hemopatch to Prevent Lymphatic Leak after Robotic Prostatectomy and Pelvic Lymph Node Dissection: A Randomized Controlled Trial

Jeremy Yuen-Chun Teoh *, Alex Qinyang Liu, Violet Wai-Fan Yuen, Franco Pui-Tak Lai, Steffi Kar-Kei Yuen, Samson Yun-Sang Chan, Julius Ho-Fai Wong, Joseph Kai-Man Li, Mandy Ho-Man Tam, Peter Ka-Fung Chiu, Samuel Chi-Hang Yee and Chi-Fai Ng

S.H. Ho Urology Center, Department of Surgery, Prince of Wales Hospital, The Chinese University of Hong Kong, Hong Kong, China
* Correspondence: jeremyteoh@surgery.cuhk.edu.hk

Simple Summary: This trial investigated the use of Hemopatch, a novel hemostatic patch, during robotic-assisted prostate and lymph node surgery for prostate cancer. The researchers hypothesize that the use of Hemopatch could decrease lymph leak from the surgical bed, which is reflected by the drain output volume. The result shows that patients who underwent surgeries with Hemopatch had a lower drain output volume in total and per day, comparatively. In conclusion, Hemopatch use should be considered in prostate cancer surgery.

Abstract: This study investigates whether the application of Hemopatch, a novel hemostatic patch, could prevent lymphatic leak after robotic-assisted radical prostatectomy (RARP) and bilateral pelvic lymph node dissection (BPLND). This is a prospective, single-center, phase III randomized controlled trial investigating the efficacy of Hemopatch in preventing lymphatic leak after RARP and BPLND. Participants were randomized to receive RARP and BPLND, with or without the use of Hemopatch, with an allocation ratio of 1:1. The primary outcome is the total drain output volume. The secondary outcomes include blood loss, operative time, lymph node yield, duration of drainage, drain output per day, hospital stay, transfusion and 30-day complications. A total of 32 patients were recruited in the study. The Hemopatch group had a significantly lower median total drain output than the control group (35 mL vs. 180 mL, $p = 0.022$) and a significantly lower drain output volume per day compared to the control group (35 mL/day vs. 89 mL/day, $p = 0.038$). There was no significant difference in the other secondary outcomes. In conclusion, the application of Hemopatch in RARP and BPLND could reduce the total drain output volume and the drain output volume per day. The use of Hemopatch should be considered to prevent lymphatic leakage after RARP and BPLND.

Keywords: Hemopatch; prostate cancer; prostatectomy; pelvic lymph node dissection; lymphatic leak

Citation: Teoh, J.Y.-C.; Liu, A.Q.; Yuen, V.W.-F.; Lai, F.P.-T.; Yuen, S.K.-K.; Chan, S.Y.-S.; Wong, J.H.-F.; Li, J.K.-M.; Tam, M.H.-M.; Chiu, P.K.-F.; et al. Hemopatch to Prevent Lymphatic Leak after Robotic Prostatectomy and Pelvic Lymph Node Dissection: A Randomized Controlled Trial. *Cancers* **2022**, *14*, 4476. https://doi.org/10.3390/cancers14184476

Academic Editors: Paula A. Oliveira, Ana Faustino and Lúcio Lara Santos

Received: 15 August 2022
Accepted: 12 September 2022
Published: 15 September 2022

Publisher's Note: MDPI stays neutral with regard to jurisdictional claims in published maps and institutional affiliations.

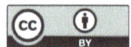

Copyright: © 2022 by the authors. Licensee MDPI, Basel, Switzerland. This article is an open access article distributed under the terms and conditions of the Creative Commons Attribution (CC BY) license (https://creativecommons.org/licenses/by/4.0/).

1. Introduction

In prostate cancer patients undergoing robot-assisted radical prostatectomy (RARP), the current European Association of Urology (EAU) prostate cancer guidelines recommend bilateral pelvic lymph node dissection (BPLND) for those with an estimated risk of occult nodal metastases exceeding 5% [1]. In a systematic review of 66 studies involving 275,269 patients, lymphadenectomy can identify node-positive patients who may benefit from adjuvant treatment [2].

BPLND in general is a well-tolerated procedure. However, when complications do occur, significant morbidity results. The benefits of BPLND must be carefully weighed against its potential complications. The most common complication of BPLND is lymphocoele formation. Small lymphatic vessels lack a muscular layer and adventitia, as opposed to blood vessels [3]. The transection of blood capillaries will lead to vasoconstriction and the eventual cessation of bleeding. This is not the case with small lymphatic vessels, and transection is likely to lead to prolonged lymphorrhoea. The incidence of lymphocoele varies from series to series, ranging from 0.8% to 33%, depending on the extent of lymphadenectomy, the surgical technique, the operative approach and the diagnostic approach [4,5]. Lymphocele formation could lead to abdominal or groin pain, abdominal swelling, lower urinary tract symptoms, bladder outlet obstruction, obstructive uropathy, infection, sepsis, lower extremity or genital oedema, deep vein thrombosis and even anastomotic disruption [6–9]. Moreover, lymphocele formation might also affect subsequent radiotherapy planning, if needed [10]. Prolonged lymphorrhoea lengthens hospital stay, places the patient at risk for nosocomial infection and has significant cost implications for the healthcare system [11].

Hemopatch is a haemostatic pad consisting of a collagen sheet derived from bovine dermis with an NHS-PEG (N-hydroxysuccinimide-functionalized pentaerythritol polyethylene glycol ether tetra-succinimidyl glutarate)-coated active surface. These two components act together to provide effective tissue adherence, sealing and haemostasis [12]. Upon tissue contact, NHS-PEG molecules on the active surface form covalent bonds with tissue proteins. Cross-linking NHS-PEG and proteins forms a hydrogel which acts as an effective tissue seal. Older-generation NHS-PEG products in the form of solutions of flowable sealants are quickly washed away by blood or other leaking body fluids, rendering them ineffective in the presence of active bleeding or fluid leakage. Hemopatch is a novel NHS-PEG delivery vehicle designed to overcome this limitation. Due to the open pore structure of the collagen, excess tissue fluids are readily absorbed, and the direct contact of NHS-PEG to the tissue surface can be achieved. The collagen pad is optimized to be soft, thin and pliable and has a high liquid absorption capacity. The pad is resorbed and replaced by the host tissue in six to eight weeks, with little tissue reaction.

We hypothesized that the application of Hemopatch to raw lymphatic tissue can prevent lymphorrhoea through its unique combination of tissue adherence, sealing and fluid absorption. This can potentially prevent lymphatic leak, reduce the drain output and facilitate earlier discharge.

2. Materials and Methods

2.1. Trial Design

This is a prospective, single-center, phase III randomized controlled trial investigating the efficacy of Hemopatch in preventing lymphatic leak after RARP and BPLND. Participants were randomized to receive RARP and BPLND, with or without the use of Hemopatch. The study was conducted at the Prince of Wales Hospital in Hong Kong from January 2020 to December 2021. The study protocol was approved by the Joint Chinese University of Hong Kong—New Territories East Cluster Clinical Research Ethics Committee (CREC Reference number: 2019.419-T). The study was registered at the US National Institutes of Health (ClinicalTrial.gov; Identifier: NCT04185922). The study was conducted in accordance with the Declaration of Helsinki and the International Conference on Harmonization, Good Clinical Practice Guidelines (ICH-GCP).

2.2. Participants

All consecutive patients with prostate cancer, indicated for RARP and BPLND, were screened for eligibility. BPLND was performed if the estimated risk of occult nodal metastases based on the Memorial Sloan Kettering Cancer Center pre-radical prostatectomy nomogram [13] was over 5% [14]. The inclusion and exclusion criteria are as follows.

Inclusion criteria
- Aged 18 years and above
- Able to give informed consent
- Suitable for minimally invasive surgery

Exclusion criteria
- Known allergy or hypersensitivity to any component of Hemopatch
- Known hypersensitivity to bovine proteins or brilliant blue
- Patients with prior pelvic radiotherapy
- Patients with non-correctable coagulopathy
- Patients who are on anticoagulants
- Contraindication to general anaesthesia
- Previous transurethral resection of prostate (TURP) or prostatic surgery
- Untreated active infection

Informed consent was obtained from the eligible study subjects before the scheduled RARP and BPLND operations.

2.3. Randomization and Blinding

Patients were randomized to receive RARP and BPLND, with or without Hemopatch, with an allocation ratio of 1:1. The randomization sequence was obtained with computer-generated random sequence numbers, with no restriction rules applied. Allocation concealment was ensured by the use of a web-based internet application to reveal randomization codes after patient recruitment. The patients were then assigned to the experimental arm or the standard arm according to the randomization codes. The operating urologist was informed of the allocated treatment arm only after BPLND had been performed. Patients receiving the treatment and investigators assessing the study outcomes were blinded from the allocated treatment arm.

2.4. Interventions

All participants received RARP and BPLND in the usual manner [15]. Each patient was first placed supine with a split leg position. Skin incisions were made to allow for the insertion of the robotic camera port, robotic instrument ports and assistant ports. The patient was then placed in a reverse Trendelenburg position, and the da Vinci Xi robotic surgical system was docked. Radical prostatectomy was performed with an anterior approach. After the prostate gland was excised, BPLND was performed with a standard template up to uretero-iliac crossing. Vesicourethral anastomosis was then performed, and a water leak test was routinely performed to ensure a water-tight anastomosis. After the vesicourethral anastomosis was completed, four pieces of Hemopatch were applied to the lymph node dissection area on each side, i.e., eight pieces in total. The distal ends at the obturator fossa and the femoral canal, along with the proximal ends at the the common iliac bifurcation and internal iliac artery, were thoroughly covered by Hemopatch (see Figure 1). The patch was kept dry until contact with the tissue. After tissue contact, pressure was applied over the pad surface for two minutes. The active comparator is standard RARP and BPLND without the use of haemostatic adjuncts, which is the standard of care at our institution. Finally, a pelvic drain was inserted before the conclusion of the operation.

2.5. Post-Operative Management

The diet was usually resumed on post-operative day 1. The pelvic drain would be removed if the output was <100 mL over the past 24 h. The patient would be discharged with a Foley catheter when the diet was well tolerated and drain was removed. The patient would return to the hospital for the removal of the urethral catheter on post-operative days 7 to 10, and this was subjected to the discretion of the operating surgeon. A further follow-up appointment was arranged one month after the operation.

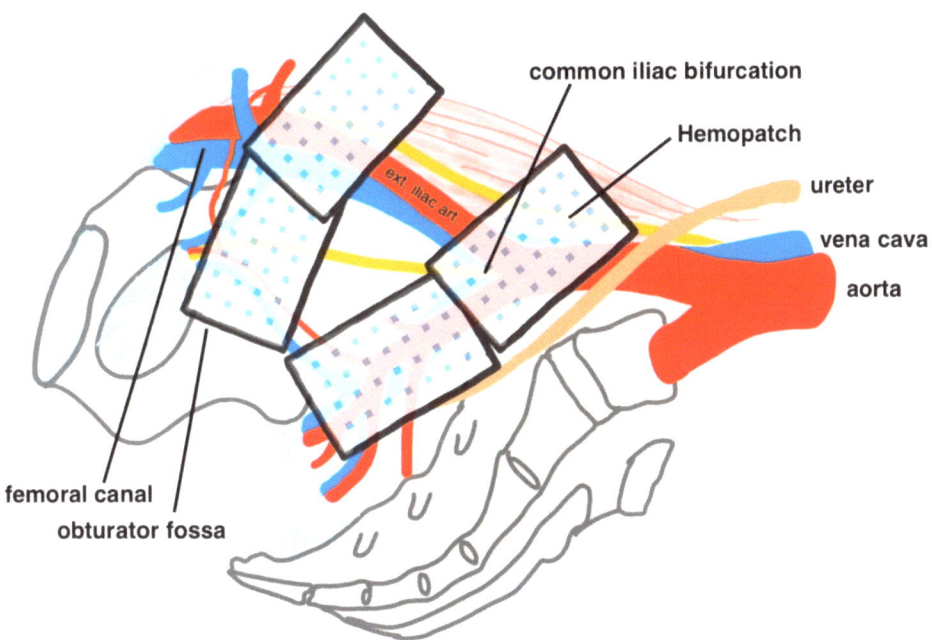

Figure 1. Hemopatch placement position diagram. Ext. iliac art. = external iliac artery.

2.6. Outcome Measures and Data Collection

The primary outcome is the total volume of drain output, which is a surrogate for lymphorrhoea. The hypothesis is that Hemopatch placement prevents lymphatic leak.

The secondary outcomes include the estimated blood loss, operative time, lymph node yield, duration of drainage, drain output per day, hospital stay, transfusion and 30-day complications.

All baseline characteristics and peri-operative complications were recorded upon the day of discharge. Any 30-day complications following the operation were recorded during the follow-up appointment. All complications were graded according to the Clavien–Dindo classification. Serious adverse events were reported until 30 days after the operation.

2.7. Sample Size

A total of 32 participants were recruited for the study, as per study protocol. Assuming a 33.3% difference in the total volume of drain output (100 mL in the Hemopatch group vs. 150 mL in the control group, with a standard deviation of 50 mL), with a two-sided significance of 0.05 and a power of 80%, 16 patients are required in each group. As the primary outcome is the total volume of drain output, which will be determined upon hospital discharge, no drop-out rate is included in the sample size calculation.

2.8. Statistical Methods

All outcome measurements were analyzed with an intention-to-treat principle. An independent samples t-test was used for parametric continuous variables; a Mann–Whitney U test was used for non-parametric continuous variables; a chi-square test was used for categorical variables. A p-value less than 0.05 is considered to be statistically significant. All statistical analyses were performed using SPSS version 23.0 (Armonk, NY, USA: IBM Corp.).

3. Results

3.1. Overview

From 28 February 2020 to 2 July 2021, 36 patients were screened for study eligibility, and 32 participants were recruited into this study. All participants were randomized and allocated into the treatment arm and the control arm, with an allocation ratio of 1:1 (Hemopatch arm: $n = 16$ vs. Control arm: $n = 16$). All participants received their allocated treatments and were followed up in our clinic after the operation. All participants were included in the final analysis. All analyses were performed by the original assigned groups. There were no losses after randomization or losses to follow-up. Figure 2 shows the CONSORT flow diagram.

Hemopatch Study Flow Diagram

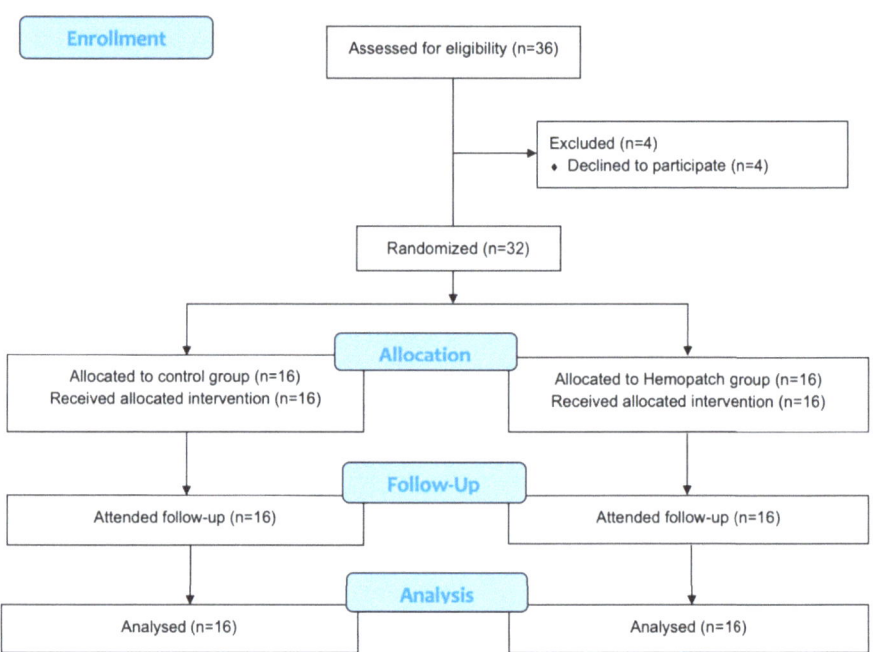

Figure 2. CONSORT flow diagram.

3.2. Patient and Disease Characteristics

The demographic and clinical characteristics of the two arms are summarized in Table 1. The mean age, weight, height and ASA grading were similar between the two groups. The baseline serum PSAs were similar: 9.0 ng/mL in the control group and 10.5 ng/mL in the Hemopatch group. The control group patients had a mean prostate volume of 53.1 cm^3 compared to 41 cm^3 in the Hemopatch group. A total of 56.3% and 68.8% of the control group and the Hemopatch group had prostate cancer with an ISUP grade group ≥ 3, respectively, and 62.5% and 56.3% of the respective arms had high-risk disease. A total of 56.3% participants in both arms had pT3 disease, and only one (6.3%) patient from the control arm was staged with pN1 disease.

Table 1. Baseline demographic and clinical characteristics.

	Control Group ($n = 16$)	Hemopatch Group ($n = 16$)
Age (year)	69 (5)	65 (6)
Weight (kg)	68.2 (10.0)	68.4 (10.2)
Height (cm)	170 (7)	170 (4)
ASA group		
ASA 1	2 (12.5%)	1 (6.3%)
ASA 2	9 (56.3%)	14 (87.5%)
ASA 3	5 (31.3%)	1 (6.3%)
ASA 4	0 (0%)	0 (0%)
Prostate volume (cm^3)	53.1 (25.8)	41.0 (22.4)
PSA (ng/mL)	9.0 (6.5)	10.5 (6.4)
ISUP ≥ 3	9 (56.3%)	11 (68.8%)
Risk category		
Low-risk disease	0 (0%)	0 (0%)
Intermediate-risk disease	6 (37.5%)	7 (43.8%)
High-risk disease	10 (62.5%)	9 (56.3%)
cT stage		
cT1	9 (56.3%)	12 (75.0%)
cT2	7 (43.8%)	4 (25.0%)
pT stage		
pT2	7 (43.8%)	7 (43.8%)
pT3a	3 (18.8%)	6 (37.5%)
pT3b	6 (37.5%)	3 (18.8%)
pN1	1 (6.3%)	0 (0%)

Continuous variables are presented as the mean (SD). Categorical variables are presented as n (%). ASA = American Society of Anaesthesiology; ISUP = International Society of Urological Pathology; PSA = Prostate-Specific Antigen.

3.3. Study Outcomes

In terms of primary outcome, the median total volumes of the drain output were 180 mL (IQR: 73–558) in the control group and 35 mL (IQR: 1–190) in the Hemopatch group. The total drain output is statistically significantly lower in the Hemopatch group ($p = 0.022$). For secondary outcomes, the Hemopatch group also demonstrated a statistically significantly lower drain output volume per day, with a median drain output per day of 35 mL/day (IQR 1–117) in the Hemopatch group compared to 89 mL/day (IQR 68–139) in the control arm ($p = 0.038$). The median duration of drainage was 2 days in the control arm and 1 day in the Hemopatch arm, and the mean duration of hospital stay was 5 days in the control arm and 3 days in the Hemopatch arm. Both drainage duration and hospitalization duration were slightly shorter in the Hemopatch arm; however, the differences did not achieve statistical significance. There are also no statistically significant differences in terms of operation time, lymph node yield, intra-operative blood loss or post-operative 30-day complications. None of the patients required transfusion post-operatively. Table 2 summarizes the primary and secondary outcome findings.

Table 2. Primary and secondary outcomes.

	Control Group (n = 16)	Hemopatch Group (n = 16)	p-Value
Primary outcome			
Total drain output (mL) *	180 (73–558)	35 (1–190)	0.022
Secondary outcomes			
Operative time (minute)	189 (45)	175 (52)	0.449
Intra-operative blood loss (mL)	272 (244)	209 (156)	0.395
Number of lymph nodes excised	13.6 (6.6)	12.69 (4.4)	0.663
Duration of drainage (day) *	2 (1–5)	1 (1–2)	0.139
Drain output per post-op day (mL/day) *	89 (68–139)	35 (1–117)	0.038
Hospital stay (day)	5 (3)	3 (1)	0.105
Transfusion	0 (0%)	0 (0%)	-
30-day complications	5 (31.3%)	3 (18.8%)	0.685

* Continuous variables are presented as means (SD) unless otherwise specified. * Continuous variables are presented as medians (IQR) and compared by the Mann–Whitney U test. Categorical variables are presented as n (%) and compared by Fisher's exact test. A two-sided p-value of <0.05 is considered statistically significant.

In the control group, five patients (31.3%) experienced complications within 30 days after operation, all being of Clavien–Dindo grade 1. These complications include right groin numbness, perineal discomfort, drain leakage, urine leak and prepuce oedema. All were conservatively managed. In the Hemopatch group, three patients (18.8%) experienced complications within 30 days, with one patient experiencing two complications. Two patients developed a Clavien–Dindo grade 2 complication of wound infection that required antibiotics use and dressing. The rest of the complications were of Clavien–Dindo grade 1, including fever and paraphimosis. The results are summarized in Table 3.

Table 3. Summary of 30-day complications.

	Control Group (n = 16)	Hemopatch Group (n = 16) *
Clavien–Dindo grade 1	5 (31.3%) i. Drain leakage (n = 1, 6.3%) ii. Perineal discomfort (n = 1, 6.3%) iii. Prepuce edema (n = 1, 6.3%) iv. Right groin numbness (n = 1, 6.3%) v. Urine leak (n = 1, 6.3%)	1 (18.8%) i. Fever (n = 1, 6.3%) ii. Paraphimosis (n = 1, 6.3%)
Calvien–Dindo grade 2	0 (0%)	2 (12.5%) i. Surgical site infection (n = 2, 12.5%)

* One patient from the Hemopatch arm was complicated with paraphimosis and wound infection.

4. Discussion

Prostate cancer is the second most common cancer affecting men globally [16], with an incidence rate that is rising with time [17]. Radical prostatectomy is recognized to be a standard modality of treatment that improves cancer-specific survival [18], and same-session BPLND is performed for those with an estimated risk of occult nodal metastases exceeding 5%, which provides valuable staging and prognostic information that cannot be matched by other available procedures [2]. However, BPLND is not without risks, with lymphocoele formation being the most common complication caused by the disruption of lymphatic drainage after pelvic lymph node dissection. Lymphocoele formation can cause compressive symptoms and infective complications and negatively affect the post-operative recovery of prostatectomy patients. Various techniques to improve lymphostasis, including bipolar diathermy, clip application [19], peritoneal flap interposition [20] and haemostatic pad application with TachoSil [21], have been explored, with no definite data to suggest the best approach.

Hemopatch is considered the second generation of advanced hemostatic pads [6]. The effectiveness of Hemopatch is largely attributed to its physical properties, which consist of a sheet-like collagen backing with a self-binding surface, with the binding agent being NHS-PEG. The design allows for a dual mechanism that allows for the rapid adherence of tissue and fluid from electrophilic cross-linking with the NHS-PEG monomers, while the collagen scaffolding would mediate intrinsic hemostatic action to form fibrin clots. By laying Hemopatch over raw lymphatic tissue, the highly porous bovine collagen sheet would allow for rapid tissue fluid absorption and increase the surface area for the delivery of NHS-PEG for sealant functions.

This is the first randomized controlled trial on the use of Hemopatch, a novel haemostatic agent composed of a bovine collagen sheet coated with NHS-PEG, in the setting of RARP with BPLND for prostate cancer patients. In this trial, the outcomes demonstrated that the application of Hemopatch to raw lymphatic tissues could reduce lymphorrhoea as shown by the lower total drain output volume and drain output volume per day when compared to the standard procedure without the use of haemostatic adjuncts. The median total drain output is only 35 mL in BPNLD with the use of Hemopatch, compared to 180 mL in the control group, showing a more-than-five-times reduction in output volume. The operative times and 30-day complications were similar between the two groups. These findings suggest that Hemopatch is a safe and effective haemostatic agent that can be laid over the ends of raw truncated lymphatic tissue after BPLND to reduce lymphorrhoea and post-operative drain output, with no additional morbidity or complication.

Hemopatch has been utilized across multiple surgical specialties [22]. In urology, a previous prospective study investigated the use of Hemopatch in laparoscopic partial nephrectomy [23,24], demonstrating its ability to help achieve haemostasis. The prospective series explored the use of Hemopatch by a single surgeon in 19 patients receiving laparoscopic partial nephrectomies (16 with zero-clamping, zero-ichemia), which showed that the application of Hemopatch successfully achieved haemostasis in all cases. However, no studies have investigated the role of Hemopatch in reducing or peventing lymphorrhoea, let alone in the RARP and BPLND setting. One randomized controlled trial of 100 patients investigated the use of TachoSil [21], a hemostatic patch comprised of a collagen sponge coated with fibrinogen and thrombin, in reducing lymphocoele formation after pelvic lymph node dissection in prostate cancer patients. The results demonstrated statistically significantly less post-operative lymphocoele on cross-sectional imaging in the TachoSil group compared to the control group.

Our study is the first to investigate the role of Hemopatch in the setting of RARP and BPLND and provides good evidence for its use given the randomized controlled design and the quasi-double blinded nature (the surgeon is left blinded for the majority of the operation until randomization). It is also the first study to demonstrate the effectiveness of Hemopatch in reducing lymphorrhoea. Another major strength of this study is the standardization of the procedure, where the Hemopatch placement position (distal ends are at the obturator fossa and the femoral canal; the proximal ends overlie the common iliac bifurcation and internal iliac artery), size and margins (Hemopatch would overlap the margins of the raw area by about 1 cm), application methods (the patch is kept dry until contact with tissue) and pressure application duration (two minutes) are clearly defined and followed. This has reduced bias and inter-surgeon variability when it comes to the application of Hemopatch.

Several limitations exist in this study. First, this is a trial conducted at a single center only; this might have affected the generalizability of the findings. Second, the sample size of the study remained small, with only 16 patients recruited into each arm, which weakened the statistical power, especially in the analysis of secondary outcomes. We have observed that both the drainage duration and hospitalization duration were shorter in the Hemopatch arm; however, the differences were not statistically significant. There are likely true differences in these areas in addition to the drain output; however, our study is underpowered to detect it. Third, our study selected drain output as a surrogate for lymphorrhoea and only followed up patients for 30 days post-operatively. This may not accurately reflect the effectiveness of Hemopatch in reducing the incidence of lymphocele formation after RARP and BPLND. The need for intervention for lymphocele was also not evaluated. To address this, future studies with larger sample sizes and longer follow-ups are needed to evaluate the relationship between Hemopatch application and lymphocele incidence. Another research gap that this study did not address is how Hemopatch performs compared to other currently available adjunctive haemostatic agents, and further study in this area is needed.

5. Conclusions

In conclusion, our study is the first randomized controlled blinded trial to demonstrate the effectiveness of Hemopatch, an NHS-PEG coated patch, in reducing the drain output volume after RARP and BPLND in prostate cancer patients. Therefore, the application of Hemopatch to raw lymphatic surfaces should be considered during RARP and BPLND.

Author Contributions: J.Y.-C.T.: Conceptualization, methodology, writing, review, editing; A.Q.L.: Analysis, writing, review, editing; V.W.-F.Y.: Analysis, data curation, project administration; F.P.-T.L.: Analysis, data curation, project administration; S.K.-K.Y.: Data acquisition, review, editing; S.Y.-S.C.: Data acquisition, review, editing; J.H.-F.W.: Data acquisition, review, editing; J.K.-M.L.: Data acquisition, review, editing; M.H.-M.T.: Data acquisition, review, editing; P.K.-F.C.: Methodology, data acquisition, review, editing; S.C.-H.Y.: Methodology, data acquisition, review, editing; C.-F.N.: Supervision, methodology, writing, review, editing. All authors have read and agreed to the published version of the manuscript.

Funding: This research received the Investigator Initiated Research Grant from Baxter International Inc., and the Hemopatch used in this study was sponsored by Baxter International Inc.

Institutional Review Board Statement: The study was conducted in accordance with the Declaration of Helsinki and approved by the Joint Chinese University of Hong Kong—New Territories East Cluster Clinical Research Ethics Committee (Protocol version 1.3; CREC Reference number: 2019.419-T). The study was registered at the US National Institutes of Health (ClinicalTrial.gov; Identifier: NCT04185922).

Informed Consent Statement: Informed consent was obtained from all subjects involved in the study.

Data Availability Statement: The data presented in this study are available on request from the corresponding author. The data are not publicly available due to the data containing patients' clinical information.

Conflicts of Interest: The Hemopatch used in this study was sponsored by Baxter International Inc. The funders had no role in the design of the study; in the collection, analyses or interpretation of data; in the writing of the manuscript; or in the decision to publish the results. The authors declare no conflict of interest.

References

1. Mottet, N.; Bellmunt, J.; Bolla, M.; Briers, E.; Cumberbatch, M.G.; De Santis, M.; Fossati, N.; Gross, T.; Henry, A.M.; Joniau, S.; et al. EAU-ESTRO-SIOG Guidelines on Prostate Cancer. Part 1: Screening, Diagnosis, and Local Treatment with Curative Intent. *Eur. Urol.* **2017**, *71*, 618–629. [CrossRef] [PubMed]
2. Fossati, N.; Willemse, P.-P.M.; Van den Broeck, T.; van den Bergh, R.C.; Yuan, C.Y.; Briers, E.; Bellmunt, J.; Bolla, M.; Cornford, P.; De Santis, M.; et al. The Benefits and Harms of Different Extents of Lymph Node Dissection During Radical Prostatectomy for Prostate Cancer: A Systematic Review. *Eur. Urol.* **2017**, *72*, 84–109. [CrossRef]
3. Breslin, J.W.; Yang, Y.; Scallan, J.P.; Sweat, R.S.; Adderley, S.P.; Murfee, W.L. Lymphatic vessel network structure and physiology. *Compr. Physiol.* **2018**, *9*, 207–299. [PubMed]
4. Gilbert, D.R.; Angell, J.; Abaza, R. Evaluation of Absorbable Hemostatic Powder for Prevention of Lymphoceles Following Robotic Prostatectomy with Lymphadenectomy. *Urology* **2016**, *98*, 75–80. [CrossRef] [PubMed]
5. Simonato, A.; Varca, V.; Esposito, M.; Venzano, F.; Carmignani, G. The Use of a Surgical Patch in the Prevention of Lymphoceles after Extraperitoneal Pelvic Lymphadenectomy for Prostate Cancer: A Randomized Prospective Pilot Study. *J. Urol.* **2009**, *182*, 2285–2290. [CrossRef]

6. Keegan, K.A.; Cookson, M.S. Complications of pelvic lymph node dissection for prostate cancer. *Curr. Urol. Rep.* **2011**, *12*, 203–208. [CrossRef]
7. Sihra, N.; Kujawa, M.; Counsell, A.; Brough, R. Post-prostatectomy lymphocoele presenting with renal failure. *Urology* **2019**, *123*, e9–e10. [CrossRef]
8. Gotto, G.T.; Yunis, L.H.; Guillonneau, B.; Touijer, K.; Eastham, J.A.; Scardino, P.T.; Rabbani, F. Predictors of symptomatic lymphocele after radical prostatectomy and bilateral pelvic lymph node dissection. *Int. J. Urol.* **2011**, *18*, 291–296. [CrossRef]
9. Mikami, H.; Ito, K.; Yoshii, H.; Kosaka, T.; Miyajima, A.; Kaji, T.; Asano, T.; Hayakawa, M. Giant lymphocele arising after extraperitoneal laparoscopic radical prostatectomy. *Hinyokika Kiyo* **2008**, *54*, 23–27.
10. Jereczek-Fossa, B.A.; Colangione, S.P.; Fodor, C.I.; Russo, S.; Cambria, R.; Zerini, D.; Bonora, M.; Cecconi, A.; Vischioni, B.; Vavassori, A.; et al. Radiotherapy in prostate cancer patients with pelvic lymphocele after surgery: Clinical and dosimetric data of 30 patients. *Clin. Genitourin. Cancer* **2015**, *13*, e223–e228. [CrossRef]
11. Waldert, M.; Remzi, M.; Klatte, T.; Klingler, H.C. FloSeal reduces the incidence of lymphoceles after lymphadenectomies in laparoscopic and robot-assisted extraperitoneal radical prostatectomy. *J. Endourol.* **2011**, *25*, 969–973. [CrossRef] [PubMed]
12. Lewis, K.M. Control of bleeding in surgical procedures: Critical appraisal of HEMOPATCH. *Med. Devices Evid. Res.* **2009**, *3*, 1–10. [CrossRef]
13. Hueting, T.A.; Cornel, E.B.; Somford, D.M.; Jansen, H.; van Basten, J.-P.A.; Pleijhuis, R.G.; Korthorst, R.A.; van der Palen, J.; Koffijberg, H. External validation of models predicting the probability of lymph node involvement in prostate cancer patients. *Eur. Urol. Oncol.* **2018**, *1*, 411–417. [CrossRef]
14. Briganti, A.; Larcher, A.; Abdollah, F.; Capitanio, U.; Gallina, A.; Suardi, N.; Bianchi, M.; Sun, M.; Freschi, M.; Salonia, A.; et al. Updated nomogram predicting lymph node invasion in patients with prostate cancer undergoing extended pelvic lymph node dissection: The essential importance of percentage of positive cores. *Eur. Urol.* **2012**, *61*, 480–487. [CrossRef] [PubMed]
15. Yip, K.H.S.; Yee, C.-H.; Ng, C.-F.; Lam, N.-Y.; Ho, K.-L.; Ma, W.-K.; Li, C.-M.; Hou, S.-M.; Tam, P.-C.; Yiu, M.-K.; et al. Robot-assisted radical prostatectomy in Hong Kong: A review of 235 cases. *J. Endourol.* **2012**, *26*, 258–263. [CrossRef]
16. Culp, M.B.; Soerjomataram, I.; Efstathiou, J.A.; Bray, F.; Jemal, A. Recent Global Patterns in Prostate Cancer Incidence and Mortality Rates. *Eur. Urol.* **2020**, *77*, 38–52. [CrossRef] [PubMed]
17. Rawla, P. Epidemiology of Prostate Cancer. *World J. Oncol.* **2019**, *10*, 63–89. [CrossRef]
18. Wilt, T.J.; Jones, K.M.; Barry, M.J.; Andriole, G.L.; Culkin, D.; Wheeler, T.; Aronson, W.J.; Brawer, M.K. Follow-up of Prostatectomy versus Observation for Early Prostate Cancer. *N. Engl. J. Med.* **2017**, *377*, 132–142. [CrossRef]
19. Stolzenburg, J.U.; Kyriazis, I.; Liatsikos, E. Postoperative Lymphocele Formation after Pelvic Lymph Node Dissection at the Time of Radical Prostatectomy Should Not Be Considered an Inevitable Consequence of the Approach. *Eur. Urol.* **2017**, *71*, 159–160. [CrossRef]
20. Lebeis, C.; Canes, D.; Sorcini, A.; Moinzadeh, A. Novel Technique Prevents Lymphoceles After Transperitoneal Robotic-assisted Pelvic Lymph Node Dissection: Peritoneal Flap Interposition. *Urology* **2015**, *85*, 1505–1509. [CrossRef]
21. Buelens, S.; Van Praet, C.; Poelaert, F.; Van Huele, A.; Decaestecker, K.; Lumen, N. Prospective Randomized Controlled Trial Exploring the Effect of TachoSil on Lymphocele Formation after Extended Pelvic Lymph Node Dissection in Prostate Cancer. *Urology* **2018**, *118*, 134–140. [CrossRef] [PubMed]
22. Lewis, K.M.; Ikeme, S.; Olubunmi, T.; Kuntze, C.E. Clinical effectiveness and versatility of a sealing hemostatic patch (Hemopatch) in multiple surgical specialties. *Expert Rev. Med. Devices* **2018**, *15*, 367–376. [CrossRef] [PubMed]
23. Imkamp, F.; Von Klot, C.; Wolters, M.; Husmann, S.; Herrmann, T.; Tolkach, Y. The role of Hemopatch in zero ischemia laparoscopic partial nephrectomy. *Eur. Urol. Suppl.* **2016**, *15*, e858. [CrossRef]
24. Imkamp, F.; Tolkach, Y.; Wolters, M.; Jutzi, S.; Kramer, M.; Herrmann, T. Initial experiences with the Hemopatch® as a hemostatic agent in zero-ischemia partial nephrectomy. *World J. Urol.* **2015**, *33*, 1527–1534. [CrossRef]

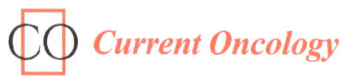 *Current Oncology*

Article

The Challenges of Patient Selection for Prostate Cancer Focal Therapy: A Retrospective Observational Multicentre Study

Alessio Paladini [1], Giovanni Cochetti [1,*], Alexandre Colau [2], Martin Mouton [2], Sara Ciarletti [1], Graziano Felici [1], Giuseppe Maiolino [1], Federica Balzarini [2], Philippe Sèbe [2] and Ettore Mearini [1]

[1] Urology Clinic, Department of Medicine and Surgery, University of Perugia, 06129 Perugia, Italy
[2] Chirurgie Urologique, Hôpital Croix Saint Simon Groupe Diaconesses, 75020 Paris, France
* Correspondence: giovanni.cochetti@unipg.it

Abstract: Increased diagnoses of silent prostate cancer (PCa) have led to overtreatment and consequent functional side effects. Focal therapy (FT) applies energy to a prostatic index lesion treating only the clinically significant PCa focus. We analysed the potential predictive factors of FT failure. We collected data from patients who underwent robot-assisted radical prostatectomy (RARP) in two high-volume hospitals from January 2017 to January 2020. The inclusion criteria were: one MRI-detected lesion with a Gleason Score (GS) of ≤7, ≤cT2a, PSA of ≤10 ng/mL, and GS 6 on a random biopsy with ≤2 positive foci out of 12. Potential oncological safety of FT was defined as the respect of clinicopathological inclusion criteria on histology specimens, no extracapsular extension, and no biochemical, local, or metastatic recurrence within 12 months. To predict FT failure, we performed uni- and multivariate logistic regression. Sixty-seven patients were enrolled. The MRI index lesion median size was 11 mm; target lesions were ISUP grade 1 in 27 patients and ISUP grade 2 in 40. Potential FT failure occurred in 32 patients, and only the PSA value resulted as a predictive parameter ($p < 0.05$). The main issue for FT is patient selection, mainly because of multifocal csPCa foci. Nevertheless, FT could represent a therapeutic alternative for highly selected low-risk PCa patients.

Keywords: prostate cancer; focal therapy; low-risk PCa; MRI; PSA

1. Introduction

Prostate cancer (PCa) is the second most common male cancer with the highest incidence in Western countries, which is partially due to the wide use of prostate-specific antigen (PSA) as the primary screening tool [1,2]. On the one hand, if the screening based on PSA has been associated with a decrease in PCa-related mortality, on the other hand, it leads to over-diagnosis and over-treatment of silent PCa at the expense of functional side effects [3]. In the era of precision medicine, the goal is to diagnose and treat only clinically significant PCa (csPCa), thus individualizing the treatments on the patient's disease characteristics.

Recent studies focused on the value of miRNAs as new tools for early cancer diagnosis, but this goal has yet to be reached [4]. Multiparametric magnetic resonance imaging (MRI) has been improving the diagnostic algorithm of csPCa; it is recommended before any prostatic biopsy, and it has been included in the protocols of active surveillance (AS) and active monitoring (AM) for PCa [2,5]. An MRI-target biopsy could improve the detection rate of ISUP grade ≥ 2 and ISUP grade ≥ 3, approximately 40% and 50%, respectively. For this reason, the EAU guidelines recommend performing naïve biopsy combining the target procedure with a systematic one [2].

Once PCa has been diagnosed, an individualised treatment respecting oncological outcomes is mandatory. For low-risk localised PCa, AS/AM is advisable for a well-informed patient who accepts the risk of progression and a strict follow-up protocol. For all the others, except the locally advanced, a local treatment, if feasible, should be proposed in personalised medicine [2,6]. Unfortunately, radical prostatectomy, even if nerve-sparing and radiotherapy, are not free of side effects [7,8]. For surgery, incontinence and erectile dysfunction rate are reported to be 31% and 38% at 12 months, respectively, if nerve-sparing techniques are performed [9,10]. Neither open, laparoscopic nor robotic approaches have demonstrated a clear superiority compared to others in terms of functional outcomes and quality of life [11,12]. Even in the case of minimally invasive surgery, patients could suffer from intra-, peri- and post-operative complications [13]. For radiotherapy, the sexual and incontinence domains show a similar result to surgery, but gastrointestinal adverse effects are predominant [2,14]. An altered functional state could impair the health-related quality of life (HRQOL), irrespective of treatment choice [15].

In particular, functional results are of paramount importance in patients who underwent radical prostatectomy for localised low- and intermediate-risk PCa because these outcomes are more emphasised. For these risk categories, focal therapy (FT) has gained increasing importance worldwide in recent years, offering an alternative to whole-gland treatment. Focal therapy (FT) for PCa applies energy to an index lesion and its surrounding margins to treat only clinically significant lesions preserving neurovascular structures close to the prostate gland [16]. The advantages of FT are exciting functional outcomes in terms of urinary continence, sexual potency and quality of life with reasonable short-term oncological safety [16]. However, FT is recommended only within the setting of clinical trials using predefined inclusion criteria and scheduled surveillance [17,18]. Population-based studies evaluating FT as a treatment for PCa are poor. Recently, Flegar et al. analysed FT cases in Germany and reported an increase from 2006 to 2008 and then a decrease until 2014. Since 2015, the overall cases of FT have shown a plateau trend [16]. The early increase in the utilization of FT is due to the development of new technologies. In contrast, the reason for the subsequent decrease in case numbers is the significant risk for tumour recurrence or progression after FT [16,19].

The current PCa diagnostic algorithm could fail to propose a focal therapy because of the risk of missing other csPCa not revealed by MRI. In this retrospective observational population-based multicentre study on patients who underwent bilateral nerve-sparing RARP for localised low-risk PCa, we analysed the preoperative patients and the disease's characteristics as potential predictive factors of FT failure.

2. Materials and Methods

In this multicentre study, we prospectively collected data from patients who consecutively underwent robot-assisted radical prostatectomy (RARP) in two high-volume tertiary hospitals (Clinica Urologica—Università degli Studi di Perugia Azienda Ospedaliera di Perugia-Italy, Service de Chirurgie Urologique Groupe Hospitalier Diaconesses Hôpital Croix Saint-Simon de Paris-France) from January 2017 to January 2020.

We performed dosages of PSA, digital rectal explorations (DREs), multiparametric-3-Tesla-MRI, MRI/ultrasound fusion guided and systematic prostatic biopsies.

We collected clinicopathological data regarding age, pre-operative PSA, prostate volume, PSA-density, clinical T stage, MRI-index lesion diameter, MRI-index lesion Prostate Imaging—Reporting and Data System version 2 (PI-RADS v2) score, Gleason score (GS) of MRI-index lesion on biopsy, Gleason score by systematic biopsy, clinical International Society of Urologic Pathologists (ISUP) grade, Gleason score and ISUP grade on histology, extracapsular-extension, PSA at 40 days and 3-6-12 months after RARP, biochemical, local or metastatic recurrence within 12 months and time to recurrence.

Inclusion criteria included patients who underwent bilateral nerve-sparing RARP with negative surgical margins, with only one MRI-detected lesion, $\leq$cT2a, PSA $\leq$ 10 ng/mL, GS $\leq$ 7 on target biopsy, GS 6 on random biopsy with $\leq$2 positives foci out 12.

We assumed the safety criteria in terms of the inclusion criteria on the final specimen, no extracapsular extension, and no biochemical, local, or metastatic recurrence within 12 months. Based on this definition, patients were divided into two groups: the first one was the FT success group, which included patients matching all of the safety criteria;

the second was the FT failure group, which consisted of those who did not match the safety criteria.

3. Results

A total of 67 patients who underwent RARP with bilateral nerve-sparing technique, matching the inclusion criteria, were enrolled. Of these, 35 patients (52.2%) were included in the FT success group and 32 (47.8%) in the FT failure group according to the potential oncological safety criteria.

Thirty-five (52.2%) had a clinical stage T1c and 32 (47.8%) cT2a. The mean age at diagnosis was 64.4 ± 6.65 years, the mean BMI 25 ± 1.56 kg/m^2, and the mean prostate volume 46.1 ± 15.5 cc without significant difference between the FT success and FT failure groups. MRI index lesion diameter, PI-RADS value, and bioptic ISUP group did not differ significantly between groups. PSA density score differed between the groups (14.8 vs. 17.8 ng/mL^2) but did not reach the statistical significance ($p = 0.10$). The mean PSA value in the FT success group was 6.14 ± 2.26 ng/mL vs 7.44 ± 1.92 ng/mL in the FT failure group, $p = 0.01$. The mean sise of the index lesion on the multiparametric MRI was 11.6 ± 4.56 mm; in twelve (17.9%) patients, the index lesion was classified as PI-RADS 3, in 33 (49.3%) as PI-RADS 4, in 22 (32.8%) as PI-RADS 5. The ISUP grade of the MRI-target lesions was 1 in 27 patients (40.3%) and 2 in 40 patients (59.7%). Clinicopathological features of the study population are shown in Table 1.

Table 1. Clinicopathologic features of our sample.

Variables *	Total (n = 67, 100%)	FT Success (n = 35, 52.2%)	FT Failure (n = 32, 47.8%)	p
Age (years)	64.4 (±6.65)	64.4 (±6.64)	64.3 (±6.77)	0.95
BMI (kg/m^2)	25.0 (±1.56)	25.1 (±1.72)	24.9 (±1.39)	0.61
CCI score	4 (5–3)	4 (5–3)	4.5 (5–3.25)	0.36
IPSS score	10 (13–7)	10 (14–7)	9.5 (12–7.25)	0.97
Prostate volume (cc)	46.1 (±15.5)	47.1 (±16.7)	45.0 (±14.2)	0.57
PSA (ng/mL)	6.76 (±2.19)	6.14 (±2.26)	7.44 (±1.92)	*0.01*
PSA density (ng/mL^2)	16.2 (±7.21)	14.8 (±8.18)	17.8 (±5.71)	0.10
MRI index lesion diameter (mm)	11.6 (±4.56)	11.8 (±4.41)	11.3 (±4.82)	0.65
PI-RADS PI-RADS 3, n (%) PI-RADS 4, n (%) PI-RADS 5, n (%)	 12 (17.9%) 33 (49.3%) 22 (32.8%)	 9 (75.0%) 16 (48.5%) 10 (45.5%)	 3 (25.0%) 17 (51.5%) 12 (54.5%)	0.21
Biopsy ISUP group ISUP 1, n (%) ISUP 2, n (%)	 27 (40.3%) 40 (59.7%)	 17 (63.0%) 18 (45%)	 10 (14.9%) 22 (55%)	0.14

* Continuous variables with normal distribution were presented as mean (±standard deviation (SD)); non-parametric categorical variables were reported as absolute and relative frequencies (n, %), and non-parametric numerical variables with median (interquartile range—IQR). In italic the significant p-value.

In the FT failure group, a second csPCa focus on the specimen was discovered in 31 patients (96.9%), an ISUP grade 3 in 8 patients (25%), ISUP grade 4 in 2 (6.25%), pT3 in 12 patients (37.5%), and biochemical recurrence in 2 patients (6.25%). The uni- and multivariate logistic regression analysis on failure therapy was performed. The PSA values of <6 and >7 ng/mL were shown to be the only predictor value of FT success and failure, respectively, both in the univariate and multivariate logistic regression analysis, Table 2. PSA value > 7 ng/mL showed a sensitivity of 62.5%, a specificity of 61.1%, and an AUC of 0.73.

Table 2. Uni- and multivariate logistic regression analysis on failure therapy.

	Univariate			Multivariate		
	HR	CI (95%)	p	HR	CI (95%)	p
Age (years)	0.99	0.92–1.07	0.95	1.01	0.93–1.11	0.77
BMI (kg/m^2)	0.92	0.67–1.26	0.61	0.96	0.65–1.43	0.85
CCI score	1.25	0.79–1.95	0.33	1.48	0.87–2.54	0.15
IPSS score	1	0.95–1.11	0.96	1.01	0.90–1.15	0.80
Prostate volume (cc)	0.99	0.96–1.02	0.57	0.95	0.86–1.04	0.27
PSA (ng/mL)	1.35	1.05–1.74	*0.02*	1.97	1.00–3.89	*0.04*
PSA density (%)	1.06	0.98–1.14	0.10	0.86	0.66–1.12	0.27
MRI index lesion diameter (mm)	0.98	0.88–1.09	0.65	0.94	0.80–1.10	0.45
PI-RADS						
PI-RADS 4 vs. PI-RADS 3	3.19	0.73–13.9	0.12	2.47	0.49–12.3	0.27
PI-RADS 5 vs. PI-RADS 3	3.60	0.76–17.0	0.10	3.59	0.44–28.7	0.23
Biopsy ISUP group (ISUP 2 vs. ISUP 1)	2.08	0.77–5.64	0.15	1.23	0.33–4.49	0.76

In italic the significant *p*-value.

4. Discussion

The definition of FT is "ablation of a cancerous lesion, diagnosed by imaging and confirmed by biopsy, with a margin of safety surrounding the target lesion" [20]. Doubts persist about the correct definition of target lesion; among experts, there is a consensus that the focus is a lesion ISUP grade $\geq$ 2, but there is no consensus that the larger lesion is the target of FT [20]. If we could treat the index lesion with a safety margin, the functional results would be preserved, and the oncological ones respected [21]. Unfortunately, although FT for PCa has been studied for more than 10 years, little is known about this procedure's optimal technology and oncological safety [15,20].

Identification of the tumour lesion and the certainty of its focal nature, the destruction of the tumour lesion with an acceptable safety margin, and a careful follow-up to diagnose the persistence or disease relapse are cornerstones of FT success.

To reach an international consensus, Van den Bos et al. proposed, as eligible criteria for FT, to include PSA levels < 15 ng/mL, clinical stage T1c-T2a, ISUP 1 or 2, life expectancy > 10 years, and any volume of the prostate gland [22]. In our study, the inclusion criteria were more restricted, enrolling only patients with low-risk PCa according to EAU criteria and those with ISUP grade 2 in a maximum of two bioptic foci. This was done to identify a category of patients with disease characteristics immediately close to those treated by active surveillance and, therefore, would have benefited more from a focal treatment. Patients with a higher risk of progression and recurrence should not be recruited since they need a lymphadenectomy for proper staging and treatment.

In our recruitment, we excluded patients with more than two positive bioptic cores because of the higher risk of BCR at 3 and 5 years, as per Truesdale et al. [23].

Perlis et al. proposed FT in selected patients with GG3-5 disease, especially in those who had particular attention to the functional outcomes or in those who had contraindications for radical treatment, be it radical prostatectomy or radiation therapy [17]. Encouraging results were highlighted in a study with selected patients affected by non-metastatic csPCa treated by HIFU. The five-year metastasis-free survival in the intermediate and high-risk groups was 99% and 97%, respectively [24]. Johnson et al. are of the opposite opinion in treating ISUP grade > 3 patients, even if highly selected. According to the authors, these patients are at high risk of persistent disease after FT because MRI has low sensitivity for identifying individual tumours foci. Approximately 22% of all PCa GG 3–5 are not correctly identified and located in the corresponding quadrant by MRI, and this percentage increases to 30% among patients with multifocal PCa. Furthermore, MRI does not reliably rule out the presence of extracapsular extension, and its diagnostic capacity appears to decrease for higher-grade lesions. In support of this, Johnson et al. reported that in their clinical experience, 48% of patients who were potential candidates for prostatic hemiablation had bilateral clinically significant disease [25]. In fact, mpMRI could omit about 20–45% of clinically significant PCa [17,26,27]. In our study, 46.3% of the patients analysed had either a second csPCa focus not detected by mpMRI or the disease had spread to the entire lobe or both. This percentage is similar to those reported in the literature showing that the inter variability is very low in the hub centres.

In the literature, however, some cases have been successfully treated. That is the case of Linder et al., who reported their promising experiences on FT laser treatment of four patients, two of which with ISUP 3. The authors described the creation of a convergent ablation with the absence of viable cells in the treated regions verified by MRI 7 days post-treatment and confirmed in the histopathology piece, but long-term data were not reported [28].

An aspect that should not be underestimated is the discrepancy between the clinical Gleason score and the pathological one. In fact, on the definitive diagnosis, about 50% of cases of upgrading in low-risk patients and up to 80% of downgrading in patients belonging to the intermediate and high-risk categories [29]. In the literature, five studies have reported a positive predictive value of <60% for detecting low-risk PCa. Although this finding can be partly explained by the fact that all studies had the lowest prevalence of low grades, it remains a surprising value [29–33]. Schiffmann et al. reported an upgrading rate of 55% for patients eligible for active surveillance and 78% for low-risk patients not eligible for active surveillance. In the same categories of patients, they reported an upstaging rate of 8% and 15%, respectively [34]. These data confirm the study by Busch et al. in which the upgrading and upstaging were 53.1% and 12.2%, respectively, for the group in active surveillance [35]. In our study, the upgrading rate was 38.1%, and for low-risk PCa patients, it was 40.7%. The possible explanation is that hub centres for PCa have the lowest rate of low-grade prostate cancer.

The lack of certainty of the disease grade and stage is a limiting factor for FT due to the risk of not respecting the oncological goal. It is necessary to assess the correct PCa grade and stage to choose the best therapeutic option. In our case, the potential success was around 52.2% and was largely influenced by radical post-prostatectomy upstaging. That underlines that a disease close to the capsule could also be poorly controlled by FT due to the lack of a safety margin, if not at the expense of the vascular-nerve bundles and a greater risk on nearby structures.

In our study, the only variable that significantly differs between groups is the PSA value, which was higher in the FT failure group. The mean value of the failure group was 7.44 ng/mL, which is only a slightly higher value. Boniol et al. reported an increasing linear risk of PCa for each percentage increase in PSA level with an odd ratio of 1.079 (95% confidence interval); however, this association is not related to a more aggressive disease [36]. Park YH et al., in their study, showed that the risk of prostate cancer was higher in men with a fluctuating PSA level and PSAV ≥ 1.0 ng/mL/yr than in those with a fluctuating PSA level and PSAV < 1.0 ng/mL/yr [37]. Moreover, patients with a positive digital rectal examination (DRE) and higher PSA levels show a higher risk of contralateral disease and may not be ideal candidates for FT [38]. These findings could explain why a small PSA level change that we found in our study could be significant. PSA density, as well, was different between groups but without significance, most likely due to the small samples. The small sample size represents the main limitation of our study.

5. Conclusions

The main issue for FT is patient selection, mainly because of multifocal csPCa foci not detected with the current diagnostic tools.

Our findings show that serum PSA could predict the success or failure of FT using a cut-off of 6 and 7 ng/mL, respectively. Further studies with a larger sample size are needed to confirm our results.

Author Contributions: Conceptualization, E.M., A.P. and P.S.; Methodology, G.C. and A.P.; Software, G.M.; Formal Analysis, G.M. and G.F.; Investigation, S.C., A.C., M.M. and F.B.; Data Curation, A.C., M.M., F.B. and G.F.; Writing—Original Draft Preparation, A.P.; Writing—Review and Editing, G.C. and E.M.; Visualization, S.C.; Supervision, E.M. and P.S. All authors have read and agreed to the published version of the manuscript.

Funding: This research received no external funding.

Institutional Review Board Statement: The study was conducted in accordance with the Declaration of Helsinki. Ethical review and approval were waived for this study due to the use of the gold standard treatment for the disease according to the European Association of Urology Guidelines.

Informed Consent Statement: Written informed consent has been obtained from the patient(s) to publish this paper.

Data Availability Statement: The data presented in this study are available on request from the corresponding author. The data are not publicly available due to privacy.

Conflicts of Interest: The authors declare no conflict of interest.

Abbreviations

PCa: prostate cancer, FT: focal therapy, GS: Gleason Score, PSA: prostate-specific antigen, csPCa clinically significant prostate cancer, MRI: magnetic resonance imaging, AS: active surveillance, AM: active monitoring, HRQOL: health-related quality of life, RARP: robot-assisted radical prostatectomy, PI-RADS v2: Prostate Imaging—Reporting and Data System version 2, ISUP: International Society of Urologic Pathologists, DRE: digital rectal examination.

References

1. Egidi, M.G.; Cochetti, G.; Guelfi, G.; Zampini, D.; Diverio, S.; Poli, G.; Mearini, E. Stability Assessment of Candidate Reference Genes in Urine Sediment of Prostate Cancer Patients for miRNA Applications. *Dis. Markers* **2015**, *2015*, 973597. Available online: http://www.hindawi.com/journals/dm/2015/973597/ (accessed on 20 May 2015). [CrossRef]
2. EAU Annual Congress. *EAU Guidelines 2020*; EAU Annual Congress: Amsterdam, The Netherlands, 2020, ISBN 978-94-92671-07-3.
3. Hayes, J.H.; Barry, M.J. Screening for Prostate Cancer with the Prostate-Specific Antigen Test. *JAMA* **2014**, *311*, 1143–1149. Available online: http://jama.jamanetwork.com/article.aspx?doi=10.1001/jama.2014.2085 (accessed on 19 March 2014). [CrossRef]
4. Cochetti, G.; de Vermandois, J.A.R.; Maulà, V.; Giulietti, M.; Cecati, M.; Del Zingaro, M.; Cagnani, R.; Suvieri, C.; Paladini, A.; Mearini, E. Role of miRNAs in prostate cancer: Do we really know everything? *Urol. Oncol. Semin. Orig. Investig.* **2020**, *38*, 623–635. Available online: https://linkinghub.elsevier.com/retrieve/pii/S1078143920300910 (accessed on 1 July 2020). [CrossRef]
5. Klotz, C.M.L. Can high resolution micro-ultrasound replace MRI in the diagnosis of prostate cancer? *Eur. Urol. Focus* **2020**, *6*, 419–423. Available online: https://linkinghub.elsevier.com/retrieve/pii/S2405456919303475 (accessed on 15 March 2020). [CrossRef]
6. Baldassarri, M.; Fallerini, C.; Cetta, F.; Ghisalberti, M.; Bellan, C.; Furini, S.; Spiga, O.; Crispino, S.; Gotti, G.; Ariani, F.; et al. Omic Approach in Non-smoker Female with Lung Squamous Cell Carcinoma Pinpoints to Germline Susceptibility and Personalized Medicine. *Cancer Res. Treat.* **2018**, *50*, 356–365. Available online: http://www.e-crt.org/journal/view.php?doi=10.4143/crt.2017.125 (accessed on 26 May 2017). [CrossRef]
7. Cochetti, G.; Boni, A.; Barillaro, F.; Pohja, S.; Cirocchi, R.; Mearini, E. Full Neurovascular Sparing Extraperitoneal Robotic Radical Prostatectomy: Our Experience with PERUSIA Technique. *J. Endourol.* **2017**, *31*, 32–37. [CrossRef]
8. Cochetti, G.; Del Zingaro, M.; Ciarletti, S.; Paladini, A.; Felici, G.; Stivalini, D.; Cellini, V.; Mearini, E. New Evolution of Robotic Radical Prostatectomy: A Single Center Experience with PERUSIA Technique. *Appl. Sci.* **2021**, *11*, 1513. [CrossRef]
9. Boni, A.; Cochetti, G.; Del Zingaro, M.; Paladini, A.; Turco, M.; de Vermandois, J.A.R.; Mearini, E. Uroflow stop test with electromyography: A novel index of urinary continence recovery after RARP. *Int. Urol. Nephrol.* **2019**, *51*, 609–615. Available online: http://link.springer.com/10.1007/s11255-019-02107-3 (accessed on 23 February 2019). [CrossRef]

10. de Carvalho, P.A.; Barbosa, J.A.; Guglielmetti, G.B.; Cordeiro, M.D.; Rocco, B.; Nahas, W.C.; Patel, V.; Coelho, R.F. Retrograde Release of the Neurovascular Bundle with Preservation of Dorsal Venous Complex During Robot-assisted Radical Prostatectomy: Optimizing Functional Outcomes. *Eur. Urol.* **2020**, *77*, 628–635. Available online: https://linkinghub.elsevier.com/retrieve/pii/S0302283818304810 (accessed on 1 May 2020). [CrossRef]
11. Yaxley, J.W.; Coughlin, G.D.; Chambers, S.K.; Occhipinti, S.; Samaratunga, H.; Zajdlewicz, L.; Dunglison, N.; Carter, R.; Williams, S.; Payton, D.J.; et al. Robot-assisted laparoscopic prostatectomy versus open radical retropubic prostatectomy: Early outcomes from a randomised controlled phase 3 study. *Lancet* **2016**, *388*, 1057–1066. Available online: https://linkinghub.elsevier.com/retrieve/pii/S014067361630592X (accessed on 10 September 2016). [CrossRef]
12. Kretschmer, A.; Bischoff, R.; Chaloupka, M.; Jokisch, F.; Westhofen, T.; Weinhold, P.; Strittmatter, F.; Becker, A.; Buchner, A.; Stief, C.G. Health-related quality of life after open and robot-assisted radical prostatectomy in low- and intermediate-risk prostate cancer patients: A propensity score-matched analysis. *World J. Urol.* **2020**, *38*, 3075–3083. Available online: http://link.springer.com/10.1007/s00345-020-03144-9 (accessed on 4 March 2020). [CrossRef] [PubMed]
13. de Vermandois, J.A.R.; Cochetti, G.; Del Zingaro, M.; Santoro, A.; Panciarola, M.; Boni, A.; Marsico, M.; Gaudio, G.; Paladini, A.; Guiggi, P.; et al. Evaluation of surgical site infection in mini-invasive urological surgery. *Open Med.* **2019**, *14*, 711–718. [CrossRef] [PubMed]
14. Tyson, M.D., II; Koyama, T.; Lee, D.; Hoffman, K.E.; Resnick, M.J.; Wu, X.C.; Cooperberg, M.R.; Goodman, M.; Greenfield, S.; Hamilton, A.S.; et al. Effect of Prostate Cancer Severity on Functional Outcomes after Localized Treatment: Comparative Effectiveness Analysis of Surgery and Radiation Study Results. *Eur. Urol.* **2018**, *74*, 26–33. Available online: https://linkinghub.elsevier.com/retrieve/pii/S0302283818301192 (accessed on 1 July 2018). [CrossRef]
15. Nahar, B.; Parekh, D.J. Focal therapy for localized prostate cancer: Where do we stand? *Eur. Urol. Focus* **2020**, *6*, 208–211. Available online: https://linkinghub.elsevier.com/retrieve/pii/S2405456919301282 (accessed on 1 May 2019). [CrossRef] [PubMed]
16. Flegar, L.; Zacharis, A.; Aksoy, C.; Heers, H.; Derigs, M.; Eisenmenger, N.; Borkowetz, A.; Groeben, C.; Huber, J. Alternative- and focal therapy trends for prostate cancer: A total population analysis of in-patient treatments in Germany from 2006 to 2019. *World J. Urol.* **2022**, *40*, 1645–1652. [CrossRef]
17. Perlis, N.; Ghai, S.; Tan, G.H.; Finelli, A. What are the limits of focal therapy for localized prostate cancer? For: GG3-5 may be considered. *Eur. Urol. Focus* **2020**, *6*, 201–202. Available online: https://linkinghub.elsevier.com/retrieve/pii/S240545691930135X (accessed on 3 May 2019). [CrossRef]
18. Mottet, N.; van den Bergh, R.C.; Briers, E.; Van den Broeck, T.; Cumberbatch, M.G.; De Santis, M.; Fanti, S.; Fossati, N.; Gandaglia, G.; Gillessen, S.; et al. EAU-EANM-ESTRO-ESUR-SIOG Guidelines on Prostate Cancer—2020 Update. Part 1: Screening, Diagnosis, and Local Treatment with Curative Intent. *Eur. Urol.* **2021**, *79*, 243–262. [CrossRef]
19. Oosterhoff, J.H.F.; Doornberg, J.N. Artificial intelligence in orthopaedics: False hope or not? A narrative review along the line of Gartner's hype cycle. *EFORT Open Rev.* **2020**, *5*, 593–603. [CrossRef]
20. Cumberbatch, M.G.; Murphy, D.G. Focal Therapy: When Nothing Is Sure, Everything Is Possible. *Eur. Urol.* **2020**, *78*, 379–380. Available online: https://linkinghub.elsevier.com/retrieve/pii/S0302283820305091 (accessed on 29 June 2020). [CrossRef]
21. Bongiolatti, S.; Corzani, R.; Borgianni, S.; Meniconi, F.; Cipollini, F.; Gonfiotti, A.; Viggiano, D.; Paladini, P.; Voltolini, L. Long-term results after surgical treatment of the dominant lung adenocarcinoma associated with ground-glass opacities. *J. Thorac. Dis.* **2018**, *10*, 4838–4848. [CrossRef]
22. Van Den Bos, W.; Muller, B.G.; Ahmed, H.; Bangma, C.H.; Barret, E.; Crouzet, S.; Eggener, S.E.; Gill, I.S.; Joniau, S.; Kovacs, G.; et al. Focal Therapy in Prostate Cancer: International Multidisciplinary Consensus on Trial Design. *Eur. Urol.* **2014**, *65*, 1078–1083. Available online: https://linkinghub.elsevier.com/retrieve/pii/S0302283814000025 (accessed on 2 January 2014). [CrossRef] [PubMed]
23. Truesdale, M.D.; Cheetham, P.J.; Hruby, G.W.; Wenske, S.; Conforto, A.K.; Cooper, A.B.; Katz, A.E. An Evaluation of Patient Selection Criteria on Predicting Progression-Free Survival after Primary Focal Unilateral Nerve-Sparing Cryoablation for Prostate Cancer. *Cancer J.* **2010**, *16*, 544–549. [CrossRef] [PubMed]
24. Guillaumier, S.; Peters, M.; Arya, M.; Afzal, N.; Charman, S.; Dudderidge, T.; Hosking-Jervis, F.; Hindley, R.G.; Lewi, H.; McCartan, N.; et al. A Multicentre Study of 5-year Outcomes Following Focal Therapy in Treating Clinically Significant Nonmetastatic Prostate Cancer. *Eur. Urol.* **2018**, *74*, 422–429. Available online: https://linkinghub.elsevier.com/retrieve/pii/S0302283818304317 (accessed on 1 June 2018). [CrossRef] [PubMed]
25. Johnson, D.C.; Reiter, R.E. Focal Therapy Should Not Be Considered for Men with Gleason Grade Group 3–5 Prostate Cancer. *Eur. Urol. Focus* **2020**, *6*, 203–204. Available online: https://linkinghub.elsevier.com/retrieve/pii/S2405456919301609 (accessed on 12 June 2019). [CrossRef]
26. Le, J.D.; Tan, N.; Shkolyar, E.; Lu, D.Y.; Kwan, L.; Marks, L.S.; Huang, J.; Margolis, D.J.; Raman, S.S.; Reiter, R.E. Multifocality and Prostate Cancer Detection by Multiparametric Magnetic Resonance Imaging: Correlation with Whole-mount Histopathology. *Eur. Urol.* **2015**, *67*, 569–576. Available online: https://linkinghub.elsevier.com/retrieve/pii/S0302283814008914 (accessed on 31 August 2014). [CrossRef] [PubMed]
27. Johnson, D.C.; Raman, S.S.; Mirak, S.A.; Kwan, L.; Bajgiran, A.M.; Hsu, W.; Maehara, C.K.; Ahuja, P.; Faiena, I.; Pooli, A.; et al. Detection of Individual Prostate Cancer Foci via Multiparametric Magnetic Resonance Imaging. *Eur. Urol.* **2019**, *75*, 712–720. Available online: https://linkinghub.elsevier.com/retrieve/pii/S0302283818309308 (accessed on 10 November 2018). [CrossRef]

28. Lindner, U.; Lawrentschuk, N.; Weersink, R.A.; Davidson, S.R.; Raz, O.; Hlasny, E.; Langer, D.L.; Gertner, M.R.; Van der Kwast, T.; Haider, M.A.; et al. Focal Laser Ablation for Prostate Cancer Followed by Radical Prostatectomy: Validation of Focal Therapy and Imaging Accuracy. *Eur. Urol.* **2010**, *57*, 1111–1114. Available online: https://linkinghub.elsevier.com/retrieve/pii/S0302283810002265 (accessed on 4 March 2010). [CrossRef]
29. Cohen, M.S.; Hanley, R.S.; Kurteva, T.; Ruthazer, R.; Silverman, M.L.; Sorcini, A.; Hamawy, K.; Roth, R.A.; Tuerk, I.; Libertino, J.A. Comparing the Gleason Prostate Biopsy and Gleason Prostatectomy Grading System: The Lahey Clinic Medical Center Experience and an International Meta-Analysis. *Eur. Urol.* **2008**, *54*, 371–381. Available online: https://linkinghub.elsevier.com/retrieve/pii/S0302283808003412 (accessed on 28 July 2022). [CrossRef]
30. Bostwick, D.G. Correlation with Grade in 316 Matched Prostatectomies. *Am. J. Surg. Pathol.* **1994**, *18*, 796–803. Available online: http://journals.lww.com/00000478-199408000-00006 (accessed on 1 August 1994). [CrossRef]
31. King, C.R. Patterns of prostate cancer biopsy grading:Trends and clinical implications. *Int. J. Cancer* **2000**, *90*, 305–311. Available online: https://onlinelibrary.wiley.com/doi/10.1002/1097-0215(20001220)90:6\T1\textless{}305::AID-IJC1\T1\textgreater{}3.0.CO;2-U (accessed on 10 January 2001). [CrossRef]
32. Narain, V.; Bianco, F.J.; Grignon, D.J.; Sakr, W.A.; Pontes, J.E.; Wood, D.P. How accurately does prostate biopsy Gleason score predict pathologic findings and disease free survival? *Prostate* **2001**, *49*, 185–190. [CrossRef] [PubMed]
33. Bott, S.R.J.; Freeman, A.A.; Stenning, S.; Cohen, J.; Parkinson, M.C. Radical prostatectomy: Pathology findings in 1001 cases compared with other major series and over time. *BJU Int.* **2005**, *95*, 34–39. [CrossRef]
34. Schiffmann, J.; Wenzel, P.; Salomon, G.; Budäus, L.; Schlomm, T.; Minner, S.; Wittmer, C.; Kraft, S.; Krech, T.; Steurer, S.; et al. Heterogeneity in D'Amico classification–based low-risk prostate cancer: Differences in upgrading and upstaging according to active surveillance eligibility. *Urol. Oncol. Semin. Orig. Investig.* **2015**, *33*, 329.e13–329.e19. Available online: https://linkinghub.elsevier.com/retrieve/pii/S1078143915001544 (accessed on 7 May 2015).
35. Busch, J.; Magheli, A.; Leva, N.; Ferrari, M.; Kramer, J.; Klopf, C.; Kempkensteffen, C.; Miller, K.; Brooks, J.D.; Gonzalgo, M.L. Higher rates of upgrading and upstaging in older patients undergoing radical prostatectomy and qualifying for active surveillance. *BJU Int.* **2014**, *114*, 517–521. [CrossRef]
36. Boniol, M.; Autier, P.; Perrin, P.; Boyle, P. Variation of Prostate-specific Antigen Value in Men and Risk of High-grade Prostate Cancer: Analysis of the Prostate, Lung, Colorectal, and Ovarian Cancer Screening Trial Study. *Urology* **2015**, *85*, 1117–1122. [CrossRef]
37. Park, Y.H.; Lee, J.K.; Jung, J.W.; Lee, B.K.; Lee, S.; Jeong, S.J.; Hong, S.K.; Byun, S.S.; Lee, S.E. Prostate cancer detection rate in patients with fluctuating prostate-specific antigen levels on the repeat prostate biopsy. *Prostate Int.* **2014**, *2*, 26–30. [CrossRef]
38. Okabe, Y.; Patel, H.D.; Rac, G.; Gupta, G.N. Multifocality of Prostate Cancer and Candidacy for Focal Therapy Based on Magnetic Resonance Imaging. *Urology* **2022**. [CrossRef] [PubMed]

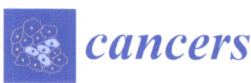 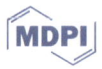

Article

Development of a Prognostic Model of Overall Survival for Metastatic Hormone-Naïve Prostate Cancer in Japanese Men

Ryunosuke Nakagawa [1], Hiroaki Iwamoto [1,*], Tomoyuki Makino [2], Renato Naito [1], Suguru Kadomoto [1], Norihito Akatani [3], Hiroshi Yaegashi [1], Shohei Kawaguchi [1], Takahiro Nohara [1], Kazuyoshi Shigehara [1], Kouji Izumi [1], Yoshifumi Kadono [1], Atsushi Takamatsu [4], Kotaro Yoshida [4] and Atsushi Mizokami [1]

1. Department of Integrative Cancer Therapy and Urology, Kanazawa University Graduate School of Medical Science, Kanazawa 920-8641, Japan
2. Department of Urology, Ishikawa Prefectural Central Hospital, Kanazawa 920-8530, Japan
3. Department of Nuclear Medicine, Kanazawa University Hospital, Kanazawa 920-8641, Japan
4. Department of Radiology, Kanazawa University Graduate School of Medical Sciences, Kanazawa 920-0934, Japan
* Correspondence: iwamoto-h@med.kanazawa-u.ac.jp

Simple Summary: Treatment strategies have changed dramatically in recent years with the development of a variety of agents for metastatic hormone-naïve prostate cancer. There is a need to identify prognostic factors for the appropriate choice of treatment for patients with hormone-naïve prostate cancer in Japanese men. Among the prostate cancer patients receiving treatment at our institution from 2000 to 2019, 198 patients with bone or visceral metastases at the initial diagnosis were included in the study. We retrospectively examined these factors of the overall survival, and identified Gleason pattern 5 content, bone scan index ≥ 1.5, and lactate dehydrogenase evels ≥ 300 IU/L as prognostic factors. Using these three factors, we developed a new prognostic model for overall survival that can more objectively predict the prognosis of patients simply and objectively.

Abstract: Background: Treatment strategies have changed dramatically in recent years with the development of a variety of agents for metastatic hormone-naïve prostate cancer (mHNPC). There is a need to identify prognostic factors for the appropriate choice of treatment for patients with mHNPC, and we retrospectively examined these factors. Methods: Patients with mHNPC treated at our institution from 2000 to 2019 were included in this study. Overall survival (OS) was estimated retrospectively using the Kaplan–Meier method, and factors associated with OS were identified using univariate and multivariate analyses. A prognostic model was then developed based on the factors identified. Follow-up was terminated on 24 October 2021. Results: The median follow-up duration was 44.2 months, whereas the median OS was 85.2 months, with 88 patients succumbing to their disease. Multivariate analysis identified Gleason pattern (GP) 5 content, bone scan index (BSI) ≥ 1.5, and lactate dehydrogenase (LDH) levels ≥ 300 IU/L as prognostic factors associated with OS. We also developed a prognostic model that classified patients with mHNPC as low risk with no factor, intermediate risk with one factor, and high risk with two or three factors. Conclusions: Three prognostic factors for OS were identified in patients with mHNPC, namely GP5 inclusion, BSI ≥ 1.5, and LDH ≥ 300. Using these three factors, we developed a new prognostic model for OS that can more objectively predict patient prognosis.

Keywords: hormone-naïve prostate cancer; prognostic model; Gleason pattern; bone scan index; lactate dehydrogenase

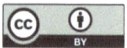

1. Introduction

Prostate cancer (PC) is the most common malignancy in men and a leading cause of cancer-related deaths in developed countries [1]. Approximately 10–20% of patients have de novo metastatic disease, with the number of patients diagnosed with metastatic PC only increasing [2]. Since 1940, the standard treatment for metastatic PC has been androgen deprivation therapy (ADT) Ref [3]. While newly diagnosed metastatic PC initially responds to ADT, it can become resistant and progress to castration-resistant PC (CRPC). Despite available treatments for CRPC, including alternative ADT [4], androgen receptor axis targeted agents (ARAT), chemotherapy [5,6], and radium-223 [7], the disease is often fatal in the end. However, six randomized trials found that the combination of drugs, such as docetaxel, abiraterone acetate, enzalutamide, and apalutamide, improved outcomes for patients with metastatic hormone-naïve PC (mHNPC) compared to ADT alone [8–14]. In Japan, abiraterone, enzalutamide, and apalutamide, have been approved for the upfront treatment of mHNPC, and have become treatment options. These reports have increased the number of treatment options for mHNPC. Interestingly, the survival benefits of these novel therapies vary depending on the extent of metastasis and severity of the cancer. The LATITUDE trial showed that the combination of abiraterone acetate and prednisolone with ADT prompted longer overall survival (OS) compared to ADT alone in high-risk mHNPC patients, although the therapeutic benefits expected in low-risk mHNPC patients remains unknown [11]. In the CHAARTED trial, the combination of prior chemotherapy with docetaxel and ADT significantly prolonged the survival of mHNPC patients; however, their subgroup analysis showed that the low-volume group exhibited no improvement in OS [10]. In other words, a certain number of patients can be expected to survive for a long time with ADT alone, and overtreatment can be minimized by identifying prognostic factors. Roy et al. created a nomogram of mHNPC patients treated with upfront ARAT [15]. Their nomogram is based on data from high-risk patients enrolled in the LATITUDE trial, and is a very effective tool because it is composed of items that are used in daily clinical practice. In this study, we retrospectively examined prognostic factors to develop a prognostic model for mHNPC patients in Japan.

2. Materials and Methods

2.1. Patient Selection

Among the PC patients receiving treatment at Kanazawa University Hospital from 2000 to 2019, 198 patients with bone or visceral metastases at the initial diagnosis were included in the study. All patients were pathologically diagnosed PC, and distant metastasis was detected through computed tomography and/or bone scans performed at the time of diagnosis.

2.2. Collection of Clinical Data

Age, Gleason pattern (GP), prostate-specific antigen (PSA), bone scan index (BSI), metastasis location, C-reactive protein (CRP), neutrophil-to-lymphocyte ratio (NLR), hemoglobin (Hb), alkaline phosphatase (ALP), and lactate dehydrogenase (LDH), were obtained from medical records and retrospectively investigated and analyzed for factors associated with OS. OS was measured from the diagnosis of PC until death or last follow-up. Follow-up was terminated on 24 October 2021.

Clinical stage was determined based on the 8th edition of the Union for International Cancer Control Tumor, Node, Metastasis classification, published in 2017. The BSI was developed as a marker of the total amount of bone metastasis using whole-body scintigraphy with 99mTc-MDP, which was calculated using the BONENAVI version 2 software program (FUJIFILM Toyama Chemical Co., Ltd., Tokyo, Japan; Exini Bone, Exini Diagnostics, Lund, Sweden) and was used herein [16]. The BSI represents the percentage of total skeletal mass taken up by the tumor, and is a reproducible quantitative expression of tumor burden seen on bone. In addition, the probability of abnormality is calculated by detecting hyperaccumulated areas in the bone scintigraphic image, thus preventing missed areas and enabling the objective evaluation of bone metastasis [17].

2.3. Statistical Analyses

OS was estimated using the Kaplan–Meier method, with differences being compared using log-rank tests. We evaluated the predictive impact of several potential factors on the OS patients using the Cox proportional hazards model. Hazard ratio (HR) and 95% confidence intervals (CI) were calculated. Thereafter, a prognostic model was developed based on the identified factors. Statistical analyses were performed using the commercially available software Prism 8 (GraphPad, San Diego, CA, USA) and the SPSS ver. 25.0 (SPSS Inc., Chicago, IL, USA), with p values of <0.05 indicating statistical significance. Nomogram was created using the R statistical software, version 3.6.3 (R Foundation for Statistical Computing, Vienna, Austria).

2.4. Ethical Considerations

This study was approved by the institutional review board of Kanazawa University Hospital (2016-328). Informed consent was obtained in the form of opt-out posted at our facility allowed by Medical Ethics Committee of Kanazawa University. All methods were performed in accordance with relevant guidelines and regulations.

3. Results

3.1. Overall Survival of Patients Classified by LATITUDE and CHAARTED Criteria

The characteristics of the 198 patients with mHNPC with bone or visceral metastases are summarized in Table 1. The median age was 71 (65–78) years, with 58.1% having lymph node metastasis, 2.5% having M1a disease, 83.3% having M1b disease, and 14.1% having M1c disease. Visceral metastases were found in the lungs (23 patients, 11.6%), liver (3 patients, 1.5%), and adrenal gland (1 patient, 0.5%). The median initial PSA was 230.5 (72.7–859.35) ng/mL, with 54.0% having Gleason score (GS) $\geq$ 9. The initial treatment consisted of combined androgen therapy (CAB) or luteinizing hormone-releasing hormone agonists alone for most patients (93.4%).

The median follow-up duration and median OS were 44.2 and 85.2 months, respectively, and 88 patients have died. The high-risk group had a significantly shorter OS (HR: 2.45, 95% CI 1.48–4.00; $p < 0.0001$) than the low-risk group based on LATITUDE criteria (Figure 1a). The median OS was 135.0 and 55.06 months in the low- and high-risk groups, respectively. Moreover, the high-volume group had a significantly shorter OS (HR: 2.55, 95% CI 1.54–4.24; $p < 0.0001$) than the low-volume group based on the CHAARTED criteria (Figure 1b). The median OS was 135.0 and 52.93 months in the low- and high-volume groups, respectively.

Table 1. Patient characteristics.

Variables	Entire Cohort (n = 198)
Age, median (range)	71 (65–78)
T stage, no (%)	
T1-2	17 (8.6)
T3	85 (42.9)
T4	77 (38.9)
Unknown	19 (9.6)
N stage, no (%)	
N0	79 (39.9)
N1	115 (58.1)
Unknown	4 (2.0)
M stage, no (%)	
M1a	5 (2.5)
M1b	165 (83.3)
M1c	28 (14.1)
Site of metastasis, no (%)	
Lymph node	116 (58.6)
Bone	188 (94.9)
Lung	23 (11.6)
Liver	3 (1.5)
Adrenal gland	1 (0.5)
Initial PSA level, ng/mL, median (range)	230.5 (72.7–859.4)
Gleason score, no (%)	
$\leq$3 + 4	10 (5.1)
4 + 3	19 (9.6)
8	52 (26.3)
$\geq$9	107 (54.0)
Unknown	10 (5.1)
Initial treatment, no (%)	
CAB	185 (93.4)
LHRH agonist	3 (1.5)
Abiraterone	1 (0.5)
Other	5 (2.5)
Unknown	4 (2.0)

PSA: prostate specific antigen; CAB: combined androgen blockade.

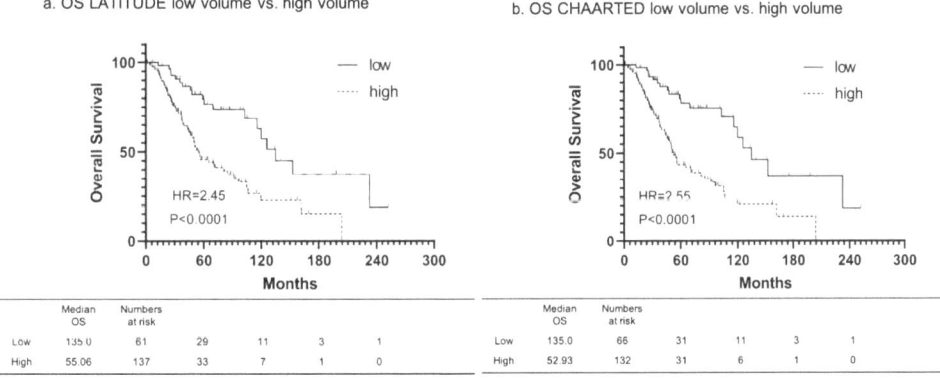

Figure 1. Kaplan-Meier showing the difference in OS classified by LATITUDE criteria, and CHAARTED criteria. (**a**) The high-risk group had a significantly shorter OS (HR: 2.45, 95% CI 1.48–4.00; $p < 0.0001$) than the low-risk group based on LATITUDE criteria. (**b**) The high-volume group had a significantly shorter OS (HR: 2.55, 95% CI 1.54–4.24; $p < 0.0001$) than the low-volume group based on the CHAARTED criteria.

3.2. Identification of Prognostic Factors in Overall Survival

Univariate analysis identified inclusion of GP 5 (HR: 2.78, 95% CI 1.72–4.47; $p < 0.001$), BSI $\geq$ 1.5 (HR: 1.91, 95% CI 1.03–3.53; $p = 0.040$), and LDH $\geq$ 300 IU/L (HR: 6.08, 95% CI 2.95–12.50; $p < 0.001$), as significant prognostic factors for OS, although age, PSA level, visceral metastasis, CRP, NLR, Hb, and ALP, were not in this cohort (Table 2). Although BSI was found to be a prognostic factor in patients with mHNPC, one other method for assessing bone metastases in prostate cancer is the extent of disease (EOD) score, proposed by Soloway et al. in 1988, and is a method for assessing bone metastasis in prostate cancer [18]. Univariate analysis of patients with low EOD scores (scores 1 and 2) and those with high EOD scores (scores 3 and 4) was performed, but it was not a significant predictor of prognosis (HR: 1.52, 95% CI 0.92–2.52; $p = 0.11$). OS was also investigated in Kaplan-Meier, but there was no significant difference between these two groups (HR: 1.49, 95% CI 0.90–2.49; $p = 0.10$) (Supplementary Figure S1).

Table 2. Univariate and multivariable analysis of prognostic factors for overall survival.

Variables	Univariate				Multivariable			
			95% CI				95% CI	
	p Value	HR	Lower	Upper	p Value	HR	Lower	Upper
Age <70 vs. $\geq$70 (years)	0.53	1.15	0.74	1.79	0.37	1.46	0.64	3.33
Include GP5	<0.001	2.78	1.72	4.47	0.045	2.77	1.03	7.49
PSA <200 vs. $\geq$200 (ng/mL)	0.40	1.21	0.78	1.86	0.32	0.55	0.17	1.78
BSI <1.5 vs. $\geq$1.5	0.04	1.91	1.03	3.53	0.033	3.48	1.10	11.00
Visceral metastasis	0.53	1.20	0.69	2.07	0.053	0.15	0.02	1.03
CRP <1.0 vs. $\geq$1.0 (mg/dL)	0.76	1.10	0.60	2.03	0.67	0.80	0.29	2.24
NLR <2.5 vs. $\geq$2.5	0.13	1.65	0.87	3.14	0.09	2.32	0.89	6.08
Hb <12 vs. $\geq$12 (g/dL)	0.35	1.35	0.72	2.56	0.64	0.79	0.29	2.15
ALP <300 vs. $\geq$300 (IU/L)	0.31	1.34	0.76	2.37	0.32	0.55	0.17	1.79
LDH <300 vs. $\geq$300 (IU/L)	<0.001	6.08	2.95	12.50	0.004	8.11	1.99	33.11

PSA: prostate specific antigen; GP: Gleason Pattern; BSI: bone scan index; CRP: C-reactive protein; NLR: neutrophil-to-lymphocyte ratio; Hb: hemoglobin; ALP: alkaline phosphatase; LDH: lactate dehydrogenase.

Multivariate analysis identified inclusion of GP 5 (HR 2.77, 95% CI 1.03–7.49; $p = 0.045$), BSI $\geq$ 1.5 (HR: 3.48, 95% CI 1.10–11.00; $p = 0.033$), and LDH $\geq$ 300 IU/L (HR: 8.11, 95% CI 1.99–33.11; $p = 0.004$), as factors associated with an increased risk of OS, similar to that in the univariate analysis. After comparing the three factors identified and detected as significant prognostic factors in both groups, OS was significantly shorter with GP 5 inclusion (HR: 2.58, 95% CI 1.72–4.47; $p < 0.001$) than with GP 5 exclusion (Figure 2a), in the BSI $\geq$ 1.5 group (HR: 3.23, 95% CI 1.77–5.89; $p = 0.037$) than in the BSI < 1.5 group (Figure 2b), and in the LDH $\geq$300 IU/L group (HR: 4.17, 95% CI 2.10–8.30; $p < 0.0001$) than in the LDH < 300 IU/L group (Figure 2c). Cancer-specific survival (CSS) was also discussed. GP5 (HR: 3.29, 95% CI 1.95–5.57; $p < 0.001$) and LDH $\geq$ 300 (HR: 7.82, 95% CI 3.71–16.48; $p < 0.001$) were risk factors in univariate analysis (Supplementary Table S1). On the other hand, BSI $\geq$ 1.5 was not a risk factor (HR: 1.61, 95% CI 0.86–3.04; $p = 0.14$). Multivariate analysis for CSS showed that only LDH $\geq$ 300 was an independent risk factor (HR: 10.14, 95% CI 2.36–43.61; $p = 0.002$).

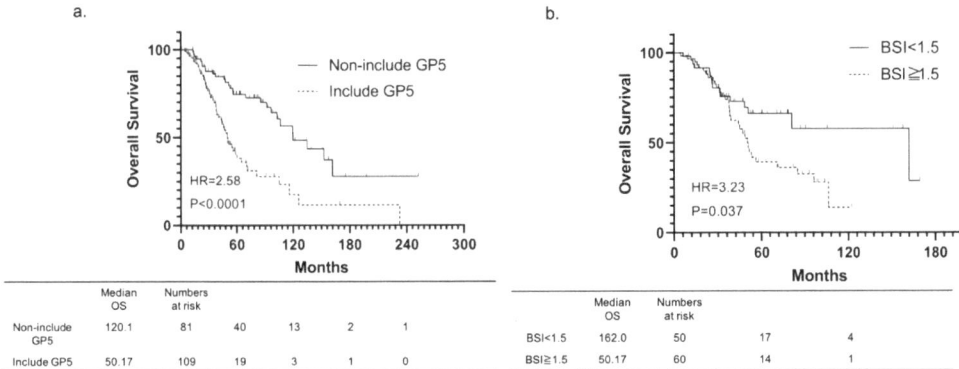
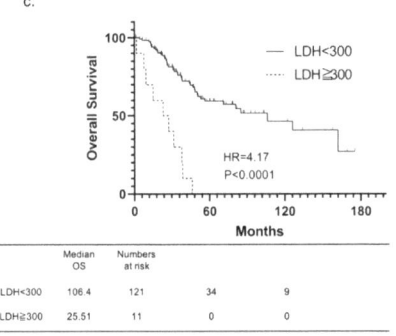

Figure 2. Kaplan-Meier showing the difference in OS stratified by inclusion of GP5, BSI ≥ 1.5, and LDH ≥ 300 IU/L. OS was significantly shorter with GP 5 inclusion (HR: 2.58, 95% CI 1.72–4.47; $p < 0.001$) than with GP 5 exclusion (**a**); in the BSI ≥ 1.5 group (HR: 3.23, 95% CI 1.77–5.89; $p = 0.037$) than in the BSI < 1.5 group (**b**); and in the LDH ≥ 300 IU/L group (HR: 4.17, 95% CI 2.10–8.30; $p < 0.0001$) than in the LDH < 300 IU/L group (**c**). Patients for whom information was available on each identified risk factors were selected. GP: Gleason pattern; BSI: bone scan index; LDH: lactate dehydrogenase.

3.3. Development of a Risk Model for Overall Survival

Patients with mHNPC were then classified into three groups according to three risk factors associated with OS. Accordingly, the low-risk group was defined as having none of the factors, the intermediate-risk group as those having one factor, and the high-risk group as those having two or three factors. The Kaplan–Meier cumulative OS is presented in Figure 3. The median OS was 162.0, 85.2, and 36.7 months in the low-risk, intermediate-risk, and high-risk group, respectively. Our findings showed that OS tended to decrease as risk increased (Log-rank test trend, $p = 0.0005$). Additionally, we have created a nomogram to predict 5-year survival using these three identified items (Supplementary Figure S2).

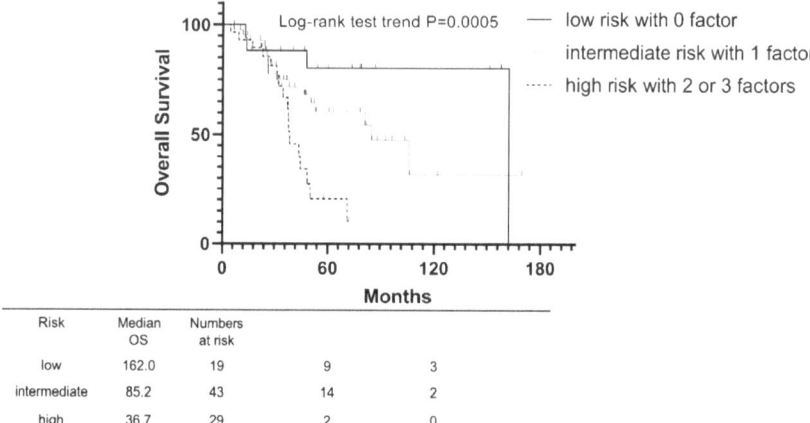

Figure 3. Kaplan-Meier estimates of cumulative OS in patients with mHNPC stratified by inclusion of GP 5, BSI ≥ 1.5, and LDH ≥ 300. Patients for whom information was available on all three identified risk factors were selected. Low risk patients had no risk factor, intermediate risk patients had one factor, and high-risk patients had two or three factors. OS tended to decrease as risk increased (Log-rank test trend, p = 0.0005). GP: Gleason pattern; BSI: bone scan index; LDH: lactate dehydrogenase.

4. Discussion

In the current study, the median OS of patients classified as high-risk based on the LATITUDE criteria was 55.06 months, which was similar to that in patients who received upfront abiraterone acetate and prednisolone in the LATITUDE study (53.3 months), despite most of the patients opting for CAB as their initial treatment [11]. Moreover, patients who were classified as high-volume according to the CHAARTED criteria had an OS of 52.93 months, which was longer than that in patients who received upfront docetaxel in the high volume arm of the CHAARTED trial (49.2 months) [10]. This may be attributed to the increased sensitivity of Asian patients with metastatic PC to castration and their significantly longer survival times compared to other ethnic groups [19]. However, it is clear whether a certain number of patients with high-volume metastases respond well to ADT. Administering ARAT, such as abiraterone acetate, or docetaxel, to such patients may cause a decrease in the patients' quality of life due to side effects, while increasing the burden of medical costs. For abiraterone, the incidence of grade 3 or 4 adverse events was 63% in the abiraterone group, compared to 48% in the placebo group [20]. We believe that this difference in incidence is not optimistic and is an impediment to the patient's quality of life. Although the CHAARTED trial did not compare docetaxel with ADT alone in terms of the incidence of adverse events [10], the fatal febrile neutropenia associated with docetaxel is a significant reduction in the quality of life of patients.

Therefore, with the emergence of various treatment options, creating a new prognostic model, identifying patients who do not respond well to ADT, and opting for upfront ARAT or chemotherapy would be very meaningful.

Various studies have been available on the prognostic factors for mHNPC. Glass et al. suggested a prognostic model, which differentiated patients into three prognosis groups based on bone metastasis localization, performance status, PSA, and GS [21]. Cooperberg et al. proposed the J-CAPRA score as a prognostic model for progression. In this model, GS, PSA, and TNM stage, are scored as factors, with difference in progression-free survival observed between the three groups of patients classified according to their model [22]. Our multivariable analysis found that the presence of GP5, BSI ≥ 1.5, and LDH ≥ 300 IU/L, were prognostic factors for mHNPC. In addition, creating a prognostic model based on these three factors and classifying the patients into three groups (low, intermediate, and high risk) resulted in differences in OS among such groups (165.0, 85.2, and 36.7 months). Roy's nomogram's composition, including LDH, bone metastases, and Gleason score, may justify our results [15]. Our identification of GP5 and their scoring item GS9-10 are strongly related and consistent. Additionally, in their nomogram, the number of skeletal lesions is one of the predictors. We believe that our predictor, BSI, is an ideal item for a more objective assessment of bone involvement.

Several reports have suggested that the inclusion of GP5 increased the aggressiveness of PC. Kryvenko et al. reported that the presence of GP5 significantly increased the risk of metastasis, prostate cancer-specific survival (PCSS), and death [23]. Tsao et al. reported that patients with GS 9–10 tended to have a greater risk of metastasis and death after local treatment compared to patients with GS8 [24]. We also looked at the International Society of Urologic Pathology (ISUP) grade groups, and grade groups 4 and 5 (GS 8–10) were also poor prognostic factors for OS in univariate analysis (HR: 3.01, 95% CI 1.43–6.34; $p = 0.004$), but they were not significant in multivariate analysis (data not shown). Huynh et al. reported that the risk of OS was significantly higher for PC with GS3+5/5+3 than for that with GS4+4 [25]. Therefore, among ISUP grade group 4 (GS 8), there is a report that the inclusion of Gleason pattern 5 affects OS, which we believe supports our results. Including the presence of GP5 as one of the prognostic factors is appropriate.

Our study identified BSI $\geq$ 1.5 as one of the prognostic factors for mHNPC. The LATITUDE criteria indicated the presence of three or more bone lesions as a high-risk factor [11]. In the CHAARTED trial, $\geq$4 bone lesions with $\geq$1 beyond the vertebral bodies and pelvis were listed as a high-volume factor [10]. In previous reports, some prognostic models have been created based on the extent of bone disease (EOD) score [18]. Shiota et al. identified EOD 4 as a risk factor for metastatic high burden for PC [26]. Akamatsu et al. listed EOD 3 or higher as a prognostic factor for OS and reported that classifying patients into three risk groups resulted in significant differences [27]. We also divided the patients into two groups with low and high EOD score and investigated their OS. However, there were no significant differences between the two groups. In our study, EOD score was not a useful prognostic factor. EOD score is based on the number of bone lesions and do not account for the size of a single bone lesion. Moreover, the lesion count may contain some subjective factors. The BSI was developed as a marker of the total amount of bone metastasis using whole-body scintigraphy with 99 mTc-MDP [28,29]. One of the major features of the BSI is that the bone scintigram can be used to objectively evaluate the degree of bone metastasis throughout the body. Poulsem et al. reported that patients with PC and metastases of BSI $\geq$ 1.0 have an increased risk of PCSS than those with BSI < 1.0 [30]. One study showed that BSI > 3.5% was a significant determinant of death in the mHNPC group and that patients with a good BSI response to treatment (>45%) had lower mortality rates than those without such a response [31]. Suzuki et al. calculated the BSI of bone lesions beyond the vertebral bodies and pelvis (bBSI) and reported that patients with PC and bone metastases of bBSI > 0.27 had a significantly shorter OS [32]. We suggest using BSI to objectively quantify the degree of bone metastasis in order to establish a more accurate prognostic model.

Another prognostic factor, serum LDH, was found to be associated with OS in patients with mHNPC. LDH is an intracellular enzyme that is widely distributed in body tissues. When one of the tissues is injured and LDH is released into the blood, the serum LDH concentration increases. LDH plays an important role in cancer metabolism [33]. Notably, LDH has been reported as a prognostic factor for metastatic PC in several studies, with our results being consistent with these reports [34,35]. In the present study, visceral metastasis was not a significant prognostic factor for OS. Several reports have also shown that visceral metastasis is not a factor associated with OS [36]. In the current study, the percentage of patients with lung metastasis was high, whereas that of other visceral metastasis, was low. One study reported that among patients with high burden metastases, those with lung metastases had better OS than those with M1b [37]. Iwamoto et al. reported that patients with PC and lung metastases only had better OS than those with visceral metastases, except for lung metastases [38]. Racial differences may be one of the reasons why visceral metastasis was not a prognostic factor [39]. This should be investigated by accumulating more cases in the future. Several risk models have been reported for Japanese patients, and these are useful risk classifications that can be very clearly stratified [26,27]. However, these risk models are somewhat complicated to stratify, and the EOD score is included as a predictor of prognosis. Our model is very important in that it is simpler and more objective in predicting patient prognosis.

In the present cohort, most patients with mHNPC were treated with CAB. The 5-year survival rate for patients classified as low risk in our proposed risk model is approximately 80%. The prognosis for this group of patients is very favorable. In the CHAARTED trial, the 5-year survival rate for patients who received upfront docetaxel in the low volume setting was approximately 70% [10], indicating that low-risk patients in our risk model have good survival outcomes with CAB alone. In the ENZAMET trial, a subgroup analysis reported a 90% 3-year survival rate in low-volume patients treated with upfront enzalutamide [12]. Our study also shows that the 3-year survival rate for low-risk patients is comparable to the ENZAMET trial. In consideration of these factors, we believe that vintage therapy for low-risk patients can never be a substitute for chemotherapy or ARAT. Ideally, this prognostic model should be used to actually make treatment choices, but this will likely be a future challenge. A larger prospective cohort study will be needed to prove this.

The current study has several limitations worth noting. This study was retrospective in nature, and treatment selection and evaluation of the effects of treatment were left to the individual physicians, which may have resulted in bias. In addition, patients included herein were all Japanese. Thus, our results may not be applicable to other races. Given that only pretreatment factors were investigated in this study, we did not examine factors that may be predictive of post-treatment outcomes, such as response to initial treatment (PSA reduction rate, time to CRPC, etc.). In addition, the patients enrolled in the study ranged from 2000 to 2019. The addition of ARAT or chemotherapy as new treatment options over the past 20 years may be one limitation when considering survival, because before the coming of ARAT or chemotherapy, patients did not have the option of receiving that treatment. Moreover, there have been International Society of Urological Pathology Consensus Conference in 2005 and 2014, where revisions were made regarding the Gleason classification. Since this is a retrospective study and the data collection for pathology results is based on medical record entries, it is possible that shifting diagnoses and definitions over time may have resulted in bias. However, in this study, we are focusing on GP 5. Since there has been no significant revision in the ISUP Consensus Conference regarding the diagnosis and definition of GP5, we do not think that it has had a significant impact on this study. Finally, the choice of sequential treatment was also left to the discretion of the physician, and the change in survival rate due to the choice of treatment after castration-resistant PC had not been investigated.

5. Conclusions

We identified three prognostic factors for OS in patients with mHNPC: GP5 inclusion, BSI ≥ 1.5, and LDH ≥ 300. Using these three factors, we developed a new prognostic model for OS that can more objectively predict the prognosis of patients simply and objectively.

Supplementary Materials: The following supporting information can be downloaded at: https://www.mdpi.com/article/10.3390/cancers14194822/s1, Figure S1: Kaplan-Meier showing the difference in OS stratified by low EOD score (score 1,2) and high EOD score (score 3,4); Figure S2: A nomogram was developed that combined the significant independent clinical variables; Table S1: Univariate and multivariable analysis of prognostic factors for cancer specific survival.

Author Contributions: Conceptualization, H.I. and K.S.; software, A.T. and K.Y.; formal analysis, R.N. (Ryunosuke Nakagawa); investigation, R.N. (Ryunosuke Nakagawa), N.A., H.Y., S.K. (Shohei

Kawaguchi) and T.N.; data curation, T.M., R.N. (Renato Naito) and S.K. (Suguru Kadomoto); writing—original draft preparation, R.N. (Ryunosuke Nakagawa); writing—review and editing, H.I.; visualization, S.K. (Shohei Kawaguchi), T.N. and K.I.; supervision, K.I., Y.K. and A.M. All authors have read and agreed to the published version of the manuscript.

Funding: This research received no external funding.

Institutional Review Board Statement: The study was conducted according to the guidelines of the Declaration of Helsinki, and approved by the institutional review board of Kanazawa University Hospital (2016-328).

Informed Consent Statement: Informed consent was obtained from all subjects involved in the study.

Data Availability Statement: The data presented in this study are available in the article and Supplementary Materials.

Conflicts of Interest: The authors declare no conflict of interest.

Ethics Statement: All procedures performed in studies involving human participants were conducted in accordance with the ethical standards of the institutional and/or national research committee and with the 1964 Helsinki Declaration and its later amendments or comparable ethical standards.

References

1. Siegel, R.L.; Miller, K.D.; Jemal, A. Cancer statistics, 2019. *CA Cancer J. Clin.* **2019**, *69*, 7–34. [CrossRef] [PubMed]
2. Yap, T.A.; Zivi, A.; Omlin, A.; de Bono, J.S. The changing therapeutic landscape of castration-resistant prostate cancer. *Nat. Rev. Clin. Oncol.* **2011**, *8*, 597–610. [CrossRef] [PubMed]
3. Huggins, C.; Hodges, C.V. Studies on prostatic cancer: I. The effect of castration, of estrogen and of androgen injection on serum phosphatases in metastatic carcinoma of the prostate. *J. Urol.* **2002**, *168*, 9–12. [CrossRef]
4. Iwamoto, H.; Kano, H.; Shimada, T.; Naito, R.; Makino, T.; Kadamoto, S.; Yaegashi, H.; Shigehara, K.; Izumi, K.; Kadonoa, Y.; et al. Effectiveness of Vintage Hormone Therapy as Alternative Androgen Deprivation Therapy for Non-metastatic Castration-resistant Prostate Cancer. *In Vivo* **2021**, *35*, 1247–1252. [CrossRef] [PubMed]
5. Tannock, I.F.; de Wit, R.; Berry, W.R.; Horti, J.; Pluzanska, A.; Chi, K.N.; Oudard, S.; Théodore, C.; James, N.D.; Turesson, I.; et al. Docetaxel plus prednisone or mitoxantrone plus prednisone for advanced prostate cancer. *N. Engl. J. Med.* **2004**, *351*, 1502–1512. [CrossRef] [PubMed]
6. Iwamoto, H.; Kano, H.; Shimada, T.; Naito, R.; Makino, T.; Kadomoto, S.; Yaegashi, H.; Shigehara, K.; Izumi, K.; Kadono, Y.; et al. Sarcopenia and Visceral Metastasis at Cabazitaxel Initiation Predict Prognosis in Patients With Castration-resistant Prostate Cancer Receiving Cabazitaxel Chemotherapy. *In Vivo* **2021**, *35*, 1703–1709. [CrossRef] [PubMed]
7. Coleman, R. Treatment of Metastatic Bone Disease and the Emerging Role of Radium-223. *Semin. Nucl. Med.* **2016**, *46*, 99–104. [CrossRef] [PubMed]
8. Kyriakopoulos, C.E.; Chen, Y.H.; Carducci, M.A.; Liu, G.; Jarrard, D.F.; Hahn, N.M.; Shevrin, D.H.; Dreicer, R.; Hussain, M.; Eisenberger, M.; et al. Chemohormonal Therapy in Metastatic Hormone-Sensitive Prostate Cancer: Long-Term Survival Analysis of the Randomized Phase III E3805 CHAARTED Trial. *J. Clin. Oncol.* **2018**, *36*, 1080–1087. [CrossRef] [PubMed]
9. Armstrong, A.J.; Szmulewitz, R.Z.; Petrylak, D.P.; Holzbeierlein, J.; Villers, A.; Azad, A.; Alcaraz, A.; Alekseev, B.; Iguchi, T.; Shore, N.D.; et al. ARCHES: A Randomized, Phase III Study of Androgen Deprivation Therapy With Enzalutamide or Placebo in Men With Metastatic Hormone-Sensitive Prostate Cancer. *J. Clin. Oncol.* **2019**, *37*, 2974–2986. [CrossRef] [PubMed]
10. Sweeney, C.J.; Chen, Y.H.; Carducci, M.; Liu, G.; Jarrard, D.F.; Eisenberger, M.; Wong, Y.N.; Hahn, N.; Kohli, M.; Cooney, M.M.; et al. Chemohormonal Therapy in Metastatic Hormone-Sensitive Prostate Cancer. *N. Engl. J. Med.* **2015**, *373*, 737–746. [CrossRef] [PubMed]
11. Fizazi, K.; Tran, N.; Fein, L.; Matsubara, N.; Rodriguez-Antolin, A.; Alekseev, B.Y.; Özgüroğlu, M.; Ye, D.; Feyerabend, S.; Protheroe, A.; et al. Abiraterone acetate plus prednisone in patients with newly diagnosed high-risk metastatic castration-sensitive prostate cancer (LATITUDE): Final overall survival analysis of a randomised, double-blind, phase 3 trial. *Lancet Oncol.* **2019**, *20*, 686–700. [CrossRef]
12. Davis, I.D.; Martin, A.J.; Stockler, M.R.; Begbie, S.; Chi, K.N.; Chowdhury, S.; Coskinas, X.; Frydenberg, M.; Hague, W.E.; Horvath, L.G.; et al. Enzalutamide with Standard First-Line Therapy in Metastatic Prostate Cancer. *N. Engl. J. Med.* **2019**, *381*, 121–131. [CrossRef]
13. Chi, K.N.; Agarwal, N.; Bjartell, A.; Chung, B.H.; Pereira de Santana Gomes, A.J.; Given, R.; Juárez Soto, Á.; Merseburger, A.S.; Özgüroğlu, M.; Uemura, H.; et al. Apalutamide for Metastatic, Castration-Sensitive Prostate Cancer. *N. Engl. J. Med.* **2019**, *381*, 13–24. [CrossRef]

14. Smith, M.R.; Hussain, M.; Saad, F.; Fizazi, K.; Sternberg, C.N.; Crawford, E.D.; Kopyltsov, E.; Park, C.H.; Alekseev, B.; Montesa-Pino, Á.; et al. Darolutamide and Survival in Metastatic, Hormone-Sensitive Prostate Cancer. *N. Engl. J. Med.* **2022**, *386*, 1132–1142. [CrossRef] [PubMed]
15. Roy, S.; Sun, Y.; Wallis, C.J.D.; Morgan, S.C.; Grimes, S.; Malone, J.; Kishan, A.U.; Mukherjee, D.; Spratt, D.E.; Saad, F.; et al. Development and validation of a multivariable prognostic model in de novo metastatic castrate sensitive prostate cancer. *Prostate Cancer Prostatic Dis.* **2022**. [CrossRef]
16. Koizumi, M.; Wagatsuma, K.; Miyaji, N.; Murata, T.; Miwa, K.; Takiguchi, T.; Makino, T.; Koyama, M. Evaluation of a computer-assisted diagnosis system, BONENAVI version 2, for bone scintigraphy in cancer patients in a routine clinical setting. *Ann. Nucl. Med.* **2015**, *29*, 138–148. [CrossRef]
17. Dennis, E.R.; Jia, X.; Mezheritskiy, I.S.; Stephenson, R.D.; Schoder, H.; Fox, J.J.; Heller, G.; Scher, H.I.; Larson, S.M.; Morris, M.J. Bone scan index: A quantitative treatment response biomarker for castration-resistant metastatic prostate cancer. *J. Clin. Oncol.* **2012**, *30*, 519–524. [CrossRef]
18. Soloway, M.S.; Hardeman, S.W.; Hickey, D.; Raymond, J.; Todd, B.; Soloway, S.; Moinuddin, M. Stratification of patients with metastatic prostate cancer based on extent of disease on initial bone scan. *Cancer* **1988**, *61*, 195–202. [CrossRef]
19. Fukagai, T.; Namiki, T.S.; Carlile, R.G.; Yoshida, H.; Namiki, M. Comparison of the clinical outcome after hormonal therapy for prostate cancer between Japanese and Caucasian men. *BJU Int.* **2006**, *97*, 1190–1193. [CrossRef]
20. Fizazi, K.; Tran, N.; Fein, L.; Matsubara, N.; Rodriguez-Antolin, A.; Alekseev, B.Y.; Özgüroğlu, M.; Ye, D.; Feyerabend, S.; Protheroe, A.; et al. Abiraterone plus Prednisone in Metastatic, Castration-Sensitive Prostate Cancer. *N. Engl. J. Med.* **2017**, *377*, 352–360. [CrossRef]
21. Glass, T.R.; Tangen, C.M.; Crawford, E.D.; Thompson, I. Metastatic carcinoma of the prostate: Identifying prognostic groups using recursive partitioning. *J. Urol.* **2003**, *169*, 164–169. [CrossRef]
22. Cooperberg, M.R.; Hinotsu, S.; Namiki, M.; Ito, K.; Broering, J.; Carroll, P.R.; Akaza, H. Risk assessment among prostate cancer patients receiving primary androgen deprivation therapy. *J. Clin. Oncol.* **2009**, *27*, 4306–4313. [CrossRef]
23. Kryvenko, O.N.; Williamson, S.R.; Schwartz, L.E.; Epstein, J.I. Gleason score 5 + 3 = 8 (grade group 4) prostate cancer-a rare occurrence with contemporary grading. *Hum. Pathol.* **2020**, *97*, 40–51. [CrossRef]
24. Tsao, C.K.; Gray, K.P.; Nakabayashi, M.; Evan, C.; Kantoff, P.W.; Huang, J.; Galsky, M.D.; Pomerantz, M.; Oh, W.K. Patients with Biopsy Gleason 9 and 10 Prostate Cancer Have Significantly Worse Outcomes Compared to Patients with Gleason 8 Disease. *J. Urol.* **2015**, *194*, 91–97. [CrossRef]
25. Huynh, M.A.; Chen, M.H.; Wu, J.; Braccioforte, M.H.; Moran, B.J.; D'Amico, A.V. Gleason Score 3 + 5 or 5 + 3 versus 4 + 4 Prostate Cancer: The Risk of Death. *Eur. Urol.* **2016**, *69*, 976–979. [CrossRef]
26. Shiota, M.; Terada, N.; Kitamura, H.; Kojima, T.; Saito, T.; Yokomizo, A.; Kohei, N.; Goto, T.; Kawamura, S.; Hashimoto, Y.; et al. Novel metastatic burden-stratified risk model in de novo metastatic hormone-sensitive prostate cancer. *Cancer Sci.* **2021**, *112*, 3616–3626. [CrossRef]
27. Akamatsu, S.; Kubota, M.; Uozumi, R.; Narita, S.; Takahashi, M.; Mitsuzuka, K.; Hatakeyama, S.; Sakurai, T.; Kawamura, S.; Ishidoya, S.; et al. Development and Validation of a Novel Prognostic Model for Predicting Overall Survival in Treatment-naïve Castration-sensitive Metastatic Prostate Cancer. *Eur. Urol. Oncol.* **2019**, *2*, 320–328. [CrossRef]
28. Nakajima, K.; Edenbrandt, L.; Mizokami, A. Bone scan index: A new biomarker of bone metastasis in patients with prostate cancer. *Int. J. Urol.* **2017**, *24*, 668–673. [CrossRef]
29. Imbriaco, M.; Larson, S.M.; Yeung, H.W.; Mawlawi, O.R.; Erdi, Y.; Venkatraman, E.S.; Scher, H.I. A new parameter for measuring metastatic bone involvement by prostate cancer: The Bone Scan Index. *Clin. Cancer Res.* **1998**, *4*, 1765–1772.
30. Poulsen, M.H.; Rasmussen, J.; Edenbrandt, L.; Høilund-Carlsen, P.F.; Gerke, O.; Johansen, A.; Lund, L. Bone Scan Index predicts outcome in patients with metastatic hormone-sensitive prostate cancer. *BJU Int.* **2016**, *117*, 748–753. [CrossRef]
31. Nakajima, K.; Mizokami, A.; Matsuyama, H.; Ichikawa, T.; Kaneko, G.; Takahashi, S.; Shiina, H.; Horikoshi, H.; Hashine, K.; Sugiyama, Y.; et al. Prognosis of patients with prostate cancer and bone metastasis from the Japanese Prostatic Cancer Registry of Standard Hormonal and Chemotherapy Using Bone Scan Index cohort study. *Int. J. Urol.* **2021**, *28*, 955–963. [CrossRef]
32. Suzuki, K.; Okamura, Y.; Hara, T.; Terakawa, T.; Furukawa, J.; Harada, K.; Hinata, N.; Fujisawa, M. Prognostic impact of bone metastatic volume beyond vertebrae and pelvis in patients with metastatic hormone-sensitive prostate cancer. *Int. J. Clin. Oncol.* **2021**, *26*, 1533–1540. [CrossRef]
33. Mongre, R.K.; Mishra, C.B.; Prakash, A.; Jung, S.; Lee, B.S.; Kumari, S.; Hong, J.T.; Lee, M.S. Novel Carbazole-Piperazine Hybrid Small Molecule Induces Apoptosis by Targeting BCL-2 and Inhibits Tumor Progression in Lung Adenocarcinoma in Vitro and Xenograft Mice Model. *Cancers* **2019**, *11*, 1245. [CrossRef]
34. Narita, S.; Hatakeyama, S.; Takahashi, M.; Sakurai, T.; Kawamura, S.; Hoshi, S.; Ishida, M.; Kawaguchi, T.; Ishidoya, S.; Shimoda, J.; et al. Clinical outcomes and prognostic factors in patients with newly diagnosed metastatic prostate cancer initially treated with androgen deprivation therapy: A retrospective multicenter study in Japan. *Int. J. Clin. Oncol.* **2020**, *25*, 912–920. [CrossRef]
35. Kobayashi, T.; Namitome, R.; Hirata, Y.U.; Shiota, M.; Imada, K.; Kashiwagi, E.; Takeuchi, A.; Inokuchi, J.; Tatsugami, K.; Eto, M. Serum Prognostic Factors of Androgen-deprivation Therapy Among Japanese Men With De Novo Metastatic Prostate Cancer. *Anticancer Res.* **2019**, *39*, 3191–3195. [CrossRef]

36. Kawahara, T.; Yoneyama, S.; Ohno, Y.; Iizuka, J.; Hashimoto, Y.; Tsumura, H.; Tabata, K.I.; Nakagami, Y.; Tanabe, K.; Iwamura, M.; et al. Prognostic Value of the LATITUDE and CHAARTED Risk Criteria for Predicting the Survival of Men with Bone Metastatic Hormone-Naïve Prostate Cancer Treated with Combined Androgen Blockade Therapy: Real-World Data from a Japanese Multi-Institutional Study. *Biomed Res. Int.* **2020**, *2020*, 7804932. [CrossRef]
37. Shiota, M.; Terada, N.; Saito, T.; Yokomizo, A.; Kohei, N.; Goto, T.; Kawamura, S.; Hashimoto, Y.; Takahashi, A.; Kimura, T.; et al. Differential prognostic factors in low- and high-burden de novo metastatic hormone-sensitive prostate cancer patients. *Cancer Sci.* **2021**, *112*, 1524–1533. [CrossRef]
38. Iwamoto, H.; Izumi, K.; Shimada, T.; Kano, H.; Kadomoto, S.; Makino, T.; Naito, R.; Yaegashi, H.; Shigehara, K.; Kadono, Y.; et al. Androgen receptor signaling-targeted therapy and taxane chemotherapy induce visceral metastasis in castration-resistant prostate cancer. *Prostate* **2021**, *81*, 72–80. [CrossRef]
39. Cooperberg, M.R.; Hinotsu, S.; Namiki, M.; Carroll, P.R.; Akaza, H. Trans-Pacific variation in outcomes for men treated with primary androgen-deprivation therapy (ADT) for prostate cancer. *BJU Int.* **2016**, *117*, 102–109. [CrossRef]

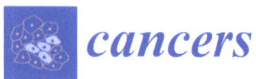

Article

Prostate-Specific Antigen Bounce after ^{125}I Brachytherapy Using Stranded Seeds with Intraoperative Optimization for Prostate Cancer

Tae Hyung Kim [1,2], Jason Joon Bock Lee [1,3] and Jaeho Cho [1,*]

1. Yonsei Cancer Center, Department of Radiation Oncology, Yonsei University College of Medicine, Seoul 03722, Korea
2. Department of Radiation Oncology, Nowon Eulji Medical Center, Eulji University School of Medicine, Seoul 01830, Korea
3. Department of Radiation Oncology, Kangbuk Samsung Hospital, Sungkyunkwan University School of Medicine, Seoul 03181, Korea
* Correspondence: jjhmd@yuhs.ac; Tel.: +82-2-2228-8095

Simple Summary: Our study investigated clinical features of prostate-specific antigen (PSA) bounce in patients undergoing brachytherapy. PSA bounce is common and discriminating between large bounces and biochemical failures is very difficult. Therefore, we suggest important points to discriminate between large bounces and biochemical failures. In addition, we aimed to examine the clinical features and details of PSA bounce in patients receiving brachytherapy.

Abstract: Prostate-specific antigen (PSA) bounce is common in patients undergoing ^{125}I brachytherapy (BT), and our study investigated its clinical features. A total of 100 patients who underwent BT were analyzed. PSA bounce and large bounce were defined as an increase of ≥ 0.2 and ≥ 2.0 ng/mL above the initial PSA nadir, respectively, with a subsequent decline without treatment. Biochemical failure was defined using the Phoenix definition (nadir +2 ng/mL), except for a large bounce. With a median follow-up of 49 months, 45% and 7% of the patients experienced bounce and large bounce, respectively. The median time to bounce was 24 months, and the median PSA value at the bounce spike was 1.62 ng/mL, a median raise of 0.44 ng/mL compared to the pre-bounce nadir. The median time to bounce recovery was 4 months. The post-bounce nadir was obtained at a median of 36 months after low-dose-rate BT. On univariate analysis, age, the PSA nadir value at 2 years, and prostate volume were significant factors for PSA bounce. The PSA nadir value at 2 years remained significant in multivariate analysis. We should carefully monitor young patients with high prostate volume having a >0.5 PSA nadir value at 2 years for PSA bounce.

Keywords: prostate cancer; brachytherapy; bounce; prognostic factor

1. Introduction

Several radiotherapeutic approaches are available for the definitive treatment of prostate cancer, including low-dose-rate (LDR) and high-dose-rate brachytherapy (BT), external beam radiotherapy (EBRT) with intensity-modulated RT, proton therapy, and even carbon ion therapy [1]. LDR-BT is a well-established standard treatment for early prostate cancer and offers excellent oncological outcomes, dosimetric advantages, and patient convenience [2–4].

Prostate-specific antigen (PSA) is a sensitive diagnostic and prognostic marker of prostate cancer. PSA bounce, a temporary increase in PSA levels and a subsequent decrease without intervention, occurs in 15–84% of men receiving ^{125}I BT [5]. Several studies and trials have demonstrated that PSA bounce after ^{125}I BT is a good prognostic factor [5,6], and young age is generally accepted as a predictive factor for PSA bounce [7,8]. In addition, few studies have investigated the difference between biochemical failure and PSA bounce [9–11], and most of them were single-center studies with several limitations. The predictive factors for PSA, as well as PSA details, remain unclear.

Therefore, this investigation aimed to examine the clinical features and details of PSA bounce in patients receiving LDR-BT.

2. Materials and Methods

2.1. Patients

From November 2012 to December 2017, 105 patients with prostate cancer underwent LDR-BT at Yonsei Cancer Center. Risk groups were defined according to the Memorial Sloan Kettering Cancer Center (MSKCC) criteria [12,13] and the D'Amico criteria [14]. Patients with localized and locally advanced disease were treated with LDR-BT, while those with metastatic disease were not. According to MSKCC risk grouping, patients with low risk and patients with intermediate to high risk whose adverse pathologic features approached that of low-risk patients were treated with LDR-BT. Patients treated with androgen deprivation therapy (ADT) before LDR-BT were included for analysis, but those who used maintenance ADT were excluded. The date of LDR-BT was day 0 of follow-up. PSA levels were measured prior to LDR-BT, every 3 months for the first year, every 6 months for 3 years, and every 12 months thereafter. Patients with a PSA follow-up duration of <2 years were excluded from the study. After exclusion, the data from 100 patients were analyzed. The procedures followed in this retrospective study were in accordance with the guidelines of the Helsinki Declaration of 1975, revised in 2000, and the study was approved by the Severance Hospital institutional review board (IRB # 4-2019-0767). Because this study was retrospective, the need for written informed consent was waived.

2.2. LDR-Brachytherapy

Preoperative treatment planning was performed based on trans-rectal ultrasonography (TRUS) images acquired during preoperative simulation. Radiation oncologist confirmed Pubic arch interference that prevents proper needle insertion into the peripheral zone of the prostate. The prostate and organs at-risk, including the urethra, bladder, rectum, and seminal vesicle, were contoured using the VariSeed software Ver. 8.0.1 (Varian Medical Systems Inc., Palo Alto, CA, USA). The prescribed dose for the prostate was 145 Gy. All patients underwent BT using stranded seeds. Post-implant computed tomography scanning was performed, and post-implant dosimetric evaluation was performed on days 0 and 30 after seed implantation. The dosimetric parameters analyzed in this study were the dose (Gy) received by 90% of the prostate gland (D90), percentage of the prostate volume receiving 100% and 150% of the prescribed peripheral dose (V100/150), and the dose (Gy) received by 90% of the urethra (D90).

2.3. Definitions of PSA Bounce

The nadir was defined as the lowest PSA value observed during the entire follow-up period after LDR-BT. The pre-bounce nadir was defined as the lowest PSA value before the bounce [15]. PSA bounce, in this study, was defined as an increase of ≥ 0.2 ng/mL above the pre-bounce nadir, with a subsequent decline without treatment [5,6]. The time before bounce was defined as the time elapsed between LDR-BT and the first PSA bounce. The bounce duration was defined as the elapsed time between the first PSA bounce and the PSA value that is less than the pre-bounce nadir. The bounce magnitude was defined as the difference in the PSA value between the pre-bounce nadir and bounce. A large PSA bounce was defined as a PSA increase ≥ 2.0 ng/mL above the nadir, with a subsequent decline to or below the initial nadir without treatment. Biochemical failure after LDR-BT was defined using the American Society for Therapeutic Radiology and Oncology Phoenix definition (nadir +2 ng/mL), except for a large PSA bounce [16].

To discriminate a large PSA bounce and biochemical failure, careful history taking was performed to determine if the condition was transient prostatitis. If acute prostatitis was suspected, anti-bacterial and anti-inflammatory drugs were administered. In addition, one or two more close follow-up with imaging studies to confirm recurrence was performed. If no signs of recurrence were present on imaging, no salvage treatment such as hormone therapy was initiated. Subsequent decrease in PSA value was considered as large PSA bounce.

PSA value decreases dramatically after initiation of ADT; therefore, its discontinuation can result in PSA elevation, which we defined as hormone withdrawal rebound. PSA bounce was determined after the PSA value showed a downward trend for patients who were treated with ADT.

2.4. Statistical Analysis

Statistical analyses were conducted using SPSS version 25.0 (IBM Corp., Armonk, NY, USA). Differences in characteristics and toxicities were compared using chi-square tests. Logistic regression modeling was performed for univariate and multivariate analyses to identify predictive factors for PSA bounce and large PSA bounce. Factors showing $p < 0.10$ in the univariate analysis were included in the multivariate analysis. Statistical significance was defined as $p < 0.05$. To assess the cutoff point of the PSA nadir value for predicting PSA bounce, receiver operating characteristic curve analysis was used and the area under the curve (AUC) was also calculated.

3. Results

3.1. Patient Characteristics

The patient characteristics are shown in Table 1. The median age was 64 years (interquartile range [IQR] 58.5–70). Most patients had Gleason 3 + 3 (55%), and 21%, 13%, and 11% of patients had Gleason 3 + 4, 4 + 3, and 4 + 4, respectively. PSA was greater than 20 ng/mL in 4% of the patients and greater than 10 ng/mL in 19%; altogether, 45%, 49%, and 6% of patients were in the low, intermediate, and high-risk groups, respectively, as per the MSKCC criteria. Seventeen patients underwent ADT before LDR-BT. Seven patients received ADT because of large prostate volume, five because of high Gleason score, and five because of delay in LDR-BT. Before LDR-BT, the mean prostate volume was 28.9 cc, and the median D90 at post-implant 0 day was 149.9 Gy. Patients who experienced PSA bounce were young ($p = 0.005$), had a large prostate volume ($p = 0.024$), and had a greater number of implanted seeds ($p = 0.03$) than those who did not.

Table 1. Patients' characteristics.

Characteristic	Total n = 100	No Bounce n = 55	PSA Bounce n = 45	p-Value
Age (years)				0.005
Range	46–82	50–82	46–77	
Median (Q1–Q3)	64 (59–70)	65 (61–73)	60 (57.5–68)	
Gleason score				0.411
6 (3 + 3)	55 (55%)	28 (50%)	27 (60%)	
7 (3 + 4)	21 (21%)	11 (20%)	10 (22%)	
7 (4 + 3)	13 (13%)	8 (15%)	5 (11%)	
8 (4 + 4)	11 (11%)	8 (15%)	3 (7%)	
T stage				0.512
T1c-T2a	79 (79%)	43 (78%)	36 (80%)	
T2b-T2c	21 (21%)	12 (22%)	9 (20%)	
Pre-BT PSA value, ng/mL				0.245
Range	2.8–32.9	3.0–20.6	2.8–32.9	
Median (Q1–Q3)	7.4 (5.5–9.7)	7.4 (5.6–9.3)	7.4 (5.4–11.9)	
Pre-BT PSA, n (%)				0.440
<10	77 (77%)	44 (80%)	33 (73%)	
10–20	19 (19%)	10 (18%)	9 (20%)	
≥20	4 (4%)	1 (2%)	3 (7%)	

Table 1. Cont.

Characteristic	Total n = 100	No Bounce n = 55	PSA Bounce n = 45	p-Value
MSKCC risk group [12]				0.815
Low	45 (45%)	25 (46%)	20 (44%)	
Intermediate	49 (49%)	26 (47%)	23 (51%)	
High	6 (6%)	4 (7%)	2 (4%)	
D'Amico risk group [14]				0.941
Low	37 (37%)	20 (36%)	17 (38%)	
Intermediate	46 (46%)	25 (46%)	21 (47%)	
High	17 (17%)	10 (18%)	7 (15%)	
ADT before BT				0.728
No	83 (83%)	45 (82%)	38 (84%)	
Yes	17 (17%)	10 (18%)	7 (16%)	
Pre-BT prostate volume, cc				0.024
Range	14.0–48.0	16.7–44.7	14.0–48.0	
Median (Q1, Q3)	28.9 (23.8–35.7)	27.1 (22.9–32.8)	31.2 (24.3–39.3)	
Number of implanted seeds				0.030
Median (Range)	76 (52–102)	74 (52–100)	80 (55–102)	
D90, Gy, median (range)	149.9 (131.0–174.9)	151.1 (131.1–173.5)	149.5 (131.0–174.9)	0.501

PSA, prostate-specific antigen; BT, brachytherapy; ADT, androgen deprivation therapy; MSKCC, Memorial Sloan Kettering Cancer Center

3.2. Analysis of Bounce Phenomenon

The median follow-up period was 49 months (24–100). Among 17 patients who underwent ADT before LDR-BT, 8 patients (47%) experienced hormone withdrawal rebound. PSA bounce occurred in 45 patients (45%), and a large PSA bounce occurred in 7 patients (7%). Figure 1 shows the PSA changes for all patients, and the PSA values of the bounce population fluctuated dynamically. In the bounce population, the median PSA value at pre-bounce nadir was 0.92 ng/mL (IQR, 0.49–1.82), and the median time to pre-bounce nadir was 10 months (IQR, 7–16). The median time to bounce was 24 months (IQR, 16–29) after LDR-BT. The median PSA value at the bounce spike was 1.62 ng/mL (IQR, 0.94–2.61), corresponding to a median raise of 0.44 ng/mL (IQR range, 0.29–0.83) compared to the pre-bounce nadir (Figure 2). The median time from PSA bounce to the date of bounce recovery was 4 months (IQR, 3–8; Figure 3). Twenty patients (46%) with a PSA bounce had a decreased PSA level within 6 months (Figure 4). The median PSA value at post-bounce nadir was 0.36 ng/mL (IQR, 0.20–0.91), obtained at a median of 36 months (IQR, 26–45) after LDR-BT.

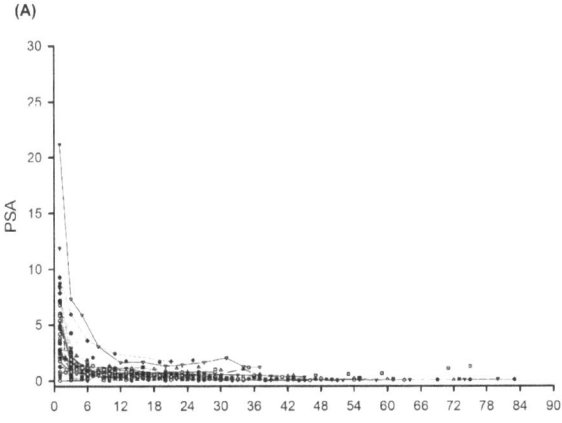

Figure 1. Cont.

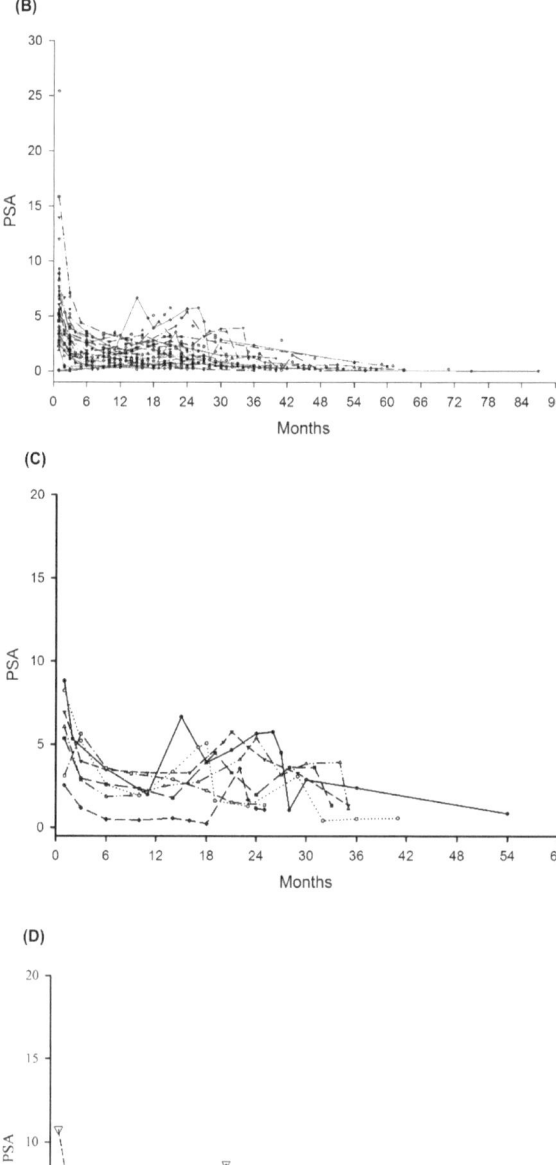

Figure 1. (**A**) PSA value for patients without bounce; (**B**) PSA value for patients with bounce; (**C**) PSA value for patients with large bounce; (**D**) PSA value for patients with failure. PSA, prostate-specific antigen.

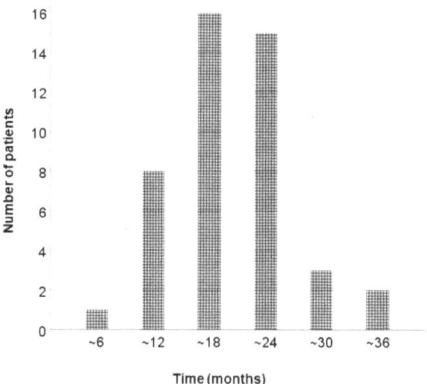

Figure 2. The period before PSA bounce. PSA, prostate-specific antigen.

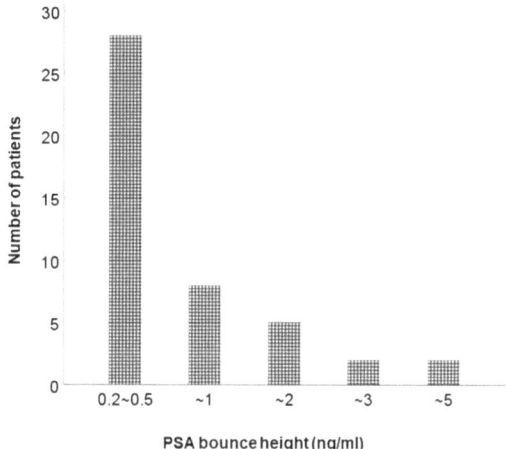

Figure 3. The PSA bounce magnitude. PSA, prostate-specific antigen.

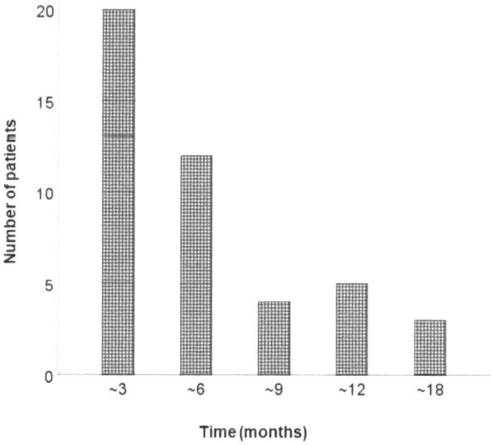

Figure 4. Time to recover from PSA bounce. PSA, prostate-specific antigen.

In the no-bounce population, the median PSA value at nadir was 0.22 ng/mL (IQR, 0.12–0.37), obtained in a median of 28 months (IQR, 20–38). There was no significant difference in the nadir values between the bounce and no-bounce populations ($p = 0.061$). The median time to obtain the nadir was significantly lower in the no-bounce population than in the bounce population ($p = 0.024$).

On univariate analysis, age at LDR-BT ($p = 0.007$), PSA nadir value at 2 years ($p < 0.001$), and prostate volume before LDR-BT ($p = 0.022$) differed significantly between the entire cohort and patients with PSA bounce. Odds ratios (ORs) were 0.928 for age at LDR-BT (95% confidence interval (CI) 0.879–0.980), 3.873 for PSA nadir value at 2 years (95% CI 1.817–8.254), and 1.064 for prostate volume before LDR-BT (95% CI 1.009–1.123). On multivariate analysis, the PSA nadir value at 2 years was the most powerful predictor of PSA bounce ($p = 0.014$; Table 2). The cut-off of PSA nadir value at 2 years was 0.5 (AUC 0.732). The rate of PSA bounce was significantly lower in patients whose PSA nadir value at 2 years was below 0.5 ng/mL (24% vs. 71%, $p < 0.001$) than in whose PSA nadir values were >0.5 ng/mL.

Table 2. The prognostic factors associated with PSA bounce.

Characteristic	Univariate Analysis			Multivariate Analysis		
	HR	95% CI	p-Value	HR	95% CI	p-Value
Age (≤60 vs. >60 years)	0.296	0.126–0.895	0.005	0.455	0.175–1.183	0.106
Gleason score (6 vs. >6)	0.691	0.312–1.534	0.364			
T stage (T1c and T2a vs. T2b and T2c)	0.896	0.339–2.366	0.824			
Pretreatment PSA value	1.052	0.968–1.143	0.230			
PSA nadir value at 2 years	3.873	1.817–8.254	<0.001	2.657	1.194–5.914	0.017
MSKCC risk group [12] (low vs. intermediate and high)	1.042	0.472–2.300	0.920			
D'Amico risk group [14] (low vs. intermediate and high)	0.941	0.416–2.127	0.884			
Hormone therapy (no vs. yes)	0.829	0.288–2.388	0.728			
Prostate volume (cc) (≤30 vs. >30)	3.083	1.358–7.003	0.007	1.940	0.772–4.875	0.106

PSA, Prostate-specific antigen; MSKCC, Memorial Sloan Kettering Cancer Center

3.3. Analysis of Large Bounce Phenomenon

Seven patients had large PSA bounces. In the large bounce population, the median PSA value at pre-bounce nadir was 1.91 ng/mL (IQR, 0.44–3.29), and the median time to pre-bounce nadir was 11 months (IQR, 7–12). The median time to large bounce was 24 months (IQR, 16–29) after LDR-BT. The median PSA value at the bounce spike was 4.84 ng/mL (IQR, 4.30–6.21), corresponding to a median raise of 2.72 ng/mL (IQR range, 2.36–3.80) compared to the pre-bounce nadir. The median time from large PSA bounce to the date of bounce recovery was 2 months. Five patients (71%) had a decreased PSA level within 3 months, and 2 patients had decreased PSA levels at 13 months and 14 months, respectively.

Univariate analysis showed that the age at LDR-BT (OR, 0.759; 95% CI, 0.640–0.900; $p = 0.001$) and PSA nadir value at 2 years (OR, 4.008; 95% CI, 1.640–9.797; $p = 0.002$) differed significantly between the whole cohort and patients with large PSA bounce. In multivariate analysis, age and the PSA nadir value at 2 years were significant prognostic factors ($p = 0.005$ and 0.029, respectively, as shown in Table 3.

Table 3. The prognostic factors associated with large PSA bounce.

Characteristic	Univariate Analysis			Multivariate Analysis		
	HR	95% CI	p-Value	HR	95% CI	p-Value
Age (≤60 vs. >60 years)	0.058	0.007–0.506	0.010	0.055	0.005–0.666	0.023
Gleason score (6 vs. >6)	0.465	0.084–2.520	0.375			
T stage (T1c and T2a vs. T2b and T2c)	1.558	0.280–8.661	0.613			
Pretreatment PSA value	1.076	0.956–1.212	0.224			
PSA nadir value at 2 years	4.008	1.640–9.797	0.002	4.961	1.448–16.998	0.011
MSKCC Risk group [12] (low vs. intermediate and high)	0.302	0.056–1.637	0.165			
D'Amico Risk group [14] (low vs. intermediate and high)	1.509	0.278–8.198	0.634			
Hormone therapy (no vs. yes)	2.080	0.369–11.738	0.407			
Prostate volume (cc) (≤30 vs. >30)	3.312	0.611–17.960	0.165			

PSA, prostate-specific antigen; MSKCC, Memorial Sloan Kettering Cancer Center

3.4. Early Clinical Outcomes

No intraprostatic gross failure or prostate cancer-related death was reported, but one regional failure and two biochemical failures were noted. One patient died 24 months after LDR-BT because of adenocarcinoma of the right upper lung, pathologically confirmed lung cancer, and non-metastatic prostate cancer. All failure patients had Gleason 4 + 3 or 4 + 4, whereas five patients (71%) with large PSA bounces had Gleason 3 + 3. Other clinical or dosimetric characteristics were similar between patients with failure and those with large PSA bounces. The median age of failure patients and large PSA bounce patients was 64 and 52 years (p = 0.008), respectively.

Two patients experienced biochemical failure at 43 and 31 months after LDR-BT. Both patients had a Gleason score of 7 (4 + 3), PSA values lower than 10 ng/mL, and clinical T2a stage. Salvage ADT was administered, and a PSA value below the nadir was achieved. One patient developed lymph node metastases. The left obturator lymph node was found 48 months after LDR-BT and treated with hypofractionated EBRT of 45 Gy in five fractions, and salvage ADT was used. After EBRT, the PSA value decreased to the undetected range, and the lymph node disappeared radiographically.

4. Discussion

In this study, with a median follow-up time of 49 months, 45%, 7%, and 3% of the patients experienced PSA bounce, large PSA bounce, and biochemical failure, respectively. Young patients (<60 years), whose PSA nadir values were >0.05 at 2 years and had large prostate volumes (>30 cc) had a high probability of having PSA bounce. Our study also showed no difference in nadir values between the bounce and no-bounce populations. The median time to obtain the nadir in the no-bounce population was significantly lower than that of the bounce population. In addition, we suggest important points to discriminate between large bounces and biochemical failures.

After successful surgery, the patient's PSA level should rapidly decrease to undetectable levels. However, BT or EBRT may take up to 5 years after treatment to achieve a final nadir in PSA. This is because of the slower tumor cell-killing process with RT, resulting in a gradual decrease in PSA [17]. Several definitions of PSA bounce have previously been used. These include an increase of ≥0.1 [18], ≥0.2 [19], 0.4 [20], 0.5 ng/mL [21], or simply an increase of any magnitude [22]. However, a PSA rise of ≥0.2 ng/mL is the most frequently used definition among those mentioned previously. One of the reasons is the need for a definition that minimizes "noise" due to laboratory testing errors. In addition, because a bounce defined as a rise of ≥0.2 ng/mL has been used by most previous publications, it allows for comparison among reports. Our study used the definition of ≥0.2 ng/mL, and the incidence of bounce was 45% in patients who received LDR-BT.

Young patients, usually younger than 65 years, experience a PSA bounce more often. A controlled study was conducted to confirm the hypothesis that a higher frequency of sexual intercourse in the young population causes a higher rate of PSA increase than in older patients [23]. Since ejaculation has been associated with transient elevation of PSA [24], a questionnaire about sexual function was administered. However, no between-group differences in sexual function were observed. An immune reaction can explain PSA bounce. Patients who experienced a PSA bounce had a higher density of cluster of differentiation (CD) 3 and CD8 lymphocyte populations within the tumor, assessed by blood samples [25]. The authors suggested that the strength of the immune response decreases with age, which can explain the decreased bounce rates in the older adult population. Furthermore, this immunologic reaction could have a systemic effect on metastasis, explaining the decrease in biological relapses and improved overall survival rate seen in the bounce population [26].

It is generally accepted that a larger prostate volume results in more frequent PSA bounces. In our study, patients with large prostate volumes had more frequent PSA bounces. According to Stock et al. [20], patients with larger prostate volumes had a 23% increased risk of bounce at 5 years after treatment. In a study by Merrick et al. [27], the transition zone volume was a predictive factor for PSA bounce but not prostate volume. The investigators stated that the increased risk of bounce might be related to the possibility that benign prostatic elements, such as benign prostatic hyperplasia, could respond to RT with different PSA kinetics than malignant cells.

When patients whose PSA nadir values increased over 2.0 ng/mL after BT, distinguishing biochemical failure and large PSA bounce is most difficult situation encountered in clinical practice because they use the same value to discriminate. However, few studies have investigated large-magnitude bounce and predictive factors for large PSA bounce. Several studies concluded that patients who experienced large PSA bounce were significantly younger than those with biochemical failure [11,28]. Herein, we suggest follow-up protocol for patients whose PSA nadir values increase over 2.0 ng/mL after BT. First, there is the possibility of transient acute prostatitis. Careful history taking and physical examination should be performed for differential diagnosis. Next, we recommend identifying recurrence through an imaging study. Finally, time of occurrence of PSA level increase could be the discrimination point between biochemical failure and large PSA bounce. PSA bounce occurs within 30 months after treatment; on the contrary, biochemical failure often occurs after 30 months post-treatment [29]. In addition, as mentioned above, younger age and PSA nadir values could be a predictive factor for large PSA bounce to ensure accurate estimation of treatment efficacy and avoid unnecessary salvage treatment.

Several studies investigated the prognostic impact of PSA bounce and found increased freedom from biochemical failure or prolonged disease specific and overall survival [26,29]. There are several reports insisting that PSA bounce after EBRT is a factor for poor prognosis [30]. In our study, the number of recurrences is too small to analyze the relation between PSA bounce and biochemical failure. However, the relation between PSA bounce and biochemical failure is debatable, and this relation will be studied by a long follow-up period with more patients treated with LDR-BT.

This study had several limitations. First, it was an institutional-based retrospective study, which introduced potential biases. Second, this study had a small sample size, which had a statistically lower power, and the follow-up period might have been short. In addition, the number of recurrences is too small to analyze the association between PSA bounce and biochemical failure. However, our study included data from treatment with the same protocol and evaluation with the same dosimetric parameters for all patients. Despite these limitations, we present lessons for follow-up patients who received LDR-BT. Patients who had PSA values lower than 0.05 2 years after LDR-BT had a low probability of PSA bounce. Furthermore, discrimination between a PSA bounce and a biochemical failure could be possible based on the time of the PSA rise after LDR-BT; a bounce occurred within 2 years, but a biochemical failure occurred after 2 years. Most bounces resolved within 6 months.

5. Conclusions

In conclusion, age at LDR-BT was a significant predictive factor for PSA bounce and a large PSA bounce. Patients with a large prostate volume before LDR-BT tended to have a PSA bounce. Therefore, we should carefully monitor patients who are young, have a high prostate volume, and have PSA nadir values more than 0.5 at 2 years for the possibility of PSA bounce.

Author Contributions: Conceptualization, T.H.K. and J.C.; methodology, T.H.K., J.J.B.L. and J.C.; validation, T.H.K. and J.J.B.L.; formal analysis, T.H.K. and J.C.; investigation, T.H.K. and J.C.; resources, J.C.; data curation, T.H.K., J.J.B.L., and J.C.; writing—original draft preparation, T.H.K.; supervision, J.C. All authors have read and agreed to the published version of the manuscript.

Funding: This research received no external funding.

Institutional Review Board Statement: The study was conducted according to the guidelines of the Declaration of Helsinki and approved by the Institutional Review Board of the Severance Hospital (IRB # 4-2019-0767).

Informed Consent Statement: The informed consent form was waived due to the retrospective nature of the study.

Data Availability Statement: The datasets generated and/or analyzed during the current study are not publicly available due to risk of personal information leakage but are available from the corresponding author on reasonable request.

Conflicts of Interest: The authors declare no conflict of interest.

References

1. Routman, D.M.; Funk, R.K.; Stish, B.J.; Mynderse, L.A.; Wilson, T.M.; McLaren, R.; Harmsen, W.S.; Mara, K.; Deufel, C.L.; Furutani, K.M.; et al. Permanent prostate brachytherapy monotherapy with I-125 for low- and intermediate-risk prostate cancer: Outcomes in 974 patients. *Brachytherapy* **2018**, *18*, 1–7. [CrossRef]
2. Crook, J.; Borg, J.; Evans, A.; Toi, A.; Saibishkumar, E.P.; Fung, S.; Ma, C. 10-year experience with i-125 prostate brachytherapy at the princess margaret hospital: Results for 1,100 patients. *Int. J. Radiat. Oncol. Biol. Phys.* **2011**, *80*, 1323–1329. [CrossRef] [PubMed]
3. Vuolukka, K.; Auvinen, P.; Palmgren, J.-E.; Voutilainen, T.; Aaltomaa, S.; Kataja, V. Long-term efficacy and urological toxicity of low-dose-rate brachytherapy (LDR-BT) as monotherapy in localized prostate cancer. *Brachytherapy* **2019**, *18*, 583–588. [CrossRef] [PubMed]
4. Kittel, J.A.; Reddy, C.A.; Smith, K.L.; Stephans, K.L.; Tendulkar, R.D.; Ulchaker, J.; Angermeier, K.; Campbell, S.; Stephenson, A.; Klein, E.A.; et al. Long-term efficacy and toxicity of low-dose-rate ^{125}I prostate brachytherapy as monotherapy in low-, intermediate-, and high-risk prostate cancer. *Int. J. Radiat. Oncol. Biol. Phys.* **2015**, *92*, 884–893. [CrossRef] [PubMed]
5. Caloglu, M.; Ciezki, J.P.; Reddy, C.A.; Angermeier, K.; Ulchaker, J.; Chehade, N.; Altman, A.; Magi-Galuzzi, C.; Klein, E.A. PSA Bounce and Biochemical Failure After Brachytherapy for Prostate Cancer: A Study of 820 Patients With a Minimum of 3 Years of Follow-Up. *Int. J. Radiat. Oncol.* **2011**, *80*, 735–741. [CrossRef] [PubMed]
6. Hinnen, K.A.; Monninkhof, E.M.; Battermann, J.J.; van Roermund, J.; Frank, S.J.; van Vulpen, M. Prostate Specific Antigen Bounce Is Related to Overall Survival in Prostate Brachytherapy. *Int. J. Radiat. Oncol.* **2011**, *82*, 883–888. [CrossRef]
7. Naghavi, A.O.; Strom, T.J.; Nethers, K.; Cruz, A.A.; Figura, N.B.; Shrinath, K.; Yue, B.; Kim, J.; Biagioli, M.C.; Fernandez, D.C.; et al. Clinical implications of a prostate specific antigen bounce after radiation therapy for prostate cancer. *Int. J. Clin. Oncol.* **2014**, *20*, 598–604. [CrossRef] [PubMed]
8. Patel, N.; Souhami, L.; Mansure, J.J.; Duclos, M.; Aprikian, A.; Faria, S.; David, M.; Cury, F.L. Prostate-specific antigen bounce after high-dose-rate prostate brachytherapy and hypofractionated external beam radiotherapy. *Brachytherapy* **2014**, *13*, 450–455. [CrossRef] [PubMed]
9. Hackett, C.; Ghosh, S.; Sloboda, R.; Martell, K.; Lan, L.; Pervez, N.; Pedersen, J.; Yee, D.; Murtha, A.; Amanie, J.; et al. Distinguishing prostate-specific antigen bounces from biochemical failure after low-dose-rate prostate brachytherapy. *J. Contemp. Brachytherapy* **2014**, *6*, 247–253. [CrossRef] [PubMed]
10. Kanzaki, H.; Kataoka, M.; Nishikawa, A.; Uwatsu, K.; Nagasaki, K.; Nishijima, N.; Hashine, K. Kinetics differences between PSA bounce and biochemical failure in patients treated with 125I prostate brachytherapy. *Jpn. J. Clin. Oncol.* **2015**, *45*, 688–694. [CrossRef] [PubMed]
11. Kubo, K.; Wadasaki, K.; Kimura, T.; Murakami, Y.; Kajiwara, M.; Teishima, J.; Matsubara, A.; Nagata, Y. Clinical features of prostate-specific antigen bounce after ^{125}I brachytherapy for prostate cancer. *J. Radiat. Res.* **2018**, *59*, 649–655. [CrossRef]

12. E Sylvester, J.; Blasko, J.C.; Grimm, P.D.; Meier, R.; A Malmgren, J. Ten-year biochemical relapse-free survival after external beam radiation and brachytherapy for localized prostate cancer: The Seattle experience. *Int. J. Radiat. Oncol.* **2003**, *57*, 944–952. [CrossRef]
13. Kim, H.; Kim, J.W.; Hong, S.J.; Rha, K.H.; Lee, C.-G.; Yang, S.C.; Choi, Y.D.; Suh, C.-O.; Cho, J. Treatment outcome of localized prostate cancer by 70 Gy hypofractionated intensity-modulated radiotherapy with a customized rectal balloon. *Radiat. Oncol. J.* **2014**, *32*, 187–197. [CrossRef] [PubMed]
14. D'Amico, A.V.; Whittington, R.; Malkowicz, S.B.; Schultz, D.; Blank, K.; Broderick, G.; Tomaszewski, J.E.; Renshaw, A.A.; Kaplan, I.; Beard, C.J.; et al. Biochemical Outcome After Radical Prostatectomy, External Beam Radiation Therapy, or Interstitial Radiation Therapy for Clinically Localized Prostate Cancer. *JAMA J. Am. Med. Assoc.* **1998**, *280*, 969–974. [CrossRef] [PubMed]
15. Charret, J.; Baumann, A.S.; Eschwege, P.; Moreau, J.L.; Bernier, V.; Falk, A.T.; Salleron, J.; Peiffert, D. Prostate-specific antigen bounce in patients treated before 60 years old by iodine 125 brachytherapy for prostate cancer is frequent and not a prognostic factor. *Brachytherapy* **2018**, *17*, 888–894. [CrossRef]
16. Roach, M.T.; Hanks, G.; Thames, H.J.; Schellhammer, P.; Shipley, W.U.; Sokol, G.H.; Sandler, H. Defining biochemical failure following radiotherapy with or without hormonal therapy in men with clinically localized prostate cancer: Recommendations of the rtog-astro phoenix consensus conference. *Int. J. Radiat. Oncol. Biol. Phys.* **2006**, *65*, 965–974. [CrossRef]
17. Crook, J.; Gillan, C.; Yeung, I.; Austen, L.; McLean, M.; Lockwood, G. PSA Kinetics and PSA Bounce Following Permanent Seed Prostate Brachytherapy. *Int. J. Radiat. Oncol.* **2007**, *69*, 426–433. [CrossRef]
18. Critz, F.A.; Williams, W.H.; Benton, J.B.; Levinson, A.K.; Holladay, C.T.; Holladay, D.A. Prostate specific antigen bounce after radioactive seed implantation followed by external beam radiation for prostate cancer. *J. Urol.* **2000**, *163*, 1085–1089. [CrossRef]
19. Ciezki, J.P.; Reddy, C.A.; Garcia, J.; Angermeier, K.; Ulchaker, J.; Mahadevan, A.; Chehade, N.; Altman, A.; Klein, E.A. PSA kinetics after prostate brachytherapy: PSA bounce phenomenon and its implications for PSA doubling time. *Int. J. Radiat. Oncol.* **2005**, *64*, 512–517. [CrossRef]
20. Stock, R.G.; Stone, N.N.; Cesaretti, J.A. Prostate-specific antigen bounce after prostate seed implantation for localized prostate cancer: Descriptions and implications. *Int. J. Radiat. Oncol. Biol. Phys.* **2003**, *56*, 448–453. [CrossRef]
21. Toledano, A.; Chauveinc, L.; Flam, T.; Thiounn, N.; Solignac, S.; Timbert, M.; Rosenwald, J.-C.; Cosset, J.-M. PSA bounce after permanent implant prostate brachytherapy may mimic a biochemical failure: A study of 295 patients with a minimum 3-year followup. *Brachytherapy* **2006**, *5*, 122–126. [CrossRef] [PubMed]
22. Reed, D.; Wallner, K.; Merrick, G.; Buskirk, S.; True, L. Clinical correlates to PSA spikes and positive repeat biopsies after prostate brachytherapy. *Urology* **2003**, *62*, 683–688. [CrossRef]
23. Mitchell, D.M.; Swindell, R.; Elliott, T.; Wylie, J.P.; Taylor, C.; Logue, J.P. Analysis of prostate-specific antigen bounce after I125 permanent seed implant for localised prostate cancer. *Radiother. Oncol.* **2008**, *88*, 102–107. [CrossRef] [PubMed]
24. Das, P.; Chen, M.-H.; Valentine, K.; Lopes, L.; A Cormack, R.; A Renshaw, A.; Tempany, C.M.; Kumar, S.; D'Amico, A.V. Using the magnitude of PSA bounce after MRI-guided prostate brachytherapy to distinguish recurrence, benign precipitating factors, and idiopathic bounce. *Int. J. Radiat. Oncol.* **2002**, *54*, 698–702. [CrossRef]
25. Yamamoto, Y.; Offord, C.P.; Kimura, G.; Kuribayashi, S.; Takeda, H.; Tsuchiya, S.; Shimojo, H.; Kanno, H.; Bozic, I.; A Nowak, M.; et al. Tumour and immune cell dynamics explain the PSA bounce after prostate cancer brachytherapy. *Br. J. Cancer* **2016**, *115*, 195–202. [CrossRef]
26. Nakai, Y.; Tanaka, N.; Asakawa, I.; Anai, S.; Miyake, M.; Morizawa, Y.; Hori, S.; Owari, T.; Fujii, T.; Yamaki, K.; et al. Prostate-specific antigen bounce after ^{125}I-brachytherapy for prostate cancer is a favorable prognosticator in patients who are biochemical recurrence-free at 4 years and correlates with testosterone. *Jpn. J. Clin. Oncol.* **2020**, *50*, 58–65. [CrossRef]
27. Merrick, G.S.; Butler, W.M.; Wallner, K.E.; Lief, J.H.; Hinerman-Mulroy, A.; Galbreath, R.W. Prostate-specific antigen (PSA) velocity and benign prostate hypertrophy predict for PSA spikes following prostate brachytherapy. *Brachytherapy* **2003**, *2*, 181–188. [CrossRef]
28. Thompson, A.; Keyes, M.; Pickles, T.; Palma, D.; Moravan, V.; Spadinger, I.; Lapointe, V.; Morris, W.J. Evaluating the phoenix definition of biochemical failure after (125)I prostate brachytherapy: Can psa kinetics distinguish psa failures from psa bounces? *Int. J. Radiat. Oncol. Biol. Phys.* **2010**, *78*, 415–421. [CrossRef]
29. Engeler, D.S.; Schwab, C.; Thöni, A.F.; Hochreiter, W.; Prikler, L.; Suter, S.; Stucki, P.; Schiefer, J.; Plasswilm, L.; Schmid, H.-P.; et al. PSA bounce after 125I-brachytherapy for prostate cancer as a favorable prognosticator. *Strahlenther. Onkol.* **2015**, *191*, 787–791. [CrossRef]
30. Hanlon, A.L.; Pinover, W.H.; Horwitz, E.M.; E Hanks, G. Patterns and fate of PSA bouncing following 3D-CRT. *Int. J. Radiat. Oncol.* **2001**, *50*, 845–849. [CrossRef]

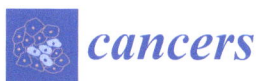

Article

Individualized Decision Making in Transperineal Prostate Biopsy: Should All Men Undergo an Additional Systematic Biopsy?

August Sigle [1,2,*], Rodrigo Suarez-Ibarrola [1], Matthias Benndorf [3], Moritz Weishaar [1], Jonathan Morlock [1], Arkadiusz Miernik [1], Christian Gratzke [1], Cordula A. Jilg [1] and Markus Grabbert [1]

[1] Department of Urology, Faculty of Medicine, Medical Center—University of Freiburg, 79106 Freiburg, Germany
[2] Berta-Ottenstein-Programme, Faculty of Medicine, University of Freiburg, 79110 Freiburg, Germany
[3] Department of Radiology, Faculty of Medicine, Medical Center—University of Freiburg, 79106 Freiburg, Germany
* Correspondence: august.sigle@uniklinik-freiburg.de; Tel.: +49-761-270-25820; Fax: +49-761-270-28960

Simple Summary: In the last few years, multiparametric magnetic resonance imaging (mpMRI) has been implemented in the diagnostic prostate cancer pathway for the identification of cancerous lesions, and consecutively, targeted fusion biopsy was implemented. In some cases, aggressive prostate cancer is missed by a targeted biopsy. To address this imperfection, additional systematic biopsy is recommended but may be harmful in terms of the additional diagnosis of indolent cancer, and the higher frequency of adverse events and resource expenditures. This study investigates whether all men should undergo an additional systematic biopsy within this clinically relevant trade-off. As a key finding, men with an mpMRI-lesion classified as PI-RADS 5 may obviate additional systematic biopsy. This was confirmed when we analyzed histopathological reclassification rates between biopsy and a subsequent radical prostatectomy.

Abstract: Background: In prostate cancer (PC) diagnosis, additional systematic biopsy (SB) is recommended to complement MRI-targeted biopsy (TB) to address the limited sensitivity of TB alone. The combination of TB+SB is beneficial for diagnosing additional significant PC (sPC) but harmful in terms of the additional diagnosis of indolent PC (iPC), morbidity, and resource expenditures. We aimed to investigate the benefit of additional SB and to identify predictors for this outcome. Methods: We analyzed the frequency of upgrading to sPC by additional SB in a retrospective single-center cohort of 1043 men. Regression analysis (RA) was performed to identify predictors for this outcome. Reclassification rates of ISUP grade groups between prostate biopsy and a subsequent radical prostatectomy were assessed. Results: Additional SB led to upgrading to sPC in 98/1043 men (9.4%) and to the additional diagnosis of iPC in 71/1043 men (6.8%). In RA, men harboring a PI-RADS 2-4 lesion were more likely to have TB results upgraded by SB ($p < 0.01$) compared to PI-RADS 5 men. When analyzing reclassification rates, additional SB reduced the upgrading to sPC from 43/214 (20.1%) to 8/214 (3.7%). In the PI-RADS 5 subgroup, this difference decreased: 4/87 (4.7%) with TB only vs. 1/87 (1.2%) with TB+SB. Conclusion: Men with a PI-RADS 5 lesion may obviate additional SB.

Keywords: prostatic neoplasms; image-guided biopsy; fusion biopsy; biopsy strategy

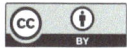

Citation: Sigle, A.; Suarez-Ibarrola, R.; Benndorf, M.; Weishaar, M.; Morlock, J.; Miernik, A.; Gratzke, C.; Jilg, C.A.; Grabbert, M. Individualized Decision Making in Transperineal Prostate Biopsy: Should All Men Undergo an Additional Systematic Biopsy? *Cancers* **2022**, *14*, 5230. https://doi.org/10.3390/cancers14215230

Academic Editor: Fumitaka Koga

Received: 15 August 2022
Accepted: 21 October 2022
Published: 25 October 2022

Publisher's Note: MDPI stays neutral with regard to jurisdictional claims in published maps and institutional affiliations.

Copyright: © 2022 by the authors. Licensee MDPI, Basel, Switzerland. This article is an open access article distributed under the terms and conditions of the Creative Commons Attribution (CC BY) license (https://creativecommons.org/licenses/by/4.0/).

1. Introduction

The significant value of MRI-targeted biopsy (TB) compared to systematic biopsy (SB) alone for the detection of clinically significant prostate cancer (sPC) has been confirmed in recent prospective clinical trials such as PROMIS [1], PRECISION [2], and MRI-FIRST [3].

However, despite the advantages of TB, such as reducing overdiagnosis of indolent cancers (iPC), morbidity, operative time, and pathologists' workload, there is a concern over the unacceptable proportion of missed high-grade cancers when SB is omitted [3]. Among the main shortcomings of TB are (1) Reading errors: Misdiagnosing lesions due to misinterpretation; (2) Presence of non-MRI visible sPC; and (3) Targeting errors by the person performing the TB [4]. A recent meta-analysis evaluating cancer detection rates (CDR) for TB versus SB found that omitting SB would miss approximately 16% of sPC [5].

Since systematic cores increase the detection of iPC [5], morbidity [6], and resource expenditures, a compromise needs to be reached to limit SB in men that are more likely to benefit from it.

There is growing interest in determining if a subgroup of men might benefit from SB in addition to TB. Previous studies have identified the clinical setting (biopsy naïve, previous negative biopsy, active surveillance), age, prostate volume, MRI-lesion volume and the PI-RADS Score [7–9] predictive for upgrading to sPC by SB. A recent study proposed patients' PI-RADS score as a promising tool to select the optimal biopsy strategy [10]. However, these findings are limited to a cohort who underwent transrectal prostate biopsy. Current guidelines favor the transperineal approach for prostate biopsy [11]. Moreover, the evaluation of reclassification rates of prostate cancer (PC) grade groups between prostate biopsy and a subsequent radical prostatectomy (RP) are missing. We aimed (1) to evaluate the frequency of upgrading to sPC by SB over TB and to identify predictors for this outcome; (2) to analyze CDRs by TB and TB+SB for transperineal prostate biopsy stratified by the identified parameters; and (3) to investigate reclassification rates of PC grade groups between prostate biopsy and a subsequent RP stratified by the identified parameters.

2. Patients and Methods

2.1. Study Population

We analyzed a retrospective single-center cohort of 1043 men (Total Cohort) who underwent prostate biopsy. The indication for biopsy was based on suspicious prostate-specific antigen (PSA) levels/dynamics, abnormal digital rectal examination, or as a part of an active surveillance routine. Men with very high PSA-levels (>20 ng/mL) and suspicion of locally advanced disease were included in this study.

Men who underwent a prostate biopsy between October 2015–May 2020 were included in the study. Men were excluded if only TB or only SB was conducted, or in the case of incomplete clinical data. Men who were diagnosed with PC and underwent RP within one year after biopsy were considered for further analysis (Prostatectomy Cohort). Data collection was approved by the local Ethics Committee (ETK 21-1191). The study was performed in accordance with the Declaration of Helsinki.

2.2. MR Imaging, Biopsy Procedure and Histopathological Analysis

All men had a pre-biopsy multiparametric magnetic resonance imaging (mpMRI) according to the current Prostate Imaging Reporting and Data System (PI-RADS) [12]. Image interpretation was performed by a group of board-certified radiologists as a part of the clinical routine and without central revision. Robot-assisted mpMRI/transrectal ultrasound fusion biopsy of the prostate (iSRobot Mona LisaTM®, Biobot Surgical, Singapore) was performed as a combined procedure of TB plus synchronous SB. The Ginsburg protocol that addresses both sides of the prostate was applied for SB planning [13]. The median total number of cores taken was 35 (interquartile range (IQR) 31–40) with a median of 31 (IQR 26–34) systematic biopsy cores.

SB was not performed blinded to MRI lesions but was planned independently from TB. Eight different surgeons performed the standardized biopsy procedures that were included in this study. Procedural details were described previously [14]. Prostate biopsy was performed in lithotomy position via the transperineal route and under general anaesthesia. Antibiotic prophylaxis and local anaesthesia were not administered.

All biopsy cores were labelled, processed and analysed individually by a group of board-certified uropathologists and according to the International Society of Urological Pathology (ISUP) standards [15].

2.3. Data collection and Statistical Analysis

Demographic and clinical data were extracted by reviewing patients' electronic medical records.

Baseline characteristics included age, previous biopsy and active surveillance status, PSA, prostate volume by MRI, mpMRI findings according to PI-RADS, zonal and side-specific information on target localization, index lesion volume, number of lesions, the number of biopsy cores and histopathological findings from prostate biopsy according to ISUP. The index lesion was defined as the lesion with the highest PI-RADS grade and in case of several equally assessed lesions the one with the largest volume was considered.

Continuous variables were described as median with interquartile range (IQR). Categorical variables were described with integers and percentages.

The primary endpoint of the study was the upgrading to sPC by additional SB. Clinically significant prostate cancer was defined as the presence of any PC classified as ISUP grade group 2 or higher. As secondary endpoints, we aimed to identify predictors for upgrading to sPC, and we assessed reclassification rates of ISUP grade groups between prostate biopsy and a subsequent RP. To identify predictors for the primary endpoint, we performed binary logistic regression analysis, including the following covariates: age, previous biopsy and active surveillance status, PSA, prostate volume, PI-RADS score, zonal and side-specific target localization, index lesion volume, number of lesions and the number of TB and SB cores. For the selection of variables in the multivariable analysis, we applied backward stepwise elimination. The binary cut-off for index lesion volume was set at 0.6 mL with respect to the variable's median. The McNemar's test was used to compare the detection rates of sPC. Moreover, we analyzed the overlap of 95% confidence intervals (CI) of the respective detection rates. p-value < 0.05 was considered statistically significant. SPSS© software (SPSS statistics 27) was used for statistical analysis.

3. Results

3.1. Study Cohort

The enrollment and outcomes are presented in Figure 1. A total of 1121 men underwent prostate biopsy at the University Hospital Freiburg, Germany between October 2015–May 2020. Thirty-four men had no TB and 44 were excluded due to missing clinical data, resulting in a total cohort of 1043 men. Among these men, 222 patients (21.3%) underwent subsequent RP. Eight men of this subgroup were excluded because the time between biopsy and surgery exceeded one year, resulting in a prostatectomy cohort of 214 men.

3.2. Baseline Characteristics

Baseline characteristics and CDRs are illustrated in Table 1. Median age and PSA were 67.0 years (interquartile range (IQR) 61.0–72.0) and 8.8 ng/mL (6.0–12.6), respectively. In the prostatectomy cohort, the median age and PSA were 67.0 years and (62.0–72.0) and 9.3 ng/mL (6.3–14.0), respectively.

3.3. Cancer Detection Rates and Upgrading in Systematic Versus MRI–Targeted Biopsy

In the total cohort 649/1043 (62.2%) men were diagnosed with PC, with 521/1043 (50.0%) men harboring sPC. The CDRs of any PC and sPC by TB/SB were 48.7%/59.5% and 40.6%/46.3%, respectively.

Additional SB led to an upgrading to sPC in 98/1043 men (9.4%). Out of these men, 70/98 (71.4%) had no PC detected by TB and 28/98 (28.6%) were upgraded from iPC. Systematic biopsy led to the additional diagnosis of iPC in 71/1043 (6.8%) men.

3.4. Regression Analysis for the Upgrading to sPC by Systematic Biopsy

To identify predictors for upgrading to sPC by SB, we calculated both univariate and multivariate regression analysis (Table 2). In univariate regression analysis, we found the PI-RADS category to be significantly associated with the study's primary endpoint: men harboring a PI-RADS lesion 2–4 were more likely to have TB results upgraded by

SB ($p < 0.01$) compared to men with a PI-RADS 5 lesion. This finding was consistent in multivariable analysis. Moreover, we found patients with non-peripheral zone lesions being less likely to be upgraded by SB (OR 0.44 (0.23–0.85; $p < 0.01$)) compared to men with lesions localized in the peripheral zone. Smaller index lesions with volumes < 0.6 mL were associated with higher rates of upgrading to sPC by SB (OR 2.15 (CI 1.38–3.34; $p < 0.01$). In addition, we found a significant association of prostate volume and the event of upgrading to sPC by SB (OR 0.99 (0.98–1.00, $p < 0.03$) in multivariate analysis.

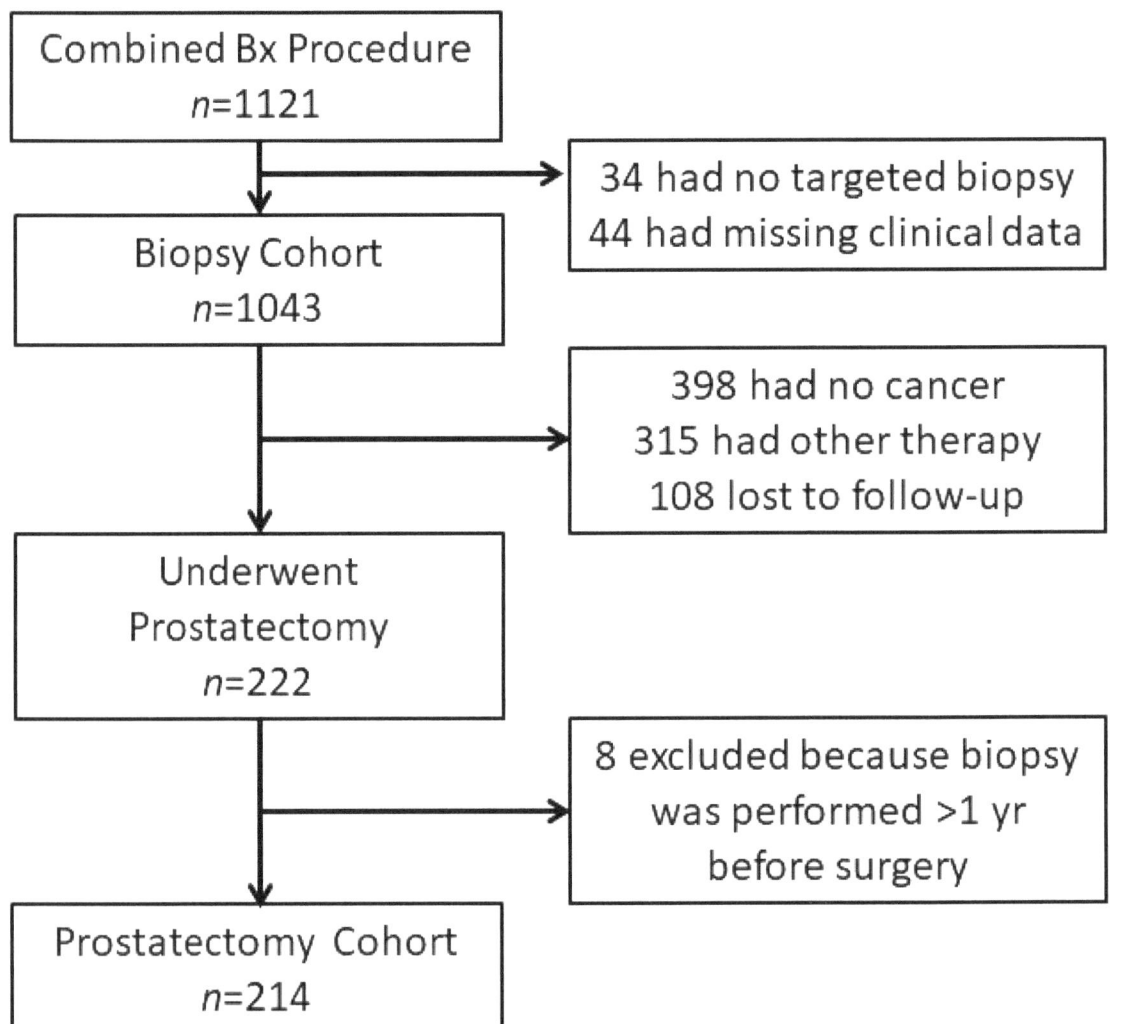

Figure 1. Enrollment and Outcomes. All included men underwent combined biopsy (Bx) procedure with a combination of MRI-targeted biopsy plus synchronous systematic biopsy. For men diagnosed with PC different treatment options were offered (active surveillance, radiotherapy, and radical prostatectomy). Men undergoing a subsequent radical prostatectomy were considered for the analysis of reclassification rates of cancer grade groups between biopsy and wholemount specimen.

Table 1. Baseline Characteristics and Cancer Detection Rates. IQR—interquartile range; PSA—prostate specific antigen; PI-RADS—Prostate Imaging Reporting and Data System; ISUP—International Society of Urological Pathology.

Characteristic	All Men	Prostatectomy Cohort
Cases, n	1043	214
Age (years), median, IQR	67.0 (61.0–72.0)	67.0 (62.0–72.0)
Previous Negative Biopsy, n (%)	244 (23.4)	43 (20.1)
Active Surveillance, n (%)	141 (13.5)	29 (13.6)
PSA (ng/mL), median, IQR	8.8 (6.0–12.6)	9.3 (6.3–14.0)
Volume (mL), median, IQR	53.0 (38.5–75.0)	47.6 (37.0–63.3)
PI-RADS, n (%)		
n/a	54 (5.2)	8 (3.7)
1	0 (0.0)	0 (0)
2	43 (4.2)	6 (2.8)
3	170 (16.3)	17 (7.9)
4	530 (50.8)	97 (43.5)
5	246 (23.6)	86 (40.2)
Target Localization, n (%)		
Unilateral	595 (57.0)	116 (54.2)
Bilateral	448 (43.0)	98 (45.8)
Non-peripheral Zone	221 (21.2)	33 (15.4)
Peripheral Zone	444 (42.6)	103 (48.1)
Bi-zonal	378 (36.2)	78 (36.4)
Index Lesion Volume (mL), median, IQR	0.58 (0.32–1.14)	0.64 (0.30–1.52)
Number of Lesions, n (%)		
1	481 (46.1)	104 (48.6)
2	394 (37.8)	80 (37.4)
3	136 (13.0)	24 (11.2)
4 or more	32 (3.1)	6 (2.8)
Number of Cores, median, IQR		
Total	35 (31–40)	34 (30–39)
From Target	5 (3–7)	4 (4–7)
Systematic	31 (26–34)	30 (25–32)
Cancer Grading according to ISUP, n (%)		
No Cancer	394 (37.8)	n/a
1	128 (12.3)	8 (3.7)
2	174 (16.7)	71 (33.2)
3	142 (13.6)	82 (38.3)
4	162 (15.5)	26 (12.1)
5	43 (4.1)	27 (12.6)

3.5. Cancer Detection Rates Stratified by PI-RADS Score

After the identification of the PI-RADS Score as a main influencing factor for the effect of SB, we stratified CDRs for TB vs. TB+SB by PI-RADS groups. The results are illustrated in Figure 2. With respect to the total cohort, the combined biopsy strategy (CB) diagnosed significantly more sPC and iPC compared to TB only (50.0% vs. 40.6%; $p < 0.001$ and 6.8% vs 2.9%, $p < 0.001$). This effect was consistent for the subgroup of men with PI-RADS 3 and PI-RADS 4 lesions, with an upgrading to sPC by SB in 20/170 (11.8%) and 62/530 (11.7%), respectively. When comparing the detection rates of sPC for CB versus TB in men classified as PI-RADS 5, there was no significant difference considering the overlap of 95% CIs: 78.0% (73.0–83.0%) for TB vs. 80.9% (75.9–85.8%) for CB. Omitting SB in men with a PI-RADS 5 lesion would have missed the diagnosis of any PC in 7/1043 (0.7%) men, with 1/1043 (0.1%) classified as ISUP 1, 3/1043 (0.3%) ISUP 2 and 3/1043 (0.3%) ISUP 3–5.

Table 2. Univariate and multivariate logistic regression analysis for upgrading to significant prostate cancer (ISUP2–5) by systematic biopsy. Backward stepwise elimination was applied for variable selection in multivariable analysis. sPC—significant prostate cancer (ISUP > 2); ISUP—International Society of Urological Pathology; OR—odds ratio; CI—confidence interval; PSA—prostate specific antigen; PI-RADS—Prostate Imaging Reporting and Data System. * $p < 0.05$; ** $p < 0.01$.

	Upgrading to sPC (ISUP2-5) by Systematic Biopsy			
	Univariate Analysis		Multivariate Analysis	
	OR (95% CI)	p	OR (95% CI)	p
Age, years	1.00 (0.97–1.03)	0.90		
Previous Negative Biopsy ≥1 vs. none	0.94 (0.58–1.52)	0.78		
Active Surveillance Yes vs. No	0.86 (0.44–1.66)	0.65		
PSA level, ng/mL	0.99 (0.94–1.04)	0.72		
Prostate volume, mL	0.99 (0.98–1.00)	0.18	0.99 (0.98–1.00)	<0.03 *
PI-RADS Score PI-RADS 5	Ref.		Ref.	
PI-RADS 4 vs.	3.70 (1.66–8.28)	<0.01 **	4.62 (2.08–10.28)	<0.01 **
PI-RADS 3 vs.	4.43 (1.82–10.79)	<0.01 **	5.54 (2.26–13.57)	<0.01 **
PI-RADS 2 vs.	5.73 (1.80–18.26)	<0.01 **	7.37 (2.41–22.53)	<0.01 **
Target Localization Unilateral vs. Bilateral	0.99 (0.64–1.54)	0.97		
Non-peripheral Zone vs. Peripheral Zone	0.44 (0.23–0.85)	<0.01 **	0.42 (0.22–0.81)	<0.01 **
Bizonal vs. Peripheral Zone	0.55 (0.33–0.90)	0.02 *	0.70 (0.44–1.20)	0.14
Index Lesion Volume <0.6 mL vs. ≥ 0.6 mL	2.15 (1.38–3.34)	<0.01 **		
Number of lesions (n) 1 vs. >1	0.99 (0.64–1.43)	0.97		
Number of Target Cores (n)	0.98 (0.89–1.07)	0.61		
Number of Systematic Cores (n)	1.03 (0.99–1.07)	0.11		

3.6. Reclassification in Subsequent Radical Prostatectomy

As a secondary endpoint, we analyzed the reclassification rates of ISUP grade groups in RP specimen with regard to the initial biopsy results (Figure 3). 214/1043 (20.5%) men of the total cohort underwent radical prostatectomy. Combined biopsy mode reduced the upgrading to sPC from 43/214 (20.1%) to 8/214 (3.7%) compared to TB only. When analyzing the subgroup of men with a PI-RADS 5 lesion, this difference decreased: 4/87 (4.7%) vs. 1/87 (1.2%).

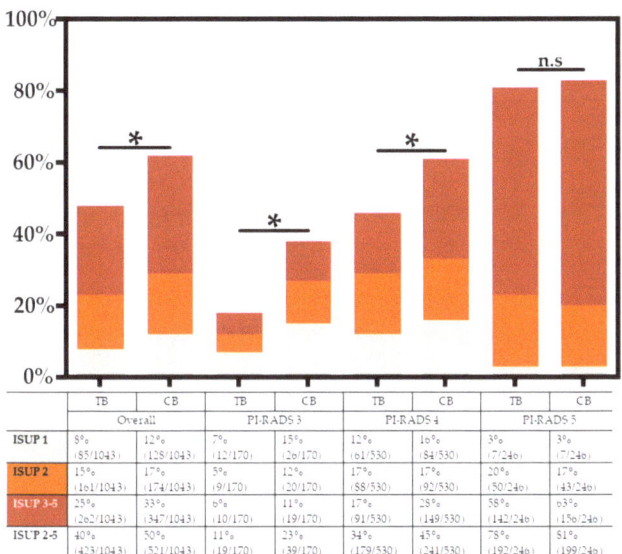

Figure 2. Cancer Detection Rates stratified by PI-RADS score and biopsy method. Additional systematic biopsy diagnosed significantly (*) more clinically significant prostate cancer (sPC) in the total cohort and in the subgroups of PI-RADS 2–4 men. For the group of men with a PI-RADS 5 lesion this difference was not statistically significant (n.s) when considering the overlap of 95% confidence intervals: sPC by TB was 78.0% (73.0–83.0%) vs. 80.9% (75.9–85.8%) for CB. TB—MRI-targeted biopsy; CB—combined biopsy = TB plus synchronous systematic biopsy.

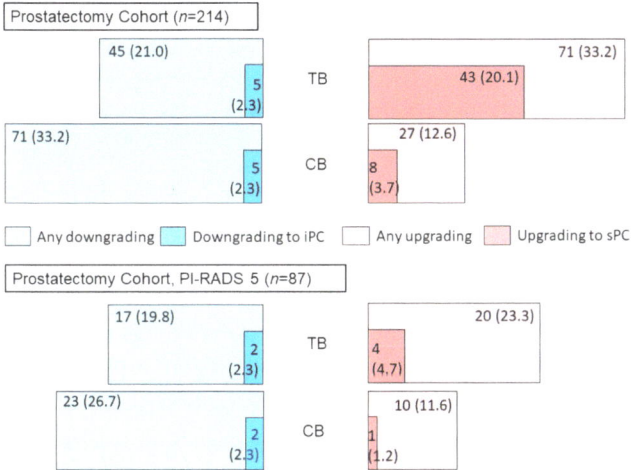

Figure 3. Reclassification rates of ISUP grade groups between prostate biopsy and a subsequent radical prostatectomy. For the whole prostatectomy cohort, combined biopsy mode (CB, MRI-targeted biopsy + synchronous systematic biopsy) reduced the upgrading to significant prostate cancer from 20.1% when considering MRI-targeted biopsy (TB) results only to 3.7%. For the subgroup of PI-RADS 5 men this effect turned neglectable (4.7% vs. 1.2%). iPC—indolent prostate cancer; sPC—significant prostate cancer; PI-RADS—Prostate Imaging Reporting and Data System; Length of bars is calculated by the respective percentages.

4. Discussion

In PC diagnosis, SB is recommended to complement TB to address the limited sensitivity of TB alone [11]. SB may be beneficial for diagnosing additional sPC but also harmful in terms of additional iPC, morbidity, and resource expenditures. This study aimed to investigate selection criteria for men who should undergo SB within this clinically relevant trade-off.

4.1. Frequency of Upgrading to sPC by Additional Systematic Biopsy

In our retrospective cohort, additional SB upgraded the diagnosis to sPC in 98/1043 (9.4%) men. Previous studies similarly reported upgrading by adding SB but varied in the frequency of this event between 1.9–11.6% [8,16,17]. A recent meta-analysis found that omitting SB would even miss approximately 16% of sPC [5]. A reason for these deviations might originate from the various SB schemes applied and the different number of cores taken. The lowest frequency of upgrading was found in a multi-centre cohort where only eight SB cores were taken per patient [16]. In contrast to this, we applied the Ginsburg Scheme for SB and sampled a median of 26 systematic cores per patient. Acknowledging a targeting error as being the main reason for missing sPC by TB [4], the effect of additional SB might be mainly dependent on the surgeon's experience. This reasoning is supported by the results of Sathianathen et al. who reported an upgrading of 11.6% by an additional 12-core SB in a cohort undergoing prostate biopsy by a group of surgeons without any experience in transperineal prostate biopsy before their study [8].

4.2. Predictors for Upgrading to sPC

When analysing predictors for the upgrading to sPC by additional SB, we found that men with PI-RADS 2-4 lesions were more likely to have their TB results upgraded by SB compared to PI-RADS 5 men. These results are in accordance with previous studies [7,18–20]. Ahdoot et al. proposed the patient's PI-RADS score as a promising tool to select the optimal biopsy strategy in terms of omitting SB in men harbouring a PI-RADS 5 lesion [10].

Moreover, we found men with small lesions (<0.6 mL) and peripheral zone lesions more likely to have their diagnosis upgraded to significant disease by additional SB. The finding that smaller lesions are more probable to be missed by TB and thus lead to upgrading by an additional SB was previously described in a small cohort [9]. Altogether the option of an extended MRI-directed biopsy scheme is discussed in the current European Association of Urology guidelines to overcome the problem of targeting errors [11].

4.3. Stratification of Cancer Detection Rates by Patient's PI-RADS Scores

Based on the finding that men harbouring PI-RADS lesions 2-4 were more likely to have their TB results upgraded by SB, we analyzed CDRs stratified by the patient's respective PI-RADS score. In our cohort, we found men with PI-RADS 3 or PI-RADS 4 lesions more likely to be upgraded to sPC by an additional SB in 11.8% and 11.7% of cases, respectively. For PI-RADS 5 men, the added value of additional SB was reduced to 2.9% and without statistical significance compared to a TB-only strategy. Our results confirm those of Ahdoot and co-workers published for a cohort of 743 men who underwent TB plus synchronous 12-core extended SB via the transrectal route: 7.5% upgrading to sPC in PI-RADS 3 men, 8.0% in PI-RADS 4 and 2.5% in PI-RADS 5 [10]. The slightly higher upgrading frequency in our study might originate from the application of the Ginsburg Scheme in our cohort, which conveys a higher number of SB cores taken.

4.4. Reclassification in Subsequent Radical Prostatectomy

Previous studies showed that CB is more predictive for a patient's true pathological grade group compared to TB alone and thus reduces diagnostic uncertainty with a consecutive decrease of both over- and undertreatment [17]. In accordance with these previously published data, we found that adding SB to TB could reduce upgrading to sPC in a subsequent radical prostatectomy from 43/214 (20.1%) to 8/214 (3.7%). When analyzing the subgroup of men with a PI-RADS 5 lesion, this difference was negligible: 4/87 (4.7%) vs. 1/87 (1.2%). To our knowledge, this is the first subgroup analysis of a biopsy cohort for upgrading to sPC with wholemount specimen as the reference standard stratified by PI-RADS groups.

4.5. Limitations and Strengths of the Study

There were several limitations to the current study that must be acknowledged. The retrospective and single-center design limits the generalizability of our results. Moreover, our data originates from a cohort from a large academic center with a high level of expertise within the radiological and urological diagnostic prostate cancer pathways, which may not reflect the reality of care.

The study's main strength is the evaluation of the additional effect of SB concerning reclassification rates in a subsequent radical prostatectomy, since this is fundamental to estimating the diagnostic uncertainty of the respective biopsy procedure. Moreover, this is the first study to evaluate the effect of additional SB stratified by PI-RADS groups in a large transperineal biopsy cohort.

4.6. Individualized Decision-Making

Our data suggest that the benefit of an additional SB in men with PI-RADS 5 lesions is limited since it only increases the rate of sPC diagnosis by 2.9%. This finding is confirmed when analyzing reclassification rates in a subsequent RP. Omitting SB in this group may result in fewer biopsy-related adverse events, a shorter operative time, lower procedure complexity, and a lower healthcare burden.

Nevertheless, the decision to perform only TB in PI-RADS 5 men must be taken individually. When considering focal therapy, CB provides information on the presence or absence of PC outside the MRI-lesion and thus is valuable for a precise surgical planning. Moreover, missing 2.9% of sPC in PI-RADS 5 men when omitting SB seems low but the risk threshold is ultimately subjective. Individual risk thresholds of both the physician and the patient must be considered when choosing the appropriate biopsy strategy.

5. Conclusions

Additional SB to complement TB conveys a trade-off between missing sPC on the one hand and the over diagnosis of iPC, and increased morbidity and resource expenditures on the other. We demonstrated that the benefit of an additional SB is small in men with a PI-RADS 5 lesion. This finding was confirmed when analyzing the diagnostic certainty of TB only versus TB+SB and comparing it with the reference standard of a subsequent radical prostatectomy. In conclusion, men with a PI-RADS 5 lesion may obviate additional SB.

Author Contributions: Conceptualization, A.S., R.S.-I. and M.G.; methodology, A.S., R.S.-I. and M.G.; formal analysis, A.S.; investigation, A.S., R.S.-I. and M.G.; resources, A.M., M.W. and J.M.; writing—original draft preparation, A.S., R.S.-I. and M.G., writing—review and editing, all authors; supervision, M.B., C.G., C.A.J., A.M. and M.G. All authors have read and agreed to the published version of the manuscript.

Funding: The article processing charge was funded by the Baden-Wuerttemberg Ministry of Science, Research and Art and the University of Freiburg in the funding programme Open Access Publishing.

Institutional Review Board Statement: The study was conducted according to the guidelines of the Declaration of Helsinki, and approved by the Institutional Review Board (or Ethics Committee) of the University of Freiburg (approval number: ETK 21-1191, date of approval: 7 April 2021).

Informed Consent Statement: In accordance with the statement of the local ethics committee, patient consent was waived due to the retrospective design of our study with a large sample size and the consecutively inadequate resource expenditure. Moreover, when only including patients with informed consent, there is a high probability of a selection bias.

Data Availability Statement: The data presented in this study are available on request from the corresponding author.

Conflicts of Interest: The authors declare no conflict of interest.

References

1. Ahmed, H.U.; El-Shater Bosaily, A.; Brown, L.C.; Gabe, R.; Kaplan, R.; Parmar, M.K.; Collaco-Moraes, Y.; Ward, K.; Hindley, R.G.; Freeman, A.; et al. Diagnostic accuracy of multi-parametric mri and trus biopsy in prostate cancer (promis): A paired validating confirmatory study. *Lancet* **2017**, *389*, 815–822. [CrossRef]
2. Kasivisvanathan, V.; Rannikko, A.S.; Borghi, M.; Panebianco, V.; Mynderse, L.A.; Vaarala, M.H.; Briganti, A.; Budäus, L.; Hellawell, G.; Hindley, R.G.; et al. Mri-targeted or standard biopsy for prostate-cancer diagnosis. *N. Engl. J. Med.* **2018**, *378*, 1767–1777. [CrossRef] [PubMed]
3. Rouvière, O.; Puech, P.; Renard-Penna, R.; Claudon, M.; Roy, C.; Mège-Lechevallier, F.; Decaussin-Petrucci, M.; Dubreuil-Chambardel, M.; Magaud, L.; Remontet, L.; et al. Use of prostate systematic and targeted biopsy on the basis of multiparametric mri in biopsy-naive patients (mri-first): A prospective, multicentre, paired diagnostic study. *Lancet Oncol.* **2019**, *20*, 100–109. [CrossRef]
4. Muthigi, A.; George, A.K.; Sidana, A.; Kongnyuy, M.; Simon, R.; Moreno, V.; Merino, M.J.; Choyke, P.L.; Turkbey, B.; Wood, B.J.; et al. Missing the mark: Prostate cancer upgrading by systematic biopsy over magnetic resonance imaging/transrectal ultrasound fusion biopsy. *J. Urol.* **2017**, *197*, 327–334. [CrossRef] [PubMed]
5. Kasivisvanathan, V.; Stabile, A.; Neves, J.B.; Giganti, F.; Valerio, M.; Shanmugabavan, Y.; Clement, K.D.; Sarkar, D.; Philippou, Y.; Thurtle, D.; et al. Magnetic resonance imaging-targeted biopsy versus systematic biopsy in the detection of prostate cancer: A systematic review and meta-analysis. *Eur. Urol.* **2019**, *76*, 284–303. [CrossRef] [PubMed]
6. Kohl, T.; Sigle, A.; Kuru, T.; Salem, J.; Rolfs, H.; Kowalke, T.; Suarez-Ibarrola, R.; Michaelis, J.; Binder, N.; Jilg, C.A.; et al. Comprehensive analysis of complications after transperineal prostate biopsy without antibiotic prophylaxis: Results of a multicenter trial with 30 days' follow-up. *Prostate Cancer Prostatic Dis.* **2022**, *25*, 264–268. [CrossRef] [PubMed]
7. Deniffel, D.; Perlis, N.; Ghai, S.; Girgis, S.; Healy, G.M.; Fleshner, N.; Hamilton, R.; Kulkarni, G.; Toi, A.; van der Kwast, T.; et al. Prostate biopsy in the era of mri-targeting: Towards a judicious use of additional systematic biopsy. *Eur. Radiol.* **2022**. [CrossRef] [PubMed]
8. Sathianathen, N.J.; Warlick, C.A.; Weight, C.J.; Ordonez, M.A.; Spilseth, B.; Metzger, G.J.; Murugan, P.; Konety, B.R. A clinical prediction tool to determine the need for concurrent systematic sampling at the time of magnetic resonance imaging-guided biopsy. *BJU Int.* **2019**, *123*, 612–617. [CrossRef] [PubMed]
9. Coker, M.A.; Glaser, Z.A.; Gordetsky, J.B.; Thomas, J.V.; Rais-Bahrami, S. Targets missed: Predictors of mri-targeted biopsy failing to accurately localize prostate cancer found on systematic biopsy. *Prostate Cancer Prostatic Dis.* **2018**, *21*, 549–555. [CrossRef] [PubMed]
10. Ahdoot, M.; Lebastchi, A.H.; Long, L.; Wilbur, A.R.; Gomella, P.T.; Mehralivand, S.; Daneshvar, M.A.; Yerram, N.K.; O'Connor, L.P.; Wang, A.Z.; et al. Using prostate imaging-reporting and data system (pi-rads) scores to select an optimal prostate biopsy method: A secondary analysis of the trio study. *Eur. Urol. Oncol.* **2022**, *5*, 176–186. [CrossRef] [PubMed]
11. Mottet, N.P.C.; van den Bergh, R.C.N.; Briers, E.; Gillessen, M.D.S.S.; Grummet, J.; van der Kwast, A.M.H.T.H.; Lam, T.B.; Mason, M.D.S.O.H.; Oprea-Lager, D.E.; Ploussard, G.; et al. EAU-EANM-ESTRO-ESUR-SIOG Guidelines on Prostate Cancer—2020. *Eur. Assoc. Urol.* **2020**, *1*, 11–143.
12. Turkbey, B.; Rosenkrantz, A.B.; Haider, M.A.; Padhani, A.R.; Villeirs, G.; Macura, K.J.; Tempany, C.M.; Choyke, P.L.; Cornud, F.; Margolis, D.J.; et al. Prostate imaging reporting and data system version 2.1: 2019 Update of prostate imaging reporting and data system version 2. *Eur. Urol.* **2019**, *76*, 340–351. [CrossRef] [PubMed]
13. Kuru, T.H.; Wadhwa, K.; Chang, R.T.M.; Echeverria, L.M.C.; Roethke, M.; Polson, A.; Rottenberg, G.; Koo, B.; Lawrence, E.M.; Seidenader, J.; et al. Definitions of terms, processes and a minimum dataset for transperineal prostate biopsies: A standardization approach of the ginsburg study group for enhanced prostate diagnostics: A standardization approach for transperineal prostate biopsies. *BJU Int.* **2013**, *112*, 568–577. [CrossRef] [PubMed]
14. Kroenig, M.; Schaal, K.; Benndorf, M.; Soschynski, M.; Lenz, P.; Krauss, T.; Drendel, V.; Kayser, G.; Kurz, P.; Werner, M.; et al. Diagnostic accuracy of robot-guided, software based transperineal mri/trus fusion biopsy of the prostate in a high risk population of previously biopsy negative men. *BioMed Res. Int.* **2016**, *2016*, 2384894. [CrossRef] [PubMed]
15. Epstein, J.I.; Allsbrook, W.C., Jr.; Amin, M.B.; Egevad, L.L.; Committee, I.G. The 2005 international society of urological pathology (isup) consensus conference on gleason grading of prostatic carcinoma. *Am. J. Surg. Pathol.* **2005**, *29*, 1228–1242. [CrossRef] [PubMed]
16. Connor, M.J.; Eldred-Evans, D.; van Son, M.; Hosking-Jervis, F.; Bertoncelli Tanaka, M.; Reddy, D.; Bass, E.J.; Powell, L.; Ahmad, S.; Pegers, E.; et al. A multicenter study of the clinical utility of nontargeted systematic transperineal prostate biopsies in patients undergoing pre-biopsy multiparametric magnetic resonance imaging. *J. Urol.* **2020**, *204*, 1195–1201. [CrossRef] [PubMed]
17. Ahdoot, M.; Wilbur, A.R.; Reese, S.E.; Lebastchi, A.H.; Mehralivand, S.; Gomella, P.T.; Bloom, J.; Gurram, S.; Siddiqui, M.; Pinsky, P.; et al. Mri-targeted, systematic, and combined biopsy for prostate cancer diagnosis. *N. Engl. J. Med.* **2020**, *382*, 917–928. [CrossRef] [PubMed]

18. Nakanishi, Y.; Ito, M.; Fukushima, H.; Yokoyama, M.; Kataoka, M.; Ikuta, S.; Sakamoto, K.; Takemura, K.; Suzuki, H.; Tobisu, K.I.; et al. Who can avoid systematic biopsy without missing clinically significant prostate cancer in men who undergo magnetic resonance imaging-targeted biopsy? *Clin. Genitourin. Cancer* **2019**, *17*, e664–e671. [CrossRef] [PubMed]
19. Drobish, J.N.; Bevill, M.D.; Tracy, C.R.; Sexton, S.M.; Rajput, M.; Metz, C.M.; Gellhaus, P.T. Do patients with a pi-rads 5 lesion identified on magnetic resonance imaging require systematic biopsy in addition to targeted biopsy? *Urol. Oncol.* **2021**, *39*, e231–e234. [CrossRef] [PubMed]
20. Gomez-Gomez, E.; Moreno Sorribas, S.; Valero-Rosa, J.; Blanca, A.; Mesa, J.; Salguero, J.; Carrasco-Valiente, J.; Lopez-Ruiz, D.; Anglada-Curado, F.J. Does adding standard systematic biopsy to targeted prostate biopsy in pi-rads 3 to 5 lesions enhance the detection of clinically significant prostate cancer? Should all patients with pi-rads 3 undergo targeted biopsy? *Diagnostics* **2021**, *11*, 1335. [CrossRef] [PubMed]

MDPI AG
Grosspeteranlage 5
4052 Basel
Switzerland
Tel.: +41 61 683 77 34

MDPI Books Editorial Office
E-mail: books@mdpi.com
www.mdpi.com/books

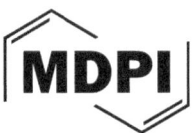

Disclaimer/Publisher's Note: The title and front matter of this reprint are at the discretion of the Topic Editors. The publisher is not responsible for their content or any associated concerns. The statements, opinions and data contained in all individual articles are solely those of the individual Editors and contributors and not of MDPI. MDPI disclaims responsibility for any injury to people or property resulting from any ideas, methods, instructions or products referred to in the content.